Disclaimer

This textbook was designed to provide a desk reference for radiologists, MRI technologists, facility managers, MRI physicists, and others. The information is current through the publication date of this textbook. MRI users are advised to check with the manufacturer of a given implant or device in order to obtain the most recent information prior to performing an MRI procedure on a patient with an implant or device in question. The content of this book is designed for general informational purposes only and is not intended to be nor should it be construed to be technical or medical advice or opinion on any specific facts or circumstances.

The author and publisher of this work disclaim any liability for the acts of any physician, individual, group, or entity acting independently or on behalf of any organization that utilizes any information for any medical procedure, activity, service, or other situation through the use of this textbook.

The content of this book makes no representations or warranties of any kind, expressed or implied, as to the information content, materials or products, included in this book. The author and publisher assume no responsibilities for errors or omissions that may include technical or other inaccuracies, or typographical errors. The author and publisher of this work specifically disclaim all representations and warranties of any kind, expressed or implied, as to the information, content, materials, or products included or referenced in this textbook.

The author and publisher disclaim responsibility for any injury and/or damage to persons or property from any of the methods, products, instructions, or ideas contained in this publication.

The author and publisher disclaim liability for any damages of any kind arising from the use of the book, including but not limited to direct, indirect, incidental, punitive and/or consequential damages.

The information and comments provided in this book are not intended to be technical or medical recommendations or advice for individuals or patients. The information and comments provided herein are of a general nature and should not be considered specific to an individual or patient, whether or not a specific patient is referenced by a physician, technologist, individual, group, or other entity seeking information.

The author and publisher assume no responsibility for the accuracy or validity of the information contained in this book nor the claims or statements of any manufacturer or website that is referenced. Manufacturers' product specifications are subject to change without notice. Always read the product labeling, instructions and warning statements thoroughly before using any medical product or similar device.

Regarding the MRI information for a given material, implant, device, or object that may be referenced herein, because of ongoing research, equipment modifications, and changes in governmental regulations, no suggested or otherwise presented product information should be used unless the reader has reviewed and evaluated the information provided with the product discussed, by reviewing the latest information provided by the manufacturer, or by reviewing the pertinent literature.

Reference Manual for Magnetic Resonance Safety, Implants, and Devices: 2010 Edition

Frank G. Shellock, Ph.D.

Adjunct Clinical Professor of Radiology and Medicine
Keck School of Medicine
University of Southern California

Director of MRI Studies of Biomimetic MicroElectronic
Systems (BMES) Implants, National Science Foundation
BMES Engineering Research Center
University of Southern California

Adjunct Professor of Clinical Physical Therapy, Division of
Biokinesiology and Physical Therapy, School of Dentistry
University of Southern California

Founder
Institute for Magnetic Resonance
Safety, Education, and Research

President
Shellock R & D Services, Inc.
Los Angeles, California

Biomedical Research Publishing Group
Los Angeles, CA

Made in the United States of America

Library of Congress Cataloging-in-Publication Data

Shellock, Frank G.

Reference Manual for Magnetic Resonance Safety, Implants, and Devices: 2010 Edition

Frank G. Shellock

p. cm.

Includes bibliographical references.

ISBN 978-0-9746410-6-5

1. Magnetic resonance imaging—Complications—Handbooks, manuals, etc. 2. Metals in medicine—Magnetic properties—Handbooks, manuals, etc. 3. Implants, Artificial—Magnetic properties—Handbooks, manuals, etc. I. Title.

[DNLM: 1. Magnetic Resonance Imaging—contraindications—handbooks. 2. Nuclear Magnetic Resonance—handbooks. 3. Metals—handbooks. 4. Implants]

Great care has been taken to assure the accuracy of the information contained in this textbook that is intended for educational and informational purposes, only. Neither the publisher nor the author assume responsibility for errors or for any consequences arising from the use of the information contained herein.

DEDICATION

To Jaana

A truly extraordinary person,
a gentle soul, and kindred spirit.

You are forever in my heart.

Contents

SECTION II
MR PROCEDURES AND IMPLANTS, DEVICES, AND MATERIALS

Acknowledgements

I am indebted to Sam Valencerina, B.S., R.T. (R)(MR), MRI Clinical Coordinator and Manager, University of Southern California, University Hospital, Los Angeles, CA, for his exceptional and most professional assistance in the evaluation of implants and devices. Special thanks to Mark Bass for his talented contributions that permit the timely publication of this textbook.

Preface

Magnetic resonance (MR) procedures continue to expand with regard to usage and complexity. Patient management and safety issues are important aspects of this diagnostic modality. Because MR technology continuously evolves, it is necessary to update, revise, and add to the safety topics in this textbook in consideration of the latest information.

This annually-revised textbook series is a comprehensive yet concise information resource that includes guidelines and recommendations for safety based on the latest peer-reviewed articles, labeling information from device manufacturers, as well as documents developed by professional organizations including the International Society for Magnetic Resonance in Medicine (ISMRM), the American College of Radiology (ACR), the Food and Drug Administration (FDA), the National Electrical Manufacturers Association (NEMA), the International Electrotechnical Commission (IEC), the Medical Devices Agency (MDA), and the International Commission on Non-Ionizing Radiation Protection (ICNIRP).

Section I presents safety guidelines and recommendations. **Section II** provides the latest information for implants, devices, and materials tested for safety in the MR environment. **"The List"** continues to grow and contains data for thousands of objects.

The clinical use of 3-Tesla MR systems for brain, musculoskeletal, body, cardiovascular, and other applications is increasing worldwide. Because prior investigations that determined safety for implants and devices used mostly MR systems operating at 1.5-Tesla or less, it is crucial to perform *in vitro* testing at 3-Tesla to characterize safety for implants, especially with regard to magnetic field interactions and, in certain cases, to assess MRI-related heating as well as alterations in the operational or functional aspects of these devices. Therefore, investigations from our group and others have evaluated safety for implants and devices at 3-Tesla. This textbook contains information for the most commonly used implants and devices tested at this static magnetic field strength.

Healthcare professionals are advised to review the terminology developed by the American Society for Testing and Materials (ASTM) International, which is currently applied to implants and devices, thus, replacing terms that were often confusing or misused. The terms, *MR Safe*, *MR Conditional*, and *MR Unsafe* are explained in this textbook. Notably, this terminology has not been applied *retrospectively* to implants and devices that previously received Food and Drug Administration (FDA) approved labeling using the terms "*MR safe*" or "*MR compatible*". Therefore, this should be understood to avoid undue confusion regarding the matter of labeling for "older" vs. "newer" implants, or for those items that have recently undergone MRI evaluations.

Appendix III, *Websites for Biomedical Companies,* lists company websites. This section has been further expanded to include additional companies to help MR healthcare professionals access the latest safety information for implants and devices.

Because of the continued concern pertaining to the use of MRI contrast agents and the association with nephrogenic systemic fibrosis (NSF), this Reference Manual provides a discussion that includes several open questions and issues. In addition, websites and links are provided to allow MR healthcare professionals to access and review the latest information on this important topic.

Frank G. Shellock, Ph.D.

Celebrating 25 Years of Service to the MRI Community

SECTION I

Guidelines and Recommendations for MR Safety

Bioeffects of Static Magnetic Fields

The introduction of MR technology as a clinical imaging modality in the early 1980s is responsible for a substantial increase in human exposure to strong static magnetic fields. Most MR systems in use today operate at fields ranging from 0.2- to 3-Tesla. According to the latest guidelines from the U.S. Food and Drug Administration, clinical MR systems using static magnetic fields up to 8.0-Tesla are considered a "non-significant risk" for adult patients. The exposure of research subjects to fields above this level requires approval of the research protocol by an Institutional Review Board and the informed consent of the subjects. Currently, the most powerful MR system in the world used for human subjects operates at a static magnetic field strength of 9.4-Tesla. Investigations by Atkinson et al. and Vaughan et al. describe findings obtained in human subjects relative to the use of the 9.4-Tesla MR system.

With respect to short-term exposures, the available information that pertains to the effects of static magnetic fields on biological tissues is extensive. Investigations include studies on alterations in cell growth and morphology, cell reproduction and teratogenicity, DNA structure and gene expression, pre- and post-natal reproduction and development, blood brain barrier permeability, nerve activity, cognitive function and behavior, cardiovascular dynamics, hematological indices, temperature regulation, circadian rhythms, immune responsiveness, processing of visual and auditory information by the brain, and other biological processes. The majority of these studies concluded that exposures to static magnetic fields produce no substantial harmful bioeffects. Although there have been reports of potentially injurious effects of static magnetic fields on isolated cells or organisms, no effect has been verified or firmly established as a scientific fact. The documented serious injuries and few fatalities that have occurred with MR system magnets were in associated with the inadvertent introduction or presence of ferromagnetic objects (e.g., oxygen tanks, wheelchairs, aneurysm clips, etc.) into the MR environment.

Regarding the effects of long-term exposures to static magnetic fields, there are several physical mechanisms of interaction between tissues and static magnetic fields that could theoretically lead to pathological changes in human subjects. However, quantitative analysis of these mechanisms indicates that they are below the threshold of significance with respect to long-term adverse bioeffects.

Presently, the peer-reviewed literature does not contain carefully controlled studies that support the absolute safety of chronic exposure to powerful magnetic fields. With the increased clinical use of interventional MR procedures, there is a critical need for such investigations. In addition, although there is no evidence for a cumulative effect of magnetic field exposure on health, further studies of the exposed populations (MR healthcare professionals, patients that undergo repeat studies, interventional MR users, etc.) will be helpful in establishing guidelines for occupational and patient exposures to powerful static magnetic fields.

REFERENCES

Atkinson IC, Renteria L, Burd H, Pliskin NH, Thulborn KR. Safety of human MRI at static fields above the FDA 8 T guideline: sodium imaging at 9.4 T does not affect vital signs or cognitive ability. J Magn Reson Imaging. 2007;26:1222-7.

Besson J, Foreman E, Eastwood L, Smith F, Ashcroft G. Cognitive evaluation following NMR imaging of the brain. Journal of Neurology, Neurosurgery, and Psychiatry 1984;47:314-316.Brockway J, Bream P. Does memory loss occur after MR imaging? Journal of Magnetic Resonance Imaging 1992;2:721-728.

Brody A, Sorette M, Gooding C, et al. Induced alignment of flowing sickle erythrocytes in a magnetic field: A preliminary report. Investigative Radiology 1985;20:560-566.

Brody A, Embury S, Mentzer W, Winkler M, Gooding C. Preservation of sickle cell blood flow pattern(s) during MR imaging: An *in vivo* study. American Journal of Roentgenology 1988; 151:139-141.

Budinger TF. Nuclear magnetic resonance (NMR) in vitro studies: known thresholds for health effects. J Comput Assisted Tomog 1981;5:800-811.

Cavin ID, Glover PM, Bowtell RW, Gowland PA. Thresholds for perceiving metallic taste at high magnetic field. J Magn Reson Imaging. 2007;26:1357-61.

Chakeres DW, de Vocht F. Static magnetic field effects on human subjects related to magnetic resonance imaging. Prog Biophys Mol Biol 2005;87:255-265.

de Vocht F, van Drooge H, Engels H, Kromhout H. Acute neurobehavior effects of xposure, health complaints and cognitive performance among employees of an MRI scanners manufacturing department. Journal of Magnetic Resonance Imaging 2006;23:197-204.

de Vocht F, Stevens T, van Wendel-de-Joode B, Engels H, Kromhout H. Acute neurobehavior effects of exposure to static magnetic fields: analysis of exposure-response relations. Journal of Magnetic Resonance Imaging 2006;23:291-297.

de Vocht F, Stevens T, Glover P, Sunderland A, Gowland P, Kromhout H. Cognitive effects of head-movements in stray fields generated by a 7 Tesla whole-body MRI magnet. Bioelectromagnetics. 2007;28:247-55.

Feychting M. Health effects of static magnetic fields--a review of the epidemiological evidence. Prog Biophys Mol Biol. 2005;87:241-6.

Fuentes MA, Trakic A, Wilson SJ, Crozier S. Analysis and measurements of magnetic field exposures for healthcare workers in selected MR environments. IEEE Trans Biomed Eng. 2008;55:1355-64.

Glover PM, Cavin I, Qian W, Bowtell R, Gowland PA. Magnetic-field-induced vertigo: a theoretical and experimental investigation. Bioelectromagnetics. 2007;28:349-61.

Hartwig V, Giovannetti G, et al. Biological effects and safety in magnetic resonance imaging: a review. Int J Environ Res Public Health. 2009;6:1778-98.

Hong CZ, Shellock FG. Short-term exposure to a 1.5 Tesla static magnetic field does not effect somato-sensory evoked potentials in man. Magnetic Resonance Imaging 1989;8:65-69.

Hsieh CH, Lee MC, Tsai-Wu JJ, Chen MH, Lee HS, Chiang H, Herbert Wu CH, Jiang CC. Deleterious effects of MRI on chondrocytes. Osteoarthritis Cartilage. 2007 Sep 3; [Epub ahead of print]

International Electrotechnical Commission (IEC), Medical Electrical Equipment, Particular requirements for the safety of magnetic resonance equipment for medical diagnosis, International Standard IEC 60601-2-33, 2002.

International Commission on Non-Ionizing Radiation Protection (ICNIRP) Statement, Medical magnetic resonance procedures: protection of patients. Health Physics 2004;87:197-216.

Innis NK, Ossenkopp KP, Prato FS, et al. Behavioral effects of exposure to nuclear magnetic resonance imaging: II. Spatial memory tests. Magnetic Resonance Imaging 1986;4:281-284.

Kannala S, et al. Occupational exposure measurements of static and pulsed gradient magnetic fields in the vicinity of MRI scanners. Phys Med Biol. 2009;54:2243-57.

Kangarlu A, Burgess RE, Zhu H, Nakayama T, Hamlin RL, Abduljahl AM, Robitaille PML. Cognitive, cardiac, and physiological safety studies in ultra high field magnetic resonance imaging. Magn Reson Imaging 1999;17:1407-1416.

Karpowicz J, Gryz K. Health risk assessment of occupational exposure to a magnetic field from magnetic resonance imaging devices. Int J Occup Saf Ergon. 2006;12:155-67.

Kay H, Herfkens R, Kay B. Effect on magnetic resonance imaging on Xenopus Laevis embryogenesis. Magnetic Resonance Imaging 1988; 6:501-506.

Laszlo J, Gyires K. 3 T homogeneous static magnetic field of a clinical MR significantly inhibits pain in mice. Life Sci. 2009;84:12-7.

Muller S, Hotz M. Human brainstem auditory evoked potentials (BAEP) before and after MR examinations. Magnetic Resonance in Medicine 1990;16:476-480.

Ossenkopp KP, Innis N, Prato F, Sestini E. Behavioral effects of exposure to nuclear magnetic resonance imaging: I. Open-field avoidance behavior an passive avoidance learning in rats. Magnetic Resonance Imaging 1986;4:275-280.

Prasad N, Wright D, Ford J, Thornby J. Safety of 4-T MR imaging: Study of effects on developing frog embryos. Radiology 1990;174:251-253.

Sakurai T, Terashima S, Miyakoshi J. Effects of strong static magnetic fields used in magnetic resonance imaging on insulin-secreting cells. Bioelectromagnetics. 2008 Jun 2. [Epub ahead of print]

Schenck JF. Health effects and safety of static magnetic fields. In: Shellock FG, ed. Magnetic resonance procedures: health effects and safety. Boca Raton, FL: CRC Press, 2001; pp. 1-30.

Schenck JF. Safety of strong, static magnetic fields. J Magn Reson Imaging 2000;12;2-19.

Schenck JF, Dumoulin CL, Redington RW, Kressel HY, Elliott RT, McDougall IL. Human exposure to 4.0-Tesla magnetic fields in a whole-body scanner. Medical Physics 1992;19:1089-1098.

Schwartz J, Crooks L. NMR imaging produces no observable mutations or cytotoxicity in mammalian cells. American Journal of Roentgenology 1982;139:583-585.

Schwenzer NF, Bantleon R, et al. Do static or time-varying magnetic fields in magnetic resonance imaging (3.0 T) alter protein-gene expression?-A study on human embryonic lung fibroblasts. J Magn Reson Imaging. 2007;26:1210-5.

Schwenzer NF, Bantleon R, Maurer B, et al. In vitro evaluation of magnetic resonance imaging at 3.0 Tesla on clonogenic ability, proliferation, and cell cycle in human embryonic lung fibroblasts. Invest Radiol. 2007;42:212-217.

Shellock FG, Crues JV. MR procedures: biologic effects, safety, and patient care. Radiology, 2004;232:635-652.

Shellock FG, Schaefer DJ, Crues JV. Exposure to a 1.5 Tesla static magnetic field does not alter body and skin temperatures in man. Magnetic Resonance in Medicine 1989;1:371-375.

Shellock FG, Schaefer DJ, Gordon CJ. Effect of a 1.5 Tesla static magnetic field on body temperature of man. Magnetic Resonance in Medicine 1986;3:644-647.

Short W, Goodwill L, Taylor C, Job C, Arthur M, Cress A. Alteration of human tumor cell adhesion by high-strength static magnetic fields. Investigative Radiology 1991;27:836-840.

Silva AK, Silva EL, Egito ES, Carrico AS. Safety concerns related to magnetic field exposure. Radiat Environ Biophys. 2006;45:245-52.

Tomasi DG, Wang R. Induced magnetic field gradients and forces in the human head in MRI. J Magn Reson Imaging. 2007;26:1340-5.

Toyomaki A, Yamamoto T. Observation of changes in neural activity due to the static magnetic field of an MRI scanner. J Magn Reson Imaging. 2007;26:1216-21

U.S. Department of Health and Human Services, Food and Drug Administration, Center for Devices and Radiological Health, Guidance for Industry and FDA Staff. Criteria for Significant Risk Investigations of Magnetic Resonance Diagnostic Devices, July 14, 2003.

Valiron O, Peris L, Rikken G, Schweitzer A, Saoudi Y, Remy C, Didier J. Cellular disorders induced by high magnetic fields. Journal of Magnetic Resonance Imaging 2005;22:334-340.

Vaughan T, DelaBarre L, Snyder C, Tian J, Akgun C, Shrivastava D, Liu W, Olson C, Adriany G, Strupp J, Andersen P, Gopinath A, van de Moortele PF, Garwood M, Ugurbil K. 9.4-T human MRI: preliminary results. Magn Reson Med. 2006;56:1274-1282.

Vecchia P, Hietanen M, et al. Guidelines on limits of exposure to static magnetic fields. International Commission on Non-Ionizing Radiation Protection. Health Physics 2009;96:504-14.

Vogl T, Pasulus W, Fuchs A, Krafczyk S, Lissner J. Influence of magnetic resonance imaging on evoked potentials and nerve conduction velocities in humans. Investigative Radiology 1991; 26:432-437.

Von Klitzing L. Do static magnetic fields of NMR influence biological signals? Clin Phys Physiol Meas 1986;7:157-160.

Weintraub MI, Khoury A, Cole SP. Biologic effects of 3 Tesla (T) MR imaging comparing traditional 1.5-T and 0.6-T in 1,023 consecutive outpatients. J Neuroimaging. 2007;17:241-5.

Weiss M, Herrick R, Tabor K, Contant C, Plishker G. Bioeffects of high magnetic fields: A study using a simple animal model. Magnetic Resonance Imaging 1992;10:689-694.

Yuh WTC, Ehrhardt JC, Fisher DJ, Shields RK, Shellock FG. Phantom limb pain induced in amputee by strong magnetic fields. J Magn Reson Imaging 1992;2:221-223.

Zaremba LA. FDA guidance for magnetic resonance system safety and patient exposures: current status and future considerations. In: Shellock FG, ed. Magnetic resonance procedures: health effects and safety. Boca Raton, FL: CRC Press, 2001; pp. 183-196.

Bioeffects of Gradient Magnetic Fields

During MR procedures, gradient or time-varying magnetic fields may stimulate nerves or muscles in patients by inducing electrical fields. This topic has been thoroughly reviewed by Schaefer et al., Nyenhuis et al., Bourland et al., and Bencsik et al. The potential for interactions between gradient magnetic fields and biologic tissue is dependent on a variety of factors including the fundamental field frequency, the maximum flux density, the average flux density, the presence of harmonic frequencies, the waveform characteristics of the signal, the polarity of the signal, the current distribution in the body, the electrical properties, and the sensitivity of the cell membrane.

GRADIENT MAGNETIC FIELD-INDUCED STIMULATION

Several investigations have characterized MR system-related, gradient magnetic field-induced stimulation in human subjects. At sufficient exposure levels, peripheral nerve stimulation is perceptible as "tingling" or "tapping" sensations. At gradient magnetic field exposure levels from 50% to 100% above perception thresholds, patients may become uncomfortable or experience pain. At extremely high levels, cardiac stimulation is a concern. However, the induction of cardiac stimulation requires exceedingly large gradient fields that are more than an order of magnitude greater than those used currently by commercially available MR systems.

With regard to gradient magnetic fields, the U.S. Food and Drug Administration considers that MR procedures using rates of change (dB/dt) sufficient to produce severe discomfort or painful nerve stimulation a significant risk. These safety standards for gradient magnetic fields associated with present-day MR systems appear to adequately protect patients from potential hazards or injuries.

Interestingly, studies performed in human subjects have indicated that anatomical sites of peripheral nerve stimulation vary depending on the activation of a specific gradient (i.e., x-, y- or, z-gradient). For example, stimulation sites for x-gradients included the bridge of the nose, left side of the thorax, iliac crest, left thigh, buttocks, and the lower back. Stimulation sites for y-gradients included the scapula, upper arms, shoulder, right side of the thorax, iliac crest, hip, hands, and upper back. Stimulation sites for z-gradients included the scapula, thorax, xyphoid, abdomen, iliac crest, and upper and lower back. Peripheral nerve stimulation sites were typically found at bony prominences. According to Schaefer et al., since bone is less conductive than the surrounding tissue, it may increase current densities in narrow regions of tissue between the bone and the skin, resulting in lower nerve stimulation thresholds than expected.

REFERENCES

Abart J, Eberhardt K, Fischer H, et al. Peripheral nerve stimulation by time-varying magnetic fields. Journal of Computer Assisted Tomography 1997; 21:532–538.

Bencsik M, Bowtell R, Bowley R. Electric fields induced in the human body by time-varying magnetic field gradients in MRI: numerical calculations and correlation analysis. Phys Med Biol. 2007;52:2337-53.

Bourland JD, Nyenhuis JA, Schaefer DJ. Physiologic effects of intense MRI gradient fields. Neuroimaging Clin North Am 1999; 9:363–377.

Budinger TF, Fischer H, Hentshel D, Reinflder HE, Schmitt F. Physiological effects of fast oscillating magnetic field gradients. Journal of Computer Assisted Tomography 1991;15:609–614.

Cohen MS, Weisskoff R, Kantor H. Sensory stimulation by time varying magnetic fields. Magn Reson 1990;14:409–414.

de Vocht F, Liket L, De Vocht A, Mistry T, Glover P, Gowland P, Kromhout H. Exposure to alternating electromagnetic fields and effects on the visual and visuomotor systems. Br J Radiol. 2007;80:822-8.

Doherty J, Whitman G, Robinson M, et al. Changes in cardiac excitability and vulnerability in NMR fields. 1985;20:129-135.

Ehrhardt JC, Lin CS, Magnotta VA, Fisher DJ, Yuh WTC. Peripheral nerve stimulation in a whole-body echo-planar imaging system. J Magn Reson Imaging 1997;7:405–409.

Fuentes MA, Trakic A, Wilson SJ, Crozier S. Analysis and measurements of magnetic field exposures for healthcare workers in selected MR environments. IEEE Trans Biomed Eng. 2008;55:1355-64.

Glover PM, Eldeghaidy S, Mistry TR, Gowland PA. Measurement of visual evoked potential during and after periods of pulsed magnetic field exposure. J Magn Reson Imaging. 2007;26:1353-6.

Ham CLG, Engels JML, van de Weil GT, Machielsen A. Peripheral nerve stimulation during MRI: effects of high gradient amplitudes and switching rates. J Magn Reson Imaging 1997;7:933–937.

Hartwig V, Giovannetti G, et al. Biological effects and safety in magnetic resonance imaging: a review. Int J Environ Res Public Health. 2009;6:1778-98.

Irnich W, Schmitt F. Magnetostimulation in MRI. Magn Reson Med 1995;33:619–623.

International Commission on Non-Ionizing Radiation Protection (ICNIRP) Statement, Medical magnetic resonance procedures: protection of patients. Health Physics 2004;87:197-216.

Kannala S, et al. Occupational exposure measurements of static and pulsed gradient magnetic fields in the vicinity of MRI scanners. Phys Med Biol. 2009;54:2243-57.

Kangarlu A, Tang L, Ibrahim TS. Electric field measurements and computational modeling at ultrahigh-field MRI. Magn Reson Imaging. 2007;25:1222-1226.

King KF, Schaefer DJ. Spiral scan peripheral nerve stimulation. J Magn Reson Imaging 2000; 12:164-170.

Li Y, Hand JW, Wills T, Hajnal JV. Numerically-simulated induced electric field and current density within a human model located close to a z-gradient coil. J Magn Reson Imaging. 2007;26:1286-95.

Mansfield P, Harvey PR. Limits to neural stimulation in echo-planar imaging. Magn Reson Med 1993; 29:746–758.

Nyenhuis JA, Bourland J, Kildishev AV, Schaefer DJ. Health effects and safety of intense gradient fields. In: Shellock FG, ed. Magnetic resonance procedures: health effects and safety. Boca Raton, FL: CRC Press, 2001; 31-54.

Nyenhuis JA, Bourland JD, Schaefer DJ. Analysis from a stimulation perspective of magnetic field patterns of MR gradient coils. J Appl Phys 1997;81:4314–4316.

Schaefer DJ, Bourland JD, Nyenhuis JA. Review of patient safety in time-varying gradient fields. J Magn Reson Imaging 2000; 12:20-29.

Schwenzer NF, Bantleon R, et al. Do static or time-varying magnetic fields in magnetic resonance imaging (3.0 T) alter protein-gene expression? A study on human embryonic lung fibroblasts. J Magn Reson Imaging. 2007;26:1210-5.

Shellock FG, Crues JV. MR procedures: biologic effects, safety, and patient care. Radiology, 2004;232:635-652.

U.S. Department of Health and Human Services, Food and Drug Administration, Center for Devices and Radiological Health, Guidance for Industry and FDA Staff. Criteria for Significant Risk Investigations of Magnetic Resonance Diagnostic Devices, July 14, 2003.

Vogt FM, Ladd ME, Hunold P, Mateiescu S, Hebrank FX, Zhang A, Debatin JF, Gohde SC. Increased time rate of change of gradient fields: Effect on peripheral nerve stimulation at clinical MR imaging. Radiology 2004;233:548-554.

Weintraub MI, Khoury A, Cole SP. Biologic effects of 3 Tesla (T) MR imaging comparing traditional 1.5-T and 0.6-T in 1,023 consecutive outpatients. J Neuroimaging. 2007;17:241-5.

Bioeffects of Radiofrequency Fields

The majority of the radiofrequency (RF) power transmitted for MR imaging or spectroscopy (including carbon decoupling, fast spin echo pulse sequences, magnetization transfer contrast pulse sequences, etc.) procedures is transformed into heat within the patient's tissue as a result of resistive losses. Not surprisingly, the bioeffects associated with exposure to RF radiation are related to the thermogenic aspects of this electromagnetic field.

Prior to 1985, there were no reports concerning the thermophysiologic responses of human subjects exposed to RF radiation during MR procedures. Since then, many investigations have characterized the thermal effects of MR procedure-related heating.

SPECIFIC ABSORPTION RATE

Thermoregulatory and other physiologic changes that a human subject exhibits in response to exposure to RF radiation are dependent on the amount of energy that is absorbed. The dosimetric term used to describe the absorption of RF radiation is the specific absorption rate (SAR). The SAR is the mass normalized rate at which RF power is coupled to biologic tissue and is typically indicated in units of watts per kilogram (W/kg). The relative amount of RF radiation that an individual encounters during an MR procedure is designated as the whole-body-averaged SAR. Other SAR levels relative to the body part exposed or peak SAR level (i.e., the amount in one gram of tissue) may also be reported by the MR system.

Measurements or estimates of SAR are not trivial, particularly in human subjects. There are several methods of determining this parameter for the purpose of RF energy dosimetry. The SAR that is produced during an MR procedure is a complex function of numerous variables including the frequency (i.e., determined by the strength of the static magnetic field of the MR system), the type of RF pulse used (e.g., 90° vs. 180° pulse), the repetition time, the type of transmit RF coil used, the volume of tissue contained within the transmit RF coil, the configuration of the anatomical region exposed, as well as other factors.

With regard to RF energy, the U.S. Food and Drug Administration currently indicates that MR procedures that exceed certain SAR values may pose significant risks (please refer to **Appendix I** to review these values).

THERMOPHYSIOLOGIC RESPONSES TO MR PROCEDURE-RELATED HEATING

Thermophysiologic responses to MR procedure-related heating depend on multiple physiologic, physical, and environmental factors. These include the duration of exposure, the rate at which energy is deposited, the response of the patient's thermoregulatory system, the presence of an underlying health condition, and the ambient conditions within the MR system.

In regards to the thermoregulatory system, when subjected to a thermal challenge, the human body loses heat by means of convection, conduction, radiation, and evaporation. Each mechanism is responsible to a varying degree for heat dissipation, as the body attempts to maintain thermal homeostasis. If the thermoregulatory effectors are not capable of totally dissipating the heat load, an accumulation or storage of heat occurs along with an elevation in local and/or overall tissue temperatures.

Various underlying health conditions may affect an individual's ability to tolerate a thermal challenge including cardiovascular disease, hypertension, diabetes, fever, old age, and obesity. In addition, medications including diuretics, beta-blockers, calcium blockers, amphetamines, and sedatives can alter thermoregulatory responses to a heat load. Importantly, certain medications have a synergistic effect with RF radiation with respect to tissue heating. The environmental conditions (i.e., ambient temperature, relative humidity, and airflow) that exist in the MR system will also affect tissue temperature changes associated with RF energy-induced heating.

The first study of human thermal responses to RF radiation-induced heating during an MR procedure was conducted by Schaefer et al. Temperature changes and other physiologic parameters were assessed in volunteer subjects exposed to a relatively high, whole-body-averaged SAR (approximately 4.0-W/kg). The data indicated that there were no excessive temperature elevations or other deleterious physiologic consequences related to exposure to RF radiation.

Several studies were subsequently conducted involving volunteer subjects and patients undergoing clinical MR procedures, with the intent of obtaining information that would be applicable to patients typically encountered in the MR setting. These investigations demonstrated that changes in body temperatures were relatively minor (i.e., less than 0.6 degrees C). While there was a tendency for statistically significant increases in skin temperatures to occur, these were of no serious physiologic consequences.

Various studies reported a poor correlation between body temperature and skin temperature changes versus whole-body-averaged SARs associated with clinical MR procedures. These findings are not surprising considering the range of thermophysiologic responses that are possible in human subjects relative to a given SAR level. For example, as previously indicated, an individual's thermoregulatory system can be greatly impacted by the presence of an underlying condition or medication that can impair the ability to dissipate heat.

An extensive investigation by Shellock et al. was conducted in volunteer subjects exposed to MR procedures performed at a whole-body-averaged SAR of 6.0-W/kg. To date, this is the highest level of RF energy that human subjects have been exposed to in associaton with MR procedures. Tympanic membrane temperature, six different skin temperatures, heart rate, blood pressure, oxygen saturation, and skin blood flow were monitored. The findings indicated that an MR procedure performed at a whole body averaged SAR of 6.0-W/kg can be physiologically tolerated by an individual with normal thermoregulatory function.

VERY-HIGH FIELD MR SYSTEMS

Many MR systems now operate at a static magnetic field strength of 3-Tesla, several operate at 4-Tesla and 7-Tesla, and one operates at 9.4-Tesla. These very-high-field MR systems are capable of depositing RF power that exceed those associated with a 1.5-Tesla MR system. Therefore, investigations are needed to characterize thermal responses in human subjects to determine potential thermogenic hazards associated with the use of these powerful MR devices, especially since frequency related differences likely exist. To date, with the exception of the work conducted by Kangarlu et al. (8-Tesla) and Shrivastava, et al. (9.4-Tesla) there have been few investigations of MR procedure-related heating performed using very-high-field MR systems.

REFERENCES

Atalar E. Radiofrequency safety for interventional MRI procedures. Acad Radiol. 2005;12:1149-1157.

Boss A, Graf H, Berger A, et al. Tissue warming and regulatory responses induced by radio frequency energy deposition on a whole-body 3-Tesla magnetic resonance imager. J Magn Reson Imaging. 2007;26:1334-9.

Bottomley PA. Turning up the heat on MRI. J Am Coll Radiol. 2008;5:853

Bottomley PA, Edelstein WA. Power deposition in whole body NMR imaging. Med Phys 1981;8: 510-512.

Budinger TF. Nuclear magnetic resonance (NMR) in vitro studies: known thresholds for health effects. J Comput Assisted Tomog 1981;5:800-811.

Drinkwater BL, Horvath SM: Heat tolerance and aging. Med Sci Sport Exer 1979;11:49-55.

Gorny KR, et al. Calorimetric calibration of head coil SAR estimates displayed on a clinical MR scanner. Phys Med Biol. 2008;53:2565-76.

Gowland PA, De Wilde J. Temperature increase in the fetus due to radio frequency exposure during magnetic resonance scanning. Phys Med Biol. 2008;53:L15-8.

Hand JW, Li Y, et al. Prediction of specific absorption rate in mother and fetus associated with MRI examinations during pregnancy. Magn Reson Med. 2006;55:883-893.

Hartwig V, Giovannetti G, et al. Biological effects and safety in magnetic resonance imaging: a review. Int J Environ Res Public Health. 2009;6:1778-98.

International Commission on Non-Ionizing Radiation Protection (ICNIRP) Statement, Medical magnetic resonance procedures: protection of patients. Health Physics 2004;87:197-216.

International Electrotechnical Commission (IEC), Medical Electrical Equipment, Particular requirements for the safety of magnetic resonance equipment for medical diagnosis, International Standard IEC 60601-2-33, 2002.

Kangarlu A, Shellock FG, Chakeres D. 8.0-Tesla MR system: Temperature changes associated with radiofrequency-induced heating of a head phantom. J Magn Reson Imaging 2003;17:220-226.

Kangarlu A, Ibrahim TS, Shellock FG. Effects of coil dimensions and field polarization on RF heating inside a head phantom. Magnetic Resonance Imaging 2005;23:53-60.

Kenny WL. Physiological correlates of heat intolerance. Sports Med 1985;2:279-286.

Jauchem JR. Effects of drugs on thermal responses to microwaves. Gen Pharmacol 1985;16:307-310.

Oh S, Webb AG, Neuberger T, Park B, Collins CM. Experimental and numerical assessment of MRI-induced temperature change and SAR distributions in phantoms and in vivo. Magn Reson Med. 2009 Sep 25 [Epub ahead of print]

Rowell LB. Cardiovascular aspects of human thermoregulation. Circ Res 1983;52:367-379.

Schaefer DJ. Health effects and safety of radiofrequency power deposition associated with magnetic resonance procedures. In: Shellock FG, ed. Magnetic resonance procedures: health effects and safety. Boca Raton, FL: CRC Press, 2001;55-74.

Shellock FG. Radiofrequency energy-induced heating during MR procedures: a review. J Magn Reson Imaging 2000;12:30-36.

Shellock FG, Crues JV. MR procedures: biologic effects, safety, and patient care. Radiology 2004;232:635-652.

Shellock FG, Crues JV. Temperature, heart rate, and blood pressure changes associated with clinical MR imaging at 1.5-T. Radiology 1987;163:259-262.

Shellock FG, Crues JV. Corneal temperature changes associated with high-field MR imaging using a head coil. Radiology 1988;167:809-811.

Shellock FG, Crues JV. Temperature changes caused by clinical MR imaging of the brain at 1.5 Tesla using a head coil. Am J Neuroradiol 1988;9:287-291.

Shellock FG, Rothman B, Sarti D. Heating of the scrotum by high-field-strength MR imaging. Am J Roentgenol 1990;154:1229-1232.

Shellock FG, Schatz CJ. Increases in corneal temperature caused by MR imaging of the eye with a dedicated local coil. Radiology 192;185:697-699.

Shellock FG, Schaefer DJ. Radiofrequency energy-induced heating during magnetic resonance procedures: laboratory and clinical experiences In: Shellock FG, ed. Magnetic resonance procedures: health effects and safety. Boca Raton, FL: CRC Press, 2001;75-96.

Shellock FG, Schaefer DJ, Crues JV. Alterations in body and skin temperatures caused by MR imaging: Is the recommended exposure for radiofrequency radiation too conservative? Br J Radiol 1989; 62:904-909.

Shellock FG, Schaefer DJ, Kanal E. Physiologic responses to MR imaging performed at an SAR level of 6.0 W/kg. Radiology 1994;192:865-868.

Shrivastava D, Hanson T, et al. Radiofrequency heating at 9.4T: in vivo temperature measurement results in swine. Magn Reson Med. 2008;59:73-8.

Shuman WP, et al. Superficial and deep-tissue increases in anesthetized dogs during exposure to high specific absorption rates in a 1.5-T MR imager. Radiology 1988;167:551-554.

Stuchly MA, Abrishamkar H, Strydom ML. Numerical Evaluation of Radio Frequency Power Deposition in Human Models during MRI. Conf Proc IEEE Eng Med Biol Soc. 2006;1:272-275.

U.S. Department of Health and Human Services, FDA, CDRH, Guidance for Industry and FDA Staff. Criteria for Significant Risk Investigations of Magnetic Resonance Diagnostic Devices, July 14, 2003.

Wang Z, Lin JC, Vaughan JT, Collins CM. Consideration of physiological response in numerical models of temperature during MRI of the human head.J Magn Reson Imaging. 2008;28:1303-1308.

Weintraub MI, Khoury A, Cole SP. Biologic effects of 3 Tesla (T) MR imaging comparing traditional 1.5-T and 0.6-T in 1,023 consecutive outpatients. J Neuroimaging. 2007;17:241-5.

Acoustic Noise
and MR Procedures*

Various types of acoustic noise are produced during the operation of an MR system. Problems associated with acoustic noise for patients and healthcare professionals include annoyance, verbal communication difficulties, heightened anxiety, temporary hearing loss and, in extreme cases, the potential for permanent hearing impairment.

Acoustic noise may pose a particular problem to specific patient groups. For example, patients with psychiatric disorders may become confused or suffer from increased anxiety as the result of exposure to loud noise. Sedated patients may experience discomfort in association with high noise levels. In addition, neonates may have adverse reactions to acoustic noise.

HEARING AND THE IMPACT OF ACOUSTIC NOISE

The human ear is a highly sensitive wide-band receiver, with the typical frequency range for normal hearing being between 20-Hz to 20,000-Hz. The ear does not tend to judge sound powers in absolute terms, but assesses how much greater one power is than another. The logarithmic decibel scale, dB, is used when referring to sound power.

Noise is defined in terms of frequency spectrum (in Hz), intensity (in dB), and time duration. Noise can be steady-state, intermittent, impulsive, or explosive. Transient hearing loss may occur following exposure to loud noise, resulting in a temporary threshold shift (i.e., a shift in audible threshold). With regard to acoustic noise associated with MR imaging, Brummett et al. reported temporary shifts in hearing thresholds in 43% of the patients scanned without ear protection and patients with improperly fitted earplugs. Recovery from the effects of noise occurs in a relatively short period of time. However, if the noise insult is particularly severe, full recovery can take up to several weeks. If the noise is sufficiently injurious, a permanent threshold shift at specific frequencies may occur.

MRI-RELATED ACOUSTIC NOISE

The gradient magnetic field is the main source of acoustic noise associated with an MR procedure. This noise occurs during the rapid alterations of currents within the gradient coils. These currents, in the presence of the strong static magnetic field of the MR system, produce significant (Lorentz) forces that act upon the gradient coils. Acoustic noise, manifested as loud tapping, knocking, chirping, or squeaking sounds, is produced when the forces cause motion or vibration of the gradient coils as they impact against their mountings which, in turn, flex and vibrate.

Alteration of the gradient output (rise time or amplitude) by modifying MR imaging parameters causes the acoustic noise to vary. Noise tends to be enhanced by decreases in section thickness, field of view, repetition time, and echo time. In addition to dependence on imaging parameters, acoustic noise is dependent on the MR system hardware, construction, and the surrounding environment. Furthermore, noise characteristics have a spatial dependence. For example, noise levels have been found to vary by as much as 10 dB as a function of patient position along the bore of the MR system. The presence and size of the patient may also affect the level of acoustic noise.

CHARACTERISTICS OF MR SYSTEM-RELATED ACOUSTIC NOISE

Gradient magnetic field-induced noise levels have been measured during a variety of pulse sequences for MR systems with static magnetic field strengths ranging from 0.35 to 4-Tesla. For example, Hurwitz et al. reported that the MR imaging-related sound levels varied from 82 to 93 dB on the A-weighted scale and from 84 to 103 dB on the linear scale.

Later studies performed using a variety of MR parameters including "worst-case" pulse sequences that applied multiple gradients simultaneously (e.g., three-dimensional, fast gradient echo techniques) reported that these are among the loudest sequences, with acoustic noise levels that ranged from 103 to 113 dB (peak) on the A-weighted scale.

Additional studies measured acoustic noise generated by echo planar imaging (EPI) and fast spin echo sequences. Echo planar sequences tend to have extremely fast gradient switching times and high gradient amplitudes. Shellock et al. reported high levels of noise ranging from 114 to 115 dBA on two different high field strength (1.5-Tesla) MR systems tested when running EPI sequences with parameters chosen to represent "worst-case" protocols. At 3-Tesla, Hattori et al. recorded sound levels that ranged from 126 to 131 dB on a linear scale, recommending the use of both earplugs and headphones for ear protection relative to the use of 3-Tesla MR systems when certain pulse sequences are used.

ACOUSTIC NOISE AND PERMISSIBLE LIMITS

In general, acoustic noise levels recorded in the MR environment have been below the maximum limits permitted by the Occupational Safety and Health Administration of the United States. This is particularly the case when one considers that the duration of exposure is an important physical factor that determines the effect of noise on hearing.

The U.S. Food and Drug Administration released guidelines for acoustic noise levels that should not be exceeded in association with the operation of MR systems, as follows (please refer to **Appendix I**):

Sound Pressure Level - Peak unweighted sound pressure level greater than 140 dB. A-weighted root mean square (rms) sound pressure level greater than 99 dBA with hearing protection in place.

While the acoustic noise levels recommended for patients undergoing MR procedures on an infrequent and short-term basis may appear to be somewhat conservative, they are deemed appropriate when one considers that individuals with underlying health conditions may have problems with noise at certain levels or frequencies. Acoustic noise produced during MR procedures represents a potential risk to such patients. As previously mentioned, the possibility exists that substantial gradient magnetic field-induced noise may produce hearing problems in patients who are susceptible to the damaging effects of loud noises.

The exposure of staff and other healthcare workers in the MR environment is also a concern (e.g., those involved in interventional MR procedures or who remain in the room for patient management reasons). Accordingly, if loud noises exist in the MR environment, staff members should routinely wear ear protection if they remain in the room during the operation of the scanner. In the United Kingdom, guidelines issued by the Department of Health recommend hearing protection be worn by staff exposed to an average of 85 dB over an eight hour day.

ACOUSTIC NOISE CONTROL TECHNIQUES

Passive noise control. The simplest and least expensive means of preventing problems associated with acoustic noise during MR procedures is to encourage the routine use of disposable earplugs or headphones. Earplugs, when properly used, can abate noise by 10 to 30 dB, which is usually an adequate amount of sound attenuation for the MR environment. The use of earplugs typically provides a sufficient decrease in acoustic noise that, in turn, is capable of preventing hearing problems. Therefore, for MR systems that generate substantial acoustic noise, patients should be required to wear these protective devices.

Unfortunately, passive noise control methods suffer from a number of limitations. For example, these devices hamper verbal communication with patients during the operation of the MR system. Additionally, standard earplugs are often too large for the ear canal of adolescents and infants. Importantly, passive noise control devices offer non-uniform noise attenuation over the hearing range. While high frequencies may be well attenuated, attenuation is often poor at low frequencies. This is problematic because, for certain pulse sequences, the low frequency range is where the peak MR imaging-related acoustic noise is generated.

Active Noise Control (ANC). A significant reduction in the level of acoustic noise caused by MR procedures has been accomplished using the active noise cancellation technique. Controlling noise from a particular source by introducing "anti-phase noise" to interfere destructively with the noise source is not a new idea. For example, Goldman et al. combined passive noise control and an active noise control system (i.e. an active system built into a headphone) to achieve an average noise reduction of approximately 14 dB.

Advances in digital signal processing technology allow efficient active noise control systems to be realized at a moderate cost. The anti-noise system involves a continuous feedback loop with continuous sampling of the sounds in the noise environment so that the gradient magnetic field-induced noise is attenuated. It is possible to attenuate the pseudo-periodic scanner noise while allowing the transmission of vocal communication or music to be maintained.

OTHER SOURCES OF MR SYSTEM-RELATED ACOUSTIC NOISE

RF hearing. When the human head is subjected to pulsed radiofrequency (RF) radiation at certain frequencies, an audible sound perceived as a click, buzz, chirp, or knocking noise may be heard. This acoustic phenomenon is referred to as "RF hearing", "RF sound" or "microwave hearing".

Thermoelastic expansion is believed responsible for the production of RF hearing, whereby there is absorption of RF energy that produces a minute temperature elevation (i.e., approximately 1×10^{-6} degrees C) over a brief time period in the tissue of the head. Subsequently, a pressure wave is induced that is sensed by the hair cells of the cochlea via bone conduction. In this manner, the pulse of RF energy is transferred into an acoustic wave within the human head and sensed by the hearing organs.

With specific reference to the operation of MR scanners, RF hearing has been found to be associated with frequencies ranging from 2.4- to 170-MHz. The gradient magnetic field-induced acoustic noise that occurs during an MR procedure is significantly louder than the sounds associated with RF hearing. Therefore, noises produced by the RF auditory phenomenon are effectively masked and not perceived by patients. Currently, there is no evidence of any detrimental health effect related to the presence of RF hearing.

Noise From Subsidiary Systems. Patient comfort fans and cryogen reclamation systems associated with superconducting magnets of MR systems are the main sources of ambient acoustic noise found in the MR environment. Acoustic noise produced by these subsidiary systems is considerably less than that caused by gradient magnetic fields.

[***Portions of this content were excerpted with permission from McJury M. Acoustic Noise and Magnetic Resonance Procedures, In: Magnetic Resonance Procedures: Health Effects and Safety, FG Shellock, Editor, CRC Press, Boca Raton, FL, 2001 and McJury M, Shellock FG. Acoustic noise and MR procedures: A review. Journal of Magnetic Resonance Imaging 12: 37-45, 2000.]**

REFERENCES

Bandettini PA, Jesmanowicz A, Van Kylen J, Birn RA and Hyde J. Functional MRI of brain activation induced by scanner acoustic noise. Magn Reson Med 1998;39:410-416.

Brummett RE, Talbot JM, Charuhas P. Potential hearing loss resulting from MR imaging. Radiology 1988;169:539-540.

Bowtell RW, Mansfield PM. Quiet transverse gradient coils: Lorentz force balancing designs using geometric similitude. Magn Reson Med 1995;34:494-497.

Chaplain GBB. Anti-noise: the Essex breakthrough. Chart Mech Engin 1983;30:41-47.

Chen CK, Chiueh TD, Chen JH. Active cancellation system of acoustic noise in MR imaging. IEEE Trans Biomed Engin 1999;46:186-190.

Cho ZH, Park SH, Kim JH, Chung SC, Chung ST, Chung JY, Moon CW, Yi JH, Wong EK. Analysis of acoustic noise in MRI. Magn Reson Imaging 1997;15:815-822.

Counter SA, Olofsson A, Grahn, Borg E. MRI acoustic noise: sound pressure and frequency analysis. J Magn Reson Imaging 1997;7:606-611.

Elliott SJ, Nelson Active noise control. IEEE Sign Proceed Magn 1983;12-35.

Elder JA. Special senses. In: United States Environmental Protection Agency, Health Effects Research Laboratory. Biological Effects of Radio frequency Radiation. EPA-600/8-83-026F, Research Triangle Park, 1984; pp. 570-571.

Goldman AM, Gossman WE, Friedlander PC. Reduction of sound levels with anti-noise in MR imaging. Radiology 1989;173:549-550.Hall DA, et al. Acoustic, psychophysical, and neuroimaging measurements of the effectiveness of active cancellation during auditory functional magnetic resonance imaging. J Acoust Soc Am. 2009;125:347-59.

Hattori Y, Fukatsu H, Ishigaki T. Measurement and evaluation of the acoustic noise of a 3 Tesla MR scanner. Nagoya J Med Sci. 2007;69:23-28.

Hedeen RA, Edelstein WA. Characteristics and prediction of gradient acoustic noise in MR imagers. Magn Reson Med 1997;37:7-10.

Hurwitz R, Lane SR, Bell RA, Brant-Zawadzki MN. Acoustic analysis of gradient-coil noise in MR imaging. Radiology 1989;173:545-548.

International Commission on Non-Ionizing Radiation Protection (ICNIRP) Statement, Medical magnetic resonance procedures: protection of patients. Health Physics 2004;87:197-216.

Leithner K, et al. Psychological reactions in women undergoing fetal magnetic resonance imaging. Obstet Gynecol. 2008;111(2 Pt 1):396-402.

Mansfield PM, Glover PM. Beaumont J Sound generation in gradient coil structures for MRI. Magn Reson Med 1998;39:539-550.

Mansfield PM, Glover PM, Bowtell RW. Active acoustic screening: design principles for quiet gradient coils in MRI. Meas Sci Technol 1994;5:1021-1025.

McJury MJ. Acoustic noise levels generated during high field MR imaging. Clinical Radiology 1995;50:331-334.

McJury M. Acoustic Noise and Magnetic Resonance Procedures. In: Magnetic Resonance Procedures: Health Effects and Safety. FG Shellock, Editor, CRC Press, Boca Raton, FL, 2001.

McJury M, Blug A, Joerger C, Condon B, Wyper D. Acoustic noise levels during magnetic resonance imaging scanning at 1.5 T. Brit J Radiol 1994;413-415.

McJury M, Shellock FG. Acoustic noise and MR procedures: A review. J Magn Reson Imaging 2000;12:37-45.

McJury M, Stewart RW, Crawford D, Toma E. The use of active noise control (ANC) to reduce acoustic noise generated during MRI scanning: some initial results. Magn Reson Imaging 1997;15:319-322.

Melnick W. Hearing loss from noise exposure. In: Harris CM, ed. Handbook of Noise Control. New York: McGraw-Hill, 1979; pp. 2.

Miller LE, Keller AM. Regulation of occupational noise. In: Harris CM, ed. Handbook of noise control. New York: McGraw-Hill, 1979; pp. 1-16.

Moelker A, Maas RA, Pattynama PM. Verbal communication in MR environments: effect of MR system acoustic noise on understanding. Radiology 2004;232:107-113.

Moelker A, Pattynama PM. Acoustic noise concerns in functional magnetic resonance imaging. Human Brain Mapping 2003;20:123-141.

More SR, Lim TC, Li M, Holland CK, Boyce S, Lee J-H. Acoustic noise characteristics of a 4 Tesla MRI scanner. Journal of Magnetic Resonance Imaging 2006;23:388-397.

Philbin MK, Taber KH, Hayman LA. Preliminary report: changes in vital signs of term newborns during MR. Am J Neuroradiol 1996;17:1033-6.

Quirk ME, Letendre AJ, Ciottone RA, Lingley JF. Anxiety in patients undergoing MR imaging. Radiology 1989;170:464-466.

Robinson DW. Characteristics of occupational noise-induced hearing loss. In: Effects of Noise on Hearing. Henderson D, Hamernik RP, Dosjanjh DS, Mills JH, Editors. Raven Press, New York, 1976; pp. 383-405.

Roschmann P. Human auditory system response to pulsed radio frequency energy in RF coils for magnetic resonance at 2.4 to 170 MHz. Magn Reson Med 1991;21:197-215.

Ruckhäberle E, et al. In vivo intrauterine sound pressure and temperature measurements during magnetic resonance imaging (1.5 T) in pregnant ewes. Fetal Diagn Ther. 2008;24:203-10.

Shellock FG, Kanal E. Policies, guidelines, and recommendations for MR imaging safety and patient management. J Magn Reson Imaging 1991;1:97-101.

Shellock FG, Morisoli SM, Ziarati M. Measurement of acoustic noise during MR imaging: Evaluation of six "worst-case" pulse sequences. Radiology 1994;191:91-93.

Shellock FG, Ziarati M, Atkinson D, Chen D-Y. Determination of gradient magnetic field-induced acoustic noise associated with the use of echo planar and three-dimensional fast spin echo techniques. J Magn Reson Imaging 1998;8:1154-1157.

Strainer JC, Ulmer JL, Yetkin FZ, Haughton VM, Daniels DL, Millen SJ. Functional MR of the primary auditory cortex: an analysis of pure tone activation and tone discrimination. Am J Roentgenol 1997;18: 601-610.

Tomasi DG, Ernst T. Echo planar imaging at 4 Tesla with minimal acoustic noise. J Magn Reson Imaging 2003;128-130.

Ulmer JL, Bharat BB, Leighton PM, Mathews VP, Prost RW, Millen SJ, Garman JN, Horzewski D. Acoustic echo planar scanner noise and pure tone hearing thresholds: the effects of sequence repetition times and acoustic noise rates. J Comp Assist Tomogr 1998;22:480-486.

U.S. Department of Health and Human Services, Food and Drug Administration, Center for Devices and Radiological Health, Radiological Devices Branch, Division of Reproductive, Abdominal, and Radiological Devices, Office of Device Evaluation. Guidance for Industry and FDA Staff. Criteria for significant Risk Investigations of Magnetic Resonance Diagnostic Devices, July 14, 2003.

Body Piercing Jewelry

Ritual or decorative body piercing is extremely popular as a form of self-expression. Different types of materials are used to make body piercing jewelry including ferromagnetic and nonferromagnetic metals, as well as non-metallic materials. The presence of body piercing jewelry that is made from ferromagnetic or conductive material of a certain shape may present a problem for a patient referred for a magnetic resonance (MR) procedure or an individual in the MR environment.

Risks include uncomfortable sensations from movement or displacement that may be mild-to-moderate depending on the site of the body piercing and the ferromagnetic qualities of the jewelry (e.g., mass, degree of magnetic susceptibility, etc.). In extreme cases, serious injuries may occur. In addition, for body piercing jewelry made from electrically conducting material, there is a possibility of MRI-related heating that could cause excessive temperature increases and burns.

Because of potential safety issues, metallic body piercing jewelry should be removed prior to entering the MR environment. However, patients or individuals with body piercings are often reluctant to remove their jewelry. Therefore, if it is not possible to remove metallic body piercing jewelry, the patient or individual should be informed regarding the potential risks. In addition, if the body piercing jewelry is made from ferromagnetic material, some means of stabilization (e.g., application of adhesive tape or bandage) should be used to prevent movement or displacement.

To avoid potential heating of body piercing jewelry made from conductive materials, the use of gauze, tape, or other similar material should be used to wrap the jewelry in such a manner as to insulate it (i.e., prevent contact) from the underlying skin is recommended. The patient should be instructed to immediately inform the MR system operator if any heating or other unusual sensation occurs in association with the body piercing jewelry.

REFERENCES

Armstrong ML, Elkins L. Body art and MRI. Am J Nurs. 2005;105:65-6.

Deboer S, Seaver M, Angel E, Armstrong M. Puncturing myths about body piercing and tattooing. Nursing. 2008;38:50-54.

Muensterer OJ. Temporary removal of navel piercing jewelry for surgery and imaging studies. Pediatrics. 2004;114:e384-6.

Shellock FG. MR safety and body piercing jewelry. Signals, No. 45, Issue 2, pp. 7, 2003.

Claustrophobia, Anxiety, and Emotional Distress in the MR Environment*

For certain patients that undergo magnetic resonance (MR) examinations, the experience may be associated with great emotional distress. Referring physicians, radiologists, and MRI technologists can best manage affected patients by understanding the etiology of the problem and knowing the appropriate maneuver or intervention to implement to counter-act the condition.

The experience of "psychological distress" in the MR environment includes all subjectively unpleasant experiences directly attributable to the procedure. Distress for the patient can range from mild anxiety that can be handled with simple reassurance, to a more serious panic attack that may require psychiatric intervention or medication. Severe psychological reactions to MR examinations, namely anxiety and panic attacks, are characterized by the rapid onset of at least four of the following: nausea, paresthesias, palpitations, chest pain, faintness, dyspnea, choking sensation, sweating, trembling, vertigo, depersonalization, and fear of losing control or dying.

Many symptoms of a panic attack mimic over-activity of the sympathetic nervous system, prompting concern that catecholamine responses may precipitate cardiac arrhythmias or ischemia in susceptible patients. However, this has not been observed in the clinical MR setting. Nevertheless, it is advisable that, in a medically unstable patient, physiologic monitoring and support be readily available.

In the mildest form, distress is the normal amount of anxiety that a person may experience when undergoing a diagnostic procedure. Moderate distress, severe enough to be described as a dysphoric psychological reaction, has been reported by as many as 65% of the patients examined by MR imaging. The most severe forms of psychological distress described by patients are anxiety, claustrophobia, or panic attacks.

Claustrophobia is a disorder characterized by the marked, persistent and excessive fear of enclosed spaces. In such affected individuals, exposure to an enclosed space such as that found with certain MR systems, almost invariably provokes an immediate anxiety response that, in its most extreme form, is indistinguishable from the panic attack described above.

The actual incidence of distress in the MR environment is highly variable across studies due to differences in outcome measures used to determine patient abnormalities. Some studies have indicated that as many as 20% of the individuals attempting to undergo MR procedures can't complete the exams secondary to serious distress such as claustrophobia or other unwanted sensations. In contrast, other investigations have reported that as few as 0.7% of individuals have incomplete or failed MR procedures due to distress.

THE IMPACT OF EMOTIONAL DISTRESS

Patient distress can contribute to adverse outcomes for the MR procedure. These adverse outcomes include unintentional exacerbation of patient distress, a compromise in the quality and, thus, the diagnostic aspects of the imaging study and decreased efficiency of the MRI facility due to delayed, prematurely terminated, or cancelled studies. Patient compliance during an MR procedure, such as the ability to remain in the MR system and to hold still long enough to complete the study, is of paramount importance to achieve a diagnostically acceptable examination. If a good quality study can't be obtained, the patient may require an invasive procedure in place of the inherently safer MR examination. Thus, for the distressed patient unable to undergo an MR procedure, there may be clinical, medico-legal, and economic related implications.

Increasing pressure to use MR system time efficiently to cover the costs of expensive diagnostic imaging equipment puts greater stress on both staff and patients. The ability of referring physicians, radiologists, and MRI technologists to detect patient distress at the earliest possible time, to discover the source of the distress, and to provide appropriate intervention can greatly improve patient comfort, quality of imaging, and efficiency of the facility.

FACTORS THAT CONTRIBUTE TO DISTRESS

Many factors contribute to distress experienced by certain patients undergoing MR procedures. Most commonly cited are concerns about the physical environment of the MR system. Also well documented is the anxiety associated with the underlying medical problem necessitating the MR examination. Certain individuals, such as those with psychiatric illnesses, may be predisposed to suffer greater distress.

The physical environment of the MR system is clearly one important source of distress. Sensations of apprehension, tension, worry, claustrophobia, anxiety, fear, and panic attacks have been directly attributed to the confining dimensions of the MR system. For example, for some scanners, the patient's face may be three to ten inches from the inner portion of the MR system, prompting feelings of uncontrolled confinement and detachment.

Similar distressing sensations have been attributed to other aspects of the MR environment including the prolonged duration of the examination, the acoustic noise, the temperature and humidity within the MR system, and the distress related to restriction of movement. Additionally, being inside of the scanner may produce a feeling of sensory deprivation, which is also known to be a precursor of anxiety states.

MR systems that have an architecture that utilizes a vertical magnetic field offer a more open design that is presumed to reduce the frequency of distress associated with MR procedures. The latest versions of these "open" MR systems, despite having static magnetic field strengths of 0.3-Tesla or lower, have improved technology (i.e., faster gradient fields, optimized surface coils, etc.) that permit acceptable image quality for virtually all types of standard, diagnostic imaging procedures. "High-field open" MR systems operating at 0.7-, 1.0- or 1.5-Tesla are now commercially available and these systems may be more acceptable to patients with feelings of distress. Also, the latest generation, high-field-strength (1.5-Tesla and 3-Tesla) MR systems have shorter and wider bore configurations that likely mitigate feelings of being enclosed or overly confined.

In 1993, a specially designed, low-field-strength (0.2-Tesla) MR system (Artoscan, Lunar Corporation/General Electric Medical Systems, Madison, WI and Esaote, Genoa, Italy) became commercially available for MR imaging of extremities. The use of this dedicated extremity MR system provides an accurate, reliable, and relatively inexpensive means (i.e., in comparison to the use of a whole-body MR system) of evaluating musculoskeletal abnormalities. In fact, utilization of this extremity MR system to assess musculoskeletal pathology is an acceptable alternative to whole-body MR systems since the diagnostic capabilities for evaluation of the knee, shoulder, and other extremities has been reported to be comparable to mid- or high-field-strength MR systems.

The architecture of the extremity MR system has no confining features or other aspects that would typically create patient-related problems. This is because only the body part that requires imaging is placed inside the bore of the magnet during the MR examination. One research study reported that 100% of the MR examinations that were initiated were completed without being interrupted or cancelled for patient-related problems. The unique design of the extremity MR system is believed to have contributed to the successful completion of the MR procedures in the patients of this study. Another dedicated-extremity MR system with an open design permits MR imaging of the shoulder. Adverse psychological reactions are sometimes associated with MR procedures simply because the examination may be perceived by the patient as a "dramatic" medical test with an associated uncertainty of outcome, such that there may be fear of the presence of disease or other condition. In fact, any type of diagnostic procedure can produce anxiety for the patient.

Patients with pre-existing psychiatric disorders may be at greater risk for experiencing distress in the MR environment. Accordingly, patients with pre-existing conditions should be identified prior to MR examinations to implement anxiety-minimizing efforts (see below). Patients with other psychiatric illnesses such as depression and any illness complicated by thought dysfunction, such as schizophrenia or manic-depressive disorder, may also be at increased risk for distress in the MR environment.

Patients with psychiatric illnesses may, under normal circumstances, be able to tolerate the MR environment without a problem, as is clear from the thousands of subjects who participate in clinical neuroimaging and functional MRI research studies each year. However, the increased stress due to their medical illness or fear of medical illness can exacerbate their psychiatric symptoms to such an extent that they may have difficulty complying with MR procedures.

TECHNIQUES TO MINIMIZE PATIENT DISTRESS

Various procedures exist to minimize distress or anxiety in patients undergoing MR procedures (Table 1). Some measures should be employed for all studies, while others may be required only if the patient experiences distress due to the factors described above.

Table 1. Techniques to manage patients with distress associated with MR procedures.

1) Prepare and educate the patient concerning specific aspects of the MR examination (e.g., MR system dimensions, gradient noise, intercom system, constant presence of the technologist etc.).
2) Allow an appropriately screened relative or friend to remain with the patient during the MR procedure.
3) Maintain verbal, visual, and/or physical contact with the patient during the MR procedure.
4) Use an appropriate stereo system to provide music to the patient.

5) Use an appropriate video monitor or goggles to provide a visual distraction to the patient.
6) Use a virtual reality environment system to provide audio and visual distraction.
7) Place the patient prone for the examination.
8) Position the patient feet-first instead of head-first into the MR system.
9) Use mirrors or prism glasses to redirect the patient's line of sight.
10) Use a blindfold so that the patient is not aware of the surroundings.
11) Use bright lights inside of the MR system.
12) Use a fan inside of the MR system.
13) Use vanilla scented oil or other similar aroma therapy.
14) Use relaxation techniques such as controlled breathing or mental imagery.
15) Use systematic desensitization.
16) Use medical hypnosis.
17) Use a sedative or other similar medication.

For All Patients Undergoing MR Procedures

Referring clinicians should take the time to explain the reason for the MR procedure and what he/she expects to learn from the results with respect to the implications for treatment and prognosis. The single most important step is to educate the patient about the aspects of the MR examination that may be challenging or difficult. This includes conveying, in terms that are understandable to the patient, the internal dimensions of the MR system, the level of gradient magnetic field-induced acoustic noise to expect, and the estimated time duration of the examination.

Studies have documented a decrease in the incidence of premature termination of MR examinations when patients were provided with detailed information about the procedures. Accordingly, patients should be provided with an appropriate brochure or video presentation supplemented by a question and answer session with an MR-trained healthcare worker prior to the examination.

Many details of patient positioning in the MR system can increase comfort and, thus, minimize distress. Taking time to ensure comfortable positioning with sufficient padding and blankets to alleviate undue discomfort or pain is also important. Adequate ear protection should be provided routinely to decrease acoustic noise from the MR system, as needed (i.e., this is typically not required for low-field-strength MR systems). Demonstration of the two-way intercom system, "squeeze ball", or other monitoring technique to reassure the patient that the MR staff is readily available during the examination is vital for proper patient management.

For Mildly-to-Moderately Distressed Patients

If a patient continues to experience distress after the afore-mentioned measures are implemented, additional interventions are required. Frequently, all that is necessary to successfully complete an MR examination is to allow an appropriately screened relative or friend to remain with the patient. A familiar person in the MR system room will often help an anxious patient develop an increased sense of security. If a supportive companion is not present, a staff member can maintain contact with the patient during the examination to decrease psychological distress.

Placing the patient prone so that the opening of the MR system can be seen will provide a sensation of being in a device that is more spacious. As such, prone positioning can alleviate the "closed-in" feelings frequently associated with being supine. Unfortunately, prone positioning may not be   practical if the patient has certain underlying medical conditions (e.g., shortness of breath, the presence of chest tubes, wearing a cervical fixation device, etc.). Another method of positioning the patient that may help is to place the individual feet-first instead of head-first into the scanner.

Mirrors or prism glasses can be used to permit the patient to maintain a vertical view of the outside of the MR system in order to minimize phobic responses. Using a blindfold or "eye pillow" (small pillow containing flax seeds) so that the patient is unaware of the close surroundings has also been suggested to be an effective technique for enabling anxious patients to successfully undergo MR procedures.

The environment of the MR system may be changed to optimize the management of apprehensive patients. For example, the presence of higher lighting levels tends to make most individuals feel less anxious. Therefore, the use of bright lights at either end and inside of the MR system can produce a less imposing environment for the patient. Using a fan inside of the scanner to increase airflow will also help reduce the sensation of confinement. In addition, aroma therapy (e.g., placing a cotton pad moistened with a few drops of lemon, vanilla, or cucumber oil in the MR system) can help reduce distress by providing the patient with a pleasant olfactory stimulation.

Specialized systems that transmit music or audio communication through headphones have been developed specifically for use with MR systems. Reports have indicated that these devices successfully reduced symptoms of anxiety in patients during MR procedures. Furthermore, it is now possible to provide visual stimulation to the patient via monitors or special goggles. Use of visual stimuli to distract patients tends to reduce distress. Finally, a system has been developed to provide a calming virtual reality environment for the patient that may likewise serve as an acceptable means of audio and visual distraction from the MR procedure (this device is frequently used for functional MRI studies).

For Severely Distressed or Claustrophobic Patients

Patients who are at high risk for severe distress in the MR environment and can be identified as such by their referring clinician or by the scheduling MR staff person should be offered the opportunity to have pre-MR procedure behavioral therapy. MR procedures conducted in patients that previously refused or were unable to tolerate the MR environment have been reported to be successfully managed using relaxation techniques, systematic desensitization, and medical hypnosis.

In the majority of MRI facilities, patients severely affected by claustrophobia, anxiety, or panic attacks in response to MR procedures usually need sedation when attempts to counteract their distress fail. Using a short-acting sedative or an anxiolytic medication may be the only means of managing a patient with a high degree of anxiety. However, the use of sedatives in patients prior to and during MR procedures may not be required in all instances, nor is it always practical.

Obviously, the use of sedation in the MR environment requires special preparation involving several important patient management considerations. For example, the time when the patient is administered the medication for optimal effect prior to the examination must be considered along with the possibility that an adverse reaction may occur. The use of acceptable monitoring equipment operated by appropriately trained and experienced healthcare professionals is required to ensure patient safety. In addition, provisions should be available for an area to permit adequate recovery of the patient after an MR procedure that involves sedation.

[*Portions of this content were excerpted with permission from Gollub RL and Shellock FG. Claustrophobia, Anxiety, and Emotional Distress in the Magnetic Resonance Environment. In, Magnetic Resonance Procedures: Health Effects and Safety. FG Shellock, Editor, CRC Press, Boca Raton, FL, 2001.]

REFERENCES

Adamietz B, Cavallaro A, et al. Tolerance of magnetic resonance imaging in children and adolescents performed in a 1.5 Tesla MR scanner with an open design Rofo. 2007;179:826-831.

Bangard C, et al. MR imaging of claustrophobic patients in an open 1.0T scanner: motion artifacts and patient acceptability compared with closed bore magnets. Eur J Radiol. 2007;64:152-7.

Bigley J, et al. Neurolinguistic programming used to reduce the need for anaesthesia in claustrophobic patients undergoing MRI. Br J Radiol. 2009. [Epub ahead of print]

Dewey M, Schink T, Dewey CF. Claustrophobia during magnetic resonance imaging: cohort study in over 55,000 patients. J Magn Reson Imaging. 2007;26:1322-7.

Eshed I, Althoff CE, Hamm B, Hermann KG. Claustrophobia and premature termination of magnetic resonance imaging examinations. J Magn Reson Imaging. 2007;26:401-404.

Gollub RL, Shellock FG. Claustrophobia, Anxiety, and Emotional Distress in the Magnetic Resonance Environment. In, Magnetic Resonance Procedures: Health Effects and Safety. FG Shellock, Editor, CRC Press, Boca Raton, FL, 2001.

Harris LM, Cumming SR, Menzies RG. Predicting anxiety in magnetic resonance imaging scans. International Journal of Behavioral Medicine 2004;11:1-7.

McGuinness TP. Hypnosis in the treatment of phobias: a review of the literature. Am J Clin Hypnosis 1984;26:261.

Murphy KJ, Brunberg JA. Adult claustrophobia, anxiety and sedation in MRI. Magnetic Resonance Imaging 1997;15:51.

Sarji SA, Abdullah BJ, Kumar G, et al. Failed magnetic resonance imaging examinations due to claustrophobia. Australas Radiol 1998;42:293.

Shellock FG. Claustrophobia, anxiety, and panic disorders associated with MR procedures, In: Magnetic Resonance: Bioeffects, Safety, and Patient Management. F.G. Shellock, and Kanal, E., Editor, Lippincott-Raven Press, New York, 1996, pp. 65

Shellock FG, Kanal E. Policies, guidelines, and recommendations for MR imaging and patient management. J. Magn. Reson. Imaging 1991;1:97.

Shellock FG, Stone KR, Resnick D, et al. Subjective perceptions of MRI examinations performed using an extremity MR system. Signals 2000;32:16.

Spouse E, Gedroyc WM. MRI of the claustrophobic patient: interventionally configured magnets. Br J Radiol. 2000;73:146-151.

Thorpe S, Salkovskis PM, Dittner A. Claustrophobia in MRI: the role of cognitions. Magn Reson Imaging. 2008;26:1081-8.

Weinreb J, Maravilla KR, Peshock R, et al. Magnetic resonance imaging: improving patient tolerance and safety. American Journal of Roentgenology 1984;143:1285.

Wollman DE, Beeri MS, Weinberger M, et al. Tolerance of MRI procedures by the oldest old. Magn Reson Imaging. 2004;22:1299-304.

Epicardial Pacing Wires and Intracardiac Pacing Wires*

Although the theoretical risk exists that MRI examinations in patients with retained temporary epicardial leads (which consist of electrically conductive material) could lead to cardiac excitation or thermal injury, such retained leads which are relatively short in length, usually do not form large loops, and are generally not believed to pose a significant hazard during MRI procedures.

Hartnell et al. reported on 51 patients with retained temporary epicardial pacing wires who underwent clinical MRI procedures. Of those patients examined with electrocardiographic monitoring, no arrhythmias were noted, and for all patients, no symptoms suggestive of arrhythmia or other cardiac dysfunction were noted (although the anatomic region examined and the RF energies used in the examinations were not specifically described). To date, there is no report of complications associated with performing MRI in a patient with retained epicardial leads.

By comparison, one *ex vivo* study of temporary intracardiac, transvenous pacing leads reported temperature increases of up to 63.1 degrees C. Preliminary results of a recent study confirmed that even unconnected temporary transvenous pacing (as well as permanent pacing) leads can undergo high temperature increases at 1.5-Tesla. In a chronic-pacemaker animal model undergoing an MRI examination at 1.5-Tesla, temperature increases of up to 20 degrees C were measured, although pathological and histological examination did not demonstrate heat-induced damage of the myocardium. The MRI conditions that generated such elevated lead temperatures included use of the body RF coil to transmit RF energy over the area of the intracardiac pacing lead (e.g., an MRI examination of the chest/thorax).

To the best of our knowledge (i.e., the Consensus Group: Levine GN, Gomes AS, Arai AE, Bluemke DA, Flamm SD, Kanal E, Manning WJ, Martin ET, Smith JM, Wilke N, Shellock FG) there are no studies assessing the safety of temporary pacemakers (lead and external pulse generator). Unlike permanent devices, temporary pacemakers use unfixed leads that are more prone to movement, longer leads that may be more prone to induction of lead currents, and a less sophisticated pulse generator, which makes these devices more susceptible to electromagnetic interference.

Thus, patients with retained temporary epicardial pacing wires are believed to be able to safely undergo MRI procedures, and these patients do not need to be routinely screened for the presence of such wires before scanning. Because of the possible risks involved with temporary-pacemaker external pulse generators, such pulse generators should not be introduced into the MRI environment.

Although temporary intracardiac, transvenous lead heating might be minimized or avoided by scanning anatomic regions above (e.g., head/brain) or below (e.g., lower extremities) the cardiac pacing leads, scanning of patients with temporary intracardiac pacing leads (without the pulse generator) is not recommended. Furthermore, because the harsh electromagnetic environment associated with the MR system can alter the operation of an external pulse generator or damage it, it may not be possible to reliably pace the patient during the MRI examination, which makes the issue of scanning a patient with a temporary intracardiac, transvenous lead irrelevant in most cases.

[Excerpted with permission from Levine GN, Gomes AS, Arai AE, Bluemke DA, Flamm SD, Kanal E, Manning WJ, Martin ET, Smith JM, Wilke N, Shellock FG. Safety of magnetic resonance imaging in patients with cardiovascular devices: an American Heart Association scientific statement from the Committee on Diagnostic and Interventional Cardiac Catheterization. Circulation 2007;116:2878-2891.]

REFERENCES

Achenbach S, Moshage W, Diem B, Bieberle T, Schibgilla V, Bachmann K. Effects of magnetic resonance imaging on cardiac pacemakers and electrodes. Am Heart J 1997;134:467-473.

Dempsey MF, Condon B, Hadley DM. Investigation of the factors responsible for burns during MRI. J Magn Reson Imaging. 2001;13:627–631.

Hartnell GG, Spence L, Hughes LA, Cohen MC, Saouaf R, Buff B. Safety of MR imaging in patients who have retained metallic materials after cardiac surgery. AJR Am J Roentgenol. 1997;168:1157–1159.

Levine GN, Gomes AS, Arai AE, Bluemke DA, Flamm SD, Kanal E, Manning WJ, Martin ET, Smith JM, Wilke N, Shellock FG. Safety of magnetic resonance imaging in patients with cardiovascular devices: an American Heart Association scientific statement from the Committee on Diagnostic and Interventional Cardiac Catheterization. Circulation 2007;116:2878-2891.

Luechinger R, Zeijlemaker VA, Pedersen EM, Mortensen P, Falk E, Duru F, Candinas R, Boesiger P. In vivo heating of pacemaker leads during magnetic resonance imaging. Eur Heart J. 2005;26:376-383.

Shellock FG, Valencerina S, Fischer L. MRI-related heating of pacemaker at 1.5- and 3-Tesla: Evaluation with and without pulse generator attached to leads. Circulation 2005;112;Supplement II:561.

Extremity MR System

In 1993, a specially designed, low-field-strength (0.2-Tesla MR system, Artoscan, Lunar Corporation Madison, WI and General Electric Medical Systems, Milwaukee, WI/Esaote, Genoa, Italy) MR system became commercially available for MR imaging of extremities. This MR system uses a small-bore permanent magnet to image feet, ankles, knees, hands, wrists, and elbows.

The ergonomic design of the extremity scanner is such that the body part of interest is placed inside the magnet bore, with the patient positioned in a seated position or supine (i.e., depending on the body part that is imaged). The entire extremity MR system has a built-in radiofrequency shield and multiple body-part-specific extremity coils.

A major advantage of this extremity MR system is that it can be sited in a relatively small space (e.g., approximately 100 square feet) without the need for a special power source, magnetic field shielding, or radiofrequency shielding. Of note is that MR imaging using the extremity MR system has been demonstrated to provide a sensitive, accurate, and reliable assessment of various forms of musculoskeletal pathology.

Because of the unique design features of the extremity MR system (which includes a low-field-strength static magnetic field with a relatively small fringe field) and in consideration of how patients are positioned for MR procedures using this device (i.e., only the body part imaged is placed within the magnet bore while the rest of the body remains outside), it may be possible to safely image patients with aneurysm clips, even if they are made from ferromagnetic materials. Furthermore, it may be possible to perform extremity MR imaging in patients with cardiac pacemakers or implantable cardioverter defibrillators (ICDs). Therefore, investigations were conducted to specifically evaluate these safety issues.

PATIENTS WITH FERROMAGNETIC ANEURYSM CLIPS

A study was performed to assess magnetic field interactions for a variety of aneurysm clips exposed to the 0.2-Tesla extremity MR system. Twenty-two different aneurysm clips were evaluated including those made from nonferromagnetic, weakly ferromagnetic, and ferromagnetic materials (e.g., a Heifetz aneurysm clip made from 17-7PH and a

Yasargil, Model FD aneurysm clip). The results indicated that none of the aneurysm clips displayed substantial magnetic field interactions in association with exposure to the 0.2-Tesla extremity MR system.

Due to the design features of the extremity MR system and in consideration of how patients are positioned during the use of this scanner (i.e., the head does not enter the magnet bore), it is considered safe to perform MR imaging in patients with the specific aneurysm clips evaluated for magnetic field interactions. These findings effectively permit an important diagnostic imaging modality to be used to evaluate patients with suspected musculoskeletal abnormalities using the Artoscan Extremity MR system.

Notably, various studies have reported that patients with Heifetz (17-7PH) and Yasargil, Model FD aneurysm clips (i.e., two of the clips evaluated in the study using the Artoscan scanner) should not undergo MR imaging using MR systems with conventional designs because of the strong attraction shown by these implants, which poses a substantial hazard to patients.

PATIENTS WITH CARDIAC PACEMAKERS AND IMPLANTABLE CARDIOVERTER DEFIBRILLATORS

In general, patients with cardiac pacemakers and implantable cardioverter defibrillators (ICDs), especially if the devices are older models (i.e., pre-1996) are generally not permitted to undergo MR procedures. However, due to the design of the Artoscan extremity MR system it may be possible to safely perform MR examinations in patients with these devices under certain conditions.

Since the magnetic fringe field of the extremity MR system is contained in close proximity to the 0.2-Tesla magnet and this scanner has an integrated Faraday cage, only the patient's examined extremity is exposed to electromagnetic fields when a procedure is performed. Notably, it is not possible for the MR system's gradient or RF electromagnetic fields to induce currents in a pacemaker or ICD because the patient's thorax (i.e., where the pacemaker or ICD is typically implanted) remains outside of the bore of the MR system.

Ex vivo experiments were conducted to assess MR safety for seven different cardiac pacemakers and seven different implantable cardioverter defibrillators manufactured by Medtronic, Inc. (Minneapolis, MN), as follows:

Device	Name	Model
Pacemaker	Elite II	7086
Pacemaker	Thera D	7944
Pacemaker	Thera D	7960I
Pacemaker	Thera DR	7962i
Pacemaker	Thera SR	8940
Pacemaker	Kappa	400
Pacemaker	Kappa	700
ICD	PCD	7217D
ICD	Jewel	7219D
ICD	Jewel Plus	7220C
ICD	Micro Jewel	7221Cx
ICD	Micro Jewel II	7223Cx
ICD	Prototype	7250G
ICD	Prototype	7271

Magnetic field interactions were assessed relative to the 0.2-Tesla static magnetic field of the extremity MR system. Additionally, the cardiac pacemakers and implantable cardioverter defibrillators were operated with various lead systems attached while immersed in a tank containing physiologic saline (i.e., this apparatus was used to simulate the thorax). This *in vitro* experimental set-up was oriented in parallel and perpendicular positions relative to the closest part of the MR system to mimic patients undergoing MR procedures using this extremity scanner.

MR studies were performed on a phantom using T1-weighted, spin echo and gradient echo pulse sequences. Various functions of the pacemakers and ICDs were evaluated before, during, and after MR imaging. The results of these tests indicated that magnetic field interactions did not present problems for the devices and the activation of the pacemakers and ICDs did not substantially affect image quality. Importantly, the operation of the extremity MR system produced no alterations in the function of the cardiac pacemakers and ICDs. Therefore, in consideration of these data and in view of how patients are positioned during MR procedures using the Artoscan extremity MR system, it should be safe to perform examinations in patients with the specific cardiac pacemakers and implantable cardioverter defibrillators evaluated in this study.

REFERENCES

Ahn JM, Sartoris DJ, Kank HS, Resnick D. Gamekeeper thumb: comparison of MR arthrography with conventional arthrography and MR imaging in cadavers. Radiology 1998;206:737-744.

Barile A, Masiocchi C, Mastantuono M, Passariello R, Satragno L. The use of a "dedicated" MRI system in the evaluation of knee joint diseases. Clinical MRI 1995;5:79-82.

Franklin PD, Lemon RA, Barden HS. Accuracy of imaging the menisci on an in-office, dedicated, magnetic resonance imaging extremity system. Am J Sports Med 1998;25:382-388.

Kersting-Sommerhoff B, Hof N, Lenz M, Gerhardt P. MRI of peripheral joints with a low-field dedicated system: a reliable and cost-effective alternative to high-field units? Eur Radiol 1996;6:561-565.

Maschicchi C. Dedicated MR system and acute trauma of the musculo-skeletal system. Eur J Radiol 1996;22:7-10.

Peterfy CG, Roberts T, Genant HK. Dedicated extremity MR imaging: an emerging technology. Radiol Clin North Am 1997;35:1-20.

Shellock FG. Magnetic Resonance Procedures: Health Effects and Safety. CRC Press, LLC, Boca Raton, FL, 2001.

Shellock FG, Bert, JM, Fritts HM, Gundry C, Easton R, Crues JV. Evaluation of the rotator cuff and glenoid labrum using a 0.2-Tesla, extremity MR system: MR results compared to surgical findings. Journal of Magnetic Resonance Imaging 2001;14:763-770.

Shellock FG, Crues JV. Aneurysm clips: Assessment of magnetic field interaction associated with a 0.2-T extremity MR system. Radiology 1998;208:407-409.

Shellock FG, O'Neil M, Ivans V, Kelly D, O'Connor M, Toay L, Crues JV. Cardiac pacemakers and implantable cardiac defibrillators are unaffected by operation of an extremity MR system. Am J Roentgenol 1999;72:165-17.

Shellock FG, Stone K, Crues JV. Development and clinical applications of kinematic MRI of the patellofemoral joint using an extremity MR system. Med Sci Sport Exerc 1999;31:788-791.

Shellock FG, Mullen M, Stone K, Coleman M, Crues JV. Kinematic MRI evaluation of the effect of bracing on patellar positions: qualitative assessment using an extremity MR system. Journal of Athletic Training 2000;35:44-49.

Guidelines for the Management of the Post-Operative Patient Referred for a Magnetic Resonance Procedure*

There is often confusion regarding the issue of performing a magnetic resonance (MR) procedure during the post-operative period in a patient with a metallic implant or device. Studies have supported that, if a metallic object is a "passive implant" (i.e., there is no electronically- or magnetically-activated component associated with the operation of the device) and it is made from nonferromagnetic material, the patient may undergo an MR procedure immediately after implantation using an MR system operating at 1.5-Tesla or less (or, the field strength that was used to test the device, including 3-Tesla). In fact, there are several reports that describe placement of vascular stents, coils, filters, and other implants using MR-guided procedures that include the use of high-field-strength (1.5- and 3-Tesla) MR systems.

Additionally, a patient or individual with a nonferromagnetic, passive implant is allowed to enter the MR environment associated with a scanner operating at 1.5-Tesla (or, the field strength that was used to test the device, including 3-Tesla) or less immediately after implantation of such an object. For an implant or device that exhibits "weakly magnetic" qualities, it may be necessary to wait a period of at least six weeks after implantation before performing an MR procedure or allowing the individual or patient to enter the MR environment. For example, certain intravascular and intracavitary coils, stents, and filters designated as "weakly magnetic" become firmly incorporated into tissue a minimum of six weeks following placement. In these cases, retentive or counter-forces provided by tissue ingrowth, scarring, or granulation serve to prevent these objects from presenting risks or hazards to patients or individuals in the MR environment.

However, patients with implants or devices that are "weakly magnetic" but rigidly fixed in the body (e.g., bone screws, other orthopedic implants, or other devices) may be studied immediately after implantation. Specific information pertaining to the recommended post-operative waiting period may be found in the labeling or product insert for an implant or device.

Special Note: If there is any concern regarding the integrity of the tissue with respect to its ability to retain the implant or object in place or the implant cannot be properly identified, the patient or individual should not be exposed to the MR environment.

[*The document, Guidelines for the Management of the Post-Operative Patient Referred for a Magnetic Resonance Procedure, was developed by the Institute for Magnetic Resonance Safety, Education, and Research (IMRSER) and published with permission.]

REFERENCES

Ahmed S, Shellock FG. Magnetic resonance imaging safety: implications for cardiovascular patients. Journal of Cardiovascular Magnetic Resonance 2001;3:171-181.

Bueker A, et al. Real-time MR fluoroscopy for MR-guided iliac artery stent placement. J Magn Reson Imaging 2000;12:616-622.

http://www.IMRSER.org; website for the Institute for Magnetic Resonance Safety, Education, and Research

Manke C, Nitz WR, Djavidani B, et al. MR imaging-guided stent placement in iliac arterial stenoses: A feasibility study. Radiology 2001;219:527-534.

Rutledge JM, Vick GW, Mullins CE, Grifka RG. Safety of magnetic resonance immediately following Palmaz stent implant: a report of three cases. Catheter Cardiovasc Interv 2001;53:519-523.

Sawyer-Glover A, Shellock FG. Pre-MRI procedure screening: recommendations and safety considerations for biomedical implants and devices. J Magn Reson Imaging 2000;12:92-106.

Shellock FG. Guidelines for the Management of the Post-Operative Patient Referred for a Magnetic Resonance Procedure. Signals, No. 47, Issue 3, pp. 14, 2003.

Shellock FG. MR safety update 2002: Implants and devices. J Magn Reson Imaging 2002;16:485-496.

Shellock FG. Magnetic Resonance Procedures: Health Effects and Safety. CRC Press, LLC, Boca Raton, FL, 2001.

Shellock FG, Cosendai G, Park S-M, Nyenhuis JA. Implantable microstimulator: magnetic resonance safety at 1.5-Tesla. Investigative Radiology 2004;39:591-594.

Shellock FG, Crues JV. MR procedures: biologic effects, safety, and patient care. Radiology, 2004;232:635-652.

Spuentrup E, et al. Magnetic resonance-guided coronary artery stent placement in a swine model. Circulation 2002;105:874-879.

Teitelbaum GP, Bradley WG, Klein BD. MR imaging artifacts, ferromagnetism, and magnetic torque of intravascular filters, stents, and coils. Radiology 1988;166:657-664.

Teitelbaum GP, Lin MCW, Watanabe AT, et al. Ferromagnetism and MR imaging: safety of cartoid vascular clamps. Am J Neuroradiol 1990;11:267-272.

Teitelbaum GP, Ortega HV, Vinitski S, et al. Low artifact intravascular devices: MR imaging evaluation. Radiology 1988;168:713-719.

Teitelbaum GP, Raney M, Carvlin MJ, et al. Evaluation of ferromagnetism and magnetic resonance imaging artifacts of the Strecker tantalum vascular stent. Cardiovasc Intervent Radiol 1989;12:125-127.

Guidelines for Screening Patients for MR Procedures and Individuals for the MR Environment*

The establishment of thorough and effective screening procedures for patients and other individuals is one of the most critical components of a program that guards the safety of all those preparing to undergo magnetic resonance (MR) procedures or to enter the MR environment. An important aspect of protecting patients and individuals from MR system-related accidents and injuries involves an understanding of the risks associated with the various implants, devices, accessories, and other objects that may cause problems in this setting. This requires constant attention and diligence to obtain information and documentation about these objects in order to provide the safest MR setting possible.

In addition, because most MR-related incidents have been due to deficiencies in screening methods and/or the lack of properly controlling access to the MR environment (especially with regard to preventing personal items and other potentially problematic objects from entering the MR system room), it is crucial to set up procedures and guidelines to prevent such incidents from occurring.

Magnetic Resonance (MR) Procedure Screening for Patients

Certain aspects of screening patients for MR procedures may take place during the scheduling process. These activities should be conducted by a healthcare worker specially trained in MR-safety (i.e., trained to understand the potential hazards and issues associated with the MR environment and MR procedures and to be familiar with the information contained on the screening forms for patients and individuals). While scheduling the patient, it may be ascertained if the patient has an implant or device that may be contraindicated or requires special attention for the MR procedure (e.g., a ferromagnetic aneurysm clip, pacemaker, neurostimulation system, etc.) or if there is a condition that needs careful consideration (e.g., the patient is pregnant, has a disability, history of renal failure, metallic foreign body, etc.). Preliminary screening helps to prevent scheduling patients that may be inappropriate candidates for MR examinations.

After preliminary screening, the patient must undergo comprehensive screening in preparation for the MR procedure. Comprehensive screening involves the use of a printed form to document the screening procedure, a review of the information on the screening form, and a verbal interview to verify the information on the form and to allow for discussion of concerns that the patient may have. An MR-safety trained healthcare professional must conduct this important aspect of patient screening.

The screening form entitled, *Magnetic Resonance (MR) Procedure Screening Form for Patients* was created in conjunction with the Medical, Scientific, and Technology Advisory Board and the Corporate Advisory Board of the Institute for Magnetic Resonance Safety, Education, and Research (IMRSER) (Figure 1). A "downloadable" version of this form may be obtained from the web sites, www.IMRSER.org and www.MRIsafety.com. This form is also available in Spanish (Figure 2, Translated by Olga Fernandez-Flygare, M.S., Brain Mapping Center, UCLA School of Medicine, Los Angeles, CA and Maelesa Rachele Oriente-Padilla', Loyola-Marymount University, Los Angeles, CA).

Page one of the screening form requests general patient-related information (name, age, sex, height, weight, etc.) as well as information regarding the reason for the MR examination and/or symptoms that may be present. Pertinent information about the patient is required not only to ensure that the medical records are up-to-date, but also in the event that the MRI facility needs to contact the referring physician for additional information regarding the examination or to verify the patient's medical condition.

The form requests information regarding a prior surgical procedure to help determine if there may be an implant or device present that could create a problem. Information is also requested pertaining to prior diagnostic imaging studies that may be helpful to review for assessment of the patient's condition.

Next, questions are posed to determine if there are issues that should be discussed with the patient prior to permitting entry to the MR environment. For example, information is requested regarding any problem with a previous MR examination, an injury to the eye involving a metallic object, or injury from a metallic foreign body. Questions are posed to obtain information about current or recently taken medications as well as the presence of drug allergies. There are also questions asked to assess past and present medical conditions that may affect the MR procedure or the use of an MRI contrast agent.

Important Information: MRI Contrast Agents and Nephrogenic Systemic Fibrosis (NSF). The American College of Radiology (ACR) Contrast Committee and the Subcommittee for MR Safety members recommend pre-screening patients prior to the administration of Gadolinium-Based MR Contrast Agents (GBMCA), as follows:

A recent (e.g., last 6 weeks) Glomerular Filtration Rate (GFR) assessment be reviewed for patients with a history of:

- Renal disease (including solitary kidney, renal transplant, renal tumor)
- Age >60 years old
- History of Hypertension
- History of Diabetes
- History of severe hepatic disease/liver transplant/pending liver transplant. For patients in this category, *only*, it is recommended that the patient's GFR assessment be nearly contemporaneous with the MR examination for which the GBMCA is to be administered.

In consideration of the above, questions are posed to the patient to determine if there are conditions that may need to be considered relative to the use of MRI contrast agents and the issue of NSF. For more information on this topic, refer to the section entitled, **MRI Contrast Agents and Nephrogenic Systemic Fibrosis (NSF)***.

At the bottom of page one, there is a section for female patients that poses questions that may impact MR procedures. For example, questions regarding the date of the last menstrual period, pregnancy or late menstrual period are included. A definite or possible pregnancy must be identified prior to permitting the patient into the MR environment so that the risk vs. the benefit of the MR procedure can be considered and discussed with the patient. MR examinations should only be performed in pregnant patients to address important clinical questions. MR facilities should have a clearly defined procedure to follow in the event that the patient has a possible or confirmed pregnancy.

Questions pertaining to the date of the last menstrual period, use of oral contraceptives or hormonal therapy, and fertility medication are necessary for female patients undergoing MR procedures that are performed to evaluate breast disease or for OB/GYN applications, as these may alter tissue contrast on MR imaging. An inquiry about breastfeeding is included in case the administration of MRI contrast media is being considered for use in nursing mothers.

Page 2 of the form has the following statement at the top of the page: "WARNING: Certain implants, devices, or objects may be hazardous to you and/or may interfere with the MR procedure (i.e., MRI, MR angiography, functional MRI, MR spectroscopy). Do not enter the MR system room or MR environment if you have any question or concern regarding an implant, device, or object. Consult the MRI Technologist or Radiologist BEFORE entering the MR system room. The MR system magnet is ALWAYS on."

Next, there is a section that lists various implants, devices, and objects to identify anything that could be hazardous to the patient undergoing the MR procedure or that may produce an artifact that could interfere with the interpretation of the MR examination. In general, these items are arranged on the checklist in order of the relative safety hazard or risk (e.g., aneurysm clip, cardiac pacemaker, implantable cardioverter defibrillator, electronic implant, etc.), followed by items that may produce imaging artifacts that could be problematic for the interpretation of the MR procedure. Additionally, questions are posed to determine if the patient has a breathing problem, movement disorder, or claustrophobia.

Figures of the human body are included on the second page of the form as a means of showing the location of any object inside of or on the body. This information allows the patient to indicate the approximate position of an object that may be hazardous or that could interfere with the interpretation of the MR procedure as a result of producing an artifact.

Page 2 of the screening form also has an *Important Instructions* section that states: "Before entering the MR environment or MR system room, you must remove all metallic objects including hearing aids, dentures, partial plates, keys, beeper, cell phone, eyeglasses, hair pins, barrettes, jewelry, body piercing jewelry, watch, safety pins, paperclips, money clip, credit cards, bank cards, magnetic strip cards, coins, pens, pocket knife, nail clipper, tools, clothing with metal fasteners, & clothing with metallic threads. Please consult the MRI Technologist or Radiologist if you have any question or concern BEFORE you enter the MR system room."

Finally, there is a statement that indicates hearing protection is "advised or required" to prevent possible problems or hazards related to acoustic noise. In general, this should not be an option for a patient undergoing an MR procedure on a high-field-strength MR system. Alternatively, it may be unnecessary for a patient to use hearing protection if undergoing an MR procedure on a low-field-strength MR system.

Importantly, undergoing previous MR procedures without incidents does not guarantee a safe subsequent MR examination. Various factors (e.g., the field strength of the MR system, the orientation of the patient, the orientation of a metallic implant or object, etc.) can substantially change the scenario. Thus, a written screening form must be completed each time a patient prepares to undergo an MR examination.

With the use of any type of written questionnaire, limitations exist related to incomplete or incorrect answers provided by the patient. For example, there may be difficulties associated with patients that are impaired with respect to their vision, language fluency, or level of literacy. Therefore, an appropriate accompanying family member or other individual (e.g., referring physician) should be involved in the screening process to verify any information that may impact patient safety. Versions of this form should also be available in other languages, as needed (i.e., specific to the demographics of the MRI facility).

In the event that the patient is comatose or unable to communicate, the written screening form should be completed by the most qualified individual (e.g., physician, family member, etc.) who has knowledge about the patient's medical history and present condition. If the screening information is inadequate, it is advisable to look for surgical scars on the patient and/or to obtain plain films of the skull and/or chest to search for implants that may be hazardous in the MR environment (e.g., aneurysm clips, cardiac pacemakers, neurostimulation systems, etc.).

Following completion of the *Magnetic Resonance (MR) Procedure Screening Form for Patients*, an MR-safety trained healthcare worker should review the form's content. Next, a verbal interview should be conducted by the MR-safety trained healthcare worker to verify the information on the form and to allow discussion of any question or concern that the patient may have. This provides a mechanism for clarification or confirmation of the answers to the questions posed to the patient so that there is no miscommunication regarding important MR safety issues. In addition, because the patient may not be fully aware of the medical terminology used for a particular implant or device, it is imperative that this particular information on the form be discussed during the verbal interview.

After the comprehensive screening procedure is completed, a patient that is transferred by a stretcher, gurney, or wheelchair to the MR system room should be checked thoroughly for metallic objects such as ferromagnetic oxygen tanks, monitors, or other objects that could pose a hazard. Obviously, only nonferromagnetic stretchers, gurneys, wheelchairs and accessories should be allowed into the MR system room.

Magnetic Resonance (MR) Environment Screening for Individuals

Before any non-patient individual (e.g., MRI technologist, physician, relative, visitor, allied health professional, maintenance worker, custodial worker, fire fighter, security officer, etc.) is allowed into the MR environment, he or she must be screened by an MR-safety trained healthcare worker. Proper screening for individuals involves the use of a printed form to document the procedure, a review of the information on the form, and a verbal interview to verify the information on the form and to allow discussion of any question or concern that the individual may have before being permitted into the MR environment.

Important Note: If for any reason the individual undergoing screening may need to enter the MR system and, thus, become exposed to the electromagnetic fields used for an MR procedure, this person must be screened using the *Magnetic Resonance (MR) Procedure Screening Form for Patients.*

In general, magnetic resonance (MR) screening forms were developed with patients in mind and, therefore, tend to pose many questions that are inappropriate or confusing to other individuals that may need to enter the MR environment. Therefore, a screening form was created specifically for individuals that need to enter the MR environment and/or MR system room. This form, entitled, *Magnetic Resonance (MR) Environment Screening Form for Individuals* was developed in conjunction with the Medical, Scientific, and Technology Advisory Board and the Corporate Advisory Board of the Institute for Magnetic Resonance Safety, Education, and Research (IMRSER) (Figure 3). A "downloadable" version of this form may be obtained from the web sites, www.IMRSER.org and www.MRIsafety.com.

At the top of this form, the following statement is displayed: "The MR system has a very strong magnetic field that may be hazardous to individuals entering the MR environment or MR system room if they have certain metallic, electronic, magnetic, or mechanical implants, devices, or objects. Therefore, all individuals are required to fill out this form BEFORE entering the MR environment or MR system room. Be advised, the MR system magnet is ALWAYS on."

The screening form for individuals requests general information (name, age, address, etc.) and poses important questions to determine if there are possible problems or issues that should be discussed with the individual prior to permitting entry to the MR environment. A warning statement is also provided on the form, as follows: "WARNING: Certain implants, devices, or objects may be hazardous to you in the MR environment or MR system room. <u>Do not enter</u> the MR environment or MR system room if you have any question or concern regarding an implant, device, or object."

In addition, there is a section that lists implants, devices, and objects to identify the presence of an object that may be hazardous to an individual in the MR environment (e.g., an aneurysm clip, cardiac pacemaker, implantable cardioverter defibrillator (ICD), electronic or magnetically activated device, metallic foreign body, etc).

Finally, there is an *Important Instructions* section on the form that states: "Remove <u>all</u> metallic objects before entering the MR environment or MR system room including hearing aids, beeper, cell phone, keys, eyeglasses, hair pins, barrettes, jewelry (including body piercing jewelry), watch, safety pins, paperclips, money clip, credit cards, bank cards, magnetic strip cards, coins, pens, pocket knife, nail clipper, steel-toed boots/shoes, and tools. Loose metallic objects are especially prohibited in the MR system room and MR environment. Please consult the MRI Technologist or Radiologist if you have any question or concern BEFORE you enter the MR system room."

The proper use of this written form along with thorough verbal screening of the individual by an MR safety trained healthcare worker will prevent accidents and injuries in the MR environment.

[***The screening forms,** *Magnetic Resonance (MR) Procedure Screening Form For Patients* **and** *Magnetic Resonance (MR) Environment Screening Form for Individuals* **were developed in conjunction with the Institute for Magnetic Resonance Safety, Education, and Research (IMRSER) and published with permission.**]

REFERENCES

http://www.IMRSER.org; website for the Institute for Magnetic Resonance Safety, Education, and Research

Kanal E, Barkovich AJ, Bell C, et al. ACR guidance document for safe MR practices: 2007. AJR Am J Roentgenol. 2007;188:1447-1474.

Sawyer-Glover A, Shellock FG. Pre-Magnetic Resonance Procedure Screening, In: Magnetic Resonance Procedures: Health Effects and Safety, FG Shellock, Editor, CRC Press, LLC, Boca Raton, FL, 2001.

Sawyer-Glover A, Shellock FG. Pre-MRI procedure screening: recommendations and safety considerations for biomedical implants and devices. J Magn Reson Imaging 2000;12: 92-106.

Shellock FG. New recommendations for screening patients for suspected orbital foreign bodies. Signals, No. 36, Issue 4, 2001, pp. 8-9.

Shellock FG. Biomedical implants and devices: assessment of magnetic field interactions with a 3.0-Tesla MR system. J Magn Reson Imaging 2002;16:721-732.

Shellock FG. MR safety update 2002: Implants and devices. Journal of Magnetic Resonance Imaging 2002;16:485-496.

Shellock FG, Crues JV. Commentary. MR safety and the American College of Radiology White Paper. American Journal of Roentgenology 2002;178:1349-1352.

Shellock FG, Crues JV. MR procedures: biologic effects, safety, and patient care. Radiology, 2004;232:635-652.

Shellock FG, Kanal E. Policies, guidelines, and recommendations for MR imaging safety and patient management. J Magn Reson Imaging 1991;1:97-101.

Shellock FG, Kanal E. Policies, guidelines, and recommendations for MR imaging safety and patient management. J Magn Reson Imaging 1991;1: 97-101.

Shellock FG, Kanal E. Magnetic Resonance: Bioeffects, Safety, and Patient Management. Second Edition, Lippincott-Raven Press, New York, 1996.

Shellock FG, Kanal E. SMRI Report. Policies, guidelines and recommendations for MR imaging safety and patient management. Questionnaire for screening patients before MR procedures. J Magn Reson Imaging 1994;4:749-751, 1994.

Shellock FG, Spinazzi A. MRI Safety Update: 2008, Part 2, Screening patients for MRI. American Journal of Roentgenology 2008;191:12-21.

Figure 1. Magnetic Resonance (MR) Procedure Screening Form For Patients (Developed in conjunction with the Institute for Magnetic Resonance Safety, Education, and Research, www.IMRSER.org)

MAGNETIC RESONANCE (MR) PROCEDURE SCREENING FORM FOR PATIENTS

Date _____/_____/_____   Patient Number _____

Name _____   Age _____ Height _____ Weight _____
        Last name   First name   Middle Initial

Date of Birth _____/_____/_____   Male ☐ Female ☐   Body Part to be Examined _____
            month   day   year

Address _____   Telephone (home) (_____) _____-_____

City _____   Telephone (work) (_____) _____-_____

State _____ Zip Code _____

Reason for MRI and/or Symptoms _____

Referring Physician _____   Telephone (_____) _____-_____

1. Have you had prior surgery or an operation (e.g., arthroscopy, endoscopy, etc.) of any kind?   ☐ No   ☐ Yes
   If yes, please indicate the date and type of surgery:
   Date _____/_____/_____   Type of surgery _____
   Date _____/_____/_____   Type of surgery _____
2. Have you had a prior diagnostic imaging study or examination (MRI, CT, Ultrasound, X-ray, etc.)?   ☐No   ☐ Yes
   If yes, please list: Body part   Date   Facility
   MRI   _____   _____/_____   _____
   CT/CAT Scan _____   _____/_____   _____
   X-Ray   _____   _____/_____   _____
   Ultrasound   _____   _____/_____   _____
   Nuclear Medicine _____ _____/_____   _____
   Other_____ _____   _____/_____

3. Have you experienced any problem related to a previous MRI examination or MR procedure?   ☐ No   ☐ Yes
   If yes, please describe: _____
4. Have you had an injury to the eye involving a metallic object or fragment (e.g., metallic slivers,
   shavings, foreign body, etc.)?   ☐ No   ☐ Yes
   If yes, please describe: _____
5. Have you ever been injured by a metallic object or foreign body (e.g., BB, bullet, shrapnel, etc.)?   ☐ No   ☐ Yes
   If yes, please describe: _____
6. Are you currently taking or have you recently taken any medication or drug?   ☐ No   ☐ Yes
   If yes, please list: _____
7. Are you allergic to any medication?   ☐ No   ☐ Yes
   If yes, please list: _____
8. Do you have a history of asthma, allergic reaction, respiratory disease, or reaction to a contrast
   medium or dye used for an MRI, CT, or X-ray examination?   ☐ No   ☐ Yes
9. Do you have anemia or any disease(s) that affects your blood, a history of renal (kidney)
   disease, renal (kidney) failure, renal (kidney) transplant, high blood pressure (hypertension),
   liver (hepatic) disease, a history of diabetes, or seizures?   ☐ No   ☐ Yes
   If yes, please describe: _____

For female patients:
10. Date of last menstrual period: _____/_____/_____   Post menopausal?   ☐ No   ☐ Yes
11. Are you pregnant or experiencing a late menstrual period?   ☐ No   ☐ Yes
12. Are you taking oral contraceptives or receiving hormonal treatment?   ☐ No   ☐ Yes
13. Are you taking any type of fertility medication or having fertility treatments?   ☐ No   ☐ Yes
    If yes, please describe: _____
14. Are you currently breastfeeding?   ☐ No   ☐ Yes

WARNING: Certain implants, devices, or objects may be hazardous to you and/or may interfere with the MR procedure (i.e., MRI, MR angiography, functional MRI, MR spectroscopy). Do not enter the MR system room or MR environment if you have any question or concern regarding an implant, device, or object. Consult the MRI Technologist or Radiologist BEFORE entering the MR system room. The MR system magnet is ALWAYS on.

Please indicate if you have any of the following:

☐ Yes ☐ No Aneurysm clip(s)
☐ Yes ☐ No Cardiac pacemaker
☐ Yes ☐ No Implanted cardioverter defibrillator (ICD)
☐ Yes ☐ No Electronic implant or device
☐ Yes ☐ No Magnetically-activated implant or device
☐ Yes ☐ No Neurostimulation system
☐ Yes ☐ No Spinal cord stimulator
☐ Yes ☐ No Internal electrodes or wires
☐ Yes ☐ No Bone growth/bone fusion stimulator
☐ Yes ☐ No Cochlear, otologic, or other ear implant
☐ Yes ☐ No Insulin or other infusion pump
☐ Yes ☐ No Implanted drug infusion device
☐ Yes ☐ No Any type of prosthesis (eye, penile, etc.)
☐ Yes ☐ No Heart valve prosthesis
☐ Yes ☐ No Eyelid spring or wire
☐ Yes ☐ No Artificial or prosthetic limb
☐ Yes ☐ No Metallic stent, filter, or coil
☐ Yes ☐ No Shunt (spinal or intraventricular)
☐ Yes ☐ No Vascular access port and/or catheter
☐ Yes ☐ No Radiation seeds or implants
☐ Yes ☐ No Swan-Ganz or thermodilution catheter
☐ Yes ☐ No Medication patch (Nicotine, Nitroglycerine)
☐ Yes ☐ No Any metallic fragment or foreign body
☐ Yes ☐ No Wire mesh implant
☐ Yes ☐ No Tissue expander (e.g., breast)
☐ Yes ☐ No Surgical staples, clips, or metallic sutures
☐ Yes ☐ No Joint replacement (hip, knee, etc.)
☐ Yes ☐ No Bone/joint pin, screw, nail, wire, plate, etc.
☐ Yes ☐ No IUD, diaphragm, or pessary
☐ Yes ☐ No Dentures or partial plates
☐ Yes ☐ No Tattoo or permanent makeup
☐ Yes ☐ No Body piercing jewelry
☐ Yes ☐ No Hearing aid
          (Remove before entering MR system room)
☐ Yes ☐ No Other implant _____
☐ Yes ☐ No Breathing problem or motion disorder
☐ Yes ☐ No Claustrophobia

Please mark on the figure(s) below the location of any implant or metal inside of or on your body.

RIGHT   LEFT   LEFT   RIGHT

⚠ **IMPORTANT INSTRUCTIONS**

Before entering the MR environment or MR system room, you must remove all metallic objects including hearing aids, dentures, partial plates, keys, beeper, cell phone, eyeglasses, hair pins, barrettes, jewelry, body piercing jewelry, watch, safety pins, paperclips, money clip, credit cards, bank cards, magnetic strip cards, coins, pens, pocket knife, nail clipper, tools, clothing with metal fasteners, & clothing with metallic threads.

Please consult the MRI Technologist or Radiologist if you have any question or concern BEFORE you enter the MR system room.

NOTE: You may be advised or required to wear earplugs or other hearing protection during the MR procedure to prevent possible problems or hazards related to acoustic noise.

I attest that the above information is correct to the best of my knowledge. I read and understand the contents of this form and had the opportunity to ask questions regarding the information on this form and regarding the MR procedure that I am about to undergo.

Signature of Person Completing Form: _____   Date ___/___/___
                                              Signature

Form Completed By: ☐ Patient ☐ Relative ☐ Nurse _____   _____
                                                      Print name   Relationship to patient

Form Information Reviewed By: _____   _____
                                      Print name   Signature

☐ MRI Technologist   ☐ Nurse   ☐ Radiologist   ☐ Other _____

Figure 2. Magnetic Resonance (MR) Procedure Screening Form For Patients: Spanish Version

---

CUESTIONARIO PREVIO A ESTUDIO CON RESONANCIA MAGNÉTICA (MR) PARA PACIENTES

Fecha ___/___/___   Número de paciente _____

Nombre _____   Edad _____ Altura _____ Peso _____
   Apellido   Primer Nombre   Segundo Nombre

Fecha de nacimiento ___/___/___   Varón ☐ Hembra ☐   Parte del cuerpo a ser examinada _____
    Mes   Dia   Año

Dirección _____   Teléfono (domicilio) (____) ____-_____

Ciudad _____   Teléfono (trabajo) (____) ____-_____

Provincia _____   Código Postal _____

Motivo para el estudio de MRI y/o sintomas _____

Médico que le refirió _____   Teléfono (____) - _____

1. Anteriormente, ¿le han hecho alguna cirugía u operación (e.g., artroscopía, endoscopía, etc.) de cualquier tipo?   ☐ No ☐ Sí
Si respondió afirmativamente, indique la fecha y que tipo de cirugía:
Fecha ___/___/___ Tipo de cirugía _____
Fecha ___/___/___ Tipo de cirugía _____
2. Anteriormente, ¿le han hecho algún estudio o exàmen de diagnóstico (MRI, CT, Ultrasonido, Rayos-X, etc.)?   ☐ No ☐ Sí
Si respondió afirmativamente, describalos a continuación:
    Parte del Cuerpo   Fecha   Lugar/Institución

Parte del Cuerpo	Fecha	Lugar/Institución
MRI	/ /	
CT/CAT	/ /	
Rayos-X	/ /	
Ultrasonido	/ /	
Medicina Nuclear	/ /	
Otro	/ /	

3. ¿Ha tenido algún problema relacionado con estudios ó procedimientos anteriores con MR?   ☐ No ☐ Sí
Si respondió afirmativamente, describalos: _____
4. ¿Se ha golpeado el ojo con un objeto ó fragmento metálico (e.g., astillas metálicas, virutas, objeto extraño, etc.)?   ☐ No ☐ Sí
Si respondió afirmativamente, describa el incidente: _____
5. ¿Ha sido alcanzado alguna vez por un objeto metálico u objeto extraño (e.g. perdigones, bala, metralla, etc.)?   ☐ No ☐ Sí
Si respondió afirmativamente, describa el incidente: _____
6. ¿Esta actualmente tomando ó ha recientemente tomado algún medicamento o droga?   ☐ No ☐ Sí
Si respondió afirmativamente, indique el nombre del medicamento: _____
7. ¿Es Ud. alérgico/a á algún medicamento?   ☐ No ☐ Sí
Si respondió afirmativamente, indique el nombre del medicamento: _____
8. ¿Tiene historia de asma, reacción alérgica, enfermedad respiratoria, ó reacción a contrastes ó tinturas usados en MRI, CT, ó Rayos-X?   ☐ No ☐ Sí
9. ¿Tiene anemia u otra enfermedad que afecte su sangre, algún episodio de enfermedad de riñón, fracaso de riñón, un transplante de riñón, hipertensión, la historia de la diabetes, relativo al higado ó de ataques epilépticos?   ☐ No ☐ Sí
Si respondió afirmativamente, describalos: _____

Para los pacientes femeninos:
10. Fecha de su último periodo menstrual: ___/___/___   En la menopausia?   ☐ No ☐ Sí
11. ¿Está embarazada ó tiene retraso con su periodo menstrual?   ☐ No ☐ Sí
12. ¿Está tomando contraceptivos orales ó recibiendo tratamiento hormonal?   ☐ No ☐ Sí
13. ¿Está tomando algún tipo de medicamento para la fertilidad ó recibiendo tratamientos de fertilidad?   ☐ No ☐ Sí
Si responde afirmativamente, describalos a continuación: _____
14. ¿Está amamantado a su bebé?   ☐ No ☐ Sí

Translated with permission 5/05 Olga Fernandez-Flygare, M.S., Brain Mapping Center, UCLA School of Medicine, Los Angeles, CA

ADVERTENCIA: Ciertos implantes, dispositivos, u objetos pueden ser peligrosos y/o pueden interferir con el procedimiento de resonancia magnética (es decir, MRI, MR angiografía, MRI funcional, MR espectroscopía). **No entre** a la sala del escáner de MR o a la zona del laboratorio de MR si tiene alguna pregunta o duda relacionadas con un implante, dispositivo, u objeto. Consulte con el técnico o radiólogo de MRI ANTES de entrar a la sala del escáner de MR. **Recuerde que el imán del sistema MR está SIEMPRE encendido.**

Por favor indique si tiene alguno de los siguientes:

☐ Sí ☐ No   Pinza(s) de aneurisma
☐ Sí ☐ No   Marcapasos cardíaco
☐ Sí ☐ No   Implante con desfibrilador para conversión cardíaca (ICD)
☐ Sí ☐ No   Implante electrónico ó dispositivo electrónico
☐ Sí ☐ No   Implante ó dispositivo activado magnéticamente
☐ Sí ☐ No   Sistema de neuroestimulación
☐ Sí ☐ No   Estimulador de la médula espinal
☐ Sí ☐ No   Electrodos ó alambres internos
☐ Sí ☐ No   Estimulador de crecimiento/fusión del hueso
☐ Sí ☐ No   Implante coclear, otológico, u otro implante del oído
☐ Sí ☐ No   Bomba de infusión de insulina ó similar
☐ Sí ☐ No   Dispositivo implantado para infusión de medicamento
☐ Sí ☐ No   Cualquier tipo de prótesis (ojo, peneal, etc.)
☐ Sí ☐ No   Prótesis de válvula cardiaca
☐ Sí ☐ No   Muelle ó alambre del párpado
☐ Sí ☐ No   Extremidad artificial ó prostética
☐ Sí ☐ No   Malla metálica (stent), filtro, ó anillo metálico
☐ Sí ☐ No   Shunt (espinal ó intraventricular)
☐ Sí ☐ No   Catéter y/u orificio de acceso vascular
☐ Sí ☐ No   Semillas ó implantes de radiación
☐ Sí ☐ No   Catéter de Swan-Ganz ó de termodilución

☐ Sí ☐ No   Parche de medicamentos (Nicotina, Nitroglicerina)
☐ Sí ☐ No   Cualquier fragmento metálico ó cuerpo extraño
☐ Sí ☐ No   Implante tipo malla
☐ Sí ☐ No   Aumentador de tejidos (e.g. pecho)
☐ Sí ☐ No   Grapas quirúrgicas, clips, ó suturas metálicas
☐ Sí ☐ No   Articulaciones artificiales (cadera, rodilla, etc.)
☐ Sí ☐ No   Varilla de hueso/coyuntura, tornillo, clavo, alambre, chapas, etc.
☐ Sí ☐ No   Dispositivo intrauterino (IUD), diafragma, ó pesario
☐ Sí ☐ No   Dentaduras ó placas parciales
☐ Sí ☐ No   Tatuaje ó maquillaje permanente
☐ Sí ☐ No   Perforación (piercing) del cuerpo
☐ Sí ☐ No   Audífono *(Quíteselo antes de entrar a la sala del escáner de MR)*
☐ Sí ☐ No   Otro implante_____
☐ Sí ☐ No   Problema respiratorio ó desorden del movimiento
☐ Sí ☐ No   Claustrofobia

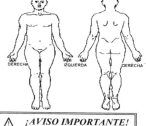

Por favor marque en la imagen de abajo la localización de cualquier implante o metal en su cuerpo.

DERECHA   IZQUIERDA   DERECHA

⚠ **¡AVISO IMPORTANTE!**

Antes de entrar a la zona de MR ó a la sala del escáner de MR, tendrá que quitarse todo objeto metálico incluyendo audífono, dentaduras, placas parciales, llaves, beeper, teléfono celular, lentes, horquillas de pelo, pasadores, todas las joyas (incluyendo "body piercing"), reloj, alfileres, sujetapapeles, clip de billetes, tarjetas de crédito ó de banco, toda tarjeta con banda magnética, monedas, plumas, cuchillos, corta uñas, herramientas, ropa con enganches de metal, y ropa con hilos metálicos.

Por favor consulte con el Técnico de MRI ó Radiólogo si tiene alguna pregunta o duda ANTES de entrar a la sala de escáner de MR.

NOTA: Es posible se le pida usar auriculares u otra protección de sus oídos durante el procedimiento de MR para prevenir problemas ó riesgos asociados al nivel de ruido en la sala del escáner de MR.

Atestiguo que la información anterior es correcta según mi mejor entender. Leo y entiendo el contenido de este cuestionario y he tenido la oportunidad de hacer preguntas en relación a la información en el cuestionario y en relación al estudio de MR al que me voy a someter a continuación.

Firma de la persona llenando este cuestionario: _____   Fecha ___/___/___
                                          Firma

Cuestionario lleno por: ☐Paciente ☐Pariente ☐Enfermera _____   _____
                                                    Nombre en letra de texto   *Relación con el paciente*

Información revisada por: _____
                        Nombre en letra de texto
☐ Técnico de MRI   ☐Enfermera   ☐ Radiólogo   ☐ Otro _____   _____
                                                                                    Firma

Translated with permission Olga Fernandez-Fygare, M.S., Brain Mapping Center, UCLA School of Medicine, Los Angeles, CA

Figure 3. Magnetic Resonance (MR) Environment Screening Form for Individuals (Developed in conjunction with the Institute for Magnetic Resonance Safety, Education, and Research, www.IMRSER.org)

MAGNETIC RESONANCE (MR) ENVIRONMENT SCREENING FORM FOR INDIVIDUALS*

The MR system has a very strong magnetic field that may be hazardous to individuals entering the MR environment or MR system room if they have certain metallic, electronic, magnetic, or mechanical implants, devices, or objects. Therefore, all individuals are required to fill out this form BEFORE entering the MR environment or MR system room. Be advised, the MR system magnet is ALWAYS on.

*NOTE: If you are a patient preparing to undergo an MR examination, you are required to fill out a different form.

Date ____ / ____ / ____   Name _____   Age _____
    month   day   year   Last Name   First Name   Middle Initial

Address _____   Telephone (home) (____) ____ - _____

City _____   Telephone (work) (____) ____ - _____

State _____   Zip Code _____

1. Have you had prior surgery or an operation (e.g., arthroscopy, endoscopy, etc.) of any kind?   ☐ No ☐ Yes
    If yes, please indicate date and type of surgery: Date ____ / ____ / ____ Type of surgery_____
2. Have you had an injury to the eye involving a metallic object (e.g., metallic slivers, foreign body)?   ☐ No ☐ Yes
    If yes, please describe:
3. Have you ever been injured by a metallic object or foreign body (e.g., BB, bullet, shrapnel, etc.)?   ☐ No ☐ Yes
    If yes, please describe:
4. Are you pregnant or suspect that you are pregnant?   ☐ No ☐ Yes

WARNING: Certain implants, devices, or objects may be hazardous to you in the MR environment or MR system room. Do not enter the MR environment or MR system room if you have any question or concern regarding an implant, device, or object.

Please indicate if you have any of the following:

☐ Yes ☐ No   Aneurysm clip(s)
☐ Yes ☐ No   Cardiac pacemaker
☐ Yes ☐ No   Implanted cardioverter defibrillator (ICD)
☐ Yes ☐ No   Electronic implant or device
☐ Yes ☐ No   Magnetically-activated implant or device
☐ Yes ☐ No   Neurostimulation system
☐ Yes ☐ No   Spinal cord stimulator
☐ Yes ☐ No   Cochlear implant or implanted hearing aid
☐ Yes ☐ No   Insulin or infusion pump
☐ Yes ☐ No   Implanted drug infusion device
☐ Yes ☐ No   Any type of prosthesis or implant
☐ Yes ☐ No   Artificial or prosthetic limb
☐ Yes ☐ No   Any metallic fragment or foreign body
☐ Yes ☐ No   Any external or internal metallic object
☐ Yes ☐ No   Hearing aid
    (Remove before entering the MR system room)
☐ Yes ☐ No   Other implant_____

⚠ **IMPORTANT INSTRUCTIONS**

Remove all metallic objects before entering the MR environment or MR system room including hearing aids, beeper, cell phone, keys, eyeglasses, hair pins, barrettes, jewelry (including body piercing jewelry), watch, safety pins, paperclips, money clip, credit cards, bank cards, magnetic strip cards, coins, pens, pocket knife, nail clipper, steel-toed boots/shoes, and tools. Loose metallic objects are especially prohibited in the MR system room and MR environment.

Please consult the MRI Technologist or Radiologist if you have any question or concern BEFORE you enter the MR system room.

I attest that the above information is correct to the best of my knowledge. I have read and understand the entire contents of this form and have had the opportunity to ask questions regarding the information on this form.

Signature of Person Completing Form: _____   Date ____ / ____ / ____
                           Signature

Form Information Reviewed By: _____
                           Print name   Signature

☐ MRI Technologist   ☐ Radiologist   ☐ Other _____

Guidelines to Prevent Excessive Heating and Burns Associated with Magnetic Resonance Procedures*

Magnetic resonance (MR) imaging is considered to be a relatively safe diagnostic modality. However, damaged radiofrequency coils, physiologic monitors, electronically-activated devices, and external accessories or objects made from conductive materials have caused excessive heating, resulting in burn injuries to patients undergoing MR procedures. Heating of implants and similar devices may also occur, but this tends be problematic primarily for objects made from conductive materials that have elongated shapes or that form loops of a certain diameter. For example, excessive MRI-related heating has been reported for leads, guidewires, certain types of catheters (e.g., catheters with thermistors or other conducting components), and certain external fixation or cervical fixation devices.

In the United States, more than 40 incidents of excessive heating have been reported in patients undergoing MR procedures that were unrelated to equipment problems or the presence of conductive external or internal implants or materials [review of data files from U.S. Food and Drug Administration, Center for Devices and Radiological Health, Manufacturer and User Facility Device Experience Database, MAUDE, http://www.fda.gov/cdrh/maude.html and U.S. Food and Drug Administration, Center for Devices and Radiological Health, Medical Device Report, (http://www.fda.gov/CDRH/mdrfile.html)]. These incidents included first, second, and third degree burns that were experienced by patients. In many of these cases, the reports indicated that the limbs or other body parts of the patients were in direct contact with transmit body radiofrequency (RF) coils or other transmit RF coils of the MR systems. In other cases, skin-to-skin contact points were suspected to be responsible for these injuries, however, the exact mechanism responsible for these incidents is unknown.

MR systems require the use of RF pulses to create the MR signal. This RF energy is transmitted through free space from the transmit RF coil to the patient. When conducting materials are placed within the RF field, a concentration of electrical currents sufficient to cause excessive heating and tissue damage may occur. The nature of high frequency electromagnetic fields is such that the energy can be transmitted across open space and through insulators. Therefore, only devices with carefully designed current paths can be made safe for use during MR procedures. Simply insulating conductive material (e.g., wire or lead) or separating it from the patient may not be sufficient to prevent excessive heating or burns from occurring for some devices.

Furthermore, certain shapes exhibit the phenomenon of "resonance" that increases their propensity to concentrate RF currents. At the operating frequencies of present day MR systems, conducting loops of tens of centimeters in size can create problems and, therefore, must be avoided, unless high impedance techniques are used to limit the RF current. Importantly, even loops that include small gaps separated by insulation may still conduct current.

To prevent patients from experiencing excessive heating and possible burns in association with MR procedures, the following guidelines are recommended:

1) Prepare the patient for the MR procedure by ensuring that there are no unnecessary metallic objects contacting the patient's skin (e.g., drug delivery patches with metallic components, jewelry, necklaces, bracelets, key chains, etc.).

2) Prepare the patient for the MR procedure by using insulation material (i.e., appropriate padding) to prevent skin-to-skin contact points and the formation of "closed-loops" from touching body parts.

3) Insulating material (minimum recommended thickness, 1-cm) should be placed between the patient's skin and transmit RF coil that is used for the MR procedure (alternatively, the transmit RF coil itself should be padded). For example, position the patient so that there is no direct contact between the patient's skin and the transmit RF body coil of the MR system. This may be accomplished by having the patient place his/her arms over his/her head or by using elbow pads or foam padding between the patient's tissue and the transmit RF body coil of the MR system. This is especially important for MR examinations that use the transmit RF body coil or other large RF coils for transmission of RF energy.

4) Use only electrically conductive devices, equipment, accessories (e.g., ECG leads, electrodes, etc.), and materials that have been thoroughly tested and determined to be safe for MR procedures.

5) Carefully follow specific MR safety criteria and recommendations for implants made from electrically-conductive materials (e.g., bone fusion stimulators, neurostimulation systems, cochlear implants, etc.).

6) Before using electrical equipment, check the integrity of the insulation and/or housing of all components including surface RF coils, monitoring leads, cables, and wires. Preventive maintenance should be practiced routinely for such equipment.

7) Remove all non-essential electrically conductive materials from the MR system (i.e., unused surface RF coils, ECG leads, EEG leads, cables, wires, etc.).

8) Keep electrically conductive materials that must remain in the MR system from directly contacting the patient by placing thermal and/or electrical insulation between the conductive material and the patient.

9) Keep electrically conductive materials that must remain within the body RF coil or other transmit RF coil of the MR system from forming conductive loops. Note: The patient's tissue is conductive and, therefore, may be involved in the formation of a conductive loop, which can be circular, U-shaped, or S-shaped.

10) Position electrically conductive materials to prevent "cross points". A cross point is the point where a cable crosses another cable, where a cable loops across itself, or where a cable touches either the patient or sides of the transmit RF coil more than once. Even the close proximity of conductive materials with each other should be avoided because cables and RF coils can capacitively-couple (without any contact or crossover) when placed close together.

11) Position electrically conductive materials to exit down the center of the MR system (i.e., not along the side of the MR system or close to the transmit RF body coil or other transmit RF coil).

12) Do not position electrically conductive materials across an external metallic prosthesis (e.g., external fixation device, cervical fixation device, etc.) or similar device that is in direct contact with the patient.

13) Allow only properly trained individuals to operate devices (e.g., monitoring equipment) in the MR environment.

14) Follow all manufacturer instructions for the proper operation and maintenance of physiologic monitoring or other similar electronic equipment intended for use during MR procedures.

15) Electrical devices that do not appear to be operating properly during the MR procedure should be removed from the patient immediately.

16) Closely monitor the patient during the MR procedure. If the patient reports sensations of heating or other unusual sensation, discontinue

the MR procedure immediately and perform a thorough assessment of the situation.

17) RF surface coil decoupling failures can cause localized RF power deposition levels to reach excessive levels. The MR system operator will recognize such a failure as a set of concentric semicircles in the tissue on the associated MR image or as an unusual amount of image non-uniformity related to the position of the RF coil.

The adoption of these guidelines will ensure that patient safety is maintained, especially as more conductive materials and electronically-activated devices are used in association with MR procedures.

[*The document, **Guidelines to Prevent Excessive Heating and Burns Associated with Magnetic Resonance Procedures,** was developed by the Institute for Magnetic Resonance Safety, Education, and Research (IMRSER) and published with permission.]

REFERENCES

Bashein G, Syrory G. Burns associated with pulse oximetry during magnetic resonance imaging. Anesthesiology 1991;75:382-3.

Brown TR, Goldstein B, Little J. Severe burns resulting from magnetic resonance imaging with cardiopulmonary monitoring. Risks and relevant safety precautions. Am J Phys Med Rehabil 1993;72:166-7.

Chou C-K, McDougall JA, Chan KW. Absence of radiofrequency heating from auditory implants during magnetic resonance imaging. Bioelectromagnetics 1997;44:367-372.

Diaz F, Tweardy L, Shellock FG. Cervical fixation devices: MRI issues at 3-Tesla. Spine (in press)

Dempsey MF, Condon B. Thermal injuries associated with MRI. Clin Radiol 2001;56:457-65.

Dempsey MF, Condon B, Hadley DM. Investigation of the factors responsible for burns during MRI. J Magn Reson Imaging 2001;13:627-631.

ECRI, Health Devices Alert. A new MRI complication? Health Devices Alert May 27, pp. 1, 1988.

ECRI. Thermal injuries and patient monitoring during MRI studies. Health Devices Alert 1991;20: 362-363.

ECRI Institute. Hazard report. Patients can be burned by damaged MRI AV entertainment systems. Health Devices. 2008;37:379-80

Finelli DA, Rezai AR, Ruggieri PM, Tkach JA, Nyenhuis JA, Hrdlicka G, Sharan A, Gonzalez-Martinez J, Stypulkowski PH, Shellock FG. MR imaging-related heating of deep brain stimulation electrodes: In vitro study. Am J Neuroradiol 2002;23:1795-1802.

Haik J, Daniel S, et al. MRI induced fourth-degree burn in an extremity, leading to amputation. Burns. 2009;35:294-6.

Hall SC, Stevenson GW, Suresh S. Burn associated with temperature monitoring during magnetic resonance imaging. Anesthesiology 1992;76:152.

Heinz W, Frohlich E, Stork T. Burns following magnetic resonance tomography study. (German) Z Gastroenterol 1999;37:31-2.

http://www.IMRSER.org; website for the Institute for Magnetic Resonance Safety, Education, and Research

International Commission on Non-Ionizing Radiation Protection (ICNIRP) Statement, Medical magnetic resonance procedures: protection of patients. Health Physics 2004;87:197-216.

International Electrotechnical Commission (IEC), Medical Electrical Equipment, Particular requirements for the safety of magnetic resonance equipment for medical diagnosis. International Standard IEC 60601-2-33, 2002.

Jones S, Jaffe W, Alvi R. Burns associated with electrocardiographic monitoring during magnetic resonance imaging. Burns 1996;22:420-421.

Kainz W. MR heating tests of MR critical implants. J Magn Reson Imaging. 2007;26:450-1

Kanal E, Barkovich AJ, Bell C, et al. ACR guidance document for safe MR practices: 2007. AJR Am J Roentgenol. 2007;188:1447-1474.

Kanal E, Shellock FG. Burns associated with clinical MR examinations. Radiology 1990;175: 585.

Kanal E, Shellock FG. Policies, guidelines, and recommendations for MR imaging safety and patient management. J Magn Reson Imaging 1992;2:247-248.

Karoo RO, Whitaker IS, Garrido A, Sharpe DT. Full-thickness burns following magnetic resonance imaging: a discussion of the dangers and safety suggestions. Plast Reconstr Surg. 2004;114:1344-1345.

Keens SJ, Laurence AS. Burns caused by ECG monitoring during MRI imaging. Anaesthesia 1996;51:1188-9.

Kim LJ, Sonntag VK, Hott JT, Nemeth JA, Klopfenstein JD, Tweardy L. Scalp burns from halo pins following magnetic resonance imaging. Case Report. Journal of Neurosurgery 2003:99:186.

Knopp MV, Essig M, Debus J, Zabel HJ, van Kaick G. Unusual burns of the lower extremities caused by a closed conducting loop in a patient at MR imaging. Radiology 1996;200:572-5.

Knopp MV, Metzner R, Brix G, van Kaick G. Safety considerations to avoid current-induced skin burns in MRI procedures. (German) Radiologe 199838:759-63.

Kugel H, Bremer C, Puschel M, Fischbach R, Lenzen H, Tombach B, Van Aken H, Heindel W. Hazardous situation in the MR bore: induction in ECG leads causes fire. Eur Radiol 2003;13:690-694.

Lange S, Nguyen QN. Cables and electrodes can burn patients during MRI. Nursing. 2006;36:18.

Mattei E, Triventi M, Calcagnini G, Censi F, Kainz W, Bassen HI, Bartolini P. Temperature and SAR measurement errors in the evaluation of metallic linear structures heating during MRI using fluoroptic probes. Phys Med Biol. 2007;52:1633-46.

Nakamura T, Fukuda K, Hayakawa K, Aoki I, Matsumoto K, Sekine T, Ueda H, Shimizu Y. Mechanism of burn injury during magnetic resonance imaging (MRI)-simple loops can induce heat injury. Front Med Biol Eng 2001;11:117-29

Nyenhuis JA, Kildishev AV, Foster KS, Graber G, Athey W. Heating near implanted medical devices by the MRI RF-magnetic field. IEEE Trans Magn 1999;35:4133-4135.

Rezai AR, Finelli D, Nyenhuis JA, Hrdlick G, Tkach J, Ruggieri P, Stypulkowski PH, Sharan A, Shellock FG. Neurostimulator for deep brain stimulation: Ex vivo evaluation of MRI-related heating at 1.5-Tesla. Journal of Magnetic Resonance Imaging 2002;15:241-250.

Ruschulte H, Piepenbrock S, Munte S, Lotz J. Severe burns during magnetic resonance examination. Eur J Anaesthesiol. 2005;22:319-320.

Schaefer DJ. Safety aspects of radio-frequency power deposition in magnetic resonance. MRI Clinics of North America 1998;6:775-789.

Schaefer DJ, Felmlee JP. Radio-frequency safety in MR examinations, Special Cross-Specialty Categorical Course in Diagnostic Radiology: Practical MR Safety Considerations for Physicians, Physicists, and Technologists, Syllabus, 87th Scientific of the Radiological Society of North America, Chicago, pp 111-123, 2001.

Shellock FG. Magnetic Resonance Procedures: Health Effects and Safety. CRC Press, LLC, Boca Raton, FL, 2001.

Shellock FG. MR safety update 2002: Implants and devices. Journal of Magnetic Resonance Imaging 2002;16:485-496.

Shellock FG. Radiofrequency-induced heating during MR procedures: A review. Journal of Magnetic Resonance Imaging 2000;12: 30-36.

Shellock FG. Guidelines to Prevent Excessive Heating and Burns Associated With Magnetic Resonance Procedures. Signals, No. 46, Issue 3, pp. 24-26, 2003.

Shellock FG. Guest Editorial. Comments on MRI heating tests of critical implants. Journal of Magnetic Resonance Imaging 2007;26:1182-1185.

Shellock FG, Crues JV. MR procedures: biologic effects, safety, and patient care. Radiology, 2004;232:635-652.

Shellock FG, Slimp G. Severe burn of the finger caused by using a pulse oximeter during MRI. American Journal of Roentgenology 1989;153:1105.

Shellock FG, Hatfield M, Simon BJ, Block S, Wamboldt J, Starewicz PM, Punchard WFB. Implantable spinal fusion stimulator: assessment of MRI safety. Journal of Magnetic Resonance Imaging 2000;12:214-223.

Smith CD, Nyenhuis JA, Kildishev AV. Health effects of induced electrical fields: implications for metallic implants. In: Shellock FG, ed. Magnetic resonance procedure: health effects and safety. Boca Raton, FL: CRC Press, 2001; 393-414.

U.S. Food and Drug Administration, Center for Devices and Radiological Health (CDRH), Medical Device Report (MDR) (http://www.fda.gov/CDRH/mdrfile.html). The files contain information from CDRH's device experience reports on devices which may have malfunctioned or caused a death or serious injury. The files contain reports received under both the mandatory Medical Device Reporting Program (MDR) from 1984 - 1996, and the voluntary reports up to June 1993. The database currently contains over 600,000 reports.

U.S. Food and Drug Administration, Center for Devices and Radiological Health (CDRH), Manufacturer and User Facility Device Experience Database, MAUDE, (http://www.fda.gov/cdrh/maude.html). MAUDE data represents reports of adverse events involving medical devices. The data consists of all voluntary reports since June, 1993, user facility reports since 1991, distributor reports since 1993, and manufacturer reports since August, 1996.

Yamazaki M, Yamada E, et al. Investigation of local heating caused by closed conducting loop at clinical MR imaging: Phantom study. Nippon Hoshasen Gijutsu Gakkai Zasshi. 2008; 20;64:883-5.

Infection Control In the MRI Environment*

The magnetic resonance (MR) imaging environment is a complex and potentially dangerous setting with respect to issues involving infection control, particularly because custodial personnel and routine cleaning equipment are not permitted to enter this setting without adhering to strict policies and procedures. Importantly, cleaning the MR system room is often the responsibility of the MR system operator, who is rarely trained or certified in infection control. Therefore, it is unreasonable to believe that the MRI environment, especially the MR system (e.g., inside the bore of the scanner, surface coils, the positioning pads/sponges, patient management accessories etc.), can be cleaned safely and effectively by untrained personnel. This important task requires specialized written procedures and training.

Patients with serious infections typically undergo diagnostic imaging during the course of their treatment. There is frequently a lack of special procedures for dealing with highly contagious patients, particularly at outpatient imaging centers and mobile centers. Contagious patients may simply be placed on the MR system table and scanned and the next patient, possibly an immunosuppressed child with a sprained knee, is put on the table directly after this infected patient without properly cleaning the properly table, pads, and sponges. Obviously, this is a serious situation that deserves attention. Therefore, radiology departments and outpatient imaging centers must take appropriate action to ensure that the MR environment is not a site for exposing patients and healthcare workers to microorganisms that are capable of causing infectious diseases.

At many MRI centers, there is a false belief that merely placing a clean sheet over the scanner table, without actually cleaning the mattress between patients, will prevent the spread of infectious agents. Of note is that placing clean sheets on a contaminated surface may contaminate the sheets and pose further infectious risk when the sheets are handled. Of further concern is that very few MRI centers clean inside of the bore of the MR system on a regular basis and the positioning pads and sponges may only be cleaned once a day.

There is also the issue of potentially spreading infectious bacteria by direct or indirect contact among the imaging staff and patients within the imaging department or center. For MR systems in mobile facilities, ensuring proper hygiene is often more difficult, since these sites may not have a sink or running water. Therefore, hand-washing between patients as well as using hand sanitizer regularly is of crucial importance.

Another overlooked area is torn and frayed positioning pads, sponges, and scanner table mattresses used in imaging departments and centers. Once the covering material has been breached, the surfaces of these items cannot be properly cleaned and should be immediately removed and replaced. It is will known that, if disinfected, a smooth surface can be repeatedly used without problems. However, for items with a porous surface (e.g., those made from "spongy" materials), the presence of infectious agents, including Methicillin-resistant Staphylococcus aureus, MRSA, can be detected even after disinfection had been performed. Thus, porous surfaces made of such materials cannot be adequately disinfected.

Protecting patients and staff takes a concerted effort by all the parties involved in the MRI facility. There is no question that infection control has not received the attention that it deserves and there is a growing concern that at least some of the spread of infectious agents could be coming from outpatient imaging centers and radiology departments in hospitals.

The following recommendations are provided for MRI facilities to address infection control standards that are used throughout the healthcare industry:

Recommendations for Infection Control in the MRI Environment

(1) Have a written infectious control policy to include cleaning procedures for the MRI environment, as well as a cleaning schedule and have it posted throughout the center.

(2) Implement a mandatory hand-washing / hand-sanitizing procedure between each patient not only for MRI healthcare workers, but also for others who come into contact with patients.

(3) Clean the MR scanner table, inside the bore of the MR system and other items that come into contact with a patient. Infection control experts recommend that this be done between each patient.

(4) Clean all positioning pads and sponges with an approved disinfectant. Infection control experts recommend cleaning after each patient.

(5) Periodically inspect the pads with a magnifying glass, particularly at the seams, to identify fraying or tearing. Replace the pads, as needed.

(6) Use pillows with a waterproof covering that is designed to be surface wiped. Replace pillows when this barrier is compromised.

(7) Promptly remove body fluids, and then disinfect all contaminated areas.

(8) If the patient has an open wound or history of infection, especially related to MRSA, gloves and gowns should be worn by all staff coming into contact with the patient. These barriers must be removed before touching other areas not coming into contact with the patient (e.g., door knobs, scanner console, computer keyboards, etc.).

(9) The scanner table, positioning sponges, and pads should be completely cleaned with disinfectant before the next patient is scanned, if this procedure is not already being performed between each patient. For patients with any known infectious process, add 10-15 minutes to the scheduled scan time to ensure that there is enough time to thoroughly clean the room and patient-related surfaces.

(10) All furniture should be periodically cleaned. Ideal surfaces are those that are waterproof and easy to clean. Infection control experts recommend that such cleaning be performed between each patient.

[Content excerpted with permission for content provided by Peter Rothschild, M.D. Louisville, KY]

REFERENCES

Brennan PJ, Abrutyn E, Developing policies and guidelines. Infec Control Hosp Epidemiol 1995; 16:512-517.

CNA, MRSA Alert: MRI infection creates new "superbug" concerns. AlertBulletin. Issue 4, 09, www.CNA.com/healthpro

Datta R, Huang SS. Risk of infection and death due to methicillin-resistant Staphylococcus aureus in long-term carriers. Clin Infect Dis. 200815;47:176-81.

Guidelines for Environmental Infection Control and Healthcare Facilities Recommendations of CDC and Healthcare Infection Control Practices Advisory Committee (HICPAC) 2003. This is available from the Center for Disease Control and Prevention, www.cdc.gov

Haley RW, Culver, DH, White JW, et al. The efficacy of infection surveilliance and control programs in preventing nosocomial infections in US hospitals. Am J Epidemiology 1985;121:182-205.

Huang SS, Datta R, Platt R. Risk of acquiring antibiotic-resistant bacteria from prior room occupants. Arch Intern Med. 2006;166:1945-51.

Huang SS, et al. Impact of routine intensive care unit surveillance cultures and resultant barrier precautions on hospital-wide methicillin-resistant Staphylococcus aureus bacteremia. Clin Infect Dis. 2006;43:971-8.

Lawton, RM, Turon, T, Cochran, RL, Cardo, D. Prepackaged hand hygiene educational tools facilitate implementation. Am J Infection Control 2006; 34: 152-154

Oie S, Yanagi C, et al. Contamination of environmental surfaces by Staphylococcus aureus in a dermatological ward and its preventive measures. J Hosp Infect. 1998;40:135-40.

Pulgliese G, Lamaberto B., Kroc KA. Development and implementation of infection control policies and procedures. In: Mayhill CG. Hospital Epidemiology and Infection Control. 2nd Ed. Philadelphia: Lippincott, Williams and Wilkins, 1999:1357-1366.

Shiomori T, et al. Evaluation of bedmaking-related airborne and surface methicillin-resistant Staphylococcus aureus contamination. J Hosp Infect. 2002;50:30-5.

Yokoe, DS, Classen, D. Improving patient safety through infection control: A new healthcare imperative. 2008;29:S3-S11.

Magnetic Resonance Imaging: Information for Patients*

What is magnetic resonance imaging (MRI)?

MRI, or magnetic resonance imaging, is a means of "seeing" inside of the body in order for doctors to find certain diseases or abnormal conditions. MRI does not rely on the type of radiation (i.e., ionizing radiation) used for an x-ray or computed tomography (CT). The MRI examination requires specialized equipment that uses a powerful, constant magnetic field, rapidly changing local magnetic fields, radiofrequency energy, and dedicated equipment including a powerful computer to create very clear pictures of internal body structures.

During the MRI examination, the patient is placed within the MR system or "scanner". The powerful, constant magnetic field aligns a tiny fraction of subatomic particles called protons that are present in most of the body's tissues. Radiofrequency energy is applied to cause these protons to produce signals that are picked up by a receiver within the scanner. The signals are specially characterized using the rapidly changing, local magnetic field and computer-processed to produce images of the body part of interest.

What is MRI used for?

MRI has become the preferred procedure for diagnosing a large number of potential problems in many different parts of the body. In general, MRI creates pictures that can show differences between healthy and unhealthy tissue. Doctors use MRI to examine the brain, spine, joints (e.g., knee, shoulder, wrist, and ankle), abdomen, pelvic region, breast, blood vessels, heart and other body parts.

Is MRI safe?

To date, over 200 million patients have had MRI examinations. MRI has been shown to be extremely safe as long as proper safety precautions are taken. In general, the MRI procedure produces no pain and causes no known short-term or long-term tissue damage of any kind.

The powerful magnetic field of the scanner can attract certain metallic objects that are "ferromagnetic", causing them to move suddenly and with great force towards the center of the MR system. This may pose a risk to the patient or anyone in the path of the object. Therefore, great care is taken to prevent ferromagnetic objects from entering the MR system room. It is vital that you remove metallic objects in advance of an MRI examination, including watches, jewelry, and items of clothing that have metallic threads or fasteners.

The MRI facility has a screening procedure that, when carefully followed, will ensure that the MRI technologist and radiologist knows about the presence of metallic implants and materials so that special precautions can be taken (see below). In some unusual cases, the examination may be canceled because of concern related to a particular implant or device. For example, if an MRI is ordered, it may be cancelled if the patient has a ferromagnetic aneurysm clip because of the risk of dislodging the clip from the blood vessel. Also, the magnetic field of the scanner can damage an external hearing aid or cause a heart pacemaker to malfunction. If you have a bullet, shrapnel, or similar metallic fragment in your body there is a potential risk that it could change position, possibly causing injury.

How to prepare for the MRI examination.

There's no special preparation necessary for the MRI examination. Unless your doctor specifically requests that you not eat or drink anything before the exam, there are no food or drink restrictions. Continue to take any medication prescribed by your doctor unless otherwise directed.

You won't be allowed to wear anything metallic during the MRI examination, so it would be best to leave watches, jewelry or anything made from metal at home. Even some cosmetics contain small amounts of metals, so it is best to not wear make-up.

In order to prevent metallic objects from being attracted by the powerful magnet of the MR system, you may receive a gown (which is advisable) to wear during your examination. Items that need to be removed before entering the MR system room include:

- Purse, wallet, money clip, credit cards, other cards with magnetic strips
- Electronic devices such as beepers or cellular phones
- Hearing aids
- Metallic jewelry, watches
- Pens, paper clips, keys, nail clippers, coins
- Hair barrettes, hairpins
- Any article of clothing that has a metallic zipper, buttons, snaps, hooks, under-wires, or metallic threads
- Shoes, belt buckles, safety pins

Before the MRI procedure, you will be asked to fill out a screening form asking about anything that might create a health risk or interfere with the examination. You will also undergo an interview by a member of the MRI facility to ensure that you understand the questions on the form. Even if you have undergone an MRI procedure before at this or another facility, you will still be asked to complete an MRI screening form.

Examples of items or things that may create a health hazard or other problem during an MRI exam include:

- Pacemaker
- Implantable cardioverter defibrillator (ICD)
- Neurostimulation system
- Aneurysm clip
- Metallic implant
- Implanted drug infusion device
- Foreign metal objects, especially if in or near the eye
- Shrapnel or bullet
- Permanent cosmetics or tattoos
- Dentures/teeth with magnetic keepers
- Other implants that involve magnets
- Medication patch (i.e., transdermal patch) that contains metallic foil

Check with the MRI technologist or radiologist at the MRI facility if you have questions or concerns about any implanted object or health condition that could impact the MRI procedure. This is particularly important if you have undergone surgery involving the brain, ear, eye, heart, or blood vessels.

Important Note: If you are pregnant or think that you could be pregnant, you must notify your physician and the radiologist or the MRI technologist at the MRI facility prior to the MRI procedure.

Before entering the MR system room, any friend or relative that might be allowed to accompany you will be asked questions to ensure that he or she may safely enter the room and will likewise be instructed to remove all metallic objects. Additionally, this individual will need to fill out a screening form.

What is the MRI examination like?

The MRI examination is performed in a special room that houses the MR system or "scanner". You will be escorted into the room by a staff member of the MRI facility and asked to lie down on a comfortably padded table that gently glides you into the scanner.

In order to prepare for the MRI examination, you may be required to wear earplugs or headphones to protect your hearing because, when certain scanners operate, they may produce loud noises. These loud noises are normal and should not worry you.

For some MRI studies, a contrast agent called "gadolinium" may be injected into a vein to help obtain a clearer picture of the body part that is undergoing examination. At some point during the procedure, a nurse or technologist will slide the table out of the scanner to inject the contrast agent. This is typically done through a small needle connected to an intravenous line that is placed in an arm or hand vein. A saline solution will drip through the intravenous line to prevent clotting until the contrast agent is injected at some point during the exam. Unlike contrast agents used in x-ray studies, MRI contrast agents do not contain iodine and, therefore, rarely cause allergic reactions or other problems.

The most important thing for you to do is to relax and remain still. Most MRI exams take between 15 to 45 minutes to complete depending on the body part imaged and how many images are needed, although some may take 60-minutes or longer. You'll be told ahead of time how long your scan is expected to take.

You will be asked to remain perfectly still during the time the imaging takes place, but between sequences some minor movement may be allowed. The MRI technologist will advise you, accordingly.

When the MRI procedure begins, you may breathe normally, however, for certain examinations it may be necessary for you to hold your breath for a short period of time.

During your MRI examination, the MR system operator will be able to speak to you, hear you, and observe you at all times. Consult the MR system operator if you have any questions or feel anything unusual.

When the MRI procedure is over, you may be asked to wait until the images are examined to determine if more images are needed. After the scan, you have no restrictions and can go about your normal activities.

Once the entire MRI examination is completed, the pictures will be reviewed by a radiologist, a specially-trained physician who is able to interpret the images for your doctor. The radiologist will send your doctor a report. You should contact your doctor to go over your results and discuss your next step.

DISCLAIMER

This information is provided for the sole purpose of educating you as to the basics of the MRI examination. You should rely on your physician, a radiologist, or an MRI technologist for specific information about your own examination.

[*Developed in conjunction with the Safety Committee of the International Society for Magnetic Resonance in Medicine, www.ISMRM.org]

Metallic Foreign Bodies and Screening

Patients and individuals with a history of being injured by a metallic foreign body such as a bullet, shrapnel, or metallic object should be thoroughly screened and evaluated prior to admission to the area of the MR system. This is particularly important because serious injury may occur as a result of movement or dislodgment of the metallic foreign body as it is attracted by the powerful magnetic field of the scanner. In addition, excessive heating may occur, although this tends to happen only if the object is made from conductive material and has an elongated shape or forms a loop with certain dimensions.

The relative risk of injury is dependent on the ferromagnetic properties of the foreign body, the geometry and dimensions of the object, the strength of the static magnetic field, and the strength of the spatial gradient of the magnet used for the MR system. Additionally, the potential for injury is related to the amount of force with which the object is fixed or retained within the tissue (i.e., counter-force or retention force may prevent movement or dislodgment) and whether or not it is positioned in or adjacent to a sensitive site of the body. These sensitive sites include vital neural, vascular, or soft tissue structures.

The use of plain film radiography is the technique of choice recommended to detect metallic foreign bodies for individuals and patients prior to admission to the MR environment. This includes screening for the presence of metallic orbital foreign bodies (see **Metallic Orbital Foreign Bodies and Screening**). The sensitivity of plain film radiography is considered to be sufficient to identify any metal with a mass large enough to present a hazard to an individual or patient in the MR environment.

REFERENCES

Boutin, R. D., Briggs, J. E., and Williamson, M. R., Injuries associated with MR imaging: survey of safety records and methods used to screen patients for metallic foreign bodies before imaging. Am J Roentgenol 1994;162:189.

Dempsey MF, Condon B, Hadley DM. Investigation of the factors responsible for burns during MRI. J Magn Reson Imaging 2001;13:627-631.

Elster, A. D., Link, K. M., and Carr, J. J., Patient screening prior to MR imaging: a practical approach synthesized from protocols at 15 U.S. medical centers. Am J Roentgenol 1994;162:195.

International Commission on Non-Ionizing Radiation Protection (ICNIRP) Statement, Medical magnetic resonance procedures: protection of patients. Health Physics 2004;87:197-216.

Jarvik JG, Ramsey JG. Radiographic screening for orbital foreign bodies prior to MR imaging: Is it worth it? Am J Neuroradiol 2000;1:245.

Mani, R. L., In search of an effective screening system for intraocular metallic foreign bodies prior to MR - An important issue of patient safety. Am J Neuroradiol 1988;9:1032.

Murphy KJ, Burnberg JA. Orbital plain film as a prerequisite for MR imaging: is a known history of injury sufficient screening criteria? Am J Roentgenol 1996;167:1053.

Otto PM, et al. Screening test for detection of metallic foreign objects in the orbit before magnetic resonance imaging. Invest Radiol 1992;27:308-311.

Seidenwurm DJ, McDonnell CH, Raghavan N, Breslau J. Cost utility analysis of radiographic screening for an orbital foreign body before MR imaging. Am J Neuroradiol 2000;21:426.

Shellock FG. Magnetic Resonance Procedures: Health Effects and Safety. CRC Press, LLC, Boca Raton, FL, 2001.

Shellock FG, Crues JV. MR procedures: biologic effects, safety, and patient care. Radiology, 2004;232:635-652.

Shellock FG, Kanal E, SMRI Safety Committee. Policies, guidelines, and recommendations for MR imaging safety and patient management. J Magn Reson Imaging 1991;1:97-101.

Williams S, Char D H, Dillon WP, Lincoff N, Moseley M. Ferrous intraocular foreign bodies and magnetic resonance imaging. Am J Ophthalmology 1998;105:398.

Zhang Y, Cheng J, et al. Tiny ferromagnetic intraocular foreign bodies detected by magnetic resonance imaging: a report of two cases. J Magn Reson Imaging. 2009;29:704-7.

Metallic Orbital Foreign Bodies and Screening

The case report in 1986 by Kelly et al. regarding a patient that sustained an orbital injury from a metallic foreign body led to substantial controversy regarding the procedure required to screen patients with suspected orbital foreign bodies prior to MR procedures. Notably, this incident is the only serious eye-related injury that has occurred in the MR environment (i.e., based on a review of the peer-reviewed literature). In consideration of this, the policy of performing radiographic screening for orbital foreign bodies in patients or individuals simply because of a history of occupational exposure to metallic fragments needs to be reconsidered.

A study by Seidenwurm et al. evaluated the practical aspects and cost-effectiveness of using a clinical versus radiographic technique to initially screen patients for orbital foreign bodies before MR procedures. The costs of screening were determined on the basis of published reports, disability rating guides, and a practice survey. A sensitivity analysis was performed for each variable. For this analysis, the benefits of screening were avoidance of immediate, permanent, nonameliorable, or unilateral blindness.

The findings of Seidenwurm et al. support the fact that the use of clinical screening before radiography increases the cost-effectiveness of foreign body screening by an order of magnitude (i.e., assuming base case ocular foreign body removal rates). From a clinical screening standpoint for a metallic foreign body located in the orbit, asking the patient "Did a doctor get it all out?" serves this purpose.

Seidenwurm et al. implemented the following policy with regard to screening patients with suspected metallic foreign bodies, "If a patient reports injury from an ocular foreign body that was subsequently removed by a doctor or that resulted in negative findings on any examination, we perform MR imaging...Those persons with a history of injury and no subsequent negative eye examination are screened radiographically." Of note is that Seidenwurm et al. has performed more than 100,000 MRI procedures under this protocol without incident.

Thus, an occupational history of exposure to metallic fragments, by itself, is insufficient to mandate radiographic orbital screening. Therefore, guidelines for foreign body screening should be based on this information and because radiographic screening before MR procedures on the basis of occupational exposure alone is neither clinically necessary nor cost-effective.

Clinical Screening Protocol. The procedure to follow with regard to patients with suspected metallic orbital foreign bodies involves asking them if they had an ocular injury. If they sustained an ocular injury, they are asked whether they had a medical examination at the time of the injury and whether they were told by the examining doctor, "It's all out." If they did not have an injury, if they were told their ophthalmologic examination was normal, and/or if the foreign body was removed entirely at the time of the injury, then they can proceed to MR imaging.

Radiographic Screening Protocol. Based on the results of the clinical screening protocol, patients are screened radiographically if they sustained an ocular injury related to a metallic foreign object and they were told that the eye examination revealed that the foreign body was not removed. In such a case, the MRI examination is postponed and the patient is scheduled for screening radiography.

In the event that the removal of the entire metallic foreign body cannot be verified or if there is insufficient information to confirm that there is no metallic foreign body present, screening radiography should be used prior to MRI.

SCREENING ADOLESCENTS FOR METALLIC ORBITAL FOREIGN BODIES

A case report by Elmquist and Shellock illustrates that special precautions are needed for screening adolescent patients prior to MR procedures. This article described an incident in which a 12-year-old patient accompanied by his parent completed all routine screening procedures prior to preparation for MR imaging of the lumbar spine. The patient and parent provided negative answers to all questions regarding prior injuries by metallic objects and the presence of metallic foreign bodies.

While entering the MR system room, the adolescent patient appeared to be anxious about the examination. He was placed in a feet-first, supine position on the MR system table and prepared for the procedure. As the patient was moved slowly toward the opening of a 1.5-Tesla MR system, he complained of a pressure sensation in his left eye. The MRI technologist immediately removed the patient from the MR environment.

Once again, the patient was questioned regarding a previous eye injury. The patient denied sustaining such an injury. Despite that patient's response, a metallic foreign body in the orbit was suspected. Therefore, plain film radiographs of the orbits were obtained and revealed a metallic foreign body in the left orbit. The patient and parent were counseled regarding the implications of future MR procedures with respect to the possibility of significant eye injury related to movement or dislodgment of the metallic object. This case demonstrates that routine safety protocols may be insufficient for adolescents referred for MR procedures. Accordingly, it is recommended that adolescents be provided with additional screening that includes private counseling about the hazards associated with the MR environment.

REFERENCES

Boutin, R. D., Briggs, J. E., and Williamson, M. R. Injuries associated with MR imaging: survey of safety records and methods used to screen patients for metallic foreign bodies before imaging. Am J Roentgenol 1994;162:189.

Elmquist, C., Shellock, F.G., and Stoller, D. Screening adolescents for metallic foreign bodies before MR procedures. J Magn Reson Imaging 1996;5:784.

Elster, A. D., Link, K. M., and Carr, J. J. Patient screening prior to MR imaging: a practical approach synthesized from protocols at 15 U.S. medical center. Am J Roentgenol 1994;162:195.

Jarvik, J. G., and Ramsey, J.G. Radiographic screening for orbital foreign bodies prior to MR imaging: Is it worth it? Am J Neuroradiol 2000;21:245.

Kanal E, Barkovich AJ, Bell C, et al. ACR guidance document for safe MR practices: 2007. AJR Am J Roentgenol. 2007;188:1447-1474.

Kelly, W. M., Pagle, P. G., Pearson, A., San Diego, A. G., and Soloman, M. A. Ferromagnetism of intraocular foreign body causes unilateral blindness after MR study. Am J Neuroradiol 1986;7: 243.

Mani, R. L. In search of an effective screening system for intraocular metallic foreign bodies prior to MR - An important issue of patient safety. Am J Neuroradiol 1988;9:1032.

Murphy, K. J., and Brunberg, J. A. Orbital plain film as a prerequisite for MR imaging: is a known history of injury sufficient screening criteria? Am J Roentgenol 1996;167:1053.

Seidenwurm, D. J., McDonnell, C. H., Raghavan, N., and Breslau, J. Cost utility analysis of radiographic screening for an orbital foreign body before MR imaging. Am J Neuroradiol 2000;21: 426.

Shellock FG. Magnetic Resonance Procedures: Health Effects and Safety. CRC Press, LLC, Boca Raton, FL, 2001.

Shellock FG. New recommendations for screening patients for suspected orbital foreign bodies. Signals, No. 36, Issue 4, pp. 8-9, 2001.

Shellock FG, Kanal E, SMRI Safety Committee. Policies, guidelines, and recommendations for MR imaging safety and patient management. J Magn Reson Imaging 1991;1:97-101.

Williams, S., Char, D. H., Dillon, W. P., Lincoff, N., and Moseley, M. Ferrous intraocular foreign bodies and magnetic resonance imaging. Am J Opthalmol 1998;05:398.

Zhang Y, Cheng J, et al. Tiny ferromagnetic intraocular foreign bodies detected by magnetic resonance imaging: a report of two cases. J Magn Reson Imaging. 2009;29:704-7.

Monitoring Patients in the MR Environment

Conventional monitoring equipment and accessories were not designed to operate in the harsh magnetic resonance (MR) environment that utilizes electromagnetic fields that can adversely affect or alter the operation of these devices. Fortunately, various monitors and other patient support devices have been developed or specially-modified to perform properly during MR procedures.

MR healthcare professionals must consider the ethical and medico-legal ramifications of providing proper patient care that includes identifying patients that require monitoring in the MR environment and following a proper protocol to ensure their safety by using appropriate equipment, devices, and accessories. The early detection and treatment of complications that may occur in high-risk, critically-ill, sedated, or anesthetized patients undergoing MR procedures can prevent relatively minor problems from becoming life-threatening situations.

GENERAL POLICIES AND PROCEDURES

Monitoring during an MR examination is indicated whenever a patient requires observations of vital physiologic parameters due to an underlying health problem or is unable to respond or alert the MRI technologist or other healthcare worker regarding pain, respiratory problem, cardiac distress, or difficulty that might arise during the examination. In addition, a patient should be monitored if there is a greater potential for a change in physiologic status during the MR procedure. Table 1 summarizes the patients that may require monitoring and support during MR procedures. Besides patient monitoring, various support devices and accessories may be needed for use in high-risk patients to ensure safety.

Because of the widespread use of MRI contrast agents and the potential for adverse effects or idiosyncratic reactions to occur, it is prudent to have appropriate monitoring equipment and accessories readily available for the proper management and support of patients who may experience side-effects. This is emphasized because adverse events, while extremely rare, may be serious or life threatening.

In 1992, the Safety Committee of the Society for Magnetic Resonance Imaging first published guidelines and recommendations concerning the monitoring of patients during MR procedures. This information indicates that all patients undergoing MR procedures should, at the very least, be visually (e.g., using a camera system) and/or verbally (e.g., intercom system) monitored, and that patients who are sedated, anesthetized, or are unable to communicate should be physiologically monitored and supported by the appropriate means.

Severe injuries and fatalities have occurred in association with MR procedures. These may have been prevented with the proper use of monitoring equipment and devices. Importantly, guidelines issued by the Joint Commission on Accreditation of Healthcare Organizations (JCAHO) indicate that patients receiving sedatives or anesthetics require monitoring during administration and recovery from these medications. Other professional organizations similarly recommend the need to monitor certain patients using proper equipment and techniques.

Table 1. Patients that require monitoring and support during MR procedures.

- Physically or mentally unstable patients.
- Patients with compromised physiologic functions.
- Patients who are unable to communicate.
- Neonatal and pediatric patients.
- Sedated or anesthetized patients.
- Patients undergoing MR-guided interventional procedures.
- Patients who may have a reaction to an MRI contrast agent.
- Critically ill or high-risk patients.

SELECTION OF PARAMETERS TO MONITOR

The proper selection of the specific physiologic parameter(s) that should be monitored during the MR procedure is crucial for patient safety. Various factors must be considered including the patient's medical history, present condition, the use of medication and possible side effects, as well as the aspects of the MR procedure to be performed. For example, if the patient receives a sedative, respiratory rate and/or oxygen saturation should be monitored. If the patient requires general anesthesia during the MR procedure, monitoring multiple physiologic parameters is required. Policies and procedures for the management of the patient in the MR environment should be comparable to those used in the operating room or critical care setting, especially with respect to monitoring and support requirements. Specific recommendations for physiologic monitoring of patients during MR procedures should be developed in consideration of "standard of care" issues as well as in consultation with anesthesiologists and other similar healthcare specialists. Notably, the Society of Anesthesiologists Task Force on Anesthetic Care for Magnetic Resonance Imaging recently presented a practice advisory on anesthetic care for patients undergoing MRI.

PERSONNEL INVOLVED IN PATIENT MONITORING

Only healthcare professionals with appropriate training and experience should be permitted to monitor patients during MR procedures. The healthcare professional must be experienced with the operation of the monitoring equipment and accessories used in the MR environment and should be able to recognize equipment malfunctions, device problems, and recording artifacts. Furthermore, the person responsible for monitoring the patient should be well-versed in screening patients for conditions that may complicate the procedure. For example, patients with asthma, congestive heart failure, obesity, obstructive sleep apnea, and other conditions are at increased risk for having problems during sedation. Also, the healthcare professional must be able to identify and manage adverse events using appropriate equipment and procedures in the MR environment.

Policies and procedures must be implemented to continue appropriate physiologic monitoring and management of the patient by trained personnel after the MR procedure is performed. This is especially needed for a patient recovering from the effects of a sedative or general anesthesia.

The monitoring of physiologic parameters and management of the patient during an MR procedure may be the responsibility of one or more individuals depending on the level of training for the healthcare worker and in consideration of the condition, medical history, and procedure that is to be performed for the patient. These individuals include anesthesiologists, nurse anesthetists, nurses, MR technologists, or radiologists.

EMERGENCY PLAN

The development, implementation, and regular practice of an emergency plan that addresses and defines the activities, use of equipment, and other pertinent issues related to a medical emergency are important for patient safety. For example, a plan needs to be developed for handling patients if there is the need to remove them from the MR system room to perform cardiopulmonary resuscitation. Obviously, taking necessary equipment such as a cardiac defibrillator, intubation instruments, or other similar devices near the MR system could pose a substantial hazard to the patients and healthcare workers if these are not safe for use in the MR environment. Healthcare professionals who are members of the cardiopulmonary resuscitation (i.e., "code blue") team must be trained to conduct their activities in the MR environment.

For out-patient or mobile MR facilities, it is necessary to educate outside emergency personnel (e.g., paramedics, firefighters, etc.) regarding the potential hazards associated with the MR environment. Typically, MRI facilities not affiliated with or in close proximity to a hospital must contact paramedics to handle medical emergencies and to transport patients to the hospital for additional care. Therefore, personnel responsible for summoning the paramedics, notifying the hospital, and performing other integral activities must be designated beforehand to avoid problems and confusion during an actual emergent event.

TECHNIQUES AND EQUIPMENT USED TO MONITOR AND SUPPORT PATIENTS

Physiologic monitoring and support of patients is not a trivial task in the MR environment. A variety of potential problems and hazards exist. Furthermore, the types of equipment for patient monitoring and support must be considered carefully and implemented properly to ensure the safety of both patients and MR healthcare professionals.

Several potential problems and hazards are associated with the performance of patient monitoring and support in the MR environment. Physiologic monitors and accessories that contain ferromagnetic components (e.g., transformers, outer casings, etc.) can be strongly attracted by the static magnetic field used of the MR system, posing a serious "missile" or projectile hazard to patients and healthcare workers.

If possible, necessary or critical devices that have ferromagnetic components should be permanently fixed to the floor and properly labeled with warning information to prevent them from being moved too close to the MR system. All personnel involved with MR procedures should be aware of the importance of the placement and use of the equipment, especially with regard to the hazards of moving portable equipment too close to the MR system.

Electromagnetic fields associated with the MR system can significantly effect the operation of conventional monitoring equipment, especially those with displays that involve electron beams (i.e., CRTs) or video display screens (with the exception of those with liquid crystal displays or LCDs). In addition, the monitoring equipment, itself, may emit spurious noise that, in turn, produces distortion or artifacts on the MR images.

Physiologic monitors that contain microprocessors or other similar components may leak RF, producing electromagnetic interference that can substantially alter MR images. To prevent adverse radiofrequency-related interactions between the MR system and physiologic monitors, RF-shielded cables, RF filters, special outer RF-shielded enclosures, or fiber-optic techniques can be utilized to prevent image-related or problems in the MR environment.

During the operation of MR systems, electrical currents may be generated in the conductive materials of monitoring equipment that are used as part of the interface to the patient. These currents can be of sufficient magnitude to cause excessive heating and thermal injury to the patient. Numerous first, second, and third degree burns have occurred in association with MR procedures that were directly attributed to the use of monitoring devices. These injuries were related to the use of electrocardiographic lead wires, plethysmographic gating systems, pulse oximeters, and other types of monitoring equipment and accessories comprised of wires, cables, or similar components made from conductive materials. Therefore, in consideration of the various problems and hazards associated with the use of monitoring equipment and accessories, it is important to follow the instructions and recommendations from the manufacturers with regard to the use of the devices in the MR environment.

Fortunately, modern-day physiologic monitoring devices have utilized fiber-optic techniques to prevent many of the afore-mentioned issues that exist with "hard-wire" cables, wires, and patient-monitor interfaces.

MONITORING EQUIPMENT AND SUPPORT DEVICES

This section describes the physiologic parameters that may be assessed in patients during MR procedures using appropriate monitoring equipment for the MR environment. In addition, various devices and accessories that are useful for the support and management of patients are presented.

Electrocardiogram and Heart Rate

Monitoring the patient's electrocardiogram (ECG) in the MR environment is particularly challenging because of the inherent distortion of the ECG waveform that occurs using MR systems operating at high field strengths. This effect is observed as blood, a conductive fluid, flows through the large vascular structures in the presence of the static magnetic field of the MR system. The resulting induced biopotential is seen primarily as an augmented T-wave amplitude, although other non-specific waveform-changes are also apparent on the ECG. Since altered T-waves or ST segments may be associated with cardiac disorders, static magnetic field-induced ECG-distortions may be problematic for certain patients. For this reason, it may be necessary to obtain a baseline recording of the ECG prior to placing the patient inside the MR system along with a recording obtained immediately after the MR procedure to determine the cardiac status of the patient.

Additional artifacts caused by the static, gradient, and RF electromagnetic fields of the MR system can severely distort the ECG, making observation of morphologic changes and detection of arrhythmias quite difficult. ECG artifacts that occur in the MR environment may be decreased substantially by implementing several simple techniques that include, the following:

- Use ECG electrodes that have minimal metal or those recommended by the manufacturer
- Select electrodes and cables that contain nonferromagnetic metals
- Place the limb electrodes in close proximity to one another
- Position the line between the limb electrodes and leg electrodes parallel to the magnetic field flux lines
- Maintain a small area between the limb and leg electrode
- Twist or braid the ECG leads
- Position the area of the electrodes near or in the center of the MR system

The use of proper ECG electrodes (i.e., those tested and deemed to be acceptable for patients) is required to ensure patient safety and proper recording of the electrocardiogram in the MR environment. Accordingly, ECG electrodes have been specially developed for use during MR procedures to protect the patient from potentially hazardous conditions. These ECG electrodes were also designed to reduce MRI-related artifacts.

Using standard ECG electrodes, leads, and cables may cause excessive heating that could burn the patient during an MR procedure. This occurs as electrical current is generated in the ECG cable or leads during the operation of the MR system. Accordingly, monitoring equipment has been modified to record the ECG while ensuring patient safety in the MR environment.

Fiber-optic ECG recording techniques may be used to prevent burns during MR procedures. For example, one such fiber-optic system acquires the ECG waveform using a special transceiver that resides in the MR system bore along with the patient and is located very near the ECG electrodes. A module digitizes and optically encodes the patient's ECG waveform and transmits it out from the MR system to the monitor using a fiber-optic cable. The use of this fiber-optic ECG technique eliminates the potential for burns associated with hard-wired ECG systems by removing the conductive patient cable and the "antenna effect" that are typical responsible for excessive heating.

Besides using an ECG monitor, the patient's heart rate may be determined continuously during the MR procedure using various types of acceptable devices including a photoplethysmograph and a pulse oximeter. A noninvasive, heart rate and blood pressure monitor (see section below) can also be utilized to obtain intermittent or semi-continuous recordings of heart rate during the MR examination.

Blood Pressure

Conventional, manual sphygmomanometers may be adapted for use during MR procedures. This is typically accomplished by lengthening the tubing from the cuff to the device so that the mercury column and other primary components may be positioned an acceptable distance (e.g., 8 to 10 feet from the bore of a 1.5-Tesla MR system) from the fringe field of the MR system.

Blood pressure measuring devices that incorporate a spring-gauge instead of a mercury column may be adversely affected by magnetic fields, causing them to work erroneously in the MR setting. Therefore, spring-gauge blood pressure devices should undergo pre-clinical testing before being used to monitor patients undergoing MR procedures.

Blood pressure monitors that use other noninvasive techniques, such as the oscillometric method, may be used to obtain semi-continuous recordings of systolic, diastolic, and mean blood pressures as well as pulse rate. These devices can be utilized to record systemic blood pressure in adult, pediatric, and neonate patients, selecting the appropriate blood pressure cuff size for a given patient. The intermittent inflation of the blood pressure cuff by an automated, noninvasive blood pressure monitor may disturb lightly sedated patients, especially infants or neonates, causing them to move and disrupt the MR procedure. For this reason, the use of a noninvasive blood pressure monitor may not be the best instrument to conduct physiologic monitoring in every patient.

Respiratory Rate and Apnea

Because respiratory depression and upper airway obstruction are frequent complications associated with the use of sedatives and anesthetics, monitoring techniques that detect a decrease in respiratory rate, hypoxemia, or airway obstruction should be used during the administration of these drugs. This is particularly important in the MR environment because visual observation of the patient's respiratory efforts is often difficult.

Respiratory rate monitoring can be performed during MR procedures by various techniques. The impedance method that utilizes chest leads and electrodes (similar to those used to record the ECG) can be used to monitor respiratory rate. This technique of recording respiratory rate measures a difference in electrical impedance induced between the leads that correspond to changes in respiratory movements. Unfortunately, the electrical impedance method of assessing respiratory rate may be inaccurate in pediatric patients because of the small volumes and associated motions of the relatively small thorax area.

Respiratory rate may also be monitored using a rubber bellows placed around the patient's thorax or abdomen (i.e., for "chest" or "belly" breathers). The bellows is attached to a pressure transducer that records body movements associated with inspiration and expiration. However, the bellows monitoring technique, like the electrical impedance method, is only capable of recording body movements associated with respiratory efforts. Therefore, these respiratory rate monitoring techniques do not detect apneic episodes related to upper airway obstruction (i.e., absent airflow despite respiratory effort) and may not provide sufficient sensitivity for assessing patients during MR procedures. For this reason, assessment of respiratory rate and identification of apnea should be accomplished using more appropriate monitoring devices.

Respiratory rate and apnea may be monitored during MR procedures using an end-tidal carbon dioxide monitor or a capnometer. These devices measure the level of carbon dioxide during the end of the respiratory cycle (i.e., end-tidal carbon dioxide). Additionally, capnometers provide quantitative data with respect to end-tidal carbon dioxide that is important for determining certain aspects of gas exchange in patients. The waveform provided on the end-tidal carbon dioxide monitors is also useful for assessing whether the patient is having difficulties breathing. The interface between the patient for the end-tidal carbon dioxide monitor and capnometer is a nasal or oro-nasal cannula that is made from plastic.

This interface prevents potential adverse interactions between the monitor and the patient during an MR procedure.

Oxygen Saturation

Oxygen saturation is a crucial variable to measure in sedated and anesthetized patients. This physiologic parameter is measured using pulse oximetry, a monitoring technique that assesses the oxygenation of tissue. Because oxygen saturated blood absorbs differing quantities of light compared with unsaturated blood, the amount of light that is absorbed by the blood can be readily used to calculate the ratio of oxygenated hemoglobin to total hemoglobin and displayed as the oxygen saturation. Additionally, the patient's heart rate may be calculated by measuring the frequency that pulsations occur as the blood moves through the vascular bed. Thus, a pulse oximeter can be used to determine oxygen saturation and pulse rate on a continuous basis by measuring the transmission of light through a vascular site such as the ear lobe, finger-tip, or toe. Notably, anesthesiologists consider the use of pulse oximetry to be the standard practice for monitoring sedated or anesthetized patients.

Commercially-available, specially-modified pulse oximeters that have hard-wire cables have been used to monitor sedated patients during MR procedures with moderate success. Unfortunately, these pulse oximeters tend to work intermittently during the operation of the MR system, primarily due to interference from the gradient and/or radio frequency electromagnetic fields. Of greater concern is the fact that pulse oximeters with hard-wire cables have been responsible for many patient burn injuries during MRI examinations, presumably as a result of excessive current being induced in the conductive cables.

Pulse oximeters have been developed that use fiber-optic technology to obtain and transmit the physiologic signals from the patient. These devices operate without interference by the electromagnetic fields used for MR procedures. It is physically impossible for a patient to be burned by the use of a fiber-optic pulse oximeter during an MR procedure because there are no conductive pathways formed by any metallic materials that connect to the patient. Several different fiber-optic pulse oximeters are commercially available for use in the MR environment.

Temperature

There are several reasons to monitor skin and/or body temperatures during MR procedures. These include recording temperatures in neonates with inherent problems retaining body heat (a tendency that is augmented during sedation or anesthesia), in patients during MR procedures that require high levels of RF power, and in patients with underlying conditions that impair their ability to dissipate heat.

Skin and body temperatures may be monitored during MR procedures using a variety of techniques. However, it should be noted that the use of hard-wire, thermistor or thermocouple-based techniques to record temperatures in the MR environment may cause artifacts or erroneous measurements due to direct heating of the temperature probes. A more appropriate, effective and easier technique of recording temperatures during MR examinations is with the use of a fluoroptic thermometry system. Notably, monitoring skin temperature, alone, is insufficient to ensure patient safety as this parameter does not provide proper information relative to deep body temperature.

The fluoroptic monitoring system has several important features that make it particularly useful for temperature monitoring during MR procedures. For example, this device incorporates fiber-optic probes that are small but efficient in carrying optical signals over long paths, it provides noise-free applications in electromagnetically hostile environments, and has fiber-optic components that will not pose a risk to patients.

Multi-Parameter Physiologic Monitoring Systems

In certain cases, it is necessary to monitor several different physiologic parameters simultaneously in patients undergoing MR procedures. While several different stand-alone units may be used to accomplish this task, the most efficient means of recording multiple parameters is by utilizing a monitoring system that permits the measurement of different physiologic functions such as heart rate, respiratory rate, blood pressure, and oxygen saturation.

Currently, there are a number of multi-parameter patient monitoring systems that are acceptable for use in the MRI environment. Typically, these devices are designed with components positioned within the MR system room and incorporate special circuitry to substantially reduce the artifacts that effect the recording of ECG and other physiologic variables, making them also useful for the performance of "gated" MR procedures.

Ventilators

Devices used for mechanical ventilation of patients typically contain mechanical switches, microprocessors, and ferromagnetic components that may be adversely effected by the electromagnetic fields used by MR systems. Ventilators that are activated by high pressure oxygen and controlled by the use of fluidics (i.e., no requirements for electricity) may still have ferromagnetic parts that can malfunction as a result of interference from MR systems.

Ventilators have been modified or specially-designed for use during MR procedures performed in adult as well as neonatal patients. These devices tend to be constructed from non-ferromagnetic materials and have undergone pre-clinical evaluations to ensure that they operate properly in the MR environment, without producing artifacts on MR images.

Additional Devices and Accessories

A variety of devices and accessories are often necessary for support and management of high-risk or sedated patients in the MR environment. Gurneys, oxygen tanks, gas regulators, stethoscopes, suction devices, infusion pumps, power injectors, and other similar devices and accessories shown to be acceptable for the MR environment may be obtained from various manufacturers and distributors. Additionally, there are gas anesthesia systems available that were designed for use in patients undergoing MR procedures.

SEDATION

Whenever sedatives are used, it is imperative to perform physiologic monitoring to ensure patient safety. In addition, it is important to have the necessary equipment readily available in the event of an emergency. These requirements should also be followed for patients undergoing sedation in the MR environment.

There is controversy regarding who should be responsible for performing sedation of patients in the MR environment. (For the sake of discussion, the terms "sedation" and "anesthesia" are used interchangeably since they are actually part of the same continuum.) Obviously, there are medical, regulatory, administrative, and financial issues to be considered.

In general, for patients with conditions that complicate sedation procedures, a nurse under the direction of an anesthesiologist or a specially trained radiologist may be responsible for preparing, sedating, monitoring, and recovering these cases. However, for patients with serious medical or other unusual problems, it is advisable to utilize anesthesia consultation to properly manage these individuals before, during, and after MR procedures.

In addition, the MRI facility should establish policies and guidelines for patient preparation, monitoring, sedation, and management during the post-sedation recovery period. These policies and guidelines should be based on standards established by the American Society of

Anesthesiologists (ASA), the American College of Radiology (ACR), the American Academy of Pediatrics Committee on Drugs (AAP-COD) and the Joint Commission on Accreditation of Healthcare Organizations (JCAHO).

Practice Guidelines for Sedation and Anesthesia from the American Society of Anesthesiologists indicate that a person must be present that is responsible for monitoring the patient if sedative or anesthetic medications are used. Furthermore, the following aspects of patient monitoring must be performed:

1) Visual monitoring
2) Assessment of the level of consciousness
3) Evaluation of ventilatory status
4) Evaluation of oxygen status assessed via the use of pulse oximetry
5) Determination of hemodynamic status via the use of blood pressure monitoring and electrocardiography if significant cardiovascular disease is present in the patient

Healthcare professionals must be able to recognize complications of sedation such as hypoventilation and airway obstruction as well as be able to establish a patent airway for postive-pressure ventilation.

Patient Preparation

Special patient screening must be conducted to identify conditions that may complicate sedation in order to properly prepare the patient for the administration of a sedative. This screening procedure should request important information from the patient that includes the following: major organ system disease (e.g., diabetes, pulmonary, cardiac, or hepatic disease), prior experience or adverse reactions to sedatives or anesthetics, current medications, allergies to drugs, and a history of alcohol, substance, or tobacco abuse.

In addition, the nothing by mouth (NPO) interval for the patient must be determined to reduce the risk of aspiration during the procedure. The ASA "Practice Guidelines Regarding Preoperative Fasting" recommend a minimum NPO periods of two hours for clear liquids, four hours for breast milk, six hours for infant formula, and six hours for a "light meal". The NPO period is extremely important because sedatives may depress the patient's gag reflex.

Administration of Sedation

A thorough discussion of sedation techniques especially with regard to the use of various pharmacologic agents is outside the scope of this monograph. Therefore, interested readers are referred to the excellent, comprehensive review of this topic written by Reinking Rothshild (2000), Dr. Reinking Rothschild is an anesthesiologist with extensive experience sedating patients in the MR environment.

Documentation

During the use of sedation, written records should be maintained that indicate the patient's vital signs as well as the name, dosage, and time of administration for all drugs that are given to the patient. The use of a time-based anesthesia-type record, such as that recommended by Reinking Rothschild (2000), is the best means of maintaining written documentation for sedation of patients in the MR environment.

Post-Sedation Recovery

After sedation, the medical care of the patient must continue. This is especially important for pediatric patients because certain medications have relatively long half-lives (e.g., chloral hydrate, pentobarbitol, etc.). Therefore, an appropriate room with monitoring and emergency equipment must be available to properly manage these patients.

Prior to allowing the patient to leave the MRI facility, the patient should be alert, oriented, and have stable vital signs. In addition, a responsible adult should accompany the patient home. Written instructions that include an emergency telephone number should be provided to the patient.

REFERENCES

American College of Radiology, ACR standard for the use of intravenous conscious sedation, and ACR standard for pediatric sedation/analgesia. In, 1998 ACR Standards, Reston, VA, American College of Radiology 1998; pp. 123.

American Academy of Pediatrics Committee on Drugs, Guidelines for monitoring and management of pediatric patients during and after sedation for diagnostic and therapeutics procedures. Pediatrics 1992;89:1100.

American Academy of Pediatrics; American Academy of Pediatric Dentistry, Cote CJ, Wilson S; Work Group on Sedation. Guidelines for monitoring and management of pediatric patients during and after sedation for diagnostic and therapeutic procedures: an update. Pediatrics. 2006;118:2587-602.

A Report by the ASA Task Force on Sedation and Analgesia by Non-Anesthesiologists. Practice guidelines for sedation and analgesia by non-anesthesiologists. Anesthesiology 1996;84:459.

Dalal PG, Murray D, Cox T, McAllister J, Snider R. Sedation and anesthesia protocols used for magnetic resonance imaging studies in infants: provider and pharmacologic considerations. Anesth Analg. 2006;103:863-8.

De Sanctis Briggs V. Magnetic resonance imaging under sedation in newborns and infants: a study of 640 cases using sevoflurane. Paediatr Anaesth. 2005;15:9-15.

Gooden CK. Anesthesia for magnetic resonance imaging. Curr Opin Anaesthesiol. 2004;17:339-42.

Holshouser, B., Hinshaw, D. B., and Shellock, F. G. Sedation, anesthesia, and physiologic monitoring during MRI. J Magn Reson Imaging 1993;3:553-558.

Kanal, E., and Shellock, F. G. Policies, guidelines, and recommendations for MR imaging safety and patient management. Patient monitoring during MR examinations. J Magn Reson Imaging 1992;2:247.

Kanal, E., and Shellock, F. G. Patient monitoring during clinical MR imaging. Radiology 1992;185:623.

Kanal E, Barkovich AJ, Bell C, et al. ACR guidance document for safe MR practices: 2007. AJR Am J Roentgenol. 2007;188:1447-1474.

McArdle, C., Nicholas, D., Richardson, C., and Amparo, E. Monitoring of the neonate undergoing MR imaging: Technical considerations. Radiology 1986;159:223.

Reinking Rothschild, D. Chapter 5, Sedation for open magnetic resonance imaging. In, Open MRI, P. A. Rothschild and D. Reinking Rothschild, Editors, Lippincott, Williams and Wilkins, Philadelphia, 2000, pp. 39.

Practice advisory on anesthetic care for magnetic resonance imaging: a report by the Society of Anesthesiologists Task Force on Anesthetic Care for Magnetic Resonance Imaging. Anesthesiology. 2009;110:459-79.

Serafini G, Ongaro L, Mori A, Rossi C, Cavalloro F, Tagliaferri C, Mencherini S, Braschi A. Anesthesia for MRI in the paediatric patient. Minerva Anestesiol. 2005;71:361-6.

Shellock, F. G., and Kanal, E. Magnetic Resonance: Bioeffects, Safety, and Patient Management. Second Edition, Lippincott-Raven Press, New York, 1996.

Shellock FG. Chapter 11, Patient monitoring in the MR environment. In: Magnetic Resonance Procedures: Health Effects and Safety. CRC Press, Boca Raton, FL, 2001, pp. 217-241.

MRI Contrast Agents and Adverse Reactions*

Gadolinium chelates have been approved for parenteral use since the late 1980s. Although these agents can be differentiated on the basis of stability, viscosity and osmolality, they cannot be differentiated on the basis of efficacy. These contrast media are extremely well tolerated by the vast majority of patients in whom they are injected. Adverse reactions are encountered with a much lower frequency than is observed after administration of iodinated contrast media.

Adverse Reactions to Gadolium Contrast Agents

The frequency of all adverse events after an injection of 0.1 or 0.2 mmol/kg ranges from 0.07–2.4 percent. The vast majority of these reactions are mild, including coldness at the injection site, nausea with or without vomiting, headache, warmth or pain at the injection site, paresthesias, dizziness, and itching. Reactions resembling an "allergic" response are very unusual and vary in frequency from 0.004–0.7 percent. A rash, hives, or urticaria are the most frequent of this group, and very rarely there may be bronchospasm. Severe, life-threatening anaphylactoid reactions are exceedingly rare (0.001–0.01 percent). In an accumulated series of 687,000 doses there were only 5 severe reactions. In another survey based on 20 million administered doses there were 55 cases of anaphylactoid shock. It would appear that, to date, only one published death has been clearly related to the administration of gadolinium-based contrast. Other deaths in other series have been ascribed to other diseases or to other drugs, or were thought to be coincidental. Clearly, fatal reactions to gadolinium agents are very rare.

Risk Factors

The frequency of adverse reactions to gadolinium contrast agents is about 2.3 to 3.7 times higher in patients with a history of reactions to iodinated contrast material and about 8 times higher in patients with a previous reaction to gadolinium-based contrast agents. Second reactions to gadolinium-based compounds tend to be more severe than the first. Persons with asthma and various allergies are also at greater risk, with reports of adverse reaction rates as high as 3.7 percent.

In the absence of any widely accepted policy for dealing with patients with prior contrast reactions (especially to gadolinium-based compounds) and the need for subsequent exposure to MR agents, it does seem prudent to at least take precautions. It should be determined if contrast material is necessary, if a different MR contrast agent could be used, and if 12–24 hours of premedication with corticosteroids and antihistamines could be initiated. This is particularly applicable in patients with prior moderate to severe reactions.

Nephrotoxicity. Gadolinium agents are considered to have no nephrotoxicity at approved dosages for MR imaging. They can be used in azotemic patients and are dialyzable. MR with gadolinium has been used instead of contrast-enhanced CT in those at risk for developing worsening renal failure if exposed to iodinated contrast material.

Gadolinium agents are radiodense and can be used for opacification in CT and angiographic examinations instead of iodinated radiographic contrast agents. However, there is controversy over whether gadolinium contrast agents are less nephrotoxic at equal-attenuating doses. Caution should be used in extrapolating the lack of nephrotoxicity of intravenous gadolinium at MR dosages to the use of gadolinium for angiographic procedures, including direct injection into the renal arteries. No assessment of gadolinium versus iodinated contrast nephrotoxicity by randomized studies of equal-attenuating doses is currently available.

Pregnancy. At doses considerably higher than recommended in humans, gadopentetate dimeglumine has been shown to retard fetal development in rats, double the incidence of post-implantation loss, and to increase the incidence of spontaneous abortion. It may also have an adverse effect on embryo-fetal development. Therefore, MR contrast using any chelate should only be performed if the potential benefit justifies the potential risk, and then only after obtaining written, informed consent.

Treatment. Treatment of moderate or severe adverse reactions to gadolinium-based contrast media is similar to that for moderate or severe reactions to iodinated contrast media. In any facility where contrast material is injected, it is imperative that personnel trained in recognizing and handling reactions and the equipment and medications to do so be on site or immediately available. Most MR facilities take the position that patients requiring treatment should be taken immediately out of the imaging room and away from the magnet so that none of the resuscitative equipment becomes a hazard.

Extravasation. The incidence of extravasation in one series of 28,000 doses was 0.05 percent. Laboratory studies in animals have demonstrated that both gadopentetate dimeglumine and gadoteridol are much less toxic to the skin and subcutaneous tissues than are equal volumes of iodinated contrast media. For these reasons the likelihood of a significant injury resulting from extravasated MR contrast agent is extremely low.

Serum Calcium Determinations

Some evidence has developed that gadolinium-based MR contrast material might interfere with total serum calcium values determined with standard colorimetric methods (Roche, Dade and Olympus). This interference is not seen using dry slide technology (Vitros). A warning from Roche Diagnostics suggested that colorimetric determination might be erroneously low, especially in patients with impaired renal function who have recently received gadolinium. It appears that the linear chelates Gd-DTPA-BMA (gado-diamide) and Gd-DTPA bis(methoxyethyl) amide (gadoversetamide) are much more likely to cause this artifact than Gd-DTPA (gadopentetate dimeglumine) or the macrocyclic chelates such as Gd-DOTA (gadoterate meglumine).

If an unexpectedly low result for serum calcium is obtained, it should be repeated two days later or checked with atomic absorption spectroscopy which is not affected by gadolinium chelates.

Off-Label Usage

Radiologists commonly use contrast media for a clinical purpose not contained in the labeling and thus commonly use contrast media off-label. Examples include MR angiography, cardiac applications, pediatric applications in patients less than two years of age, and usage in patients with renal failure.

[*American College of Radiology, Manual on Contrast Media, 5th Edition, 2004; Reprinted with permission of the American College of Radiology. No other representation of this article is authorized without express, written permission from the American College of Radiology. Also, please see the new version of this document Manual on Contrast Media, Version 6, 2008 – full version available at www.acr.org]

REFERENCES

Cochran ST, Bomyea K, Sayre JW. Trends in adverse events after IV administration of contrast media. AJR 2001; 176:1385–1388.

Cohan RH, Ellis JH, Garner WL. Extravasation of radiographic contrast material: recognition, prevention, and treatment. Radiology 1996;200:593–604.

Cohan RH, Leder RA, Herzberg AJ et al. Extravascular toxicity of two magnetic resonance contrast agents: preliminary experience in the rat. Invest Radiol 1991; 26:224–226.

Goldstein HA, Kashanian FK, Blumetti RF, et al. Safety assessment of gadopentetate dimeglumine in U.S. clinical trials. Radiology 1990;174:17–23.

Haustein J, Laniado M, Niendorf HP, et al. Triple-dose versus standard-dose gadopen-tetate dimeglumine: a randomized study in 199 patients. Radiology 1993;186:855–860.

Jordan RM, Mintz RD. Fatal reaction to gadopentetate dimeglumine. AJR 1995;164:743–744.

Lin J, Idee JM, Port M, et al. Interference of magnetic resonance imaging contrast agents with the serum calcium measurement technique using colorimetric reagents. J Pharm Biomed Anal 1999; 21:931–943.

McAlister WH, McAlister VI, Kissane JM. The effect of Gd-dimeglumine on subcutaneous tissues: a study with rats. AJNR 1990;11:325–327.

Murphy KJ, Brunberg JA, Cohan RH. Adverse reactions to gadolinium contrast media: a review of 36 cases. AJR 1996;167:847–849.

Murphy KP, Szopinski KT, Cohan RH, et al. Occurrence of adverse reactions to gadolinium based contrast material and management of patients at increased risk: a survey of the American Society of Neuroradiology Fellowship Directors. Acad Radiol 1999;6:656–664.

Niendorf HP, Brasch RC. Gd-DTPA tolerance and clinical safety. In: Brasch RC, Drayer BP, Haughton VM, et al, eds. MRI contrast enhancement in the central nervous system: a case study approach. New York, NY: Raven, 1993:11–21.

Niendorf HP, Haustein J, Conelius I, et al. Safety of gadolinium-DTPA: extended clinical experience. Magn Reson Med 1991;22:222–228.

Nelson KL, Gifford LM, Lauber-Huber C, et al. Clinical safety of gadopentetate dime-glumine. Radiology 1995;196:439–443.

Nyman U, Elmstahl B, Leander P, et al. Are gadolinium-based contrast media really safer than iodinated media for digital subtraction angiography in patients with azotemia? Radiology 2002; 223:311–318.

Olukotun AY, Parker JR, Meeks MJ, et al. Safety of gadoteridol injection: U.S. clinical trial experience. J Magn Reson Imaging 1995;5:17–25.

Omohundro JE, Elderbrook MK, Ringer TV. Laryngospasm after administration of gado pentetate dimeglumine. J Magn Reson Imaging 1992;2:729–730.

Runge VM, Bradley WG, Brant-Zawadzki MN, et al. Clinical safety and efficacy of gadoteridol: a study in 411 patients with suspected intracranial and spinal disease. Radiology 1991; 181:701–709.

Runge VM. Safety of approved MR contrast media for intravenous injection. J Magn Reson Imaging 2000;212:205–213.

Runge VM. Safety of magnetic resonance contrast media. Top Magn Reson Imaging 2001;12:309-314.

Salonen OL. Case of anaphylaxis and four cases of allergic reaction following Gd-DTPA administration. J Comput Assist Tomogr 1990;14:912–913.

Shellock FG, Hahn HP, Mink JH, et al. Adverse reaction to intravenous gadoteridol. Radiology 1993;189:151–152.

Spinosa DJ, Kaufmann JA, Hartwell GD. Gadolinium chelates in angiography and interventional radiology: a useful alternative to iodinated contrast media for angiography. Radiology2002;223:319-325.

Takebayashi S, Sugiyama M, Nagase M, et al. Severe adverse reaction to IV gadopentetate dimeglumine. AJR 1993;160:659.

Tardy B, Guy C, Barral G, et al. Anaphylactic shock induced by intravenous gadopentetate dimeglumine. Lancet 1992;339:494.

Tishler S, Hoffman JC. Anaphylactoid reactions to IV gadopentetate dimeglumine. AJNR 1990; 11:1167.

Weiss KL. Severe anaphylactoid reaction after IV Gd-DTPA. Magn Reson Imaging 1990;8:817–818.

Witte RJ, Anzai LL. Life-threatening anaphylactoid reaction after intravenous gadoteridol administration in a patient who had previously received gadopentetate dimeglumine. AJNR 1994;15:523–524.

MRI Contrast Agents and Breast Feeding Mothers*

Administration of a gadolinium-based MRI contrast agent occasionally is indicated for an imaging study in a woman who is breast-feeding. Both the patient and the patient's physician may have concerns regarding potential toxicity to the infant from contrast media that is excreted into the breast milk.

The literature on the excretion into breast milk of gadolinium-based MRI contrast agents and the gastrointestinal absorption of these agents from breast milk is limited. A review of the literature, however, reveals important facts: (1) less than 1% of the administered maternal dose of contrast agent is excreted into breast milk; and (2) less than 1% of the contrast medium in breast milk ingested by an infant is absorbed from the gastro-intestinal tract. Therefore, the expected dose of contrast medium absorbed by an infant from ingested breast milk is extremely low.

The Committee on Drugs and Contrast Media of the American College of Radiology (ACR) has discussed this issue extensively and has prepared the following summary information and recommendations.

Gadolinium-based MRI Contrast Agents and Breast Feeding Mothers

Background. Gadolinium compounds are safe and useful as magnetic resonance imaging (MRI) contrast agents. Although free gadolinium is neurotoxic when complexed to one of a variety of chelates, it is safe for use in adults and children. These hydrophilic gadolinium chelate agents have pharmacokinetic properties very similar to those of iodinated X-ray contrast media. Like iodinated contrast agents, gadolinium contrast agents have a plasma half-life of approximately 2 hours and are nearly completely cleared from the bloodstream within 24 hours.

Less than 0.04% of the intravascular dose given to the mother is excreted into the breast milk in the first 24 hours. Because less than 1% of the contrast medium ingested by the infant is absorbed from its gastrointestinal tract, the expected dose absorbed by the infant from the breast milk is less than 0.0004% of the intravascular dose given to the mother. Even in the extreme circumstance of a mother weighing 150 kg and receiving a dose of 0.2 mmol/kg, the absolute amount of gadolinium excreted in the breast milk in the first 24-hours after administration would be no more than 0.012 mmol. Thus, the dose of gadolinium absorbed from the gastrointestinal tract of a breast-feeding infant weighing 1,500 grams or more would be no more than 0.00008 mmol/kg, or 0.04% (four ten-thousandths) of the permitted adult or pediatric (2 years of age or older) intravenous dose of 0.2 mmol/kg. The potential risks to the infant include direct toxicity (including toxicity from free gadolinium, because it is unknown how much, if any, of the gadolinium in breast milk is in the unchelated form) and allergic sensitization or reaction, which are theoretical concerns but have not been reported.

Recommendation. Review of the literature shows no evidence to suggest that oral ingestion by an infant of the tiny amount of gadolinium contrast agent excreted into breast milk would cause toxic effects. Therefore, the available data suggest that it is safe for the mother and infant to continue breast-feeding after receiving such an agent.

If the mother remains concerned about any potential ill effects, she should be given the opportunity to make an informed decision as to whether to continue or temporarily abstain from breast-feeding after receiving a gadolinium contrast agent. If the mother so desires, she may abstain from breast-feeding for 24 hours with active expression and discarding of breast milk from both breasts during that period. In anticipation of this, she may wish to use a breast pump to obtain milk before the contrast study to feed the infant during the 24-hour period following the examination.

[*American College of Radiology, Manual on Contrast Media, 5th Edition, 2004; Reprinted with permission of the American College of Radiology. No other representation of this article is authorized without express, written permission from the American College of Radiology. <u>Also, please see the new version of this document Manual on Contrast Media, Version 6, 2008 – full version available at www.acr.org</u>]

REFERENCES

American College of Radiology, Manual on Contrast Media, 5th Edition, 2004.

Ilett KF, Hackett LP, Paterson JW, et al. Excretion of metrizamide in milk. Br J Radiol 1981;54:537–538.

Johansen JG. Assessment of a non-ionic contrast medium (Amipaque) in the gastrointestinal tract. Invest Radiol 1978;13:523–527.

Kubik-Huch RA, Gottstein-Aalame NM, Frenzel T, et al. Gadopentetate dimeglumine excretion into human breast milk during lactation. Radiology 2000;216:555–558.

Nielsen ST, Matheson I, Rasmussen JN, et al. Excretion of iohexol and metrizoate in human breast milk. Acta Radiol 1987;28:523–526.

Rofsky NM, Weinreb JC, Litt AW. Quantitative analysis of gadopentetate dimeglumine excreted in breast milk. J Magn Reson Imaging 1993;3:131–132.

Schmiedl U, Maravilla KR, Gerlach R, et al. Excretion of gadopentetate dimeglumine in human breast milk. American Journal of Roentgenology 1990;154:1305–1306.

Shellock FG, Kanal E. Safety of magnetic resonance imaging contrast agents. Journal of Magnetic Resonance Imaging 1999;10:477-484.

Weinmann HJ, Brasch RC, Press WR, et al. Characteristics of gadolinium-DTPA complex: a potential NMR contrast agent. American Journal of Roentgenology 1984;142: 619–624.

MRI Contrast Agents and Pregnant Patients*

Studies of low molecular weight water-soluble extracellular substances such as gadolinium-based magnetic resonance imaging (MRI) contrast agents in pregnancy have been limited, and effects on the human embryo or fetus are unknown. A standard gadolinium-based MRI contrast agent has been shown to cross the placenta in primates and appear within the fetal bladder within 11 minutes after intravenous administration. It must be assumed that all gadolinium-based contrast media behave in a similar fashion and cross the blood-placental barrier into the fetus.

After entering the fetal blood stream, these agents will be excreted via the urine into the amniotic fluid and be subsequently swallowed by the fetus. It is then possible that a small amount will be absorbed from the gut of the fetus and the rest eliminated back into the amniotic fluid, the entire cycle being repeated innumerable times.

In the study in primates, placental enhancement could be detected up to two hours following the intravenous administration of gadopentetate dimeglumine. When gadopentetate dimeglumine was injected directly into the amniotic cavity, it was still conspicuous at one hour after administration. There are no data available to assess the rate of clearance of contrast agents from the amniotic fluid.

The American College of Radiology (ACR) Committee on Drugs and Contrast Media has reviewed this issue extensively and has prepared the following summary of information and recommendations.

Gadolinium-Based MRI Contrast Agents and Pregnant Patients

It is known that gadolinium-based MR contrast media cross the human placenta and into the fetus when given in clinical dose ranges. No adequate and well-controlled teratogenic studies of the effects of these agents in pregnant women have been performed. The ACR recommends that all imaging facilities should have policies and procedures to reasonably attempt to identify pregnant patients prior to the performance of the MR exam, and before the use of MRI contrast media in these patients. The ACR has issued a White Paper on MR safety in pregnancy and related issues that is also consistent with the ACR Committee on Drugs and Contrast Media's recommendation for MRI contrast media.

While there is no compelling evidence of teratogenicity or other adverse effect on the fetus of MR imaging or of gadolinium-based MRI contrast agents, neither the safety of the MR environment nor the safety of the MRI contrast agents in pregnant patients has been established. It is therefore prudent for pregnant patients at any stage of pregnancy to be informed of the risk-benefit ratio that may warrant the performance of an MR scan with or without contrast media. The radiologist should confer with the referring physician and document the following in the radiology report or the patient's medical record:

1) The information requested from the MR study cannot be acquired using other nonionizing radiation imaging modalities (e.g., ultrasonography).

2) That the information needed affects the care of the patient and fetus during the pregnancy.

3) That the referring physician is of the opinion that it is not prudent to wait to obtain this information until after the patient is no longer pregnant.

It is recommended that the pregnant patient undergoing an MR examination with contrast material provide informed consent to document that she understands the risk/benefits of the MR procedure to be performed, and the alternative diagnostic options available to her (if any), and that she wishes to proceed.

[*Excerpted with permission from Runge VM. Chapter 12, Safety of Magnetic Resonance Contrast Agents. In: Magnetic Resonance Procedures: Health Effects and Safety. CRC Press, Boca Raton, FL, 2001, pp. 241-260 and the American College of Radiology, Manual on Contrast Media, 5th Edition, 2004; Reprinted with permission of the American College of Radiology. No other representation of this article is authorized without express, written permission from the American College of Radiology. Also, please see the new version of this document Manual on Contrast Media, Version 6, 2008 – full version available at www.acr.org]

REFERENCES

American College of Radiology, Manual on Contrast Media, 5th Edition, 2004.

Kanal E, Barkovich AJ, Bell C, et al. ACR guidance document for safe MR practices: 2007. AJR Am J Roentgenol. 2007;188:1447-1474.

Panigel M, Wolf G, Zeleznick A. Magnetic resonance imaging of the placenta in rhesus monkeys, Macaca mulatta. J Med Primatol 1988;17:3–18.

Runge VM. Chapter 12, Safety of Magnetic Resonance Contrast Agents. In: Magnetic Resonance Procedures: Health Effects and Safety. CRC Press, Boca Raton, FL, 2001, pp. 241-260.

Shellock FG, Kanal E. Safety of magnetic resonance imaging contrast agents. Journal of Magnetic Resonance Imaging 1999;10:477-484.

MRI Contrast Agent: MultiHance Frequently Asked Questions

QUESTION: How does the safety profile of MultiHance compare to the other currently available gadolinium-based contrast agents.

ANSWER: The safety profile of MultiHance is similar to that of the other approved gadolinium agents. As stated in the American College of Radiology Manual on Contrast Media, gadolinium-containing contrast media are extremely well tolerated by the vast majority of patients in whom they are injected. Clinical studies have been performed comparing the safety profiles of other gadolinium-based contrast agents and MultiHance. In these studies the frequency and type of adverse reactions seen after the two agents were similar.

QUESTION: Do the container closure or formulation of MultiHance contain latex?

ANSWER: No.

QUESTION: Since the MultiHance package insert contains a contraindication for use in patients with known allergic or hypersensitivity reactions to gadolinium or any other ingredient, can we use MultiHance in patients who developed a sensitivity reaction such as hives after administration of another gadolinium-based contrast agent?

ANSWER: No. It is advisable to seek a different modality anytime a patient exhibits sensitivity to a component of a drug. However, please note that this type of a statement is made in all of the gadolinium agent package inserts. It is contained in the contraindications section of the last two agents approved by the FDA (MultiHance and OptiMARK) and it is contained in the warnings section of the earlier approved agents (ProHance, Magnevist, and Omniscan). There is no evidence that adverse reactions are more frequent or more serious with the more recently approved agents.

QUESTION: Should breastfeeding be discontinued after administration of MultiHance?

ANSWER: The MultiHance package insert suggests that breastfeeding be discontinued for approximately 24 hours after administration of MultiHance. There is similar language in the package inserts of the other approved gadolinium contrast agents.

QUESTION: Is there any information about the safe use of MultiHance for MR arthrography procedures?

ANSWER: Currently there is no literature describing MultiHance use for MR arthrography. This is not an approved indication for any gadolinium contrast agent, however numerous protocols for this procedure have been published.

QUESTION: Is there any information available about the use of MultiHance in patients with renal impairment?

ANSWER: The MultiHance package insert CLINICAL PHARMACOLOGY section contains a sub-section entitled "Pharmacokinetics in Special Populations. Renal Impairment" stating that: "the overall extent of elimination of gadobenate was not influenced by impaired renal function. Also, no differences were noted in patients with renal impairment in the rate and type of adverse events reported compared with healthy volunteers, and no deterioration in renal function was observed in this population following the administration of MULTIHANCE. Therefore, dosage adjustment is not recommended". These recommendations are based on studies with MultiHance conducted in patients with varying degrees of renal impairment and in patients on hemodialysis.

QUESTION: For what indications has MultiHance been studied that are not contained in the package insert?

ANSWER: Liver Imaging, Magnetic Resonance Angiography (MRA), Body/MRA, Breast Imaging, MRI/Acute Myocardial Infarction, CNS Imaging in pediatric patients.

QUESTION: Why doesn't MultiHance have a pediatric imaging indication in the US?

ANSWER: No safety concerns have been raised about the use of MultiHance in children. In fact, MultiHance is approved for use in pediatric patients in Canada. To date, the safety and efficacy of MultiHance has been evaluated in 174 children between the age of 6 months and 16 years (Ref Colosimo, Ped Radiol 2005). In addition, the pharmacokinetics of MultiHance in children was studied in 25 subjects. This can be compared to the 173 patients that were enrolled in clinical trials with Omniscan. The safety profile of MultiHance in children was found to be equal to that of Magnevist and the pharmacokinetics were found to be similar to those in adult patients. The FDA has requested that a larger population of children be studied before granting the pediatric indication in the US. The manufacturer of MultiHance (Bracco Diagnostics Inc.) decided to launch the product for adults in the US while obtaining the additional requested data in pediatric patients.

QUESTION: The package insert states that once MultiHance is filled into a plastic syringe, it should be used immediately. Is there a reason that is specific to MultiHance that would require this precaution?

ANSWER: There are no data that suggests that MultiHance acts any differently than the other gadolinium-based contrast agents when exposed to plastic syringes. In fact, the OptiMARK package insert contains the same statement. The FDA now requires that this precaution be placed in the IV administered contrast agent labeling. The reason for the statement is that it is possible for extractable contaminants to leach from the plastic used to make the syringe. Unless there is stability data for all commercially available plastic syringes that proves otherwise, the precaution is required. The Magnevist package insert contains the statement "After Magnevist injection is drawn into the syringe the solution should be used immediately." The ProHance and Omniscan package inserts contain this statement as well. This statement is found in the PRECAUTIONS –General section of these package inserts.

QUESTION: Can MultiHance be double dosed as is sometimes done with ProHance or Omniscan?

ANSWER: Currently MultiHance is approved in the U.S. at a dose of 0.1 mmo/kg body weight. Due to the higher relaxivity of MultiHance it may not be necessary to give higher doses in certain applications. Several reports in the literature describe the use of dosages greater than that indicated in the DOSAGE AND ADMINISTRATION section of the MultiHance package insert. In a comprehensive safety assessment published in 2000, Kirchin and colleagues found no increase in the rate of adverse events in patients given higher doses of MultiHance.

QUESTION: What is the potential for MultiHance interaction with drugs which undergo a similar hepatobiliary elimination?

ANSWER: Following IV injection, Gd-BOPTA, the active ingredient of MultiHance, is internalized by hepatocytes through a passive mechanism (simple diffusion though the hepatocyte cell membrane) and a small percentage is actively excreted via the ATP-dependent export pump for anionic conjugates MRP2 (multidrug resistance-associated protein 2, also known as multi-specific organic anion transport system, cMOAT), located in the apical membranes of hepatocytes. MRP2 functions as the major exporter of organic anions from the liver into the bile, such as conjugated bilirubin. Gd-BOPTA, even in patients with reduced liver function, had no impact on the elimination of conjugated bilirubin, although conjugated bilirubin can be only eliminated by the MRP2.

The following drugs with substantial hepatic excretion via the MRP2 and a narrow therapeutic window have been used in combination with

MultiHance in clinical trials: daunorubicin, doxorubicin, epirubicin, glyburide (glibenclamide), tamoxifen, taxol, and taxotere. The most frequent concomitant use was of glyburide (43 patients). No adverse events suggestive of hypoglycemia, cholestatic jaundice, agranulocytosis, or aplastic and/or hemolytic anemia (indicative of overdosing of glyburide) were observed. The magnitude of the changes in conjugated bilirubin in these patients was negligible and similar to that observed in patients who did not take drugs competing for the MRP2. No adverse events suggestive of increased blood levels of the anthracyclines or the taxanes (cardiac toxicity, bone marrow depression), nor of increased blood levels of tamoxifen (flushes, nausea, vomiting, or thromboembolic complications) were noted. No other serious clinical adverse events or significant ECG and laboratory abnormalities were reported for these patients. Out of approximately 1.3 million patients exposed to MultiHance to date, no data suggest that Gd-BOPTA interferes with the uptake or metabolism of any drug or biological agent.

This may be explained by the fact that: a) only single administrations of MultiHance are used; b) a small percentage of the injected dose of Gd-BOPTA (0.6-4%) is excreted into the bile; c) most drugs competing for the the MRP2 can also be eliminated by other liver transporters (e.g., MDR1, MRP1, and BCRP); d) MRP2 is not only expressed on the hepatocytes, but also on enterocytes of the proximal small intestine, and proximal renal tubular cells; e) anthracyclines and taxanes lead to overexpression of MDR1, MRP1 and MRP2 in hepatic and non-hepatic tissues, like cancer tissues, small intestine, kidney, and others. In view of the available data, MultiHance is not expected to interfere with the elimination of drugs with a narrow therapeutic window which are excreted via the MRP2 pathway, nor to affect the course of treatment with these drugs.

QUESTION: Can anaphylactic reactions occur in patients who are hypersensitive to benzyl alcohol?

ANSWER: Hypersensitivity to benzyl alcohol is mainly described in the literature in the form of contact dermatitis following external administration (delayed-type dermatitis). No one has ever shown a correlation between a contact allergy (delayed type, cell-mediated) to benzyl alcohol and systemic reactions (immediate type, not cell-mediated) following parenteral administration. Important: benzyl alcohol is present in many drug formulations, has been administered in millions and millions of people, but the literature reports only 3 reports of possible hypersensitivity following parenteral administration, and none of them was an anaphylactic or anaphylactoid reaction.

Hypersensitivity to gadolinium chelates is more frequent and much more clinically important than possible hypersensitivity to benzyl alcohol. Serious and life threatening hypersensitivity reactions to gadolinium chelates are well documented and may occur with any gadolinium agent. Such documentation for benzyl alcohol is difficult if not impossible to find. Vials of MultiHance may contain only minute traces of benzyl alcohol.

QUESTION: Does MultiHance affect colorimetric assays for serum calcium?

ANSWER: No. It is well known that some gadolinium chelates, notably gadodiamide (Omniscan) and gadoversetamide (OptiMARK), may interfere with the colorimetric determination of serum calcium or other metal or metabolites. The mechanism of this interference appears to be related to the propensity of the agent to de-chelate once injected. According to Bracco Diagnostics Inc., the manufacturer of MultiHance, this agent has been thoroughly evaluated for potential interference in colorimetric assay tests in two separate batteries of test and no interference was demonstrated. The assays tested included: Albumin (BCG method), Alkaline Phosphatase (AP), Bilirubin (total) (DPD method), Calcium (O-CPC method), Chloride, Cholesterol (CHOD-PAP method), Creatine kinase (CK) (NAC-activated) Creatinine, Glucose, Glutamate oxalacetate transaminase (GOT or ASAT), Glutamate phosphate transinase (GPT or ALAT), Iron (ferrozin-method), Lactate dehydrogenase (LDH) (optimized UV test), Phosphate (direct phosphomolybdate method), Sodium/potassium, Total proteins (Biuret method), Triglycerides (GPO-PAP method), and Urea.

REFERENCES

Shellock FG, Parker JR, Pirovano G, Shen N, Venetianer C, Kirchin MA, Spinazzi A. Safety characteristics of gadobenate dimeglumine: Clinical experience from intra- and interindividual comparison studies with gadopentate dimeglumine. Journal of Magnetic Resonance Imaging 2006;24:1378-1285.

Shellock FG, Parker J, Spinazzi A. Safety of gadobenate dimeglumine: summary of findings from clinical studies and post-marketing surveillance. Investigative Radiology 2006;41:500-509.

MRI Contrast Agents and Nephrogenic Systemic Fibrosis (NSF)*

Nephrogenic systemic fibrosis (NSF), also known as nephrogenic fibrosing dermopathy, is a rare, relatively recent diagnosis, whose natural history is not well understood.

The evidence to date is:

- NSF is a systemic fibrosing disorder with its most prominent and visible effects in the skin, but other signs and symptoms may be present (e.g., muscle hardening and/or weakness, as well as burning, itching, or severe sharp pains in areas of involvement)(1-4);
- So far, it has occurred only in patients with severe or end-stage renal failure, acute or chronic (stages 4 or 5, according to the classification of the National Kidney Foundation)(1-4);
- NSF appears to affect males and females in approximately equal numbers (1);
- NSF has been confirmed in children and the elderly, but tends to affect the middle-aged most commonly (1);
- NSF has been identified in patients from a variety of ethnic backgrounds and from North America, Europe, and Asia (1);
- There is no definitive cure. There are some anecdotal reports describing at least partial responses to various therapies such as plasmapheresis, extracorporeal photopheresis, sodium thiosulphate, and thalidomide (1, 2). The disease is progressive. NSF can be fulminant in approximately 5% of cases and can be fatal (1).
- NSF may occur after exposure to gadolinium-based contrast agents in patients with, acute or chronic severe renal insufficiency (glomerular filtration rate <30 mL/min/1.73 m^2), or acute renal insufficiency of any severity due to the hepato-renal syndrome or in the perioperative liver transplantation period (3-16). To date, there is no evidence that other patient groups are at risk.

- Recent reports have strongly correlated the development of NSF with exposure to gadolinium-containing MRI contrast agents;
- To date, the majority of NSF cases have been reported in association with the administration of Omniscan (gadodiamide, GE Healthcare), and the second highest number of cases of NSF has been reported in association with the administration of Magnevist (gadopentetate dimeglumine, Bayer Healthcare).
- Several cases followed the administration of high doses of the product or repeated contrast-enhanced MR exams (high single or cumulative doses);
- In the vast majority of cases (approx. 90%), NSF develops in the first 6 months after the last exposure to a gadolinium chelate (80% in the first three months). Some reports suggest the development of NSF at 9 months, 12 months or even 2 years after the exposure to a gadolinium chelates. Gadolinium may be found in the skin of patients with impaired renal function up to 11 months after the administration of Omniscan (gadodiamide).

Open questions regarding MRI contrast agents and NSF include the following:

- Does the entire gadolinium chelate molecule, the excess chelate or free gadolinium trigger NSF?
- How can gadolinium chelates, excess chelate or free gadolinium trigger NSF?
- If free gadolinium in skin may trigger the disease, is the risk of NSF lower with more stable chelates?
- Why has NSF developed in only 3-5% of patients with GFR < 30 mL/min after the administration of Omniscan? The incidence of NSF following exposure to other gadolinium chelates is unknown.
- What are the concomitant risk factors?
- Preventative measures: Any?
- Post-contrast dialysis: Does it help? If so, when?

[*Special thanks to Alberto Spinazzi, M.D., Senior Vice President, Group Regulatory and Medical Affairs, Bracco Diagnostics, Inc. For additional information, please refer to the following comprehensive review Shellock FG, Spinazzi A. MRI Safety Update: 2008, Part 1, MRI contrast agents and nephrogenic systemic fibrosis. American Journal of Roentgenology 2008;191:1-11. This article is available as a free downloadable PDF file at http://www.ajronline.org/]

REFERENCES

(1) Yerram P, Saab G, Karuparthi PR, Hayden MR, Khanna R. Nephrogenic Systemic Fibrosis: A Mysterious Disease in Patients with Renal Failure— Role of Gadolinium-Based Contrast Media in Causation and the Beneficial Effect of Intravenous Sodium Thiosulfate. Clin J Am Soc Nephrol 2007; 2: 258-263.

(2) Richmond H, Zwerner J, Kim Y, Fiorentino D. Nephrogenic Systemic Fibrosis. Relationship to Gadolinium and Response to Photopheresis. Arch Dermatol. 2007;143(8):1025-1030

(3) Grobner T (2006) Gadolinium—a specific trigger for the development of nephrogenic fibrosing dermopathy and nephrogenic systemic fibrosis? Nephrol Dial Transplant 2006; 21: 1104–1108.

(4) Marckmann P, Skov L, Rossen K et al. Nephrogenic systemic fibrosis: suspected etiological role of gadodiamide used for contrast-enhanced magnetic resonance imaging. J Am Soc Nephrol 2006 17: 2359–2362.

(5) Khurana A, Runge VM, Narayanan M, Greene JF., Nickel AE. Nephrogenic Systemic Fibrosis A Review of 6 Cases Temporally Related to Gadodiamide Injection (Omniscan). Invest Radiol 2007; 42: 139–145.

(6) Broome DR, Girguis MS, Baron PW, Cottrell AC, Kjellin I, Kirk GA. Gadodiamide-associated nephrogenic systemic fibrosis: why radiologists should be concerned. Am J Roentgenol 2007 Feb; 188(2): 586-92.

(7) Sadowski EA, Bennett LK, Chan MR, Wentland AL, Garrett AL, Garrett RW, Djamali A. Nephrogenic Systemic Fibrosis: Risk factors and incidence estimation. Radiology 2007 April; 243(1): 148-157.

(8) Lin S-P, Brown JJ, MR Contrast Agents: Physical and Pharmacologic Basics. J Magn Reson Imag 2007; 25: 884-899.

(9) Pedersen M. Safety update on the possible causal relationship between gadolinium-containing MRI agents and nephrogenic systemic fibrosis. J Magn Reson Imag 2007; 25: 881-883.

(10) Lim YL, Lee HY, Low SCS, Chan LP, Goh NSG, Pang SM. Possible role of gadolinium in nephrogenic systemic fibrosis: report of two cases and review of the literature. Clin Exp Dermatol 2007; doi: 10.1111/j.1365-2230.2007.02412.x (E-pub ahead of print).

(11) Bongartz G. Imaging in the time of NFD/NSF: do we have to change our routines concerning renal insufficiency? Magn Reson Mater Phy 2007; 20: 57-62.

(12) Pryor JG, Poggioli G, Galaria N, Gust A, Robison J, Samie F, Hanjani NM, Scott GA. Nephrogenic systemic fibrosis: A clinicopathologic study of six cases. J Am Acad Dermatol 2007; 57: 105-111.

(13) Kanal E, Barkovich AJ, Bell C, et al. ACR guidance document for safe MR practices: 2007. AJR Am J Roentgenol. 2007;188:1447-1474.

(14) Othersen JB, Maize JC, Woolson RF, Budisavljevic MN. Nephrogenic systemic fibrosis after exposure to gadolinium in patients with renal failure. Nephrol Dial Transplant. 2007;22:3179-85.

(15) Todd DJ, et al. Cutaneous changes of nephrogenic systemic fibrosis. Arthritis Rheumatism 2007;56: 3433-3441

(16) Thakral C, et al. Long-term retention of gadolinium in tissues from nephrogenic systemic fibrosis patient after multiple gadolinium-enhanced MRI scans: case report and implications. Contrast Media Mol Imaging Contrast Media Mol Imaging. 2007;2:199-205.

ADDITIONAL PERTINENT REFERENCES

Abujudeh HH, Kaewlai R, et al. Nephrogenic systemic fibrosis after gadolinium exposure: Case series of 36 patients. Radiology 2009;253:81-99.

Altun E, Martin DR, et al. Nephrogenic systemic fibrosis: change in incidence following a switch in gadolinium agents and adoption of a gadolinium Policy--report from two U.S. universities. Radiology. 2009 Sep 29. [Epub ahead of print]

Altun E, Semelka RC, Cakit C. Nephrogenic systemic fibrosis and management of high-risk patients. Acad Radiol. 2009;16:897-905.

Cowper SE. Nephrogenic systemic fibrosis: an overview. J Am Coll Radiol. 2008;5:23-8.

Dawson P. Nephrogenic systemic fibrosis: possible mechanisms and imaging management strategies. JMRI 2008;28:792-804.

Heinz-Peer G, Neruda A, et al. Prevalence of NSF following intravenous gadolinium-contrast media administration in dialysis patients with endstage renal disease. Eur J Radiol. 2009 Jul 18. [Epub ahead of print]

Hope TA, High WA, et al. Nephrogenic systemic fibrosis in rats treated with erythropoietin and intravenous iron. Radiology. 2009;253:390-8.

Idee JM, Port M, et al. Involvement of gadolinium chelates in the mechanism of nephrogenic systemic fibrosis: an update. Radiol Clin North Am. 2009;47:855-69.

Juluru K, Vogel-Claussen J, et al. MR imaging in patients at risk for developing nephrogenic systemic fibrosis: protocols, practices, and imaging techniques to maximize patient safety. Radiographics. 2009;29:9-22.

Karcaaltincaba M, Oguz B, Haliloglu M. Current status of contrast-induced nephropathy and nephrogenic systemic fibrosis in children. Pediatr Radiol. 2009;39 Suppl 3:382-4.

Kuo PH. Gadolinium-containing MRI contrast agents: important variations on a theme for NSF. J Am Coll Radiol. 2008;5:29-35.

Marckmann P, Skov L. Nephrogenic systemic fibrosis: clinical picture and treatment. Radiol Clin North Am. 2009;47:833-40.

Morris MF, Zhang Y, et al. Features of nephrogenic systemic fibrosis on radiology examinations. AJR 2009;193:61-9.

Prince MR, Zhang H, et al. Incidence of nephrogenic systemic fibrosis at two large medical centers. Radiology. 2008;248:807-16.

Shellock FG, Spinazzi A. MRI Safety Update: 2008, Part 1, MRI contrast agents and nephrogenic systemic fibrosis. American Journal of Roentgenology. 2008;191:1-11.

Sieber MA, et al. Gadolinium-based contrast agents and their potential role in the pathogenesis of nephrogenic systemic fibrosis: the role of excess ligand. J Magn Reson Imaging. 2008;27:955-62.

So K, Macquillan GC, et al. Malignant fibrous histiocytoma complicating nephrogenic systemic fibrosis post liver transplantation. Intern Med J. 2009;39:613-7.

Spinazzi A, Kirchin MA, Pirovano G. Nephrogenic systemic fibrosis: the need for accurate case reporting. J Magn Reson Imaging. 2009;29:1240.

Thakral C, Abraham JL. Nephrogenic systemic fibrosis: histology and gadolinium detection. Radiol Clin North Am. 2009;47:841-53.

Thomsen HS. How to avoid nephrogenic systemic fibrosis: current guidelines in Europe and the United States. Radiol Clin North Am. 2009;47:871-5.

Thomsen HS. Nephrogenic systemic fibrosis: history and epidemiology. Radiol Clin North Am. 2009;47:827-31.

Weinreb JC, Kuo PH. Nephrogenic systemic fibrosis. Magn Reson Imaging Clin N Am. 2009;17:159-67.

Wertman R, at al. Risk of nephrogenic systemic fibrosis: evaluation of gadolinium chelate contrast agents at four American universities. Radiology. 2008;248:799-806.

Wollanka H, Weidenmaier W, Giersig C. NSF after Gadovist exposure: a case report and hypothesis of NSF development. Nephrol Dial Transplant. 2009 Sep 19, [Epub ahead of print]

MRI Contrast Agents and NSF: Websites and Links to Obtain Current Information*

American College of Radiology
http://www.acr.org/
http://www.acr.org/SecondaryMainMenuCategories/quality_safety/
MRSafety.aspx

The International Center for Nephrogenic Fibrosing Dermopathy Research (ICNFDR)
http://www.icnfdr.org/

International Society for Magnetic Resonance in Medicine
http://ismrm.org/
http://ismrm.org/special/FDA.htm

Medicines and Healthcare products Regulatory Agency
http://www.mhra.gov.uk/home/idcplg?IdcService=SS_GET_PAGE&
useSecondary=true&ssDocName=CON2031543&ssTargetNodeId=221

United States Food and Drug Administration
http://www.fda.gov/cder/drug/infopage/gcca/qa_20061222.htm
http://www.fda.gov/cder/drug/advisory/gadolinium_agents.htm
http://www.fda.gov/bbs/topics/NEWS/2007/NEW01638.html
http://www.fda.gov/cder/drug/infopage/gcca/qa_200705.htm
http://www.fda.gov/cder/drug/infopage/gcca/default.htm
http://www.fda.gov/cder/drug/advisory/gadolinium_agents_20061222.htm

[*For additional information, please refer to the following comprehensive review Shellock FG, Spinazzi A. MRI Safety Update: 2008, Part 1, MRI contrast agents and nephrogenic systemic fibrosis. American Journal of Roentgenology 2008;191:1-11. This article is available as a free downloadable PDF file at http://www.ajronline.org/]

Pregnant Patients and MR Procedures*

Magnetic resonance (MR) imaging has been used to evaluate obstetrical, placental, and fetal abnormalities in pregnant patients for more than 25 years. MR imaging is recognized as a beneficial diagnostic tool and is utilized to assess a wide range of diseases and conditions that affect the pregnant patient as well as the fetus.

Initially, there were substantial technical problems with the use of MR imaging primarily due to image degradation from fetal motion. However, several technological improvements, including the development of high-performance gradient systems and rapid pulse sequences, have provided major advances especially useful for imaging pregnant patients. Thus, MR imaging examinations for obstetrical and fetal applications may now be accomplished routinely in the clinical setting.

PREGNANCY AND MR SAFETY

The use of diagnostic imaging is often required in pregnant patients. Thus, it is not surprising, that the question of whether or not a patient should undergo an MR examination during pregnancy will often arise. Unfortunately, there have been few studies directed toward determining the relative safety of using MR procedures in pregnant patients. Safety issues include possible bioeffects of the static magnetic field of the MR system, risks associated with exposure to the gradient magnetic fields, the potential adverse effects of radiofrequency (RF) energy, and possible adverse effects related to the combination of these three electromagnetic fields.

MR environment-related risks are difficult to assess for pregnant patients due to the number of possible permutations of the various factors that are present in this setting (e.g., differences in field strengths, pulse sequences, exposure times, etc.). This becomes even more complicated since new hardware and software is developed for MR systems on an on-going basis.

There have been a number of laboratory and clinical investigations conducted to determine the effects of using MR imaging during pregnancy. Most of the laboratory studies showed no evidence of injury or harm to the fetus, while a few studies reported adverse outcomes for laboratory animals. However, whether or not these findings can be extrapolated to human subjects is debatable.

By comparison, there have been relatively few studies performed in pregnant human subjects exposed to MR imaging or the MR environment. Each investigation reported no adverse outcomes for the subjects. For example, Baker et al. reported no demonstrable increase in disease, disability, or hearing loss in 20 children examined *in utero* using echo-planar MRI for suspected fetal compromise. Myers et al. reported no significant reduction in fetal growth vs. matched controls in 74 volunteer subjects exposed *in utero* to echo-planar MRI performed at 0.5-Tesla. A survey of reproductive health among 280 pregnant MR healthcare professionals performed by Kanal et al. showed no substantial increase in common adverse reproductive outcomes.

With regard to the publications to date, there are discrepancies with respect to the experimental findings of the effects of electromagnetic fields used for MR procedures and the pertinent safety aspects of pregnancy. These discrepancies may be explained by a variety of factors, including the differences in the scientific methodology used, the type of organism examined, and the variance in exposure duration, as well as the conditions of the exposure to the electromagnetic fields. Additional investigations are warranted before the risks associated with exposure to MR procedures can be absolutely known and properly characterized.

GUIDELINES FOR THE USE OF MR PROCEDURES IN PREGNANT PATIENTS

As stated in the Policies, Guidelines, and Recommendations for MR Imaging Safety and Patient Management issued by the Safety Committee of the Society for Magnetic Resonance Imaging in 1991, "MR imaging may be used in pregnant women if other nonionizing forms of diagnostic imaging are inadequate or if the examination provides important information that would otherwise require exposure to ionizing radiation (e.g., fluoroscopy, CT, etc.). Pregnant patients should be informed that, to date, there has been no indication that the use of clinical MR imaging during pregnancy has produced deleterious effects." This policy has been adopted by the American College of Radiology and is considered to be the "standard of care" with respect to the use of MR procedures in pregnant patients. Importantly, this information applies to MR systems operating up to and including 3-Tesla.

Thus, MR procedures may be used in pregnant patients to address important clinical problems or to manage potential complications for the patient or fetus. The overall decision to utilize an MR procedure in a pregnant patient involves answering a series of important questions including, the following:

- Is sonography satisfactory for diagnosis?
- Is the MR procedure appropriate to address the clinical question?
- Is obstetrical intervention prior to the MR procedure a possibility? That is, is termination of pregnancy a consideration? Is early delivery a consideration?

With regard to the use of MR procedures in pregnant patients, this diagnostic technique should not be withheld for the following cases:

- Patients with active brain or spine signs and symptoms requiring imaging.
- Patients with cancer requiring imaging.
- Patients with chest, abdomen, and pelvic signs and symptoms of active disease when sonography is non-diagnostic.
- In specific cases of suspected fetal anomaly or complex fetal disorder.

[*Portions of the content on this topic were excerpted with permission from Colletti P M. Magnetic Resonance Procedures and Pregnancy, In: Magnetic Resonance Procedures: Health Effects and Safety, FG Shellock, Editor, CRC Press, Boca Raton, FL, 2001.]

REFERENCES

Baker, P.N., Johnson IR, Harvey PR, et al, A three-year follow-up of children imaged *in utero* with echo-planar magnetic resonance. Am J Obstet Gynecol 170, 32-33, 1994.

Benson, R.C., Colletti, P.M., Platt, L.D., et al, MR imaging of fetal anomalies. Am. J. Roentgenol., 156, 1205, 1991.

Brown, C.E.L., and Weinreb, J.C., Magnetic resonance imaging appearance of growth retardation in a twin pregnancy. Obstet. Gynecol. 71, 987, 1988.

Carnes, K.I., and Magin, R.L., Effects of in utero exposure to 4.7 T MR imaging conditions on fetal growth and testicular development in the mouse. Magn. Reson. Imaging, 14, 263, 1996.

Carswell, H., Fast MRI of fetus yields considerable anatomic detail. Diag. Imaging, Nov, 11-12, 1988.

Chen MM, Coakley FV, et al. Guidelines for computed tomography and magnetic resonance imaging use during pregnancy and lactation. Obstet Gynecol. 2008;112 (2 Pt 1):333-40.

Colletti, P.M., Computer-assisted imaging of the fetus with magnetic resonance imaging. Comput. Med. Imaging Graph., 20, 491, 1996.

Colletti, P.M., and Platt, L.D., When to use MRI in obstetrics. Diag. Imaging, 11, 84, 1989.

Colletti, P.M., and Sylvestre, P.B., Magnetic resonance imaging in pregnancy. MRI Clin. N. Am., 2, 291, 1994.

De Wilde JP, Rivers AW, Price DL. A review of the current use of magnetic resonance imaging in pregnancy and safety implications for the fetus. Prog Biophys Mol Biol. 2005;87:335-353.

Dinh, D.H., et al. The use of magnetic resonance imaging for the diagnosis of fetal intracranial anomalies. Child Nerv. Syst., 6, 212, 1990.

Dunn, R.S., and Weiner, S.N., Antenatal diagnosis of sacrococcygeal teratoma facilitated by combined use of Doppler sonography and MR imaging. Am. J. Roentgenol., 156,1115, 1991.

Fitamorris-Glass, R., Mattrey, R.F., Cantrell, C.J., Magnetic resonance imaging as an adjunct to ultrasound in oligohydramnio. J Ultrasound Med. 8,159, 1989.

Fraser, R., Magnetic resonance imaging of the fetus. Initial experience [letter]. Gynecol. Obstet. Invest., 29, 255, 1990.

Garcia-Bournissen F, Shrim A, Koren G. Safety of gadolinium during pregnancy. Can Fam Physician. 2006 Mar;52:309-10.

Gardens AS, Weindling AM, Griffiths RD, et al, Fast-scan magnetic resonance imaging of fetal anomalies. Br J Obstet Gynecol 98,1217-1222, 1991

Hand JW, Li Y, et al. Prediction of specific absorption rate in mother and fetus associated with MRI examinations during pregnancy. Magn Reson Med. 2006;55:883-893.

Hill MC, Lande IM, Larsen JW Jr, Prenatal diagnosis of fetal anomalies using ultrasound and MRI. Radiol Clin North Am 26,287-307, 1988

Horvath L, Seeds JW, Temporary arrest of fetal movement with pancuronium bromide to enable antenatal magnetic resonance imaging of holosencephaly. Am. J. Roentgenol., 6,418-420, 1989

Heinrichs, W.L., et al., Midgestational exposure of pregnant BALB/c mice to magnetic resonance imaging conditions. Magn Reson Imaging, 6,305, 1988.

Huisman TA. Fetal magnetic resonance imaging. Semin Roentgenol. 2008;43:314-36.

International Commission on Non-Ionizing Radiation Protection Statement, Medical magnetic resonance procedures: protection of patients. Health Physics 2004;87:197-216.

Jackson HA, Panigrahy A. Fetal magnetic resonance imaging: the basics. Pediatr Ann. 2008;37:388-93.

Junkermann H. Indications and contraindications for contrast-enhanced MRI and CT during pregnancy. Radiologe. 2007;47:774-7.

Kanal E, Barkovich AJ, Bell C, et al. ACR guidance document for safe MR practices: 2007. AJR Am J Roentgenol. 2007;188:1447-1474.

Kanal, E., Gillen, J., Evans, J.A., et al, Survey of reproductive health among female MR workers. Radiology, 187,395, 1993.

Kanal, E, Shellock, F.G., and Sonnenblick, D., MRI clinical site safety: Phase I results and preliminary data. Magn. Reson. Imaging 7[Suppl] 1, 106, 1988.

Kay, H.H., Herfkens, R.J., and Kay, B.K., Effect of magnetic resonance imaging on Xenopus laevis embryogenesis. Magn. Reson. Imaging, 6, 501-6, 1988.

Lenke RR, et al. Use of pancuronium bromide to inhibit fetal movement during magnetic resonance imaging. J. Reprod. Med. 34,315-317, 1989

Leithner K, et al. Psychological reactions in women undergoing fetal magnetic resonance imaging. Obstet Gynecol. 2008;111(2 Pt 1):396-402.

Levine D. Obstetric MRI. J Magn Reson Imaging 2006;24:1-15

Malko, J.A., Constatinidis, I, Dillehay, D., et al., Search for influence of 1.5 T magnetic field on growth of yeast cells. Bioelectromagnetics, 15, 495, 1987.

Mansfield P, Stehling MK, Ordidge RJ, et al. Study of internal structure of the human fetus in utero at 0.5-T. Br J Radiol 13,314-318, 1990

McCarthy, S.M., Stark, D.D., Filly, R.A., et al. Uterine neoplasms: MR imaging. Radiology, 170, 125, 1989.

McCarthy SM, Filly RA, Stark DD, et al, Magnetic resonance imaging of fetal anomalies

McRobbie, D., and Foster, M.A., Pulsed magnetic field exposure during pregnancy and implications for NMR foetal imaging. A study with mice. Magn. Reson. Imaging, 3, 231, 1985.

Myers, C., Duncan, K.R., Gowland, P.A., et al., Failure to detect intrauterine growth restriction following in utero exposure to MRI. Br J Radiol, 71, 549, 1998.

Murakami, J., et al. Fetal developmet of mice following intrauterine exposure to a static magnetic field of 6.3-T. Magn. Reson. Imaging, 10, 433, 1992.

Nara, V.R., Howell, R.W., Goddu, S.M., et al., Effects of a 1.5T static magnetic field on spermatogenesis and embryogenesis in mice. Invest. Radiology 31, 586, 1996.

Oto A. MR imaging evaluation of acute abdominal pain during pregnancy. Magn Reson Imaging Clin N Am. 2006;14:489-501.

Ruckhäberle E, et al. In vivo intrauterine sound pressure and temperature measurements during magnetic resonance imaging (1.5 T) in pregnant ewes. Fetal Diagn Ther. 2008;24:203-10.

Shellock FG, Crues JV. MR procedures: biologic effects, safety, and patient care. Radiology, 2004;232:635-652.

Shellock, F.G., and Kanal, E., Policies, guidelines, and recommendations for MR imaging safety and patient management. J. Magn. Reson. Imaging, 1, 97, 1991.

Shellock, F.G., and Kanal, E. Magnetic resonance procedures and pregnancy. In, Magnetic Resonance Bioeffects, Safety, and Patient Management. Second Edition, Lippincott-Ravin, Philadelphia, New York, 1996, Chapter 4, pp. 49.

Smith FW, Kent C, Abramovich DR, et al. Nuclear magnetic resonance imaging – a new look at the fetus. Br J Gynaecol 92,1024-1033, 1985

Smith FW, Sutherland HW. Magnetic resonance imaging: The use of the inversion recovery sequence to display fetal morphology. Br J Radiol 61,338-341, 1988.

Stark, D.D., McCarthy, S.M., Filly, R.A., et al. Pelvimetry by magnetic resonance imaging. Am. J. Roentgenol., 144, 947, 1985.

Tesky, G.C., et al. Survivability and long-term stress reactivity levels following repeated exposure to nuclear magnetic resonance imaging procedures in rats. Physiol. Chem. Phys. Med. NMR, 19, 43, 1987.

Tyndall, D.A., MRI effects on the teratogenicity of x-irradiation in the C57BL/6J mouse. Magn. Reson. Imaging, 8, 423, 1990.

Tyndall, R.J., and Sulik, K.K., Effects of magnetic resonance imaging on eye development in the C57BL/6J mouse. Teratology, 43, 263, 1991.

Tyndall, D.A., MRI effects on craniofacial size and crown-rump length in C57BL/6J mice in 1.5 T fields. Oral Surg. Oral Med. Oral Pathol. 76, 655, 1993.

Yip, Y.P., et al. Effects of MR exposure at 1.5 T on early embryonic development of the chick. J. Magn. Reson. Imaging, 4, 742, 1994.

Yip, Y.P., et al. Effects of MR exposure on axonal outgrowth in the sympathetic nervous system of the chick. J. Magn. Reson. Imaging, 4, 457, 1995.

Yip, Y.P., et al. Effects of MR exposure on cell proliferation and migration of chick motor neurons. J. Magn. Reson. Imaging, 4,799, 1994.

Vadeyar, S.H., et al., Effect of fetal magnetic resonance imaging on fetal heart rate patterns. Am. J. Obstet. Gynecol., 182, 666, 2000.

Webb JA, et al. Members of Contrast Media Safety Committee of European Society of Urogenital Radiology (ESUR). The use of iodinated and gadolinium contrast media during pregnancy and lactation. Eur Radiol. 2005;15:1234-40.

Weinreb, JC et al., Pelvic masses in pregnant patients, MR and US imaging. Radiology, 159, 717, 1986.

Weinreb JC, Lowe T, Santos-Ramos R, et al. Magnetic resonance imaging in obstetric diagnosis. Radiology 154,157-161, 1985.

Wenstrom KD, Williamson RA, Weiner CP, et al. Magnetic resonance imaging of fetuses with intracranial defects. Obstet Gynecol., 77,529-532, 1991.

Wilcox, A., Weinberg, C., O'Connor J, et al. Incidence of early loss of pregnancy. New Engl. J. Med., 319,189-194, 1988.

Williamson, RA, Weiner CP, Yuh WTC, et al. Magnetic resonance imaging of anomalous fetuses. Obstet Gynecol 71,952, 1988.

Pregnant Technologists and Other Healthcare Workers in the MR Environment

Due to the concern with regard to pregnant technologists and other healthcare workers in the MR environment, a survey of reproductive health among female MR system operators was conducted by Kanal et al. Questionnaires were sent to female MR technologists and nurses at the majority of the MRI facilities in the United States. The questionnaire addressed menstrual and reproductive experiences as well as work activities. This study attempted to account for known potential confounding variables (e.g., age, smoking, alcohol use) for this type of data.

Of the 1,915 completed questionnaires analyzed, there were 1,421 pregnancies: 280 occurred while working as an MR employee (technologist or nurse), 894 while employed at another job, 54 as a student, and 193 as a homemaker. Five categories were analyzed that included spontaneous abortion rate, pre-term delivery (less than 39 weeks), low birth weight (less than 5.5 pounds), infertility (taking more than eleven months to conceive), and gender of the offspring.

The data indicated that there were no statistically significant alterations in the five areas studied for MR healthcare professionals relative to the same group studied when they were employed elsewhere, prior to becoming MR healthcare employees. Additionally, adjustment for maternal age, smoking, and alcohol use failed to markedly change any of the associations. Menstrual regularity, menstrual cycle, and related topics were also examined in this study. These included inquiries regarding the number of days of menstrual bleeding, the heaviness of the bleeding, and the time between menstrual cycles.

Admittedly, this is a difficult area to objectively examine because it depends on both subjective memory and the memory of the respondent for a given topic. Subjective memory is often inadequate. Nevertheless, the data suggested that there were no clear correlations between MR workers and specific modifications of the menstrual cycle.

The data from this extensive epidemiological investigation were reassuring insofar as that there did not appear to be deleterious effects from exposure to the static magnetic field of the MR system. Therefore, a policy is recommended that permits pregnant technologists and healthcare workers to perform MR procedures, as well as to enter the MR system room, and attend to the patient during pregnancy, regardless of the trimester. Importantly, technologists and healthcare workers should not remain within the MR system room or magnet bore during the actual operation of the scanner.

This later recommendation is especially important for those healthcare workers involved in patient management or interventional MR-guided examinations and procedures, since it may be necessary for them to be directly exposed to the MR system's electromagnetic fields at levels similar to those used for patients. These recommendations are not based on indications of adverse effects, but rather, from a conservative point of view and the feeling that there are insufficient data pertaining to the effects of the other electromagnetic fields of the MR system to support or allow unnecessary exposures.

REFERENCES

Evans JA, Savitz DA, Kanal E, Gillen J. Infertility and pregnancy outcome among magnetic resonance imaging workers. J Occu Med 1993;12:1191-1195.

International Commission on Non-Ionizing Radiation Protection (ICNIRP) Statement, Medical magnetic resonance procedures: protection of patients. Health Physics 2004;87:197-216.

Kanal E, Gillen J, Evans J, Savitz D, Shellock FG. Survey of reproductive health among female MR workers. Radiology 1993;187:395-399.

Shellock FG. Magnetic Resonance Procedures: Health Effects and Safety. CRC Press, LLC, Boca Raton, FL, 2001.

Shellock FG, Kanal E. Policies, guidelines, and recommendations for MR imaging safety and patient management. J Magn Reson Imaging 1991;1: 97-101.

Prevention of Missile
Effect Accidents

The "missile effect" refers to the capability of the fringe field of an MR system to attract a ferromagnetic object, drawing it rapidly into the scanner by considerable force. The missile effect can pose a significant risk to the patient inside the MR system and/or anyone in the path of the projectile. Therefore, a strict policy must be established by the MRI facility to detect metallic objects prior to allowing individuals or patients to enter the MR environment. In addition, to guard against accidents from metallic projectiles, the immediate area around the MR system should be clearly demarcated, labeled with appropriate danger signs, and secured by trained staff aware of proper MR safety procedures.

For patients preparing to undergo MR examinations, all metallic or other potentially problematic personal belongings (i.e., hearing aids, analogue watches, beepers, cell phones, jewelry, etc.) and devices must be removed as well as clothing items that have metallic fasteners or other metallic components (e.g., threads). The most effective means of preventing a ferromagnetic object from inadvertently becoming a missile and to ensure that no inappropriate objects enter the MR environment is to require the patient to wear a gown for the MR examination.

Non-ambulatory patients must only be allowed to enter the area of the MR system using a nonferromagnetic wheelchair or nonferromagnetic gurney. Wheelchairs and gurneys should also be inspected for the presence of a ferromagnetic oxygen tank, IV pole, or other similar problematic component or accessory before allowing the patient into the MR setting. Fortunately, there are many commercially-available devices that are appropriate for use to transport and support patients in the MR environment.

Any individual accompanying the patient must be required to remove all metallic objects or other problematic items before entering the MR area and should undergo a careful and thorough screening procedure. All hospital and outside personnel that may need to enter the MR environment periodically or in response to an emergency (e.g., custodial staff, maintenance workers, housekeeping staff, bioengineers, nurses, security officers, fire fighters, etc.) should be educated about the potential hazards associated with the MR system. These individuals should, likewise, be instructed to remove inappropriate objects before entering the MR environment.

Many serious incidents have occurred when individuals who were unaware of the powers of the MR system entered the MR environment with items such as oxygen tanks, wheel chairs, scissors, hand guns, monitors, and other similar objects.

In 2001, the first fatal accident occurred that illustrated the importance of careful attention to preventing ferromagnetic objects from entering the MR environment. In this widely publicized incident, a young patient suffered a blow to the head from a ferromagnetic oxygen tank that became a projectile in the presence of a 1.5-Tesla MR system.

While MR safety guidelines and procedures are well known, accidents related to the missile effect continue to occur. Guidelines for preventing these hazards are presented in Table 1.

Table 1. Guidelines for preventing hazards related to missile effects.*

1) Appoint a safety officer or other appropriately trained person to be responsible for ensuring that proper procedures are in effect, enforced, and updated to ensure safety in the MR environment.
2) Establish and routinely review safety policies and procedures and assess the level of compliance by all staff members.
3) Provide all MR staff, along with other personnel who may need to enter the MR environment (e.g., transport personnel, security officers, housekeeping staff, maintenance workers, fire department personnel, etc.) with formal training on MR safety. This should be done on a regular basis, especially for all new orientees.
4) Emphasize to all personnel that the MR system's powerful static magnetic field is always "on" and treat the MR environment, accordingly.
5) Don't allow equipment and devices containing ferromagnetic components into the MR environment, unless they have been tested and labeled "MR-safe" or "MR-conditional".
6) Adhere to restrictions provided by suppliers regarding the use of MR-safe and/or MR-conditional equipment and devices in the MR environment.
7) Maintain a list of MR-safe and MR-conditional equipment, including restrictions for use. This list should be kept and updated in every MRI facility by the MR safety officer (refer to www.MRIsafety.com for comprehensive information).

8) Bring non-ambulatory patients into the MR environment using a nonmagnetic wheelchairs or gurneys. Ensure that no oxygen tanks, sandbags with metal shot, or other ferromagnetic objects are concealed under blankets or sheets or stowed away on the transport equipment.

9) Ensure that IV poles accompanying patients into the MR environment are nonferromagnetic.

10) Carefully screen all individuals entering the MR environment to identify magnetic objects in their bodies (e.g., implants, bullets, shrapnel, etc.), on their bodies (e.g., hair pins, brassieres, buttons, zippers, jewelry, clothing with metallic threads), or attached to their bodies (e.g., body piercing jewelry, body modification implants, halo vests, cervical fixation devices, external fixation systems, prosthetic appliances). Ferromagnetic objects on or attached to the bodies of patients, family members, or staff members should be removed, if feasible, before the individuals enter the MR environment. Additional attention must also be given to items that are made from conducting metals, as these may pose hazards under certain conditions.

11) Have patients wear hospital gowns without metallic fasteners for MR procedures. Clothing that contains metallic objects or threads that may pose a hazard in the MR environment.

[*Adapted and published permission from ECRI Report, 2001 and Shellock FG, 2001; updated 2007.]

REFERENCES

Chaljub G, et al. Projectile cylinder accidents resulting from the presence of ferromagnetic nitrous oxide or oxygen tanks in the MR suite. American Journal of Roentgenology 2001;177:27-30.

Colletti PM. Size "H" oxygen cylinder: accidental MR projectile at 1.5-Tesla. Journal of Magnetic Resonance Imaging 2004;19:141-143.

ECRI. Patient Death Illustrates the Importance of Adhering to Safety Precautions in Magnetic Resonance Environments. ECRI, Plymouth Meeting, PA, Aug. 6, 2001.

Kanal E, Barkovich AJ, Bell C, et al. ACR guidance document for safe MR practices: 2007. AJR Am J Roentgenol. 2007;188:1447-1474.

International Commission on Non-Ionizing Radiation Protection (ICNIRP) Statement, Medical magnetic resonance procedures: protection of patients. Health Physics 2004;87:197-216.

Joint Commission on Accreditation of Healthcare Organizations, USA. Preventing accidents and injuries in the MRI suite. Sentinel Event Alert. 2008 Feb 14; 1-3.

Shellock FG. Magnetic Resonance Procedures: Health Effects and Safety. CRC Press, LLC, Boca Raton, FL, 2001.

Signs to Help Control Access to the MR Environment

To guard against accidents and injuries to patients and other individuals as well as damage to magnetic resonance (MR) systems, the general and immediate areas associated with the scanner (also referred to as the MR environment) must have supervised and controlled access. Supervised and controlled access involves having MR safety-trained personnel present at all times during the operation of the facility to ensure that no unaccompanied or unauthorized individuals are allowed to enter the MR environment. MR safety-trained personnel should be responsible for performing comprehensive screening of patients and other individuals before allowing them to enter the MR system room. The area should be secured and/or controlled by appropriate means when MR safety-trained personnel are not present.

Importantly, it is necessary to educate and train individuals who need to enter the MR environment on a regular basis or responding to an emergency (e.g., custodial workers, transporters, security personnel, firefighters, nurses, anesthesiologists, etc.) regarding the potential hazards related to the powerful magnetic field of the MR system. Unfortunately, even with proper MR safety procedures in place, many individuals and patients have inadvertently "wandered" unattended into the MR environment, and these situations have resulted in problematic or disastrous consequences.

As one means of helping to control access to the MR environment, the area must be clearly demarcated and labeled with prominently displayed signs to make all individuals and patients aware of the risks associated with the MR system. Access to the MR environment must also be monitored and controlled on a continuous basis.

Signs with appropriate content and information were designed to promote a safe MR environment. According to the U.S. Food and Drug Administration document entitled, Guidance for the Submission Of Premarket Notifications for Magnetic Resonance Diagnostic Devices (issued November 14, 1998), Attachment B, states: "The controlled access area should be labeled "Danger - High Magnetic Field" at all entries." Also, this FDA document indicates, "Operators should be warned by appropriate signs about the presence of magnetic fields and their force and torque on magnetic materials, and that loose ferrous objects should be excluded."

"DANGER" Sign

In consideration of the above, the sign used for the MRI environment states:

DANGER!

Additionally, to inform everyone about the powerful static magnetic field associated with the MR system, especially individuals unacquainted with MR technology, the following information is prominently shown on this sign:

RESTRICTED ACCESS
STRONG MAGNETIC FIELD
THIS MAGNET IS ALWAYS ON!

With respect to the information for implants and devices, in addition to cardiac pacemakers, implantable cardioverter defibrillators (ICDs) are also potentially hazardous for patients and individuals in the MR environment. Therefore, this information is included on the sign used for the MR environment. Notably, the peer-reviewed literature has reported that many types of metallic implants are acceptable for patients undergoing MR procedures, while others are not. As such, this information is clarified on the current sign, with individuals and patients informed to consult MRI professionals if there are questions regarding this matter, as follows:

"Persons with certain metallic, electronic, magnetic, or mechanically-activated implants, devices, or objects may not enter this area. Serious injury may result. Do not enter this area if you have any question regarding an implant, device, or object. Consult the MRI Technologist or Radiologist."

Finally, the sign also states:

"Objects made from ferrous materials must not be taken into this area. Serious injury or property damage may result. Electronic objects such as hearing aids, cell phones, and beepers may also be damaged."

Many individuals fail to realize that the MR system's static magnetic field is always on. In fact, investigations of accidents that involved relatively large ferromagnetic objects like oxygen cylinders, chairs, IV poles, and wheelchairs revealed that the offending hospital personnel thought that the powerful magnetic field was activated *only* during the MR procedure. Therefore, a smaller sign or decal is particularly useful to emphasize the potentially hazardous nature of the MR environment, which states:

DANGER! THIS MAGNET IS ALWAYS ON!

Sign Placement. The strategic placement of signs in and around the MR environment is crucial to ensure that all individuals and patients see them before entering this area. In general, a sign should be placed on the door or entrance to MR system room and near or on the doorframe to be viewed by individuals and patients, especially if the door to the MR system room is open.

[*To obtain the afore-mentioned signs designed to help control access to the MR environment, please visit www.Magmedix.com]

REFERENCES

U. S. Department Of Health and Human Services, Center for Devices and Radiological Health Food and Drug Administration, the document entitled, Guidance for the, Submission Of Premarket Notifications for Magnetic Resonance Diagnostic Devices, Issued November 14, 1998.

Tattoos, Permanent Cosmetics, and Eye Makeup

Traditional (i.e., decorative) and cosmetic tattoo procedures have been performed for thousands of years. In the United States, cosmetic tattoos or "permanent cosmetics" are used to reshape, recolor, recreate, or modify eye shadow, eyeliner, eyebrows, lips, beauty marks, and cheek blush. Additionally, permanent cosmetics are often used aesthetically to enhance nipple-areola reconstruction procedures.

Unfortunately, there is much confusion regarding the overall safety aspects of permanent cosmetics. For example, based on a few reports of symptoms localized to the tattooed area during MR imaging, many radiologists have refused to perform examinations on individuals with permanent cosmetics, particularly tattooed eyeliner. This undue and unwarranted concern for possible adverse events prevents patients with cosmetic tattoos access to an important diagnostic imaging technique.

While it is well-known that permanent cosmetics and tattoos may cause artifacts and both cosmetic and decorative tattoos may be associated with relatively minor, short-term cutaneous reactions, the exact frequency and severity of soft tissue reactions or other problems related to MR imaging and cosmetic tattoos while unknown, is considered to be quite low.

In 2002, Tope and Shellock conducted a study to determine the frequency and severity of adverse events associated with MR imaging in a population of subjects with permanent cosmetics. A questionnaire was distributed to clients of cosmetic tattoo technicians. This survey asked study subjects for demographic data, information about their tattoos, and for their experiences during MR imaging procedures. Results from 1,032 surveys were tabulated. One hundred thirty-five (13.1%) study subjects underwent MR imaging after having permanent cosmetics applied. Only two individuals (1.5%) experienced problems associated with MR imaging. One subject reported a sensation of "slight tingling" and the other reported a "burning" sensation. Both incidents were transient and did not prevent the MR procedures from being performed. Based on these findings and additional information in the peer-reviewed literature, it appears that MR imaging may be performed in patients with permanent cosmetics without serious soft tissue reactions or adverse events.

Therefore, the presence of permanent cosmetics should not prevent a patient from undergoing MR imaging.

Before undergoing an MR procedure, the patient should be asked if he or she has ever had a permanent coloring technique (i.e., tattooing) applied to the body. This includes cosmetic applications such as eyeliner, lip-liner, lip coloring, as well as decorative designs. This question is necessary because of the associated imaging artifacts and, more importantly, because a small number of patients (fewer than 10 documented cases) have experienced transient skin irritation, cutaneous swelling, or heating sensations at the site of the permanent colorings in association with MR procedures (review of Medical Device Reports, 1985 to 2009).

Interestingly, decorative tattoos tend to cause worse problems (including first- and second-degree burns) for patients undergoing MR imaging compared to those that have been reported for cosmetic tattoos. With regard to decorative tattoos, a letter to the editor described a second-degree burn that occurred on the skin of the deltoid from a decorative tattoo. The authors suggested that "the heating could have come either from oscillations of the gradients or, more likely from the RF-induced electrical currents". However, the exact mechanism(s) responsible for complications or adverse events in the various cases that have occurred related to decorative tattoos is unknown.

Additionally, Kreidstein et al. reported that a patient experienced a sudden burning pain at the site of a decorative tattoo while undergoing MR imaging of the lumbar spine using a 1.5-Tesla MR system. Swelling and erythema was resolved within 12 hours, without evidence of permanent sequelae. The tattoo pigment used in this case was ferromagnetic, which possibly explained the symptoms experienced by the patient. Surprisingly, in order to permit the MRI examination, an excision of the tattooed skin was performed.

The authors of this report stated, "Theoretically, the application of a pressure dressing of the tattoo may prevent any tissue distortion due to ferromagnetic pull". (However, this relatively benign procedure was not attempted for this patient.) The authors also indicated that, "In some cases, removal of the tattoo may be the most practical means of allowing MRI".

Kanal and Shellock (1998) commented on this report in a letter to the editor, suggesting that the response to this situation was "rather aggressive". Clearly the trauma, expense, and morbidity associated with excision of a tattoo far exceed those that may be associated with ferromagnetic tattoo interactions. A firmly applied pressure bandage may be used if there is concern related to "movement" of the ferromagnetic particles in the tattoo pigment. Additionally, direct application of a cold compress to the site of a tattoo would likely mitigate any heating sensation that may occur in association with MR imaging.

Artifacts. Imaging artifacts associated with permanent cosmetics and certain types of eye makeup have been reported. These artifacts are predominantly associated with the presence of pigments that use iron oxide or other type of metal and occur in the immediate area of the applied pigment or material. As such, tattoo- and makeup-related MR imaging artifacts should not prevent a diagnostically adequate MR imaging procedure from being performed, especially in consideration that careful selection of imaging parameters may easily minimize artifacts related to metallic materials.

The only possible exception to this is if the anatomy of interest is in the *exact* same position of where the tattoo was applied using an iron oxide-based pigment. For example, Weiss et al. reported that heavy metal particles used in the pigment base of mascara and eyeliner tattoos, have a paramagnetic effect that causes alteration of the local magnetic field in adjacent tissues. Changes in the MR signal pattern may result in distortion of the globes. In some cases, the artifact and distortion may mimic actual ocular disease, such as a ciliary body melanoma or cyst.

GUIDELINES AND RECOMMENDATIONS

In consideration of the available literature and experience pertaining to MR procedures and patients with permanent cosmetics and tattoos, guidelines to manage these individuals include, the following:

1) The screening form used for patients should include a question to identify the presence of permanent cosmetics or decorative tattoos.
2) Before undergoing an MR procedure, the patient should be asked if he or she had a permanent coloring technique (i.e., tattooing) applied to any part of the body. This includes cosmetic applications such as eyeliner, lip-liner, lip coloring, as well as decorative designs.
3) The patient should be informed of the potential risks associated with the site of the tattoo.
4) The patient should be advised to immediately inform the MRI technologist regarding any unusual sensation felt at the site of the tattoo in association with the MR procedure.
5) The patient should be closely monitored using visual and auditory means throughout the operation of the MR system to ensure safety. In the event that the patient reports a problem, the MR examination

must be stopped immediately and an investigation conducted to ensure patient safety.

6) As a precautionary measure, a cold compress (e.g., wet washcloth) may be applied to the tattoo site during the MR procedure.

In addition to the above, information and recommendations have been provided for patients by the United States Food and Drug Administration, Center for Food Safety and Applied Nutrition, Office of Cosmetics and Colors Fact Sheet, as follows: "... the risks of avoiding an MRI when your doctor has recommended one are likely to be much greater than the risks of complications from an interaction between the MRI and tattoo or permanent makeup. Instead of avoiding an MRI, individuals who have tattoos or permanent makeup should inform the radiologist or technician of this fact in order to take appropriate precautions, avoid complications, and assure the best results."

REFERENCES

Becker H. The use of intradermal tattoo to enhance the final result of nipple-areola reconstruction. Plast Reconstr Surg 1986;77:673.

Carr JJ. Danger in performing MR imaging on women who have tattooed eyeliner or similar types of permanent cosmetic injections. AJR Am J Roentgenol 1995;165:1546-1547.

Gomey M. Tattoo pigments, patient clothing, and magnetic resonance imaging. Risk Management Bulletin #12748-8/95, The Doctors' Company, Napa, CA. August, 1995.

Halder RM, Pham HN, Hreadon JY, Johnson HA. Micropigmentation for the treatment of vitiligo. J Dermatol Surg Oncol 1989;15:1092-1098.

Jackson JG, Acker H. Permanent eyeliner and MR imaging. (letter) AJR Am J Roentgenol 1987;149:1080.

Kanal E, Barkovich AJ, Bell C, et al. ACR guidance document for safe MR practices: 2007. AJR Am J Roentgenol. 2007;188:1447-1474.

Kanal E, Shellock FG. MRI interaction with tattoo pigments. (letter) Plast Reconstr Surg 1998;101:1150-1151.

Klitscher D, Blum J, Kreitner KF, Rommens PM. MRT-induced burns in tattooed patients. Case report of a traumatic surgery patient. Unfallchirurg 2005;108:410-414.

Kreidstein ML, Giguere D, Freiberg A. MRI interaction with tattoo pigments: case report, pathophysiology, and management. Plast Reconstr Surg 1997;99:1717-1720.

Lund A, Nelson ID, Wirtschafter ID, Williams PA. Tattooing of eyelids: magnetic resonance imaging artifacts. Ophthalmic Surg 1986;17:550-553.

Morishita Y, Miyati T, et al. Influence of mechanical effect due to MRI-magnet on tattoo seal and eye makeup. Nippon Hoshasen Gijutsu Gakkai Zasshi. 2008;64:587-90.

Sacco D, et al. Artifacts caused by cosmetics in MR imaging of the head. Am J Roentgenol 1987;148:1001-1004.

Shellock FG. Magnetic Resonance Procedures: Health Effects and Safety, CRC Press, LLC, Boca Raton, FL, 2001.

Tattoos. FDA Medical Bulletin 1994;24:8.

Tope WD, Shellock FG. Magnetic resonance imaging and permanent cosmetics (tattoos): survey of complications and adverse events. J Magn Reson Imaging 2002;15:180-184.

Vahlensieck M. Tattoo-related cutaneous inflammation (burn grade I) in a mid-field MR scanner. (letter) Eur Radiol 2000;10:97.

Wagle WA, Smith M. Tattoo-induced skin burn during MR imaging. (letter) Am J Roentgenol 2000: 174:1795.

Weiss RA, Saint-Louis LA, Haik BG, McCord CD, Taveras JL. Mascara and eye-lining tattoos: MRI artifacts. Ann Ophthalmology 1989;21:129-131.

Terminology for Implants and Devices

MRI Labeling Information for Implants and Devices: Explanation of Terminology*

Summary Statement. This Editorial presents the recommendations from the Food and Drug Administration for MR safety terminology and labeling for medical devices and provides an explanation of how this information is applied.

The magnetic resonance (MR) environment may pose risks or problems to patients with certain implants and other medical devices primarily due to factors that include electromagnetic field interactions, MRI-related heating, and the creation of artifacts (1-5). In addition, for electrically-activated implants and other medical devices, there are concerns that the MR system may affect the operation of the medical device and/or to induce currents in the device (1-3, 5). With the growing use of MRI in the 1990s, the Food and Drug Administration (FDA) recognized the need for standardized tests to address MRI safety issues for implants and other medical devices (4, 6). Thus, over the years, test methods have been developed by various organizations including the American Society for Testing and Materials (ASTM) International (formerly the American Society for Testing and Materials), with an ongoing commitment to ensure patient safety in the MR environment (7-10).

The FDA is responsible for reviewing the MR terminology and labeling that manufacturers provide to their devices. The MR terminology, as it pertains to performing MR examinations in patients with implants and other medical devices, has continued to evolve to keep pace with advances in MRI technology (4, 6, 11). Unfortunately, members of the MRI community frequently do not always understand the terms that are used and are often confused by the conditions that are specified in "MR Conditional" labeling. This lack of understanding may result in patients with implants being exposed to potentially hazardous MRI conditions or in inappropriately preventing them from undergoing needed MRI examinations. Importantly, there is now new labeling terminology, which is associated with expanded labeling information. Therefore, the goal of this Editorial is to present background information about the terms used for MRI labeling of implants and other medical devices, to define the current terms, and to illustrate the use of the new labeling by providing a sample label with a detailed explanation of how the terminology is used.

Prior Terminology

In 1997, the FDA's Center for Devices and Radiological Health (CDRH) first proposed terms to be used to label MRI information for medical devices, which was presented in the draft document, "A Primer on Medical Device Interactions with Magnetic Resonance Imaging Systems (6). These terms were defined, as follows (6):

MR Safe: This term indicates that the device, when used in the MR environment, has been demonstrated to present no additional risk to the patient, but may affect the quality of the diagnostic information.

MR Compatible: This term indicates that the device, when used in the MR environment, is MR Safe and has been demonstrated to neither significantly affect the quality of the diagnostic information nor have its operations affected by the MR device."

This document further stated that, "The use of the terms, "MR Compatible" and "MR Safe" without specification of the MR environment in which the device was tested should be avoided since interpretation of these claims may vary and are difficult to substantiate rigorously. Statements such as "intended for use in the MR environment" or similar claims along with appropriate qualifying information are preferred (i.e. test conditions should be specifically stated)(6)." Here, the term "MR environment" encompasses the static, gradient (time-varying), and RF electromagnetic fields that may impact an implant or device.

Using this terminology, MRI testing of an implant or device for "MR safety" involved *in vitro* assessments of static magnetic field interactions, MRI-related heating, and, in some cases, induced electrical currents (i.e., from gradient magnetic fields), while "MR compatibility" testing required all of these as well as characterization of artifacts. In addition, it may have been necessary to evaluate the effect of various MRI conditions on the functional or operational aspects of an implant or device (2, 3, 4, 6, 7-10).

Revised Terminology

In time, it became apparent that the terms, "MR Safe" and "MR Compatible" were confusing and often used interchangeably or incorrectly (2-4, 11, 12). In particular, the terms were sometimes used without including the list of conditions for which the device had been demonstrated to be safe, in some cases inappropriately giving the impression that the device is "safe" or "compatible" in all MR environments. Therefore, in an effort to develop more appropriate terminology and, more importantly, because the misuse of these terms could result in serious accidents for patients and others in the MR environment, the MR Task Group of ASTM International Committee F04 on Medical and Surgical Materials and Devices developed standard ASTM F2503 which includes a new set of MR labeling terms with associated icons (4). The new terms defined in ASTM F2503 (released in August 2005) and currently recognized by the FDA are (11, 13), as follows:

MR Safe - an item that poses no known hazards in all MRI environments. Using the terminology, "MR Safe" items are non-conducting, non-metallic, and non-magnetic items such as a plastic Petri dish. An item may be determined to be MR Safe by providing a scientifically based rationale rather than test data.

MR Conditional - an item that has been demonstrated to pose no known hazards in a specified MR environment with specified conditions of use. "Field" conditions that define the MR environment include static magnetic field strength, spatial gradient, dB/dt (time rate of change of the magnetic field), radio frequency (RF) fields, and specific absorption rate (SAR). Additional conditions, including specific configurations of the item (e.g., the routing of leads used for a neurostimulation system), may be required.

For MR Conditional items, the item labeling includes results of testing sufficient to characterize the behavior of the item in the MR environment. In particular, testing for items that may be placed in the MR environment should address magnetically induced displacement force and torque, and RF heating. Other possible safety issues include but are not limited to, thermal injury, induced currents/voltages, electromagnetic compatibility, neurostimulation, acoustic noise, interaction among devices, and the safe functioning of the item and the safe operation of the MR system. Any parameter that affects the safety of the item should be listed and any condition that is known to produce an unsafe condition must be described.

MR Unsafe - an item that is known to pose hazards in all MRI environments. MR Unsafe items include magnetic items such as a pair of ferromagnetic scissors.

Associated Icons. In addition to the terms, MR Safe, MR Conditional, and MR Unsafe, the ASTM International MR marking standard introduced corresponding icons, consistent with international standards for colors and shapes of safety signs (13). These icons are intended for use on items that may be brought into or near the MR environment as well as in product labeling for implants and other medical devices. The icons may be reproduced in color or in black and white, however, the use of color is encouraged because of the added visibility (13).

The "MR Safe" icon consists of the letters 'MR' in green in a white square with a green border, or the letters 'MR' in white within a green square. The "MR Conditional" icon consists of the letters 'MR' in black inside a yellow triangle with a black border. The "MR Unsafe" icon consists of the letters 'MR' in black on a white field inside a red circle with a diagonal red band. Importantly, for "MR Conditional" items, the item's labeling must include the parameters and results used for testing that are sufficient to characterize the behavior of the item in the MRI environment (13).

Further details and a comprehensive discussion of the labeling applied to passive implants are presented in the recent FDA document, "Guidance for Industry and FDA Staff - Establishing Safety and Compatibility of Passive Implants in the Magnetic Resonance (MR) Environment" (11).

Use of Terminology: Reasons for Confusion

Because of the variety of MR systems and MR conditions in clinical use today (e.g., ranging from 0.2- to 9.4-Tesla), the current terminology is intended help elucidate labeling matters for medical devices and other items that may be used in the MR environment to ensure the safe use of MRI technology. However, it should be noted that this updated terminology has not been applied *retrospectively* to the many implants and devices that previously received FDA approved labeling using the terms "MR Safe" or "MR Compatible" (in general, this applies to those objects tested prior to the release of the ASTM International standard for labeling, around August 2005).

Therefore, this important point must be understood to avoid undue confusion regarding the matter of the labeling that has been applied to previously tested implants (i.e., labeled as "MR safe" or "MR Compatible") versus those that have recently undergone MRI testing (i.e., now labeled as "MR Conditional")(2, 3).

The labeling for medical devices that were **appropriately** labeled using the historical definitions for MR Safe or MR Compatible, **including the list of conditions** for which the device has been determined to be safe or compatible, is still accurate. Indeed, part of the confusion that exists on this matter is due to the use coexistence of the newer terminology with the prior labeling terminology.

In order to eliminate this ongoing confusion, in 2005 FDA recognized the new set of terms in ASTM F2503 and asks manufacturers to use them for all new products. When manufacturers make a submission to FDA for an existing device, FDA requests the manufacturers of these previously approved devices update their labeling to use the new MR safety terminology. Labeling information for implants and other medical devices has been compiled and is available in published and on-line formats (2, 14). Specific testing and labeling for active implants (e.g., those involving electronics) is currently being developed by an ISO (International Standards Organization) – IEC (International Electrotechnical Commission) joint working group.

MR Conditional Labeling Information: Explanation of the Content

In addition to the frequent problems associated with understanding the MRI labeling, the actual content of the label is often misunderstood with respect to the conditions indicated for a given implant that is labeled "MR Conditional". Therefore, the following is an example of "MR Conditional" labeling for an implant, *Example Implant*, along with an explanation of the content, provided for each aspect of the label (1-4, 11, 13) (**Table 1**):

MRI Information

Non-clinical testing has demonstrated the Example Implant is MR Conditional. It can be scanned safely under the following conditions:

-Static magnetic field of 3-Tesla

This is the static magnetic field for which the implant gave acceptable test results, generally the largest static magnetic field used for testing the implant. In some cases the labeling will state, "Static magnetic field of 3-Tesla or less" or "Static magnetic field of 3-Tesla, *only"* or *"static magnetic field of 1.5-Tesla or 3-Tesla."* Therefore, carefully reading and implementing this portion of the labeling for the implant is advised in order to avoid possible injuries to patients.

-Spatial gradient field of 720-Gauss/cm or less.

This is a frequently misinterpreted parameter because the MRI user sees the term "gradient field" and presumes that it refers to the time-varying or gradient fields used during MR imaging. However, the term, "**spatial gradient field**" for medical device labeling relates to the rate at which the static magnetic field strength changes over space per unit length (thus, indicated as dB/dx or, in this case, as 720-Gauss/cm for this example). Notably, the point of the highest spatial magnetic gradient is the position where translational attraction (i.e., determined using the deflection angle method) is typically assessed for an implant or device, according to ASTM F2052 - 06e1. The MR system manufacturer is able to provide spatial gradient magnetic field information for a particular MR system or it may determined using a Gauss meter.

<u>-Maximum MR system reported, whole body averaged specific absorption rate (SAR) of 2-W/kg for 15-minutes of scanning.</u>

Confusion commonly exists with respect to this stated parameter insofar as the term "scanning" is presumed to apply to the entire MRI procedure when, in fact, it applies to only each particular pulse *sequence* that is used and, of course, multiple sequences are utilized when performing the MRI examination. Therefore, to adequately safeguard the patient, the whole body averaged SAR for each scan sequence must be maintained at or below 2-W/kg for each scan sequence.

<u>-In non-clinical testing, the Example Implant produced a temperature rise of less than 2.0°C at a maximum MR system reported, whole body averaged specific absorption rate (SAR) of 2- W/kg for 15 minutes of MR scanning in a (static magnetic field strength _____) (model _____) (MR system manufacturer _____) (software version _____) MR scanner.</u>

The labeling for the implant has additional information with respect to the temperature rise that is associated with certain MRI parameters, that is based on the findings obtained in the MRI-related heating test. Therefore, as seen in this example, the expected "worst case" temperature rise is 2.0 degrees C or less during MRI performed at a whole body averaged SAR of 2-W/kg for 15-min., using a particular MR system type (i.e., with the make, model, and software of the scanner indicated). The MR system reported, whole body averaged SAR of 2-W/kg is the level specified in the ASTM F2182 - 02a and is the level commonly reported in device labeling, although higher or lower SAR levels may also be indicated. (It should be noted that, in this labeling section, certain labels for implants and other medical devices may state that this information applies to the use of a particular type of transmit RF coil that should be used, such as a transmit body or transmit head RF coil.)

Image Artifact

MR image quality may be compromised if the area of interest is in the same area or relatively close to the position of the device. Therefore, it may be necessary to optimize MR imaging parameters for the presence of this implant.

This is a common statement for many different implants and devices. Since the size of the artifact for an implant or device may impact the diagnostic use of MR imaging, information is typically provided in the label that characterizes the size and shape of the artifacts associated with certain pulse sequences (e.g., T1-weighted spin echo and gradient echo), according to ASTM F2119 - 07 or an equivalent method. For devices with a lumen (e.g., stent), the labeling may indicate whether the lumen is obscured by the size of the artifact.

The FDA also recommends that the patient register the conditions under which their MR Conditional implant can be scanned safely with the MedicAlert Foundation or other equivalent organization, and so the device labeling may include contact information for MedicAlert (11).

Table 1. Example of MRI labeling information for a medical implant or device.

MRI Information

Non-clinical testing has demonstrated the Example Implant is MR Conditional. It can be scanned safely under the following conditions:

- Static magnetic field of 3-Tesla.
- Spatial gradient field of 720-Gauss/cm or less.
- Maximum MR system reported, whole body averaged specific absorption rate (SAR) of 2-W/kg for 15-minutes of scanning.
- In non-clinical testing, the Example Implant produced a temperature rise of less than 2.0°C at a maximum MR system reported, whole body averaged specific absorption rate (SAR) of 2- W/kg for 15 minutes of MR scanning in a (static magnetic field strength _____) (model _____) (MR system manufacturer _____) (software version _____) MR scanner.

Image Artifact

MR image quality may be compromised if the area of interest is in the same area or relatively close to the position of the device. Therefore, it may be necessary to optimize MR imaging parameters for the presence of this implant.

Summary and Conclusions

This Editorial presents current FDA recommendations for MR safety terminology and labeling for implants and other medical devices and provides an explanation of how this information may be applied. Notably, the specific content of the MR labeling may take other forms (especially for electrically active implants and devices) as the format continues to be refined by the FDA in an ongoing effort to properly communicate this information to ensure patient safety.

REFERENCES

(1) Shellock FG, Crues JV. MR procedures: biologic effects, safety, and patient care. Radiology, 2004; 232:635-652.

(2) Shellock FG. Reference Manual for Magnetic Resonance Safety Implants and Device: 2009 Edition. Biomedical Research Publishing Group, Los Angeles, CA, 2009.

(3) Shellock FG, Spinazzi A. MRI Safety Update: 2008, Part 2, Screening patients for MRI. American Journal of Roentgenology 2008;191:12-21.

(4) Woods TO. Standards for medical devices in MRI: present and future. J Magn Reson Imaging. 2007; 26:1186-9.

(5) Levine GN, Gomes AS, Arai AE, Bluemke DA, Flamm SD, Kanal E, Manning WJ, Martin ET, Smith JM, Wilke N, Shellock FG. Safety of magnetic resonance imaging in patients with cardiovascular devices: an American Heart Association Scientific Statement from the Committee on Diagnostic and Interventional Cardiac Catheterization. Circulation 2007; 116:2878-2891.

(6) United States Food and Drug Administration, Center for Devices and Radiological Health, A Primer on Medical Device Interactions with Magnetic Resonance Imaging Systems. http://www.fda.gov/cdrh/ode/primerf6.html, 1997.

(7) American Society for Testing and Materials (ASTM) International, Designation: ASTM F2052 - 06e1, Standard Test Method for Measurement of Magnetically Induced Displacement Force on Medical Devices in the Magnetic Resonance Environment. ASTM International, West Conshohocken, PA.

(8) American Society for Testing and Materials (ASTM) International, Designation: ASTM F2213-06, Standard Test Method for Measurement of Magnetically Induced Torque on Medical Devices in the Magnetic Resonance Environment. ASTM International, West Conshohocken, PA.

(9) American Society for Testing and Materials (ASTM) International, Designation: ASTM F2119 – 07, Standard Test Method for Evaluation of MR Image Artifacts from Passive Implants. ASTM International, West Conshohocken, PA.

(10) American Society for Testing and Materials (ASTM) International, Designation: ASTM F2182 - 02a, Standard Test Method for Measurement of Radio Frequency Induced Heating Near Passive Implants During Magnetic Resonance Imaging. ASTM International, West Conshohocken, PA.

(11) Guidance for Industry and FDA Staff - Establishing Safety and Compatibility of Passive Implants in the Magnetic Resonance (MR) Environment. Document issued on: August 21, 2008; http://www.fda.gov/cdrh/osel/guidance/1685.html

(12)Shellock FG, Crues JV. Commentary: MR safety and the American College of Radiology White Paper. American Journal of Roentgenology 2002; 178:1349-1352.

(13) American Society for Testing and Materials (ASTM) International, Designation: F2503-08, Standard Practice for Marking Medical Devices and Other Items for Safety in the Magnetic Resonance Environment. ASTM International, West Conshohocken, PA.

(14) http://www.mrisafety.com/ accessed June, 2009.

[Portions of this content were excerpted with permission from Shellock FG, Woods TO, Crues JV. MRI Labeling Information for Implants and Devices: Explanation of Terminology. Radiology 2009;253:26-30. This full-length article may be downloaded from www.IMRSER.org]

SECTION II

MR Procedures and Implants, Devices and Materials

General Information

Magnetic resonance (MR) procedures may be contraindicated for patients primarily because of risks associated with movement or dislodgment of a ferromagnetic biomedical implant, material, or device. There are other possible hazards and problems related to the presence of a metallic object that include induction of currents (e.g., in materials that are conductors), excessive heating, changes in the operational aspects of the device, and the misinterpretation of an imaging artifact as an abnormality.

Induced Electrical Currents. The potential for MR procedures to injure patients by inducing electrical currents in conductive materials or devices such as gating leads, indwelling catheters with metallic components (e.g., thermodilution catheters), guide wires, pacemakers, implantable cardioverter defibrillators, neurostimulation systems, disconnected or broken surface coils, external fixation devices, cervical fixation devices, cochlear implants, infusion pumps, or improperly used physiologic monitors has been previously reported. Recommendations have been presented to protect patients from injuries related to induced currents that may develop during MR procedures.

Heating. Temperature increases produced in association with MR procedures have been studied using *ex vivo* techniques to evaluate various metallic implants, devices, and objects of a variety of different sizes, shapes, and metallic compositions. In general, reports have indicated that only minor temperature changes occur in association with MR procedures involving relatively small metallic objects that are "passive" implants (i.e., those that are not electronically-activated), including implants such as aneurysm clips, hemostatic clips, prosthetic heart valves, vascular access ports, and similar devices. Therefore, heat generated during an MR procedure involving a patient with a metallic "passive" implant does not appear to be a substantial hazard. In fact, to date, there has been no report of a patient being seriously injured as a result of excessive heat that developed in a relatively small "passive" metallic implant or device.

However, MRI-related heating is potentially problematic for implants that have an elongated shape or those that form a conducting loop of a certain diameter. For example, substantial heating can occur under some MR conditions for objects that form resonant conducting loops or for elongated implants (e.g., wires) that form resonant antennae.

Artifacts. The type and extent of artifacts caused by the presence of metallic implants, materials, and devices have been described and tend to be easily recognized on MR images. Artifacts and image distortion associated with metallic objects are predominantly caused by a disruption of the local magnetic field that perturbs the relationship between position and frequency. Additionally, artifacts associated with metallic objects may be caused by gradient switching due to the generation of eddy currents.

The relative amount of artifact seen on an MR image is dependent on the magnetic susceptibility, quantity, shape, orientation, and position of the object in the body as well as the technique used for imaging (i.e., the specific pulse sequence parameters) and the image processing method. An artifact caused by the presence of a metallic object in a patient during MR imaging is seen typically as a signal void or loss and may include a local or regional distortion of the image. In some cases, there may be areas of high signal intensity seen along the edges of the signal void.

Magnetic Field Interactions. Numerous studies have assessed magnetic field interactions for implants, materials, devices, and objects by measuring deflection forces, translational attraction, torque or other interactions associated with the static magnetic fields of MR systems. These investigations demonstrated that, for certain implants, MR procedures may be performed safely in patients with metallic objects that are nonferromagnetic or "weakly" ferromagnetic (i.e., only minimally attracted by the magnetic field in relation to its *in vivo* application), such that the associated magnetic field interactions are insufficient to move or dislodge them, *in situ*. Furthermore, the "intended *in vivo* use" of the implant or device must be taken into consideration, because this can impact whether or not a given object is acceptable for a patient undergoing an MR procedure. For example, sufficient counter-forces may exist to retain even a ferromagnetic implant, *in situ*.

In general, each implant, material, device, or object (particularly those made from unknown materials) should be evaluated using *ex vivo* techniques before allowing an individual or patient with the object to enter the MR environment and/or before performing the MR procedure. By following this guideline, the relative magnetic susceptibility for an object may be determined so that a competent decision can be made concerning possible risks associated with exposure to the MR system. Because movement or dislodgment of an implanted metallic object in a patient undergoing an MR procedure is the primary mechanism responsible for an injury, this aspect of testing is considered to be of utmost importance and should involve the use of an MR system operating at an appropriate static magnetic field strength. As previously mentioned, it may also be necessary to assess MRI-related heating for a given implant.

Various factors influence the risk of performing an MR procedure in a patient with a metallic object including the strength of the magnetic field, the magnetic susceptibility of the object, the mass of the object, the geometry of the object, the location and orientation of the object *in situ*, the presence of retentive mechanisms (i.e., fibrotic tissue, bone, sutures, etc.) and the length of time the object has been in place. These factors should be carefully considered before subjecting a patient or individual with a ferromagnetic object to an MR procedure or allowing entrance to the MR environment. This is particularly important if the object is located in a potentially dangerous area of the body such as a vital neural, vascular, of soft tissue structure where movement or dislodgment could injure the patient.

Furthermore, in certain cases, there is a possibility of changing the operational or functional aspects of the implant or device as a result of exposure to the electromagnetic fields of the MR system. Therefore, this important aspect must be evaluated using comprehensive testing techniques to verify that MR conditions will not impact the operation of a given implant or device.

Notably, patients with certain implants or devices that have relatively strong ferromagnetic qualities may be safely scanned using MR procedures because the objects are held in place by sufficient retentive forces that prevent them from being moved or dislodged. This is, with reference to the "intended *in vivo* use" of an implant or device. For example, there is an interference screw (i.e., the Perfix Interference Screw) used for reconstruction of the anterior cruciate ligament that has been demonstrated to be highly ferromagnetic. However, once this implant is screwed into the patient's bone, this prevents it from being moved, even if the patient is exposed to a 1.5-Tesla MR system. Other implants that exhibit substantial ferromagnetic qualities may likewise be safe for patients undergoing MR procedures under highly specific conditions as a result of the presence of counter-forces that prevent movement of these objects.

MR systems with very low (0.2-Tesla or less) or very high (9.4-Tesla) static magnetic fields are currently used for clinical and research applications. Considering that most metallic objects evaluated for magnetic field interactions were assessed at 1.5-Tesla, an appropriate variance or modification of the information provided regarding the safety of performing an MR procedure in a patient with a metallic object may exist when an MR system with a lower or higher static magnetic field strength is used. That is, it may be acceptable to adjust safety recommendations depending on the static magnetic field strength and other aspects of a given MR system. Obviously, performing an MR procedure using a 0.2-Tesla MR system has different risk implications for a patient with a ferromagnetic object compared with using a 9.4-Tesla MR system.

Information Pertaining to Implants, Materials, Devices and Objects. The information contained in this textbook is a compilation of the current data available relative to the assessment of magnetic field interactions, MRI-related heating, and other tests conducted on implants, materials, and devices and is based primarily on published reports in the peer-reviewed literature. This compilation also includes unpublished data acquired from *ex vivo* testing conducted on implants and devices using standardized or well-accepted techniques. Furthermore, MRI-related information obtained from manufacturers (e.g., the Product Insert or Instructions for Use information) is provided for various implants and devices.

Although every attempt was made to provide comprehensive and accurate information, there are many other implants, materials, devices, and objects in existence that remain to be evaluated with regard to the MR environment. In addition, new or updated information may exist for a given implant, especially those that are electronically-activated, since test procedures used to assess these devices continues to evolve. Therefore, to ensure the safety of an individual or patient in the MR environment or undergoing an MR procedure, MR healthcare professionals should follow the guideline whereby MR procedures should only be performed in a patient with a metallic object that has been previously tested and demonstrated to be safe. A similar guideline should be followed with regard to whether or not to allow an individual with an implant or device to enter the MR environment. Finally, for electronically-activated implants, the most current safety guidelines must be obtained and followed. Therefore, the MR healthcare professional is advised to confirm the latest MRI labeling information with the respective manufacturer prior to performing an MRI examination on the patient.

Terminology Applied to Implants and Devices

To ensure the proper understanding of the terminology applied to implants and devices, please review the following section in this textbook:

- **Terminology for Implants and Devices**

REFERENCES

American Society for Testing and Materials (ASTM) International, Designation: F2503-05. Standard Practice for Marking Medical Devices and Other Items for Safety in the Magnetic Resonance Environment. ASTM International, West Conshohocken, PA, 2005.

American Society for Testing and Materials (ASTM) Designation: F 2052. Standard test method for measurement of magnetically induced displacement force on passive implants in the magnetic resonance environment. In: Annual Book of ASTM Standards, Section 13, Medical Devices and Services, Volume 13.01 Medical Devices; Emergency Medical Services. West Conshohocken, PA, 2002; pp. 1576-1580.

Arena L, Morehouse HT, Safir J. MR imaging artifacts that simulate disease: how to recognize and eliminate them. Radiographics 1995;15:1373-1394.

Calcagnini G, et al. In vitro investigation of pacemaker lead heating induced by magnetic resonance imaging: role of implant geometry. J Magn Reson Imaging. 2008;28:879-86.

Davis PL, Crooks L, Arakawa M, et al. Potential hazards in NMR imaging: heating effects of changing magnetic fields and RF fields on small metallic implants. AJR Am J Roentgenol 1981;137:857-860.

Dempsey MF, Condon B, Hadley DM. Investigation of the factors responsible for burns during MRI. J Magn Reson Imaging 2001;13:627-631.

Diaz F, Tweardy L, Shellock FG. Cervical fixation devices: MRI issues at 3-Tesla. Spine (in press)

Graf H, Steidle G, Martirosian P, Lauer UA, Schick F. Metal artifacts caused by gradient switching. Magnetic Resonance in Medicine 2005;54;231-234.

Kanal E, Barkovich AJ, Bell C, et al. ACR guidance document for safe MR practices: 2007. AJR Am J Roentgenol. 2007;188:1447-1474.

Kainz W. MR heating tests of MR critical implants. J Magn Reson Imaging. 2007;26:450-1.

Levine GN, Gomes AS, Arai AE, Bluemke DA, Flamm SD, Kanal E, Manning WJ, Martin ET, Smith JM, Wilke N, Shellock FG. Safety of magnetic resonance imaging in patients with cardiovascular devices: an American Heart Association scientific statement from the Committee on Diagnostic and Interventional Cardiac Catheterization. Circulation 2007;116:2878-2891.

Masaki F, Shuhei Y, Riko K, Yohjiro M. Iatrogenic second-degree burn caused by a catheter encased tubular braid of stainless steel during MRI. Burns. 2007;33:1077-9.

Mattei E, Triventi M, Calcagnini G, Censi F, Kainz W, Bassen HI, Bartolini P. Temperature and SAR measurement errors in the evaluation of metallic linear structures heating during MRI using fluoroptic probes. Phys Med Biol. 2007;52:1633-46.

Neufeld E, Kuhn S, Szekely G, Kuster N. Measurement, simulation and uncertainty assessment of implant heating during MRI. Phys Med Biol. 2009;54:4151-69.

Nordbeck P, Fidler F, et al. Spatial distribution of RF-induced E-fields and implant heating in MRI. Magn Reson Med. 2008;60:312-9.

Nordbeck P, Weiss I, Ehses P, et al. Measuring RF-induced currents inside implants: Impact of device configuration on MRI safety of cardiac pacemaker leads. Magn Reson Med. 2009;61:570-8.

Nyenhuis JA, Kildishev AV, Foster KS, Graber G, Athey W. Heating near implanted medical devices by the MRI RF-magnetic field. IEEE Trans Magn 1999;35:4133-4135.

Nyenhuis JA, Park SM, Kamondetdacha R, Amjad A, Shellock FG, Rezai A. MRI and implanted medical devices: basic interactions with an emphasis on heating. IEEE Transactions on Device and Materials Reliability 2005;5:467-478.

Rezai AR, Baker K, Tkach J, Phillips M, Hrdlicka G, Sharan A, Nyenhuis J, Ruggieri P, Henderson J, Shellock FG. Is magnetic resonance imaging safe for patients with neurostimulation systems used for deep brain stimulation (DBS)? Neurosurgery 2005;57:1056-1062.

Roguin A, et al. Magnetic resonance imaging in individuals with cardiovascular implantable electronic devices. Europace. 2008;10:336-46.

Schenck JF. Chapter 1, Health Effects and Safety of Static Magnetic Fields. In: Magnetic Resonance Procedures: Health Effects and Safety. CRC Press, LLC, Boca Raton, FL, 2001; pp. 1-31.

Shellock FG. Magnetic Resonance Procedures: Health Effects and Safety. CRC Press, LLC, Boca Raton, FL, 2001.

Shellock FG. Guest Editorial. Comments on MRI heating tests of critical implants. Journal of Magnetic Resonance Imaging 2007;26:1182-1185.

Shellock FG. Excessive temperature increases in pacemaker leads at 3-T MR imaging with a transmit-received head coil. Radiology 2009;251:948-949.

Shellock FG. Biomedical implants and devices: assessment of magnetic field interactions with a 3.0-Tesla MR system. J Magn Reson Imaging 2002;16:721-732.

Shellock FG. MR safety update 2002: Implants and devices. J Magn Reson Imaging 2002;16:485-496.

Shellock FG. Surgical instruments for interventional MRI procedures: assessment of MR safety. J Magn Reson Imaging 2001;13:152-157.

Shellock FG, Crues JV. High-field strength MR imaging and metallic biomedical implants: an *ex vivo* evaluation of deflection forces. AJR Am J Roentgenol 1988;151:389-392.

Shellock FG, Crues JV. MR procedures: biologic effects, safety, and patient care. Radiology, 2004;232:635-652.

Shellock FG, Kanal E. Magnetic Resonance: Bioeffects, Safety, and Patient Management. Second Edition, Lippincott-Raven Press, New York, 1996.

Shellock FG, Mink JH, Curtin S, et al. MRI and orthopedic implants used for anterior cruciate ligament reconstruction: assessment of ferromagnetism and artifacts. J Magn Reson Imaging 1992;2:225-228.

Shellock FG, Spinazzi A. MRI Safety Update: 2008, Part 2, Screening patients for MRI. American Journal of Roentgenology 2008;191:12-21.

Shellock FG, Tkach JA, Ruggieri PM, Masaryk TJ, Rasmussen P. Aneurysm clips: evaluation of magnetic field interactions and translational attraction using "long-bore" and "short-bore" 3.0-Tesla MR systems. Am J Neuroradiology 2003;24:463-471.

Shellock FG, Tkach JA, Ruggieri PM, Masaryk TJ. Cardiac pacemakers, ICDs, and loop recorder: Evaluation of translational attraction using conventional ("long-bore") and "short-bore" 1.5- and 3.0-Tesla MR systems. Journal of Cardiovascular Magnetic Resonance 2003;5:387-397.

Shellock FG, Woods TO, Crues JV. MRI Labeling Information for Implants and Devices: Explanation of Terminology. Radiology 2009;253:26-30.

Shinbane J, Colletti P, Shellock FG. MR in patients with pacemakers and ICDs: Defining the Issues. Journal of Cardiovascular Magnetic Resonance 2007;9:5-13.

Smith CD, Kildishev AV, Nyenhuis JA, Foster KS, Bourland JD, Interactions of MRI magnetic fields with elongated medical implants. J Appl Physics 2000; 87:6188-6190.

Smith CD, Nyenhuis JA, Kildishev AV. Chapter 16. Health effects of induced electrical currents: Implications for implants. In: Magnetic resonance: Health Effects and Safety, FG Shellock, Editor, CRC Press, Boca Raton, FL, 2001; pp. 393-413.

Stradiotti P, et al. Metal-related artifacts in instrumented spine. Techniques for reducing artifacts in CT and MRI: state of the art. Eur Spine J. 2009;18 Suppl 1:102-8.

Tandri H, et al. Determinants of gradient field-induced current in a pacemaker lead system in a magnetic resonance imaging environment. Heart Rhythm. 2008;5:462-8.

Woods TO. Guidance for Industry and FDA Staff - Establishing Safety and Compatibility of Passive Implants in the Magnetic Resonance (MR) Environment. Document issued on: August 21, 2008; http://www.fda.gov/cdrh/osel/guidance/1685.html

Woods TO. Standards for medical devices in MRI: present and future. J Magn Reson Imaging. 2007;26:1186-9.

Yang CW, Liu L, et al. Magnetic resonance imaging of artificial lumbar disks: safety and metal artifacts. Chin Med J (Engl). 2009;20;122:911-6.

3-Tesla MR Safety Information for Implants and Devices

Because previous investigations performed to evaluate MR safety issues for implants and devices used mostly scanners with static magnetic fields of 1.5-Tesla or less, it is crucial to perform *ex vivo* testing at 3-Tesla to determine possible risks for these objects, especially with respect to magnetic field interactions. Importantly, a metallic object that displayed "weakly" ferromagnetic qualities in association with a 1.5-Tesla MR system may exhibit substantial magnetic field interactions during exposure to a 3-Tesla scanner.

Furthermore, for elongated devices or those that form a loop of a certain diameter, the effects of MRI-related heating may be substantially different. For example, evidence from a study conducted by Shellock et al. reported that significantly *less* MRI-related heating occurred at 3-Tesla/128-MHz (MR system reported whole body averaged SAR, 3-W/kg) versus 1.5-Tesla/64-MHz (MR system reported whole body averaged SAR, 1.4-W/kg) for a pacemaker lead (same lead length, positioning, etc.). This phenomenon, whereby less heating was observed at 3-Tesla/128-MHz vs. 1.5-Tesla/64-MHz, has also been observed for external fixation devices, Foley catheters with temperature sensors, neurostimulation systems, relatively long vascular stents, and other objects (Unpublished Observations, F.G. Shellock, 2008). Therefore, it is crucial to conduct *ex vivo* testing to assess magnetic field interactions and, for certain devices, MRI-related heating, to identify potentially hazardous objects prior to subjecting individuals to the MR environment or patients to an MR examination at 3-Tesla.

Magnetic Field Interactions at 3-Tesla. From a magnetic field interaction consideration, translational attraction and/or torque may cause movement or dislodgment of a ferromagnetic implant resulting in an uncomfortable sensation or injury to a patient or individual. Translational attraction is dependent on the strength of the static magnetic field, the spatial magnetic gradient, the mass of the object, the shape of the object, and its magnetic susceptibility. The effects of translational attraction on external and implanted ferromagnetic objects are predominantly responsible for possible hazards in the immediate area of the MR system.

That is, as one moves closer to the MR system or is moved into the scanner for an examination. An evaluation of torque is also important for a metallic object, especially if it has an elongated configuration. Qualitative and quantitative techniques have been used to determine magnetic field-related torque for implants and devices.

From a practical consideration, in addition to the findings for translational attraction and torque, the "intended *in vivo* use" of the implant or device must be considered as well as mechanisms that may provide retention of the object *in situ* (e.g., implants or devices held in place by sutures, granulation or ingrowth of tissue, fixation devices, or by other means) with regard to potential risks for a given metallic object (for further information on this topic, please refer to the prior section in this textbook, **General Information).**

Long-Bore vs. Short-Bore 3-Tesla MR Systems. Different magnet designs exist for commercially available 3-Tesla MR systems, including configurations that are conventional "long-bore" scanners and "short-bore" systems. Because of physical differences in the position and magnitude of the highest spatial magnetic gradient for different magnets, measurements of deflection angles for implants using long-bore vs. short-bore MR systems can produce substantially different results for deflection angle measurements (i.e., translational attraction), as reported by Shellock et al. Studies conducted using 3-Tesla MR systems indicated that, in general, there were significantly ($p < 0.01$) higher deflection angles measured for implants in association with exposure to short-bore vs. the long-bore MR systems. The differences in deflection angle measurements for the metallic objects were related to differences in the highest spatial magnetic gradients for short-bore vs. long-bore scanners.

The safety implications are primarily for magnetic field-related translational attraction with respect to short-bore versus long-bore 3-Tesla MR systems. For example, the deflection angle measured for an implant on a short-bore can be substantially higher (and thus, potentially unsafe from a magnetic field interaction consideration) compared to the deflection angle measured on a long-bore MR system. Therefore, safety information for measurements of magnetic field interactions for metallic objects must be considered with regard to the specific type of MR system used for the evaluation or, more accurately, with respect to the level of the highest spatial gradient fields that were used for the tests.

Heating of Implants and Devices at 3-Tesla. *Ex vivo* testing has been used to evaluate MRI-related heating for various metallic implants, materials, devices, and objects of a variety of sizes, shapes, and metallic compositions. In general, reports have indicated that only minor temperature changes occur in association with MR procedures involving metallic objects that are relatively small passive implants (e.g., those that are not electronically-activated). Therefore, heat generated during an MR procedure performed at 3-Tesla involving a patient with relatively small, passive metallic implant does not appear to be a substantial hazard.

However, because excessive heating and burns have occurred in association with implants and devices that have elongated configurations or that form conducting loops, patients with these objects should not undergo MR procedures at 3-Tesla until *ex vivo* heating assessments are performed to determine the relative risks. *Ex vivo* investigations have demonstrated that excessive heating may occur for certain implants related to MRI performed at 3-Tesla.

REFERENCES

American Society for Testing and Materials (ASTM) Designation: F 2052. Standard test method for measurement of magnetically induced displacement force on passive implants in the magnetic resonance environment. In: Annual Book of ASTM Standards, Section 13, Medical Devices and Services, Volume 13.01 Medical Devices; Emergency Medical Services. West Conshohocken, PA, 2002; pp. 1576-1580.

Davis P L, Crooks L, Arakawa M, et al. Potential hazards in NMR imaging: heating effects of changing magnetic fields and RF fields on small metallic implants. AJR Am J Roentgenol 1981;137:857-860.

Dempsey MF, Condon B, Hadley DM. Investigation of the factors responsible for burns during MRI. J Magn Reson Imaging 2001;13:627-631.

Diaz F, Tweardy L, Shellock FG. Cervical fixation devices: MRI issues at 3-Tesla. Spine (in press)

Edwards M-B, Draper ERC, Hand JW, Taylor KM, Young IR. Mechanical testing of human cardiac tissue: some implications for MRI safety. Journal of Cardiovascular Magnetic Resonance 2005;7:835-840.

Gimbel JR. Magnetic resonance imaging of implantable cardiac rhythm devices at 3-Tesla. Pacing Clin Electrophysiol. 2008;31:795-801.

Hennemeyer CT, Wicklow K, Feinberg DA, Derdeyn CP. In vitro evaluation of platinum Guglielmi detachable coils at 3-T with a porcine model: safety issues and artifacts. Radiology 2001;219:732-737.

Martin AD, Driscoll CL, Wood CP, Felmlee JP. Safety evaluation of titanium middle ear prostheses at 3-Tesla. Otolaryngol Head Neck Surg 2005;132:537-42.

Medtronic Heart Valves, Medtronic, Inc., Minneapolis, MN, Permission to publish 3-Tesla MR testing information for Medtronic Heart Valves provided by Kathryn M. Bayer, Senior Technical Consultant, Medtronic Heart Valves, Technical Service.

Nyehnuis JA, Kildishev AV, Foster KS, Graber G, Athey W. Heating near implanted medical devices by the MRI RF-magnetic field. IEEE Trans Magn 1999;35:4133-4135.

Schenck JF. Chapter 1, Health Effects and Safety of Static Magnetic Fields. In: Magnetic Resonance Procedures: Health Effects and Safety. CRC Press, LLC, Boca Raton, FL, 2001; pp. 1-31.

Shellock FG Radiofrequency-induced heating during MR procedures: A review. J Magn Reson Imaging 2000;12:30-36.

Shellock FG. MR safety update 2002: Implants and devices. J Magn Reson Imaging 2002;16:485-496.

Shellock FG. Biomedical implants and devices: assessment of magnetic field interactions with a 3.0-Tesla MR system. J Magn Reson Imaging 2002;16:721-732.

Shellock FG. Begnaud J, Inman DM. VNS Therapy System: *In vitro* evaluation of MRI-related heating and function at 1.5- and 3-Tesla. Neuromodulation 2006;9:204-213.

Shellock FG. Forder J. Drug eluting coronary stent: *In vitro* evaluation of magnetic resonance safety at 3-Tesla. Journal of Cardiovascular Magnetic Resonance 2005;7:415-419.

Shellock FG, Woods TO, Crues JV. MRI labeling information for implants and devices: Explanation of terminology. Radiology 2009;253:26-30.

Shellock FG, Gounis M, Wakhloo A. Detachable coil for cerebral aneurysms: *In vitro* evaluation of magnet field interactions, heating, and artifacts at 3-Tesla. American Journal of Neuroradiology 2005;26:363-366.

Shellock FG, Habibi R, Knebel J. Programmable CSF shunt valve: *In vitro* assessment of MRI safety at 3-Tesla. American Journal of Neuroradiology 2006;27:661-665.

Shellock FG, Wilson SF, Mauge CP. Magnetically programmable shunt valve: MRI at 3-Tesla. Magnetic Resonance Imaging 2007;25:1116-21.

Shellock FG, Tkach JA, Ruggieri PM, Masaryk TJ. Cardiac pacemakers, ICDs, and loop recorder: Evaluation of translational attraction using conventional ("long-bore") and "short-bore" 1.5- and 3.0-Tesla MR systems. Journal of Cardiovascular Magnetic Resonance 2003;5:387-397.

Shellock FG, Tkach JA, Ruggieri PM, Masaryk T, Rasmussen P. Aneurysm clips: evaluation of magnetic field interactions and translational attraction using "long-bore" and "short-bore" 3.0-Tesla MR systems. American Journal of Neuroradiology 2003;24:463-471.

Shellock FG, Valencerina S. Septal repair implants: evaluation of MRI safety at 3-Tesla. Magnetic Resonance Imaging 2005;23:1021-1025.

Shellock FG, Valencerina S, Fischer L. MRI-related heating of pacemaker at 1.5- and 3-Tesla: Evaluation with and without pulse generator attached to leads. Circulation 112;Supplement II:561, 2005.

Shellock FG. Valencerina S. *In vitro* evaluation of MRI issues at 3-Tesla for aneurysm clips: findings and information that pertain to 154 additional aneurysm clips. American Journal of Neuroradiology (in press)

Smith CD, Kildishev AV, Nyenhuis JA, Foster KS, Bourland JD, Interactions of MRI magnetic fields with elongated medical implants. J Appl Physics 2000;87:6188-6190.

Smith CD, Nyenhuis JA, Kildishev AV. Chapter 16. Health effects of induced electrical currents: Implications for implants. In: Magnetic resonance: health effects and safety, FG Shellock, Editor, CRC Press, Boca Raton, FL, 2001; pp. 393-413.

Sommer T, Maintz D, Schmiedel A, et al. High field MR imaging: magnetic field interactions of aneurysm clips, coronary artery stents and iliac artery stents with a 3.0 Tesla MR system. Rofo Fortschr Geb Rontgenstr Neuen Bildgeb Verfahr 2004;176:731-8.

Woods TO. Standards for medical devices in MRI: present and future. J Magn Reson Imaging. 2007;26:1186-9.

Woods TO. Guidance for Industry and FDA Staff - Establishing Safety and Compatibility of Passive Implants in the Magnetic Resonance (MR) Environment. Document issued on: August 21, 2008; http://www.fda.gov/cdrh/osel/guidance/1685.html

AccuRx Constant Flow Implantable Pump and DuraCath Intraspinal Catheter

AccuRx Constant Flow Implantable Pump. The AccuRx Constant Flow Implantable Pump (Advanced Neuromodulation Systems, Plano, TX) is an implantable device that stores and dispenses medication at a constant factory-set flow rate to a specific site. The pumps are available in a range of flow rates to allow physicians to tailor therapy to the needs of the patient.

The AccuRx Constant Flow Implantable Pump consists of a single sealed chamber formed between a rigid titanium shell and a polymeric diaphragm. The chamber holds the drug to be infused. The diaphragm exerts pressure on the medication causing it to flow out of the chamber through a series of filters and a flow restrictor, and then out the catheter (see DuraCath Intraspinal Catheter information below) to the delivery site. The AccuRx Constant Flow Implantable Pump is refilled through a raised refill port in the center of the titanium shell. Refilling the pump expands the diaphragm outward and starts the pump on the next cycle of drug infusion.

DuraCath Intraspinal Catheter. The DuraCath Intraspinal Catheter (Advanced Neuromodulation Systems, Plano, TX) is designed for long-term intraspinal (epidural or intrathecal) implantation. The trimmable, flexible, elastic radiopaque catheter incorporates insertion depth markings and a removable guide wire to facilitate implantation. This catheter has a closed tip and multiple side-exit channels to facilitate dispersion of the drug to reduce the probability of catheter tip complications. There are one- and two-piece versions of the DuraCath Intraspinal Catheter to suite a variety of clinical needs. The DuraCath Intraspinal Catheter is made from silicone and has a small connector made from 316L stainless steel.

MAGNETIC RESONANCE IMAGING (MRI) INFORMATION

Exposure of the AccuRx Constant Flow Implantable Pump and DuraCath Intraspinal Catheter to magnetic resonance imaging (MRI) fields of 1.5-Tesla has demonstrated no impact on pump or catheter performance and a limited effect on the quality of the diagnostic information. Testing performed on the AccuRx Constant Flow Implantable Pump and DuraCath Intraspinal Catheter has established the following with regard to MRI safety and diagnostic issues:

Static Magnetic Field. Testing demonstrated that a 1.5-Tesla magnetic resonance environment produced no measurable magnetic field interactions (i.e., translational attraction and torque) for the AccuRx Constant Flow Implantable Pump and DuraCath Intraspinal Catheter.

Heating During MRI. Testing demonstrated that little heating occurred for the AccuRx Constant Flow Implantable Pump in association with MR imaging conducted using an excessive amount of RF energy (i.e., a whole-body averaged specific absorption rate of 1.5 W/kg). Furthermore, heating was considered to be physiologically inconsequential and will not pose an additional risk to the patient undergoing an MR procedure under the conditions used for the evaluation. In the unlikely event that the patient experiences warmth near the pump, the MR procedure should be stopped immediately.

Peripheral Nerve Stimulation. The presence of the AccuRx Constant Flow Implantable Pump may cause a one-fold increase (doubling) of the induced gradient current in tissues near the device. This increase in the induced gradient current is similar to that already present elsewhere in the body (e.g., at bone-tissue interfaces) and, as such, will not cause nerve stimulation. In the unlikely event that the patient reports stimulation during the scan, the MR procedure should be stopped immediately.

REFERENCE

AccuRX Constant Flow Implantable Pumps, Technical Manual, Advanced Neuromodulation Systems, Inc., Plano, TX.

ActiFlo Indwelling Bowel Catheter System

The ActiFlo Indwelling Bowel Catheter System (also known as the Zassi Bowel Management System, Hollister, Libertyville, IL) is intended for diversion of fecal matter to minimize external contact with the patient's skin, to facilitate the collection of fecal matter for patients requiring stool management, to provide access for colonic irrigation and to administer enema/medications. This system consists of three main parts: the catheter, the collection bag, and the irrigation bag. The insertion end of the catheter contains a retention cuff and an intraluminal balloon, each with its own Luer connector used for inflation and deflation. A third connector provides a way to administer medications into the rectum and provides access for colonic irrigation. The ActiFlo Indwelling Bowel Catheter System allows stool to drain directly from the rectum into a closed or drainable collection bag.

MRI Information

The ActiFlo Indwelling Bowel Catheter System was determined to be MR conditional according to the terminology specified in the ASTM International, Designation: F2503-05. Standard Practice for Marking Medical Devices and Other Items for Safety in the Magnetic Resonance Environment:

Non-clinical testing demonstrated that this product is MR Conditional according to the following conditions:

-Static magnetic field of 3-Tesla or less

-Highest spatial gradient magnetic field of 720-Gauss/cm or less

Important note: A metallic spring used for this device is located outside of the patient's body during the intended *in vivo* use of this product. Therefore, the only possible MRI-related issue pertains to magnetic field interactions. Heating and artifacts are of no concern. As such, the assessment of magnetic field interactions for this product specifically involved evaluations of translational attraction and torque in relation to exposure to a 3-Tesla MR system, *only*. Evaluations of MRI-related heating and artifacts were not conducted and are unnecessary.

REFERENCE

http://www.hollister.co.za/us/

ActiPatch

ActiPatch (BioElectronics, Frederick, MD) is a medical, drug-free device that delivers pulsed electromagnetic frequency therapies to accelerate healing of soft tissue injuries. The ActiPatch has an embedded battery-operated microchip that delivers continuous pulsed therapy to reduce pain and swelling.

MRI and the ActiPatch

The ActiPatch must be removed prior to performing an MRI procedure to prevent possible damage to this device and the potential risk of excessive heating.

REFERENCE

http://www.bioelectronicscorp.com/

Alsius Intravascular Temperature Management

Alsius Corporation products are designed for placement in the central venous system. Via a proprietary, "closed loop" internal cooling circuit, the catheter cools or warms the patient's blood as it circulates past the catheter. The catheters (Cool Line, Icy, and Fortius) are attached to the CoolGard 3000 Thermal Regulation System, an electronic cooling system that regulates the cooling performance of the catheter via remote sensing of the patient's temperature. Alsius catheters are also designed to facilitate critical care management with features similar to those found in conventional central venous catheters.

CoolGard 3000. All Alsius heat exchange catheters connect to the CoolGard 3000 Thermal Regulation System, which achieves and maintains a target temperature input by the user. It remotely senses changes in patient core temperature and automatically adjusts the temperature of the circulating saline within the catheter (0-42°C), providing consistent maintenance of temperature. The CoolGard 3000 represents a powerful platform for current and future temperature management therapies as they are developed.

Cool Line Catheter. The Cool Line Catheter is inserted into the subclavian or jugular vein and resides in the superior vena cava. The Cool Line Catheter incorporates two proprietary, MicroTherm balloons which have sterile temperature-controlled saline flowing within a closed-loop design enabling direct heat exchange with the central circulation. The Cool Line Catheter combines temperature control and central venous catheter capabilities.

Icy Catheter. The Icy catheter is inserted into the femoral vein and resides in the inferior vena cava.

Fortius Catheter. The Fortius catheter is inserted percutaneously into the femoral vein residing in the inferior vena cava, just below the heart. The Fortius catheter provides maximum heat exchange power with minimum time to target temperature. This catheter incorporates a proprietary serpentine cooling balloon design to provide the ultimate solution for endovascular cooling therapy.

MRI Information

The following models of Alsius Heat Exchange catheters have been determined to be MR-safe:

1) Cool Line
2) Icy
3) Fortius

Magnetic resonance imaging (MRI) procedures must be performed according to the following guidelines:

Through non-clinical testing, these catheters were shown to be MR safe* at a field strength of 1.5 Tesla or less and a maximum whole body averaged specific absorption rate (SAR) of 2.0 W/kg for 20 minutes of MRI. MRI at 1.5-Tesla (highest spatial gradient, 2.4 Tesla/meter) or less may be performed immediately following the insertion of the one of these catheters.

MR image quality may be compromised if the area of interest is in the exact same area or relatively close to the position of these catheters. Therefore, it may be necessary to optimize the MRI parameters for the presence of these metallic devices.

IMPORTANT NOTE: The Alsius CoolGard 3000 system is NOT MRI Safe NOR Compatible NOR Intended for Use in an MRI environment. The Catheter should be disconnected from the System prior to moving the patient to the MRI facility.

[*Note the use of the term "MR Safe". These products underwent testing and labeling prior to the implementation of the current terminology. For further explanation, please refer to the section in this textbook, entitled: **Terminology for Implants and Devices.**]

REFERENCE

http://www.alsius.com

Ambulatory Infusion Systems

Ambulatory Infusion Systems (Smiths Medical) are designed to help healthcare providers administer medications accurately, monitor patient's response to therapy, stimulate early clinical assessment and facilitate patient recovery. These devices include the following:

CADD – 1 Ambulatory Infusion Pump
CADD – Legacy 1 Ambulatory Infusion Pump
CADD – Legacy Ambulatory Infusion Pump
CADD – Legacy PCA Ambulatory Infusion Pump
CADD – Legacy PLUS Ambulatory Infusion Pump
CADD – Micro Ambulatory Infusion Pump
CADD – MS 3 Ambulatory Infusion Pump
CADD – PCA Ambulatory Infusion Pump
CADD – PLUS Ambulatory Infusion Pump
CADD – Prizm PCS Ambulatory Infusion Pump
CADD – Prizm PCS II Ambulatory Infusion Pump
CADD – Prizm VIP Ambulatory Infusion Pump
CADD – Solis Ambulatory Infusion Pump
CADD – TPN Ambulatory Infusion Pump

MRI Information
Regarding the pump used for each device, the Operator's Manual states: "Magnetic fields produced by magnetic resonance imaging (MRI) equipment may adversely affect the operation of the pump. Remove the pump from the patient during MRI procedures and keep it at a safe distance from magnetic energy."

REFERENCES

http://www.smiths-medical.com/
http://www.smiths-medical.com/education-resources/downloads/infusion-systems/infusion-systems-downloads.html

Aneurysm Clips

The surgical management of intracranial aneurysms and arteriovenous malformations (AVMs) by the application of aneurysm clips is a well-established procedure. The presence of an aneurysm clip in a patient referred for an MR procedure represents a situation that requires the utmost consideration because of the associated risks.

Certain types of intracranial aneurysm clips (e.g., those made from martensitic stainless steels such as 17-7PH or 405 stainless steel) are a contraindication to the use of MR procedures because excessive, magnetically induced forces can displace these implants and cause serious injury or death. By comparison, aneurysm clips classified as "nonferromagnetic" or "weakly ferromagnetic" (e.g., those made from Phynox, Elgiloy, austentitic stainless steels, titanium alloy, or commercially pure titanium) are acceptable for patients undergoing MR procedures (additional information on performing MR procedures in patients with aneurysm clips is provided in the section entitled, **Extremity MR System***).

[For the sake of discussion, the term "weakly magnetic" refers to metal that may demonstrate some extremely low ferromagnetic qualities using highly sensitive measurements techniques (e.g., vibrating sample magnetometer, superconducting quantum interference device or SQUID magnetometer, etc.) and as such, may not be technically referred to as being "nonmagnetic." All metals possess some degree of magnetism, such that no metal is entirely "nonmagnetic".]

MR procedures have been used to evaluate patients with certain types of aneurysm clips. Becker et al., using MR systems that ranged from 0.35 to 0.6-Tesla, studied three patients with nonferromagnetic aneurysm clips (one patient, Yasargil, 316 LVM stainless steel; two patients, Vari-Angle McFadden, MP35N; 316 LVM) and one patient with a ferromagnetic aneurysm clip (Heifetz aneurysm clip) without incident. Dujovny et al. similarly reported no adverse effects in patients with nonferromagnetic aneurysm clips that underwent procedures using 1.5-Tesla MR systems.

Pride et al. performed a study in patients with nonferromagnetic aneurysm clips that underwent MR imaging. There were no adverse outcomes for the patients, confirming that MR procedures can be performed safely in patients with nonferromagnetic clips. Brothers et al.

also demonstrated that MR imaging at 1.5-Tesla can be performed safely in patients with nonmagnetic aneurysm clips. This report was particularly important because, according to Brothers et al., MR imaging was found to be better than CT in the postoperative assessment of aneurysm patients, especially with regard to showing small zones of ischemia.

To date, only one ferromagnetic aneurysm clip-related fatality has been reported in the peer-reviewed literature. According to this report, the patient became symptomatic at a distance of approximately 1.2-meters from the bore of the MR system, suggesting that translational attraction of the aneurysm clip was likely responsible for dislodgment of this implant.

This incident was the result of erroneous information pertaining to the type of aneurysm clip that was present in the patient. That is, the clip was thought to be a nonmagnetic Yasargil aneurysm clip (Aesculap Inc., Central Valley, PA) and turned out to be a magnetic Vari-Angle clip (Codman & Shurtleff, Randolf, MA).

There has never been a report of an injury to a patient or individual in the MR environment related to the presence of an aneurysm clip made from a nonmagnetic or "weakly" magnetic material. In fact, there have been cases in which patients with ferromagnetic aneurysm clips (based on the extent of the artifact seen during MR imaging or other information) have undergone MR procedures without sustaining injuries (Personal communications, D. Kroker, 1995; E. Kanal, 1996; A. Osborne, 2002).

In these cases, the aneurysm clips were exposed to magnetic-induced translational attraction and torque associated with MR systems that had static magnetic fields of up to 1.5-Tesla. Although these cases do not prove or suggest safety, they do demonstrate the difficulty of predicting the outcome for patients with ferromagnetic aneurysm clips that undergo MR procedures. Variables to consider include the size, shape (especially the length of the blade), mass and material of the aneurysm clip.

There is controversy regarding the amount of ferromagnetism that needs to be present in an aneurysm clip to constitute a hazard for a patient in the MR environment. Consequently, this issue has not only created problems for MR healthcare professionals but for manufacturers of aneurysm clips, as well.

For example, MR healthcare professionals performing tests on aneurysm clips similar to the method described in the report by Kanal et al. (1996) presumably identified the presence of magnetic field interactions and returned several clips made from Phynox to the manufacturer (Personal Communication, Aesculap, Inc., South San Francisco, CA, 1997). However, the testing method used by Kanal et al. (1996) was admittedly crude and developed to primarily obtain rapid, qualitative screening data for large numbers of aneurysm clips to determine if quantitative assessments were necessary. Importantly, the test technique used by Kanal et al. (1996) may be problematic and yield spurious results, especially if the aneurysm clip has a shape or configuration that is somewhat "unstable" (Unpublished Observations, F.G. Shellock, 1997). For example, aneurysm clips with blades that are bayonet, curved, or angled shapes are less stable on a piece of plate glass (i.e., using the testing method described by Kanal et al.) when placed in certain orientations compared with aneurysm clips with blades that are straight.

A variety of more appropriate testing techniques have been developed and utilized over the years to evaluate the relative amount of ferromagnetism present for implants and devices prior to allowing patients with these objects to enter the MR environment. In 2002, the American Society for Testing and Materials (ASTM) provided recommendations for testing passive implants that involves the use of the deflection angle test, originally described by New et al., to assess translational attraction. Additionally, the U.S. Food and Drug Administration recommends that an evaluation of torque should be performed on aneurysm clips. Thus, procedures such as the deflection angle test and some form of evaluation of torque (qualitative or quantitative) are the most appropriate means of determining which specific aneurysm clip may present a hazard to a patient or individual in the MR environment.

Aneurysm Clips and MRI Procedures: Guidelines. In consideration of the knowledge pertaining to aneurysm clips, the following guidelines are recommended with regard to performing an MR procedure in a patient with an aneurysm clip or before allowing an individual with an aneurysm clip into the MR environment:

1) Specific information (i.e., manufacturer, type or model, material, lot and serial numbers) about the aneurysm clip must be known, especially with respect to the material used to make the aneurysm clip, so that only patients or individuals with nonferromagnetic or weakly ferromagnetic clips are allowed into the MR environment. The manufacturer provides this information in the labeling of the aneurysm clip. The implanting surgeon is responsible for properly recording and communicating this information in the patient's or individual's records.

2) An aneurysm clip that is in its original package and made from Phynox, Elgiloy, MP35N, titanium alloy, commercially pure titanium or other material known to be nonferromagnetic or weakly

ferromagnetic does not need to be evaluated for ferromagnetism. Aneurysm clips made from nonferrromagnetic or "weakly" ferromagnetic materials in original packages do not require testing of ferromagnetism because the manufacturers ensure the pertinent MR safety or conditional aspects of these clips and, therefore, are responsible for the accuracy of the labeling.

3) If the aneurysm clip is not in its original package and/or properly labeled, it should undergo testing for magnetic field interactions following appropriate testing procedures to determine if it is safe or unsafe for the MR environment.

4) The radiologist and implanting surgeon are responsible for evaluating the information pertaining to the aneurysm clip, verifying its accuracy, obtaining written documentation, and deciding to perform the MR procedure after considering the risk vs. benefit aspects for a given patient.

5) Consideration must be give to the static magnetic field strength that is to be used for the MRI procedure and the strength of the static magnetic field that was used to test magnetic field interactions for the aneurysm clip in question.

MRI at 3-Tesla and Aneurysm Clips. Many aneurysm clips have been tested for magnetic field interactions in association with 3-Tesla MR systems (refer to **The List** for information for aneurysm clips tested at 3-Tesla). Findings for these specific implants indicated that they either exhibited no magnetic field interactions or relatively minor or "weak" magnetic field interactions. Accordingly, these particular aneurysm clips are considered acceptable for patients undergoing MR procedures using MR systems operating at 3-Tesla or less.

Yasargil Aneurysm Clips (Information dated 11/11/09 - Aesculap Inc., Center Valley, PA)

Aesculap currently markets two lines of YASARGIL aneurysm clips, one from a cobalt-chrome alloy ("Phynox") and one from a titanium alloy. Phynox clips have been available since 1983 and have catalog numbers that begin with "FE". Titanium clips have been available since 1997 and have catalog numbers that begin with "FT". All "FE" and "FT" model YASARGIL aneurysm clips are non-ferromagnetic and may be safely exposed to MRI. Both implant materials have been tested and proven MR-safe as per ASTM-2052-02 up to 3.0 Tesla*.

Prior to 1985, Aesculap distributed various models of aneurysm clips manufactured from stainless steel. These aneurysm clips were identified with the letters "FD" and have not been proven safe under exposure to

MRI. For this reason, **Aesculap <u>does not</u> recommend the use of MRI on a patient implanted with a YASARGIL aneurysm clip identified with the letters "FD".**

For additional information, please refer to the following three scientific publications:

1)   Dujovny, M., et. al. (1985). *Aneurysm clip motion during magnetic resonance imaging: in vivo experimental study with metallurgical factor analysis, Journal of Neurosurgery,. 17(4), 543-548.*

2)   *Shellock, F.G, Kanal, E.,. (1998). Aneurysm clips: evaluation of MR imaging artifacts at 1.5. Radiology, 209(2), 563-566.*

3)   Romner, B., et. al. (1989).   *Magnetic resonance imaging and aneurysm clips, Journal of Neurosurgery, 70(3), 426-431.*

*These Aesculap devices were cleared by FDA as "MR-Safe" per ASTM-2052-02. Due to a change in definition within this standard (F 2503-2005-08), these devices are now termed as "MR Conditional" by ASTM. The FDA has not mandated a revision to our labeling because the device material and performance have not changed.

Aneurysm Clips, Codman & Shurtleff, Inc., a Johnson & Johnson Company, Raynham, MA

Recently, three different MP35N aneurysm clips (Codman Slim-Line Aneurysm Clip, Straight, Blade length 25-mm; Codman Slim-Line Aneurysm Clip Graft, 5-mm Diameter X 5-mm width; Codman Slim-Line Aneurysm Clip, Reinforcing 30-degree angle, 6-mm X 18-mm; Codman & Shurtleff, Inc., a Johnson & Johnson Company, Raynham, MA) underwent MRI testing that represented the largest mass for 155 additional clips made from MP35N. The clips were evaluated at 3-Tesla for magnetic field interactions, heating, and artifacts. Each aneurysm clip showed relatively minor magnetic field interactions that will not cause movement *in situ*. Heating was not excessive (highest temperature change, < 1.8°C). Artifacts may create issues if the area of interest is in the same area or close to the aneurysm clip. The results of this investigation demonstrated that it would be acceptable (i.e., "MR conditional" using current terminology) for patients with these aneurysm clips to undergo MRI at 3-Tesla or less. Notably, in consideration of the sizes of the clips that underwent testing, these findings pertain to 155 additional aneurysm clips made from the same material, which includes the following:

Codman Slim-Line Aneurysm Clip
Codman AVM Micro Clip
Codman Slim-Line Aneurysm Clip Graft
Codman Slim-Line Mini Aneurysm Clip
Codman Slim-Line Temporary Vessel Aneurysm Clip

The following is the MRI labeling for these aneurysm clips approved by the Food and Drug Administration:

Magnetic Resonance Imaging Information

Non-clinical testing of representative configurations of **Codman Slim-Line Aneurysm, Mini, Micro and Graft Clips** (Codman Slim-Line Clips) up to 25-mm in blade length has demonstrated that they are **MR Conditional.** A patient with one such clip up to 25-mm in blade length (i.e., Codman Slim-Line Aneurysm, Mini, Micro and Graft Clips (Codman Slim-Line Clips) can be scanned safely, immediately after placement under the following conditions.

3.0 Tesla Systems:

- Static magnetic field of 3.0 Tesla.
- Spatial gradient magnetic field of 720 Gauss/cm or less.
- Maximum MR system reported, whole-body-averaged specific absorption rate (SAR) of 3.0 W/kg for 15 minutes of scanning (i.e., per pulse sequence).

MRI Related Heating

MRI related heating was assessed for the representative configurations of the Codman clips (up to 25-mm in blade length) following guidelines provided in ASTM F2182-02a. A maximum temperature change equal to or less than 1.8 ° C was observed during testing (parameters listed below).

Parameters:

- Maximum MR system-reported, whole-body-averaged SAR of 3.0 W/kg (associated calorimetry measured whole body averaged value of 2.8 W/kg).
- 15-minute duration MR scanning (i.e., per pulse sequence).
- 3 Tesla MR System (EXCITE MR Scanner, Software G3 .0-052B, General Electric Healthcare, Milwaukee, WI) using a transmit/receive RF body coil.

Artifact Information

Artifacts were assessed for representative clip configurations using T1-weighted spin echo (T1-SE) and gradient echo (GRE) pulse sequences following methods similar to the guidelines provided in ASTM F2119-07. The 25-mm blade-length aneurysm clip imaged using a GRE pulse sequence produced an artifact that extended approximately 5-cm from the clip in the parallel (long-axis) imaging plane. The void size corresponding to this artifact was approximately 1251-mm^2. MR image quality may be compromised if the area of interest is in the exact location or within a few centimeters of the Codman Slim-Line Clip. In general, the GRE pulse sequence produced larger artifacts than the T1-SE sequence for each clip. However, MRI artifacts can be minimized by careful selection of pulse sequence parameters.

MRI at 8.0-Tesla and Aneurysm Clips. *Ex vivo* testing has been conducted to identify potentially hazardous implants and devices using an 8-Tesla MR system. The first investigation to determine magnetic field interactions for aneurysm clips exposed to the 8.0-Tesla MR system was conducted by Kangarlu and Shellock.

Twenty-six different aneurysm clips were tested for magnetic field interactions using previously-described techniques. These implants were specifically selected for this investigation because they represent various types of clips used for temporary or permanent treatment of aneurysms or arteriovenous malformations. Additionally, these aneurysm clips were reported previously to be safe for patients undergoing MR procedures using MR systems with static magnetic field strengths of 1.5-Tesla or less.

According to the results, six aneurysm clips (i.e., type, model, blade length) made from stainless steel alloy (Perneczky) and Phynox (Yasargil, Models FE 748 and FE 750) displayed deflection angles above 45 degrees (i.e., referring to the guideline stated by the American Society for Testing and Materials, ASTM) and relatively high qualitative torque values. These findings indicated that these specific aneurysm clips may be unsafe for individuals or patients in an 8.0-Tesla or higher MR environment.

Aneurysm clips made from commercially pure titanium (Spetzler), Elgiloy (Sugita), titanium alloy (Yasargil, Model FE 750T), and MP35N (Sundt) displayed deflection angles less than 45 degrees (i.e., referring to the ASTM guideline) and qualitative torque values that were relatively minor. Accordingly, these aneurysm clips are considered to be acceptable for patients or individuals exposed to an 8.0-Tesla MR system.

As previously indicated, at 1.5-Tesla, aneurysm clips that are considered to be acceptable for patients or others in the MR environment include those made from commercially pure titanium, titanium alloy, Elgiloy, Phynox, and austentic stainless steel. By comparison, findings from the 8.0-Tesla study indicated that deflection angles for the aneurysm clips made from commercially pure titanium and titanium alloy ranged from 5 to 6 degrees, suggesting that these aneurysm clips would be safe for patients or individuals in the 8.0-Tesla MR environment. However, deflection angles for aneurysm clips made from Elgiloy ranged from 36 to 42 degrees, such that further consideration must be given to the specific type of Elgiloy clip that is present. For example, an Elgiloy clip that has a greater mass than those tested in this study may exceed a deflection angle of 45 degrees (i.e., referring to the ASTM guideline of 45 degrees or less being acceptable for translational attraction) in association with an 8.0-Tesla MR system.

Depending on the actual dimensions and mass, an aneurysm clip made from Elgiloy may or may not be acceptable for a patient or individual in the 8.0-Tesla MR environment. Notably, the results of this investigation are specific to the types of intracranial aneurysm clips that underwent testing (i.e., with regard model, shape, size, blade length, material, etc.) as well as the spatial gradient associated with the 8.0-Tesla MR system.

Effects of Long-Term and Multiple Exposures to the MR System. MR testing procedures used for aneurysm clips over the past few years would result in the potential for reintroduction of aneurysm clips into strong magnetic fields several times prior to implantation into the patient. Furthermore, there are patients with implanted aneurysm clips previously tested and designated as "MR-safe" or "MR-conditional" that have undergone repeated exposures to strong magnetic fields during follow-up MR examinations.

A concern has emerged that a potential alteration in the magnetic properties of pre-or post-implanted aneurysm clips may occur that results from long-term or multiple exposures to strong magnetic fields. Long-term or multiple exposures to strong magnetic fields (such as those associated with MR imaging systems) have been suggested to grossly "magnetize" aneurysm clips, even if they are made from nonferromagnetic or weakly ferromagnetic materials. This could present a substantial hazard to an individual in the MR environment. Therefore, an *in vitro* investigation was conducted to study intracranial aneurysm clips prior to and following long-term and multiple exposures to 1.5-Tesla MR systems. This was done to quantify possible alterations in the magnetic properties of these aneurysm clips.

Aneurysm clips made from Elgiloy, Phynox, titanium alloy, commercially pure titanium, and austenitic stainless steel were tested in association with long-term and multiple exposures to 1.5-Tesla MR systems. The findings indicated that there was a lack of response to the magnetic field exposure conditions that were used, such that long-term or multiple exposures to 1.5-Tesla MR systems should not result in significant changes in their magnetic properties.

Artifacts Associated with Aneurysm Clips. An additional problem related to aneurysm clips is that artifacts produced by these metallic implants may substantially detract from the diagnostic aspects of MR procedures. MR imaging, MR angiography, and functional MRI are frequently used to evaluate the brain or cerebral vasculature of patients with aneurysm clips. For example, to reduce morbidity and mortality after subarachnoid hemorrhage, it is imperative to assess the results of the surgical treatment of cerebral aneurysms.

The extent of the artifact produced by a given aneurysm clip will have a direct effect on the diagnostic aspects of the MR procedure. Therefore, an investigation was conducted to characterize artifacts associated with aneurysm clips made from nonferromagnetic or weakly ferromagnetic materials. Five different aneurysm clips made from five different materials were evaluated in this investigation, as follows:

1) Yasargil, Phynox (Aesculap, Inc., Central Valley, PA),
2) Yasargil, titanium alloy (Aesculap, Inc., Central Valley, PA),
3) Sugita, Elgiloy (Mizuho American, Inc., Beverly, MA),
4) Spetzler Titanium Aneurysm Clip, commercially pure titanium (Elekta Instruments, Inc., Atlanta, GA), and
5) Perneczky, cobalt alloy (Zepplin Chirurgishe Instrumente, Pullach, Germany).

These aneurysm clips were selected for testing because they are made from nonferromagnetic or weakly ferromagnetic materials. These aneurysm clips have been previously reported to be acceptable for patients in the 1.5-Tesla MR environment and, as such, are often found in patients referred for MR procedures.

MR imaging artifact testing revealed that the size of the signal voids were directly related to the type of material (i.e., the magnetic susceptibility) used to make the particular clip. Arranged in decreasing order of artifact size, the materials responsible for the artifacts associated with the aneurysm clips were, as follows: Elgiloy (Sugita), cobalt alloy (Perneczky), Phynox (Yasargil), titanium alloy (Yasargil), and commercially pure titanium (Spetzler). These results have implications when one considers the various critical factors that are responsible for the decision to use a particular type of aneurysm clip (e.g., size, shape, closing force, biocompatibility, corrosion resistance, material-related effects on diagnostic imaging examinations, etc.).

An aneurysm clip that causes a relatively large artifact is less desirable because it can impact the diagnostic capabilities of the MR procedure if the area of interest is in the immediate location of where the aneurysm clip was implanted. Fortunately, aneurysm clips exist that are made from materials (i.e., commercially pure titanium and titanium alloy) that created minimal artifacts.

Burtscher et al. conducted additional artifact research with the intent of determining the extent to which titanium aneurysm clips could improve the quality of MR imaging compared to stainless steel aneurysm clips and to assess whether the associated artifacts could be reduced by controlling MR imaging parameters. The results of this investigation indicated that the use of titanium aneurysm clips reduced MR artifacts by approximately 60% compared to stainless steel aneurysm clips. MR imaging artifacts were further reduced by using spin echo pulse sequences with high bandwidths or, if necessary, gradient echo pulse sequences with a low echo times (TE).

REFERENCES

American Society for Testing and Materials (ASTM) Designation: F 2052. Standard test method for measurement of magnetically induced displacement force on passive implants in the magnetic resonance environment. In: Annual Book of ASTM Standards, Section 13, Medical Devices and Services, Volume 13.01 Medical Devices; Emergency Medical Services. West Conshohocken, PA, 2002, pp. 1576-1580.

Becker RL, Norfray JF, Teitelbaum GP, et al. MR imaging in patients with intracranial aneurysm clips. Am J Roentgenol 1988;9:885-889.

Brothers MF, Fox AJ, Lee DH, Pelz DM, Deveikis JP. MR imaging after surgery for vertebrobasilar aneurysm. Am J Neuroradiol 1990;11:149-161.

Brown MA, Carden JA, Coleman RE, et al. Magnetic field effects on surgical ligation clips. Magn Reson Imaging 1987;5:443-453.

Burtscher IM, Owman T, Romner B, Stahlberg F, Holtas S. Aneurysm clip MR artifacts. Titanium versus stainless steel and influence of imaging parameters. Acta Radiology 1998;39:70-76.

Dujovny M, Kossovsky N, Kossowsky R, et al. Aneurysm clip motion during magnetic resonance imaging: *in vivo* experimental study with metallurgical factor analysis. Neurosurgery 1985;17:543-548.

Kanal E, Barkovich AJ, Bell C, et al. ACR guidance document for safe MR practices: 2007. AJR Am J Roentgenol. 2007;188:1447-1474.

FDA stresses the need for caution during MR scanning of patients with aneurysm clips. In: Medical Devices Bulletin, Center for Devices and Radiological Health. March, 1993;11:1-2.

Johnson GC. Need for caution during MR imaging of patients with aneurysm clips [Letter]. Radiology 1993;188:287.

Kanal E, Shellock FG. MR imaging of patients with intracranial aneurysm clips. Radiology 1993;187:612-614.

Kanal E, Shellock FG. Aneurysm clips: effects of long-term and multiple exposures to a 1.5-Tesla MR system. Radiology 1999;210:563-565.

Kanal E, Shellock FG, Lewin JS. Aneurysm clip testing for ferromagnetic properties: clip variability issues. Radiology 1996;200:576-578.

Kangarlu A, Shellock FG. Aneurysm clips: evaluation of magnetic field interactions with an 8.0-T MR system. J Magn Reson Imaging 2000;12:107-111.

Klucznik RP, Carrier DA, Pyka R, Haid RW. Placement of a ferromagnetic intracerebral aneurysm clip in a magnetic field with a fatal outcome. Radiology 1993;187:855-856.

Lauer UA, Graf H, Berger A, Claussen CD, Schick F. Radio frequency versus susceptibility effects of small conductive implants-a systematic MRI study on aneurysm clips at 1.5 and 3 T. Magn Reson Imaging 2005;23:563-9.

New PFJ, Rosen BR, Brady TJ, et al. Potential hazards and artifacts of ferromagnetic and nonferromagnetic surgical and dental materials and devices in nuclear magnetic resonance imaging. Radiology 1983;147:139-148.

Olsrud J, Latt J, Brockstedt S, Romner B, Bjorkman-Burtscher IM. Magnetic resonance imaging artifacts caused by aneurysm clips and shunt valves: dependence on field strength (1.5 and 3 T) and imaging parameters. J Magn Reson Imaging 2005;22:433-7.

Pride GL, Kowal J, Mendelsohn DB, Chason DP, Fleckenstein JL. Safety of MR scanning in patients with nonferromagnetic aneurysm clips. J Magn Reson Imaging 2000;12:198-200.

Shellock FG. Magnetic Resonance Procedures: Health Effects and Safety. CRC Press, LLC, Boca Raton, FL, 2001.

Shellock FG. Magnetic resonance procedures and aneurysm clips: A review. Signals, No. 33, Issue 2, pp. 17-20, 2000.

Shellock FG. Biomedical implants and devices: assessment of magnetic field interactions with a 3.0-Tesla MR system. J Magn Reson Imaging 2002;16:721-732.

Shellock FG, Tkach JA, Ruggieri PM, Masaryk T, Rasmussen P. Aneurysm clips: evaluation of magnetic field interactions and translational attraction using "long-bore" and "short-bore" 3.0-Tesla MR systems. American Journal of Neuroradiology 2003;24:463-471.

Shellock FG, Crues JV. High-field strength MR imaging and metallic biomedical implants: an *ex vivo* evaluation of deflection forces. Am J Roentgenol 1988;151:389-392.

Shellock FG, Crues JV. Aneurysm clips: Assessment of magnetic field interaction associated with a 0.2-T extremity MR system. Radiology 1998;208:407-409.

Shellock FG, Kanal E. Aneurysm clips: Evaluation of MR imaging artifacts at 1.5-Tesla. Radiology 1998;209:563-566.

Shellock FG, Kanal E. Magnetic Resonance: Bioeffects, Safety, and Patient Management. Second Edition, Lippincott-Raven Press, New York, 1996.

Shellock FG, Kanal E. Yasargil aneurysm clips: evaluation of interactions with a 1.5-Tesla MR system. Radiology 1998;207:587-591.

Shellock FG, Shellock VJ. MR-compatibility evaluation of the Spetzler titanium aneurysm clip. Radiology 1998;206:838-841.

Shellock FG. Valencerina S. *In vitro* evaluation of MRI issues at 3-Tesla for aneurysm clips: findings and information that pertain to 154 additional aneurysm clips. American Journal of Neuroradiology (in press)

Baha, Bone Conduction Implant

What is Baha?

The Baha system (Cochlear Americas, Englewood, Colorado) utilizes the body's natural ability to conduct sound. Bone, like air, conducts sound vibrations. For people with hearing loss, this provides another pathway to perceive sound.

Typical hearing aids rely on air conduction and a functioning middle ear. In cases where the middle ear function may be blocked, damaged or occluded, the Baha system may be a better option as it bypasses the middle ear altogether. Instead, sound is sent around the damaged or problematic area, naturally stimulating the cochlea through bone conduction. Once the cochlea receives these sound vibrations, the organ 'hears' in the same manner as through air conduction; the sound is converted into neural signals and is transferred to the brain, allowing a Baha recipient to perceive sound.

How does it work?

We receive sound in two ways, by air conduction via the ear canal, eardrum, and ossicles, and by bone conduction. Bone conduction transmits sound directly though the bones in the jaw and skull, bypassing the outer and middle ear.

In most cases, those with a hearing loss will be fitted with traditional air conduction devices. Typically, these hearing aids are placed inside the ear canal or behind the ear. However, some people are unable to benefit from this type of device.

The Baha system, which is based on bone conduction, utilizes a titanium implant, which is placed in the skull bone behind the ear. An abutment connects the sound processor with the implant in the bone. This creates direct (percutaneous) bone conduction. In contrast, traditional bone conductors connect indirectly to the bone through unbroken skin (transcutaneous) and work by exerting pressure against the skull.

Direct bone conduction, provided by Baha, gives improved access to sound when compared to traditional bone conductors since sound is not weakened when passing through the skin. This unique hearing treatment is the only system of its kind cleared by the U.S. Food and Drug Administration (FDA) to treat hearing loss.

One reason the Baha system works so well is due to its simple design. The Baha system combines a sound processor with an abutment and a small titanium implant. The implant is placed behind the non-functioning ear. Surgery is minor, and Baha recipients report a wide range of advantages over other hearing devices.

MRI INFORMATION

Can I wear the sound processor if I have to undergo an MRI?

The sound processor should be removed prior to undergoing an MRI, but the titanium implant will not pose any risk. Cochlear (Cochlear Americas, Englewood, Colorado) provides wearers with MRI and security check information card.

[MR healthcare professionals are advised to contact the respective manufacturer in order to obtain the latest safety information to ensure patient safety relative to the use of an MR procedure.]

REFERENCE

http://www.cochlearamericas.com/

Biopsy Needles, Markers, and Devices

Magnetic resonance (MR) imaging has been used to guide tissue biopsy and apply markers for many years. These specialized procedures require tools that are acceptable for use with MR systems. Many commercially available biopsy needles, markers, and devices (i.e., guide wires, stylets, marking wires, marking clips, biopsy guns, etc.) have been evaluated with respect to producing artifacts and being safe with MR procedures. The results have indicated that most of the commercially available biopsy needles, markers, and devices are not useful for MR-guided biopsy procedures due to the presence of excessive ferromagnetism and the associated artifacts that may limit or obscure the area of interest.

For many of the commercially available devices, studies have reported that the presence of ferromagnetic biopsy needles and lesion marking wires in a tissue phantom used for testing produced such substantial artifacts that they would not be useful for MR-guided procedures. Needles or devices containing any type of ferromagnetic material tend to have too much magnetic susceptibility to allow effective use for MR-guided procedures. Fortunately, several needles, markers, and devices have been constructed using materials with low magnetic susceptibility specifically for use in MR-guided procedures.

Although most of the biopsy guns tested for magnetic field interactions and artifacts were found to be ferromagnetic, since they are not used in the immediate area of the target tissue, artifacts associated with these devices are unlikely to affect the resulting images during MR-guided biopsy procedures. Nevertheless, the presence of ferromagnetism may preclude the optimal use of most biopsy guns in the MR environment, especially if a 3-Tesla scanner is being used for the procedure. Currently, there are several commercially available biopsy devices, including vacuum-assisted systems, developed specifically for use in MR-guided procedures.

REFERENCES

Causer PA, Piron CA, Jong RA, et al. MR imaging-guided breast localization system with medial or lateral access. Radiology. 2006;240:369-79.

Chen X, Lehman CD, Dee KE. MRI-guided breast biopsy: clinical experience with 14-gauge stainless steel core biopsy needle. AJR Am J Roentgenol. 2004;182:1075-80.

Daniel BL, Freeman LJ, Pyzoha JM, et al. An MRI-compatible semiautomated vacuum-assisted breast biopsy system: initial feasibility study. J Magn Reson Imaging. 2005;21:637-44.

Hall WA, Galicich W, Bergman T, Truwit CL. 3-Tesla intraoperative MR imaging for neurosurgery. J Neurooncol. 2006;77:297-303.

Lehman CD, Eby PR, Chen X, Dee KE, Thursten B, McCloskey J. MR imaging-guided breast biopsy using a coaxial technique with a 14-gauge stainless steel core biopsy needle and a titanium sheath. AJR Am J Roentgenol. 2003;181:183-5.

Lewin JS, et al. Needle localization in MR-guided biopsy and aspiration: Effect of field strength, sequence design, and magnetic field orientation. AJR Am J Roentgenol 1996;166:1337-1341.

Lufkin R, Layfield L. Coaxial needle system of MR- and CT-guided aspiration cytology. J Computer Assist Tomogr 1989;13:1105-1107.

Lufkin R, Teresi L, Hanafee W. New needle for MR-guided aspiration cytology of the head and neck. AJR Am J Roentgenol 1987;149:380-382.

Moscatel M, Shellock FG, Morisoli S. Biopsy needles and devices: assessment of ferromagnetism and artifacts during exposure to a 1.5-Tesla MR system. J Magn Reson Imaging 1995;5:369-372.

Shellock FG. Magnetic Resonance Procedures: Health Effects and Safety. CRC Press, LLC, Boca Raton, FL, 2001.

Shellock FG, Kanal E. Magnetic Resonance: Bioeffects, Safety, and Patient Management. Second Edition, Lippincott-Raven Press, New York, 1996.

Shellock FG, Shellock VJ. Additional information pertaining to the MR-compatibility of biopsy needles and devices. J Magn Reson Imaging 1996;6:411.

Shellock FG, Shellock VJ. Metallic marking clips used after stereotactic breast biopsy: *ex vivo* testing of ferromagnetism, heating, and artifacts associated with MRI. AJR Am J Roentgenol 1999;172:1417-1419.

Veltman J, Boetes C, Wobbes T, Blickman JG, Barentsz JO. Magnetic resonance-guided biopsies and localizations of the breast: initial experiences using an open breast coil and compatible intervention device. Invest Radiol. 2005;40:379-84.

Zangos S, Herzog C, Eichler K, et al. MR-compatible assistance system for punction in a high-field system: device and feasibility of transgluteal biopsies of the prostate gland. Eur Radiol. 2007;17:1118-24.

Bone Fusion Stimulator/Spinal Fusion Stimulator

The implantable bone fusion or spinal fusion stimulator (EBI, LLC., Biomet, Inc.) is designed for use as an adjunct therapy to a spinal fusion procedure. The implantable spinal fusion stimulator consists of a direct current generator with a lithium iodine battery and solid-state electronics encased in a titanium shell, partially-coated with platinum that acts as an anode. The generator is implanted beneath the skin and muscle near the vertebral column and provides the full-rated current for approximately 24 to 26 weeks. The use of this electronic implant provides a faster consolidation of the bone grafts, leading to higher fusion rates and improved surgical outcomes, along with a reduced need for orthopedic instrumentation.

Studies using excessively-high electromagnetic fields under highly-specific experimental conditions and modeling scenarios for the lumbar/torso area (i.e., 1.5-Tesla MR system, excessive exposures to RF fields, excessive exposures to gradient magnetic fields, etc.) have demonstrated that the implantable spinal fusion stimulator will not present a hazard to a patient undergoing MR imaging with respect to movement, heating, or induced electrical fields during the use of conventional MR techniques.

Additionally, there was no evidence of malfunction of the implantable spinal fusion stimulator based on *in vitro* and *in vivo* experimental findings. These studies addressed the use of conventional pulse sequences and parameters with an acknowledgement that echo planar techniques or imaging parameters that require excessive RF power will have different implications and consequences for the patient with an implantable spinal fusion stimulator.

To date, MR examinations have been performed in many patients (conceivably, using MR imaging conditions that involved a wide-variety of imaging parameters and conditions) with implantable spinal fusion stimulators with no reports of substantial adverse events (based on a review of data obtained through the Freedom of Information Act and Unpublished Observations, Simon BJ, EBI, LLC, Parsippany, NJ).

In an *in vivo* study, there were no reports of immediate or delayed (minimum of one month follow up) adverse events from patients with implantable spinal fusion stimulators who underwent MR imaging at 1.5-Tesla. Each patient was visually inspected following the MRI study and there was no evidence of excessive heating (i.e., change in skin color or other similar response).

One patient indicated a sensation of "warming" felt at the site of the stimulator, however, this feeling was described as minor and the MR examination was completed without further indication of unusual sensations or problems. Of further note is that there were no reports of excessive heating or neuromuscular stimulation in association with the presence of the implantable spinal fusion stimulators in patients that underwent MR procedures.

Chou et al. conducted a thorough investigation of the effect of heating of the implantable spinal fusion stimulator associated with MR imaging. This work was performed using a human phantom during MR procedures involving a relatively high exposure to RF energy (i.e., at whole body averaged specific absorption rates of approximately 1.0-W/kg). Fluoroptic thermometry probes were placed at various positions on and near the cathodes, leads, and the stimulator for each experiment to record temperature changes.

The phantom used by Chou et al. did not include the effects of blood flow, which obviously would help dissipate heating that may occur during MR imaging and, therefore, it further represents an excessive RF exposure condition. With the implantable spinal fusion stimulator in place and the leads intact, the maximum temperature rise after 25 minutes of scanning occurred at the center of the stimulator and was less than 2 degrees C.

The temperature rise at the cathodes was less than 1 degree C. When the stimulator was removed, the maximum temperature rise was less than 1.5 degrees C, recorded at the tip of the electrode with insignificant temperature changes occurring at the cathode. These temperature changes are within physiologically acceptable ranges for the tissues where the implantable spinal fusion stimulator is implanted, especially considering that the temperatures for muscle and subcutaneous tissues are at levels that are known to be several degrees below the normal core temperature of 37 degrees C.

Chou et al. also investigated heating of the tips of broken leads of the implantable spinal fusion stimulator (this device was the same as that which underwent testing in the present study). Temperature changes occurred in localized regions that were within a few millimeters of the cut ends of the leads, with maximum temperature increases that ranged from 11 to 14 degrees C.

If these levels of temperatures occurred during MR imaging, the amount of possible tissue damage would be comparable in characteristics and clinical significance to a small electrosurgical lesion and would likely occur in the scar tissue that typically forms around the implanted leads. Additionally, the potential for tissue damage is only theoretical and a brief temperature elevation around a broken lead, over an approximated volume of 2- to 3-mm radius may not be clinically worse than the scar tissue that forms over the leads during implantation. Fortunately, broken leads are rare, occurring in approximately 10 out of the 70,000 devices implanted over the last ten years (Personal Communication, Simon BJ, EBI, LLC, Parsippany, NJ).

Based on findings from the various investigations that have been conducted, RF energy-induced heating during MR imaging does not appear to present a major problem for a patient with the implantable spinal fusion stimulator, as long as there is no broken lead. Accordingly, the integrity of the leads should be assessed using a radiograph prior to the MR procedure.

MRI Safety Information - SpF-XL IIb
SpF-XL IIb Model

Safety information for the use of Magnetic Resonance Imaging (MRI) procedures (i.e., imaging, angiography, functional imaging, spectroscopy, etc.) pertains to shielded MRI systems with static magnetic fields of 1.5 Tesla or less (maximum spatial gradient 450 gauss/cm), gradient magnetic fields of 20 Tesla/second or less, and a maximum whole body averaged Specific Absorption Rate (SAR) of 1.1 W/kg for 25 minutes of imaging. The effects of MRI procedures using MR systems and conditions above these levels have not been determined.

The **SpF** devices have been determined to be MR safe, thereby (when used in the MRI environment) there is no additional risk to the patient, but may affect image quality. MRI procedures must only be performed according to the following guidelines:

- Plain films (radiographs) must be obtained to assess the site of the implanted **SpF** prior to the MRI examination to verify that there are no broken leads present.
- If this cannot be reliably determined, then the potential risks and benefits to the patient requiring the MRI examination must be

carefully assessed in consideration of the possibility of excessive heating to develop in the leads.

- The patient must be continuously observed during the MRI procedure and instructed to report any unusual sensations including any feelings of warming, burning, or neuromuscular excitation or stimulation.
- If these occur, the MRI procedure must be discontinued.

Static Magnetic Field of MR Systems

A patient with a **SpF** may safely undergo an MRI procedure using a shielded MR system with a static magnetic field of 1.5 Tesla or less (maximum spatial gradient 450 gauss/cm)

Gradient Magnetic Fields of MR Systems

Pulse sequences (e.g., echo planar imaging techniques or other rapid imaging pulse sequences), gradient coils or other techniques, and procedures that exceed a gradient magnetic field of 20 Tesla/second must not be used for MRI procedures. The use of unconventional or non-standard MRI techniques must be avoided. Standard or conventional pulse sequences (e.g., spin echo, fast spin echo, gradient echo, etc.) may be used for MRI examinations.

Radio Frequency (RF) Fields of MR Systems

MRI procedures must not exceed exposures to RF fields greater than a whole body averaged specific absorption rate (SAR) of 1.1 W/kg for 25 minutes of imaging. The use of unconventional or non-standard MRI techniques must be avoided.

MRI Artifacts

Artifacts for the **SpF** have been characterized using a 1.5 Tesla MR system (maximum spatial gradient 450 gauss/cm) and various pulse sequences. Based on this information, implantation of the **SpF** (i.e., with reference to the center of the device) a distance of at least 5-8 cm from the imaging area of interest is likely to maintain the diagnostic quality of the MRI examination. Artifact size is dependent on the type of pulse sequence used for imaging (e.g., larger for gradient echo pulse sequences and smaller for fast spin echo pulse sequences), the direction of the frequency encoding direction (larger if the frequency encoding direction is perpendicular to the device and smaller if it is parallel to the device), and the size of the field of view. Positional errors and artifacts on MR images may be larger for MR systems with static magnetic field strengths greater than 1.5 Tesla or smaller for MR systems with lower static magnetic fields strengths using the same imaging parameters.

Implant the **SpF** as far as possible from the spinal canal and bone graft is desirable since this will decrease the possibility that artifacts will affect this area of interest on MRI examinations. The use of fast spin echo pulse sequences will minimize the amount of artifact associated with the presence of the **SpF** compared to the use of other imaging techniques.

Nerve Excitation

The cathodes of the implantable spinal fusion stimulator must be positioned a minimum of 1 cm from nerve roots to reduce the possibility of nerve excitation during a MRI procedure.

Torque

To minimize the possibility of magnetically induced torque during MR imaging, the stimulator should be oriented with its broad face (36 mm x 23 mm plane) parallel to the body and to the static field lines inside the bore.

MRI Safety Information - SpF PLUS-Mini
SpF PLUS-Mini 60μA/W and 60μA/M

Safety information for the use of Magnetic Resonance Imaging (MRI) procedures (i.e., imaging, angiography, functional imaging, spectroscopy, etc.) pertains to shielded MRI systems with static magnetic fields of 1.5 Tesla or less (maximum spatial gradient 250 gauss/cm), gradient magnetic fields of 20 Tesla/second or less, and a maximum whole body averaged Specific Absorption Rate (SAR) of 1.1 W/kg for 25 minutes of imaging. The effects of MRI procedures using MR systems and conditions above these levels have not been determined.

The **SpF** devices have been determined to be MR safe, thereby (when used in the MRI environment) there is no additional risk to the patient, but may affect image quality. MRI procedures must only be performed according to the following guidelines:

- Plain films (radiographs) must be obtained to assess the site of the implanted **SpF** prior to the MRI examination to verify that there are no broken leads present.
- If this cannot be reliably determined, then the potential risks and benefits to the patient requiring the MRI examination must be carefully assessed in consideration of the possibility of excessive heating to develop in the leads.

- The patient must be continuously observed during the MRI procedure and instructed to report any unusual sensations including any feelings of warming, burning, or neuromuscular excitation or stimulation.
- If these occur, the MRI procedure must be discontinued.

Static Magnetic Field of MR Systems

A patient with a **SpF** may safely undergo an MRI procedure using a shielded MR system with a static magnetic field of 1.5 Tesla or less (maximum spatial gradient 250 gauss/cm)

Gradient Magnetic Fields of MR Systems

Pulse sequences (e.g., echo planar imaging techniques or other rapid imaging pulse sequences), gradient coils or other techniques, and procedures that exceed a gradient magnetic field of 20 Tesla/second must not be used for MRI procedures. The use of unconventional or non-standard MRI techniques must be avoided. Standard or conventional pulse sequences (e.g., spin echo, fast spin echo, gradient echo, etc.) may be used for MRI examinations.

Radio Frequency (RF) Fields of MR Systems

MRI procedures must not exceed exposures to RF fields greater than a whole body averaged specific absorption rate (SAR) of 1.1 W/kg for 25 minutes of imaging. The use of unconventional or non-standard MRI techniques must be avoided.

MRI Artifacts

Artifacts for the **SpF** have been characterized using a 1.5 Tesla MR system (maximum spatial gradient 250 gauss/cm) and various pulse sequences. Based on this information, implantation of the **SpF** (i.e., with reference to the center of the device) a distance of at least 5-8 cm from the imaging area of interest is likely to maintain the diagnostic quality of the MRI examination. Artifact size is dependent on the type of pulse sequence used for imaging (e.g., larger for gradient echo pulse sequences and smaller for fast spin echo pulse sequences), the direction of the frequency encoding direction (larger if the frequency encoding direction is perpendicular to the device and smaller if it is parallel to the device), and the size of the field of view. Positional errors and artifacts on MR images may be larger for MR systems with static magnetic field strengths greater than 1.5 Tesla or smaller for MR systems with lower static magnetic fields strengths using the same imaging parameters.

Implant the **SpF** as far as possible from the spinal canal and bone graft is desirable since this will decrease the possibility that artifacts will affect this area of interest on MRI examinations. The use of fast spin echo pulse sequences will minimize the amount of artifact associated with the presence of the **SpF** compared to the use of other imaging techniques.

Nerve Excitation

The cathodes of the implantable spinal fusion stimulator must be positioned a minimum of 1 cm from nerve roots to reduce the possibility of nerve excitation during a MRI procedure.

Torque

To minimize the possibility of magnetically induced torque during MR imaging, the stimulator should be oriented with its broad face (36 mm x 23 mm plane) parallel to the body and to the static field lines inside the bore.

[MR healthcare professionals are advised to contact the respective manufacturer in order to obtain the latest safety information to ensure patient safety relative to the use of an MR procedure.]

REFERENCES

http://www.biomet.com/spine/mriInfo.cfm?pdid=3

Chou C-K, McDougall JA, Chan KW. RF heating of implanted spinal fusion stimulator during magnetic resonance imaging. IEEE Trans Biomed Engineering 1997;44:357-373.

Shellock FG. Magnetic Resonance Procedures: Health Effects and Safety. CRC Press, LLC, Boca Raton, FL, 2001.

Shellock FG, Hatfield M, Simon BJ, Block S, Wamboldt J, Starewicz PM, Punchard WFB. Implantable spinal fusion stimulator: assessment of MRI safety. J Magn Reson Imaging 2000;12:214-223.

Bravo pH Monitoring System

Indications for Use. The Bravo pH Monitoring System with Accessories (Medtronic, Inc., Minneapolis, MN) is intended to be used for gastroesophageal pH measurement and monitoring of gastric reflux. The pH probe (capsule) can be delivered and placed endoscopically or with standard manometric procedures. The pH Software Analysis Program is intended to record, store, view and analyze gastroesophageal pH data.

Warnings and Precautions. Potential complications associated with gastrointestinal endoscopy include but are not limited to: perforation, hemorrhage, aspiration, fever, infection, hypertension, respiratory arrest, cardiac arrhythmia or arrest. Potential complications associated with nasal intubation include but are not limited to: sore throat, trauma to nasopharynx or bloody nose. Complications associated with the Bravo System include premature detachment of the capsule, failure of the capsule to slough off in a timely period, or discomfort associated with the capsule requiring endoscopic removal.

The Bravo pH Capsule with Delivery System is a single use, disposable device. Reuse or any other misuse of a Bravo pH Capsule with Delivery System will result in an increased potential for damage to the device and ancillary equipment.

Prior to use, all equipment for the procedure should be examined carefully to verify proper function.

MRI Information
Patients are restricted from undergoing an MRI study within 30 days of the Bravo procedure.

[MR healthcare professionals are advised to contact the respective manufacturer in order to obtain the latest safety information to ensure patient safety relative to the use of an MR procedure.]

REFERENCE

http://www.medtronic.com/physician/gastro/disclosure.html

Breast Tissue Expanders and Implants

Adjustable breast tissue expanders and mammary implants are utilized for breast reconstruction following mastectomy, for the correction of breast and chest-wall deformities and underdevelopment, for tissue defect procedures, and for cosmetic augmentation. These devices are typically equipped with either an integral injection site or a remote injection dome that is utilized to accept a needle for placement of saline for expansion of the prosthesis intra-operatively and/or postoperatively.

There are many different types of breast tissue expanders. For example, the Becker and the Siltex prostheses provide a choice of a standard injection dome or a micro-injection dome. The Radovan expander is indicated for temporary implantation only. The injection port for this device contains 316L stainless steel to guard against piercing the injection port by the needle used to fill the implant.

Notably, there are various breast tissue expanders that have magnetic ports to allow for a more accurate detection of the injection site. These devices are substantially attracted to the static magnetic fields of MR systems and, therefore, may be uncomfortable, injurious, or contraindicated for patients undergoing MR procedures. One such device is the Contour Profile Tissue Expander (Mentor, Santa Barbara, CA), which contains a magnetic injection dome and is considered to be unsafe for an MR examination.

Breast tissue expanders with magnetic ports produce relatively large artifacts on MR images and, as such, assessment of the breast using MR imaging is problematic. Importantly, there may be a situation during which a patient is referred for MR imaging for the determination of breast cancer or a breast implant rupture, such that the presence of the metallic artifact could obscure the precise location of the abnormality. In view of this possibility, it is recommended that a patient with a breast tissue expander that has a metallic component be identified prior to MRI so that the radiologist is aware of the potential problems related to the generation of artifacts as well as a possible injury.

McGhan Medical Breast Tissue Expanders and MRI Issues. McGhan Medical Breast Tissue Expanders are intended for temporary subcutaneous implantation to develop surgical flaps and additional tissue coverage (Product Information, Style 133 Family of Breast Tissue Expanders with MAGNA-SITE Injection Sites, McGhan Medical/INAMED Aesthetics, Santa Barbara, CA). These breast tissue expanders are constructed from silicone elastomer and consist of an expansion envelope with a textured surface, and a MAGNA-SITE integrated injection site. The expanders are available in a wide range of styles and sizes to meet diverse surgical needs. Specific styles include: Style 133 FV with MAGNA-SITE injection site, Style 133 LV with MAGNA-SITE injection site, Style 133 MV with MAGNA-SITE injection site.

The MAGNA-SITE injection site and MAGNA-FINDER external locating device contain rare-earth, permanent magnets for an accurate injection system. When the MAGNA-FINDER is passed over the surface of the tissue being expanded, its rare-earth, permanent magnet indicates the location of the MAGNA-SITE injection site.

The Product Information document for the McGhan Medical Breast Tissue Expanders (Style 133 Family of Breast Tissue Expanders with MAGNA-SITE Injection Sites, McGhan Medical/INAMED Aesthetics, Santa Barbara, CA) states: "DO NOT use MAGNA-SITE expanders in patients who already have implanted devices that would be affected by a magnetic field (e.g., pacemakers, drug infusion devices, artificial sensing devices). DO NOT perform diagnostic testing with Magnetic Resonance Imaging (MRI) in patients with MAGNA-SITE expanders in place."

Furthermore, in the Warnings section of the Product Information document, the following is indicated: "Diagnostic testing with Magnetic Resonance Imaging (MRI) is contraindicated in patients with MAGNA-SITE expanders in place. The MRI equipment could cause movement of the MAGNA-SITE breast tissue expander, and result in not only patient discomfort, but also expander displacement, requiring revision surgery. In addition, the MAGNA-SITE magnet could interfere with MRI detection capabilities."

Therefore, MR procedures are deemed unsafe for patients with the McGhan Medical Breast Tissue Expanders, Style 133 Family of Breast Tissue Expanders with MAGNA-SITE Injection Sites (McGhan Medical/INAMED Aesthetics, Santa Barbara, CA).

Zegzula et al. presented a case of bilateral tissue expander infusion port dislodgment associated with an MRI examination. The report involved a 56-year-old woman that underwent bilateral mastectomy and immediate reconstruction with McGhan BIOSPAN tissue expanders. As noted, these implants contain the "MAGNA-SITE" components. Several weeks postoperatively the patient underwent MR imaging of her spine. Subsequently, the infusion ports could not be located with the finder magnet (used to re-fill the tissue expander). A chest radiograph was obtained that demonstrated bilateral dislodgment of the infusion ports. Surgical removal and replacement of the tissue expanders were required. This incident emphasizes that all patients undergoing tissue expansion with implants that contain magnetic ports should be thoroughly warned about the potential hazards of MR imaging.

In another incident involving a tissue expander, Duffy and May reported a case of a woman who developed a burning sensation at the site of the tissue expander during an MR procedure. The sensation resolved rapidly once the scan was discontinued. The implications of the symptoms for in this case are unclear. Nevertheless, a patient with a tissue expander that requires an MR procedure should be alerted to the possibility of localized symptoms in the region of the implant during scanning.

REFERENCES

Duffy FJ Jr, May JW Jr. Tissue expanders and magnetic resonance imaging: the "hot" breast implant. Ann Plast Surg 1995;5:647-9.

Fagan LL, Shellock FG, Brenner RJ, Rothman B. Ex vivo evaluation of ferromagnetism, heating, and artifacts of breast tissue expanders exposed to a 1.5-T MR system. J Magn Reson Imaging 1995;5:614-616.

Liang MD, Narayanan K, Kanal E. Magnetic ports in tissue expanders: a caution for MRI. Magn Reson Imaging 1989;7:541-542.

Product Information, Style 133 Family of Breast Tissue Expanders with Magna-Site Injection Sites, McGhan Medical/INAMED Aesthetics, Santa Barbara, CA.

Shellock FG, Kanal E. Magnetic Resonance: Bioeffects, Safety, and Patient Management. Second Edition, Lippincott-Raven Press, New York, 1996.

Zegzula HD, Lee WP. Infusion port dislodgment of bilateral breast tissue expanders after MRI. Ann Plast Surg 2001;46:46-8.

Cardiac Pacemakers and Implantable Cardioverter Defibrillators

Cardiac pacemakers and implantable cardioverter defibrillators (ICDs) are crucial implanted devices for patients with heart conditions and serve to maintain quality of life and substantially reduce morbidity. Expanded indications for cardiac pacemakers and ICDs (e.g., heart failure, obstructive sleep apnea, and other conditions) emphasize that an increasing number of patients will be treated with these devices. Currently, these cardiovascular implants are considered a relative contraindication for patients referred for MR procedures Additionally, individuals with cardiac pacemakers and ICDs should be prevented from entering the MR environment because of potential risks. For additional information on this important topic, please refer to the following sections: **Cardiac Pacemaker: EnRhythm MRI SureScan Pacing System** and **Extremity MR System**.

Cardiac pacemakers and ICDs have been suggested to present potential problems to patients undergoing MR procedures from various mechanisms, including:

1) Movement of the pulse generator or lead(s);
2) Temporary or permanent modification of the function of the device;
3) Inappropriate sensing, triggering, or activation of the device;
4) Excessive heating of the leads; and
5) Induced currents in the leads.

The effects of the MR environment and MR procedures on the functional and operational aspects of cardiac pacemakers and ICDs vary, depending on several factors including the type of device, how the device is programmed, the static magnetic field strength of the MR system, and the imaging conditions used for the procedure (i.e., the anatomic region imaged, type of surface coil used, the pulse sequence, amount of radiofrequency energy used, etc.). Notably, most of the data concerning the deleterious effects of MR imaging on cardiac pacemakers involved the use of older versions (i.e., pre-1996) of these devices.

Recently, many compelling reports have been published concerning "modern-day" pacemakers (i.e. devices with decreased ferromagnetic components and more sophisticated circuitry) that indicate that certain patients may undergo MR examinations without harmful effects by following specific guidelines to minimize or prevent risks. Thus, there is growing evidence that it may be possible to perform MR procedures safely in patients with cardiovascular devices under highly controlled conditions (see below).

Implantable cardioverter defibrillators (ICDs) are medical devices designed to automatically detect and treat episodes of ventricular fibrillation, ventricular tachycardias, bradycardia, and other conditions. When a problem is identified, the device can deliver defibrillation, cardioversion, antitachycardia pacing, bradycardia pacing, or other therapy.

In general, exposure to an MR system or to an MR procedure has similar effects on an ICD as that previously described for a cardiac pacemaker, since some of the basic components are comparable. However, there are several unique aspects of ICDs that impact the possible safe performance of MR procedures in patients with these devices. Therefore, patients and individuals with these devices are generally not allowed to enter the MR environment. In addition, since ICDs also have electrodes placed in the myocardium, patients are typically not permitted to undergo MR examinations because of the inherent risks related to the presence of these conductive materials.

Similar to cardiac pacemakers, it is anticipated that, in lieu of developing a truly acceptable ICD for the MR environment, safety criteria may be determined for "modern-day" ICDs that entail using specialized programming, monitoring procedures, and MR conditions to allow patients to undergo MR examinations safely. Several recent studies have described patients with ICDs examined by MR imaging without serious problems.

However, potential problems remain for these cardiovascular devices, as indicated by recent reports by Gimbel (2009) and Mollerus et al. (2009), such that extreme caution must be exercised when scanning patients, even with "modern" cardiac pacemakers and ICDs.

Growing Evidence for Performing MR Procedures in Nonpacemaker Dependent Patients

Harmful effects related to performing MRI procedures in patients with cardiac pacemakers have been documented. Notably, in virtually every case involving a fatality, the patient apparently entered the MR environment without the staff knowing a cardiac pacemaker was present. Importantly, these deaths were poorly characterized, no electrocardiographic data were available for review, it was unknown whether these patients were pacemaker dependent, and the actual cause or mechanism of death were not confirmed. By comparison, no irreversible harm has been reported when patients with cardiac pacemakers were carefully monitored during MR procedures and/or the devices underwent reprogramming prior to the scans.

Regardless of the known hazards of subjecting a patient with a cardiac pacemaker to the MR environment, numerous patients (700+) have now undergone MR imaging during purposeful, monitored procedures performed in order to conduct necessary diagnostic examinations. These patients were safely and successfully imaged using MR systems operating at static magnetic fields ranging from 0.35- to 3-Tesla without serious adverse events.

In consideration of the above, there is increasing evidence from *in vitro*, laboratory, and clinical studies that strict restrictions prohibiting MR procedures in patients with "modern" cardiac pacemakers and ICDs may be modified. Similar to performing MR procedures in patients with other electronically-activated devices (e.g., bone fusion stimulators, cochlear implants, neurostimulation systems, programmable injusion pumps, etc.), scanning patients with cardiac pacemakers and ICDs involves following highly specific procedures to ensure patient safety.

Interestingly, a recent study by Gimbel (2008) reported scanning patients with cardiac pacemakers at 3-Tesla with no restrictions placed on pacemaker dependency, region scanned, device type, or manufacturer. This somewhat limited experience suggested that patients may undergo carefully tailored 3-Tesla MRI scans when pre-MRI reprogramming of the device occurs in conjunction with extensive monitoring, supervision, and follow-up.

Proposed Guidelines for Performing MRI in Nonpacemaker Dependent Patients

Guidelines have been presented by Martin et al. (2004), Roquin et al. (2004), Loewy et al. (2004), the American College of Radiology (2007) and the American College of Cardiology/American Heart Association (2007) with regard to performing MR procedures in nonpacemaker dependent patients. These guidelines include, the following:

- Establish a risk-benefit ratio for the patient
- Obtain written and verbal informed consent

- Pretest pacemaker functions using appropriate equipment outside of the MR environment
- A cardiologist/electrophysiologist should decide whether it is necessary to program the pacemaker prior to the MR examination
- A cardiologist/electrophysiologist with Advanced Cardiac Life Support (ACLS) training must be in attendance for the entire MRI examination
- The patient should be monitored continuously during the MR procedure (e.g., blood pressure, pulse rate, oxygen saturation, and ECG)
- Appropriate personnel, a crash cart, and defibrillator must be available throughout the procedure to address an adverse event
- Maintain visual and voice contact throughout the procedure with the patient
- Instruct the patient to alert the MR system operator of any unusual sensations or problems so that, if necessary, the MR system operator can immediately terminate the procedure
- After the MRI examination, a cardiologist/electrophysiologist should interrogate the pacemaker to confirm that the function is consistent with the pre-examination state

MRI at 1.5 and 3-Tesla and Cardiac Pacemakers and ICDs: Magnetic Field Interactions

As previously discussed, one important safety aspect of the MR environment on cardiac pacemakers and ICDs is related to magnetic field interactions. Component parts of pacemakers and ICDs, such as batteries, reed-switches, or transformer core materials may contain ferromagnetic materials. Therefore, substantial magnetic field interactions may exist, causing these implants to move or be uncomfortable for patients or individuals. Therefore, as an important part of evaluating pacemakers and ICDs, tests for magnetic field interactions have been conducted using MR systems operating at static magnetic field strengths ranging from 0.2-Tesla (i.e., the dedicated-extremity MR system) to 3-Tesla.

Luechinger et al. investigated magnetic field interactions for thirty-one cardiac pacemakers and thirteen ICDs in association with exposure to a 1.5-Tesla MR system (Gyroscan ACS NT, Philips Medical Systems, Best, The Netherlands). The investigators reported that "newer" cardiac pacemakers had relatively low magnetic force values compared to older devices. With regard to ICDs, with the exception of one newer model (GEM II, 7273 ICD, Medtronic, Inc., Minneapolis, MN), all ICDs showed relatively high magnetic field interactions. Luechinger et al.

concluded that modern-day pacemakers present no safety risk with respect to magnetic field interactions at 1.5-Tesla, while ICDs could pose problems due to strong magnet-related mechanical forces.

The clinical use of 3-Tesla MR systems for brain, musculoskeletal, body and cardiovascular applications is increasing. Because previous investigations performed to determine MR safety for pacemakers and ICDs used MR systems with static magnetic fields of 1.5-Tesla or less, it is crucial to perform *ex vivo* testing at 3-Tesla to characterize magnetic field-related safety for these implants, with full appreciation that additional MR safety issues exist for these devices, as described-above.

An important aspect of determining magnetic field interactions for metallic implants involves the measurement of translational attraction. Translational attraction is assessed for metallic implants using the standardized deflection angle test recommended by the American Society for Testing and Materials (ASTM) International. According to ASTM International guidelines, the deflection angle for an implant or device is generally measured at the point of the "highest spatial gradient" for the specific MR system used for testing. Notably, the deflection angle test is commonly performed as an integral part of safety testing for metallic implants and devices.

Various types of magnets exist for commercially available 1.5- and 3-Tesla MR systems, including magnet configurations that are used for conventional "long-bore" scanners and newer "short-bore" systems. Because of physical differences in the position and magnitude of the highest spatial gradient for different magnets, measurements of deflection angles for implants using long-bore vs. short-bore MR systems can produce substantially different results for magnetic field-related translational attraction, as reported by Shellock et al.

The implications are primarily for magnetic field-related translational attraction with regard to long-bore vs. short-bore 3-Tesla MR systems (with short-bore scanners producing greater translational attraction for a given implant). Therefore, a study was conducted on fourteen different cardiac pacemakers and four ICDs to evaluate translational attraction for these devices in association with long-bore and short-bore 1.5- and 3-Tesla MR systems. Deflection angles were measured based on guidelines from the ASTM International.

In general, deflection angles for the cardiovascular implants that underwent evaluation were significantly (p<0.01) higher on 1.5- and 3-Tesla short-bore scanners compared to long-bore MR systems. For the 1.5-Tesla MR systems, three cardiac pacemakers (Cosmos, Model 283-01

Pacemaker, Intermedics, Inc., Freeport, TX; Nova Model 281-01 Pacemaker, Intermedics, Inc., Freeport, TX; Res-Q ACE, Model 101-01 Pacemaker; Intermedics, Inc., Freeport, TX) exhibited deflection angles greater than 45 degrees (i.e., exceeding the recommended ASTM International criteria) on both long-bore and short-bore 1.5-Tesla MR systems. The findings indicated that these devices are potentially problematic for patients from a magnetic field interaction consideration.

With regard to the 3-Tesla MR systems, seven implants exhibited deflection angles greater than 45 degrees on the long-bore 3-Tesla scanner, while 13 exhibited deflection angles greater than 45 degrees on the short-bore 3-T MR system (refer to **The List** for information on the cardiac pacemakers and ICDs that underwent testing). Importantly, the findings for magnetic field-related translational attraction were substantially different comparing the long-bore (i.e., lower values) and short-bore (i.e., higher values) MR systems.

As stated, other factors exist that may impact MR safety for these cardiac pacemakers and ICDs. Therefore, regardless of the fact that magnetic field interactions may not present a risk for some of the cardiovascular implants that have been tested, these potentially hazardous mechanisms must be considered carefully for these devices.

[MR healthcare professionals are advised to contact the respective manufacturer in order to obtain the latest safety information to ensure patient safety relative to the use of an MR procedure.]

REFERENCES

Achenbach S, Moshage W, et al. Effects of magnetic resonance imaging on cardiac pacemakers and electrodes. Am Heart J 1997;134:467-473.

Alagona P, Toole JC, et al. Nuclear magnetic resonance imaging in a patient with a DDD pacemaker. Pacing Clin Electrophysiol 1989;12:619 (letter).

American Society for Testing and Materials (ASTM) Designation: F 2052. Standard test method for measurement of magnetically induced displacement force on passive implants in the magnetic resonance environment. In: Annual Book of ASTM Standards, Section 13, Medical Devices and Services, Volume 13.01 Medical Devices; Emergency Medical Services. West Conshohocken, PA, 2002, pp. 1576-1580.

Anfinsen OG, Berntsen RF, Aass H, Kongsgaard E, Amlie JP. Implantable cardioverter defibrillator dysfunction during and after magnetic resonance imaging. Pacing Clin Electrophysiol 2002;25:1400-1402.

Bailey SM, Gimbel JR, Ruggieri PM, Tchou PJ, Wilcoff BL. Magnetic resonance imaging (MRI) of the brain in pacemaker dependent patients. Pacing and Clinical Electrophysiology 2005;2:S128.

Bhachu DS, Kanal E. Implantable pulse generators (pacemakers) and electrodes: safety in the magnetic resonance imaging scanner environment. J Magn Reson Imaging 2000; 12:201-204.

Bonnet CA, Elson JJ, Fogoros RN. Accidental deactivation of the automatic implantable cardioverter defibrillator. Am Heart J 1990;3:696-697.

Calcagnini G, et al. In vitro investigation of pacemaker lead heating induced by magnetic resonance imaging: role of implant geometry. J Magn Reson Imaging. 2008;28:879-86.

Del Ojo JL, Moya F, et al. Is magnetic resonance imaging safe in cardiac pacemaker recipients? Pacing Clin Electrophysiol 2005;28:274-8.

Duru F, Luechinger R, Scheidegger MB, Luscher TF, Boesiger P, Candinas R. Pacing in magnetic resonance imaging environment: clinical and technical considerations on compatibility. Eur Heart J 2001;22:113-124.

Duru F, Luechinger R, Candinas R. MR imaging in patients with cardiac pacemakers. Radiology 2001;219:856-858.

Erlebacher JA, Cahill PT, Pannizzo F, Knowles RJR. Effect of magnetic resonance imaging on DDD pacemakers. Am J Cardio 1986;57:437-440.

Faris OP, Shein M. Food and Drug Administration perspective: Magnetic resonance imaging of pacemaker and implantable cardioverter-defibrillator patients. Circulation 2006;114:1232-1233.

Fetter J, Aram G, Holmes DR, Gray JE, Hayes DL. The effects of nuclear magnetic resonance imagers on external and implantable pulse generators. Pacing Clin Electrophysiol 1984;7:720-727.

Fiek M, Remp T, Reithmann C, Steinbeck G. Complete loss of ICD programmability after magnetic resonance imaging. Pacing Clin Electrophysiol 2004;27:1002-4.

Fontaine JM, Mohamed FB, Gottlieb C, Callans DJ, Marchlinski FE. Rapid ventricular pacing in a pacemaker patient undergoing magnetic resonance imaging. Pacing Clin Electrophysiol 1998;21:1336-1339.

Garcia-Bolao I, Albaladejo V, et al. Magnetic resonance imaging in a patient with a dual chamber pacemaker. Acta Cardiol 1998;53:33-35.

Gimbel JR. Unexpected asystole during 3T magnetic resonance imaging of a pacemaker dependent patient with a 'modern' pacemaker. Europace. 2009;11:1241-2.

Gimbel JR. Letter to the Editor. Pacing Clin Electrophysiol 2003;26:1.

Gimbel JR. Magnetic resonance imaging of implantable cardiac rhythm devices at 3-Tesla. Pacing Clin Electrophysiol. 2008;31:795-801.

Gimbel JR. Implantable pacemaker and defibrillator safety in the MR environment: new thoughts for the new millennium. RSNA Special Cross-Specialty Categorical Course in Diagnostic Radiology: Practical MR Safety Considerations for Physicians, Physicists, and Technologists 2001;69-76.

Gimbel JR, Johnson D, Levine PA, Wilkoff BL. Safe performance of magnetic resonance imaging on five patients with permanent cardiac pacemakers. Pacing Clin Electrophysiol 1996;19:913-919.

Gimbel JR, Kanal E, Schwartz KM, Wilkoff BL. Outcome of magnetic resonance imaging (MRI) in selected patients with implantable cardioverter defibrillators (ICDs). Pacing Clin Electrophysiol 2005;28:270-3.

Goldsher D, Amikam S, Boulos M, et al. Magnetic resonance imaging for patients with permanent pacemakers: initial clinical experience. Isr Med Assoc J 2006;8:91-94.

Hayes DL, Holmes DR, Gray JE. Effect of 1.5 Tesla nuclear magnetic resonance imaging scanner on implanted permanent pacemakers. J Am Coll Cardiol 1987;10:782-786.

Heatlie G, Pennell DJ. Cardiovascular magnetic resonance at 0.5-T in five patients with permanent pacemakers. J Cardiovasc Magn Reson. 2007;9:15-9.

Holmes DJ, Hayes DL, Gray JE, Merideth J. The effects of magnetic resonance imaging on implantable pulse generators. Pacing Clin Electrophysiol 1986;9:360-370.

Inbar S, Larson J, et al. Case report: nuclear magnetic resonance imaging in a patient with a pacemaker. Am J Med Sci 1993;3:174-175.

Irnich W, Irnich B, et al. Do we need pacemakers resistant to magnetic resonance imaging? Europace. 2005;7:353-65.

International Commission on Non-Ionizing Radiation Protection (ICNIRP) Statement, Medical magnetic resonance procedures: protection of patients. Health Physics 2004;87:197-216.

Juralti NM, Sparker J, Gimbel JR, et al. Strategies for the safe performance of magnetic resonance imaging in selected pacemaker patients (abstract) Circulation 2001;104 (Suppl.):3020.

Kanal E, Barkovich AJ, Bell C, et al. ACR guidance document for safe MR practices: 2007. AJR Am J Roentgenol. 2007;188:1447-1474.

Lauck G, von Smekal A, Wolke S, Seelos KC, Jung W, Manz M, et al. Effects of nuclear magnetic resonance imaging on cardiac pacemakers. Pacing Clin Electrophysiol 1995;18:1549-55.

Levine PA. Industry Viewpoint: St. Jude Medical: Pacemakers, ICDs and MRI. Pacing and Clinical Electrophysiology 2005;28:266.

Levine GN, Gomes AS, Arai AE, Bluemke DA, Flamm SD, Kanal E, Manning WJ, Martin ET, Smith JM, Wilke N, Shellock FG. Safety of magnetic resonance imaging in patients with cardiovascular devices: an American Heart Association scientific statement from the Committee on Diagnostic and Interventional Cardiac Catheterization. Circulation 2007;116:2878-2891.

Loewy J, Loewy A, Kendall EJ. Reconsideration of pacemakers and MR imaging. Radiographics 2004;24:1257-1268.

Luechinger RC. Safety Aspects of Cardiac Pacemakers in Magnetic Resonance Imaging. Swiss Institute of Technology, Zurich, Dissertation, 2002

Luechinger RC, Duru F, Zeijlemaker VA, Scheidegger MB, Boesiger P, Candinas R. Pacemaker reed-switch behavior in 0.5, 1.5, and 3.0 Tesla magnetic resonance units: Are reed switches always closed in strong magnetic fields? Pacing Clin Electrophysiol 2002;25:1419-1423.

Luechinger RC, Duru F, Scheidegger MB, Boesiger P, Candinas R. Force and torque effects of a 1.5 Tesla MRI scanner on cardiac pacemakers and ICDs. Pacing Clin Electrophysiol 2001;24:199-205.

Luechinger R, Zeijlemaker VA, Pedersen EM, Mortensen P, Falk E, Duru F, Candinas R, Boesiger P. *In vivo* heating of pacemaker leads during magnetic resonance imaging. Eur Heart J 2005;26:376-83.

Martin TE, Coman JA, Shellock FG, Pulling C, Fair R, Jenkins K. Magnetic resonance imaging and cardiac pacemaker safety at 1.5-Tesla. Journal of the American College of Cardiology 2004;43:1315-1324.

Mollerus M, et al. Ectopy in patients with permanent pacemakers and implantable cardioverter-defibrillators undergoing an MRI scan. Pacing Clin Electrophysiol. 2009;32:772-8.

Naehle CP, et al. Evaluation of cumulative effects of MR imaging on pacemaker systems at 1.5 Tesla. Pacing Clin Electrophysiol. 2009 Sep 30. [Epub ahead of print]

Naehle CP, Meyer C, et al. Safety of brain 3-T MR imaging with transmit-receive head coil in patients with cardiac pacemakers: pilot prospective study with 51 examinations. Radiology. 2008;249:991-1001.

Naehle CP, Strach K, et al. Magnetic resonance imaging at 1.5-T in patients with implantable cardioverter-defibrillators. J Am Coll Cardiol. 2009;54:549-55.

Nazarian S, Halperin HR. How to perform magnetic resonance imaging on patients with implantable cardiac arrhythmia devices. Heart Rhythm. 2009;6:138-43.

Nazarian S, Roguin A, et al.. Clinical utility and safety of a protocol for noncardiac and cardiac magnetic resonance imaging of patients with permanent pacemakers and implantable-cardioverter defibrillators at 1.5 Tesla. Circulation 2006;114:1277-1284.

Nordbeck P, Weiss I, Ehses P, et al. Measuring RF-induced currents inside implants: Impact of device configuration on MRI safety of cardiac pacemaker leads. Magn Reson Med. 2009;61:570-8.

Pavlicek W, Geisinger M, et al. The effects of nuclear magnetic resonance on patients with cardiac pacemakers. Radiology 1983;147:149-153.

Pulver AF, Puchalski MD, et al. Safety and imaging quality of MRI in pediatric and adult congenital heart disease patients with pacemakers. Pacing Clin Electrophysiol. 2009;32:450-6.

Roguin A, et al. Magnetic resonance imaging in individuals with cardiovascular implantable electronic devices. Europace. 2008;10:336-46.

Roguin A, Donahue JK, Bomma CS, Bluemke DA, Halperin HR. Cardiac magnetic resonance imaging in a patient with implantable cardioverter-defibrillator. Pacing Clin Electrophysiol 2005;28:336-8.

Roguin A, Zviman M, et al. Modern pacemaker and implantable cardioverter-defibrillator systems can be MRI-safe. Circulation 2004;110:475-482.

Schmiedel A, et al. Magnetic resonance imaging of the brain in patients with cardiac pacemakers. In-vitro- and in-vivo-evaluation at 1.5 Tesla. Rofo 2005;177:731-44.

Shellock FG. Guest Editorial. Comments on MRI heating tests of critical implants. Journal of Magnetic Resonance Imaging 2007;26:1182-1185.

Shellock FG. Excessive temperature increases in pacemaker leads at 3-T MR imaging with a transmit-received head coil. Radiology 2009;251:948-949.

Shellock FG. Cardiac pacemakers: growing evidence for MRI safety. Signals, No. 48, Issue 1, pp. 14-15, 2004.

Shellock FG, Magnetic Resonance Procedures: Health Effects, Safety, and Patient Management CRC Press, LLC, Boca Raton, FL, 2001.

Shellock FG, Crues JV. MR procedures: biologic effects, safety, and patient care. Radiology 2004;232:635-652.

Shellock FG, Fieno DS, Thomson TJ, Talavage TM, Berman DS. Cardiac pacemaker: *in vitro* assessment of MR safety at 1.5-Tesla. American Heart Journal 2006;151:436-443.

Shellock FG, Fischer L, Fieno DS. Cardiac pacemakers and implantable cardioverter defibrillators: in v*itro* evaluation of MRI safety at 1.5-Tesla. Journal of Cardiovascular Magnetic Resonance 2007;9:21-31.

Shellock FG, O'Neil M, Ivans V, Kelly D, O'Connor M, Toay L, Crues JV. Cardiac pacemakers and implantable cardiac defibrillators are unaffected by operation of an extremity MR system. AJR Am J Roentgenol 1999;72:165-170.

Shellock FG, Tkach JA, Ruggieri PM, Masaryk TJ. Cardiac pacemakers, ICDs, and loop recorder: Evaluation of translational attraction using conventional ("long-bore") and "short-bore" 1.5- and 3.0-Tesla MR systems. Journal of Cardiovascular Magnetic Resonance 2003;5:387-397.

Shellock FG, Valencerina S, Fischer L. MRI-related heating of pacemaker at 1.5- and 3-Tesla: Evaluation with and without pulse generator attached to leads. Circulation 112;Supplement II:561, 2005.

Shinbane J, Colletti P, Shellock FG. MR in patients with pacemakers and ICDs: Defining the issues. Journal of Cardiovascular Magnetic Resonance 2007;9:5-13.

Sommer T, Vahlhaus C, et al. MR imaging and cardiac pacemakers: in vitro evaluation and in vivo studies in 51 patients at 0.5 T. Radiology 2000;215:869-879.

Sommer T, Naehle CP, Yang A, Zeijlemaker V, et al. Strategy for safe performance of extrathoracic magnetic resonance imaging at 1.5 Tesla in the presence of cardiac pacemakers in non-pacemaker-dependent patients: a prospective study with 115 examinations. Circulation 2006;114:1285-92

Sutton R, Kanal E, Wilkoff BL, et al. Safety of magnetic resonance imaging of patients with a new Medtronic EnRhythm MRI SureScan pacing system: clinical study design. Trials. 2008 Dec 2;9:68.

Tandri H, et al. Determinants of gradient field-induced current in a pacemaker lead system in a magnetic resonance imaging environment. Heart Rhythm. 2008;5:462-8

Vahlhaus C, Sommer T, et al. interference with cardiac pacemakers by magnetic resonance imaging: Are there irreversible changes at 0.5 Tesla? Pacing Clin Electrophysiol 2001;24(Pt. I):489-95.

Wollmann C, Grude M, et al. Safe performance of magnetic resonance imaging on a patient with an ICD. Pacing Clin Electrophysiol 2005;28:339-42.

Zimmermann BH, Faul DD. Artifacts and hazards in NMR imaging due to metal implants and cardiac pacemakers. Diagn Imaging Clin Med 1984;53:53-56.

Cardiac Pacemaker: EnRhythm MRI SureScan Pacing System

A new cardiac pacemaker has been developed that permits MRI procedures to be performed in patients by following specific labeling requirements (http://www.medtronic.com/mrisurescan). The EnRhythm MRI SureScan Pacing System (Medtronic, Inc., Minneapolis, MN; Note: the Advisa MRI SureScan Pacing System is also now available but not in the United States) was designed to minimize the potential interactions with the electromagnetic fields used for MR systems. Comprehensive labeling information must be reviewed and adhered to ensure patient safety and includes, but is not limited to:

MRI conditions for use

Non-clinical testing has demonstrated that the SureScan pacing system is safe for use in the MRI environment when used according to the *Instructions for Use*. The SureScan pacing system can be scanned in patients under these conditions:

- Closed bore, cylindrical magnet, clinical MRI systems with a static magnetic field of 1.5 Tesla (T) must be used.
- Gradient systems with maximum gradient slew rate performance per axis of ≤ 200 T/m/s must be used.
- Whole body averaged specific absorption rate (SAR) as reported by the MRI equipment must be ≤ 2.0 W/kg; head SAR as reported by the MRI equipment must be < 3.2 W/kg.
- Patients and their implanted systems must be screened per the contraindications in Section 4 of the *Instructions for Use*.
- Transmit/receive and transmit-only coils (local, volume, interventional, or surface) must not be placed within the isocenter landmark exclusion zone as described in Section 7 of the *Instructions for Use*. Receive-only coils are permissible.
- Proper patient monitoring must be provided as described in Section 6.3 of the *Instructions for Use*.
- The patient position restrictions described in Section 7 of the *Instructions for Use* must be followed.

- The implanted system must consist solely of a SureScan device and SureScan leads as described in Section 8.1 of the *Instructions for Use.*

The EnRhythm MRI SureScan Pacing System is commercially available in Europe but is not currently available for sale in the United States. In the United States the device is limited by federal law to investigational use only.

For more information please visit **http://www.medtronic.com/mrisurescan**

[MR healthcare professionals are advised to contact the respective manufacturer in order to obtain the latest safety information to ensure patient safety relative to the use of an MR procedure.]

REFERENCES

http://www.medtronic.com/mrisurescan

Instructions for Use, SURESCAN MRI procedural information for EnRhythm MRI SureScan EMDR01, CapSureFix MRI 5 086MRI, Medtronic, Inc., Minneapolis, MN

Sutton R, Kanal E, Wilkoff BL, et al. Safety of magnetic resonance imaging of patients with a new Medtronic EnRhythm MRI SureScan pacing system: clinical study design. Trials. 2008 Dec 2;9:68.

Cardiovascular Catheters and Accessories

Cardiovascular catheters and accessories are indicated for use in the assessment and management of critically-ill or high-risk patients including those with acute heart failure, cardiogenic shock, severe hypovolemia, complex circulatory abnormalities, acute respiratory distress syndrome, pulmonary hypertension, certain types of arrhythmias and other various medical emergencies. In these cases, cardiovascular catheters are used to measure intravascular pressures, intracardiac pressures, cardiac output, and oxyhemoglobin saturation. Secondary indications include venous blood sampling and therapeutic infusion of solutions or medications. In addition, some cardiovascular catheters are designed for temporary cardiac pacing and intra-atrial or intraventricular electrocardiographic monitoring.

Because patients with cardiovascular catheters and associated accessories may require evaluation using MR procedures or these devices may be considered for use during MR-guided procedures, it is imperative that a thorough *ex vivo* assessment of MR-safety be conducted for these devices to ascertain the potential risks of their use in the MR environment. For example, MR imaging, angiography, and spectroscopy procedures may play an important role in the diagnostic evaluation of these patients. Furthermore, the performance of certain MR-guided interventional procedures may require the utilization of cardiovascular catheters and accessories to monitor patients during biopsies, interventions, or treatments.

There is at least one report of a cardiovascular catheter (Swan-Ganz Triple Lumen Thermodilution Catheter) that "melted" in a patient undergoing MR imaging. This catheter contained a wire made from a conductive material that was considered to be responsible for this problem. Thus, there are realistic concerns pertaining to the use of similar devices in patients undergoing MR examinations. Therefore, an investigation was performed using *ex vivo* testing techniques to evaluate various cardiovascular catheters and accessories with regard to magnetic field interactions, heating, and artifacts associated with MR imaging.

A total of fifteen different cardiovascular catheters and accessories (Abbott Laboratories, Morgan Hill, CA) were selected for evaluation because they represent a wide-variety of the styles and types of devices that are commonly-used in the critical care setting (i.e., the basic structures of these devices are comparable to those made by other manufacturers). Of these devices, the 3-Lumen CVP Catheter, CVP-PVC Catheter (used for central venous pressure monitoring, administration of fluids, and venous blood sampling; polyurethane and polyvinyl chloride, respectively), Thermoset-Iced, and Thermoset-Room (used as accessories for determination of cardiac output using the thermodilution method; plastic), and Safe-set with In-Line Reservoir (used for in-line blood sampling; plastic) were determined to have no metallic components (Personal communications, Ann McGibbon, Abbott Laboratories, 1997). Thus, these devices were deemed safe for patients undergoing MR procedures and were not included in the overall *ex vivo* tests for MR safety. The remaining ten devices were evaluated for the presence of potential problems in the MR environment.

Excessive heating of implants or devices made from conductive materials has been reported to be a hazard for patients who undergo MR procedures. This is particularly a problem for a device that is a certain length or in the form of a loop or coil because, under certain conditions, current can be induced during operation of the MR system, to the extent that a first, second or third-degree burn can be produced.

Additional physical factors responsible for this hazard have not been identified or well-characterized (i.e., the imaging parameters, specific gradient field effects, size of the loop associated with excessive heating, etc.). For this reason, the afore-mentioned study examining cardiovascular catheters and accessories did not attempt to investigate the effect of various "coiled" catheter shapes on the development of substantial heating during an MR procedure, especially since there are many factors in addition to the shape or configuration of the catheter with a conductive component that can also influence the amount of heating that occurs during an MR procedure.

The thermodilution Swan-Ganz catheter and other similar cardiovascular catheters have nonferromagnetic materials that include conductive wires. A report indicated that a portion of a Swan-Ganz thermodilution catheter that was outside the patient melted during MR imaging. It was postulated that the high-frequency electromagnetic fields generated by the MR system caused eddy current-induced heating of either the wires within the thermodilution catheter or the radiopaque material used in the construction of the catheter.

This incident suggests that patients with this catheter or similar device that has conductive wires or other component parts, could be potentially injured during an MR procedure. Furthermore, heating of the wire or lead of a temporary pacemaker (e.g., the RV Pacing Lead) is of at least a theoretical concern for any similar wire in the bore of an MR system. Cardiac pacemaker leads are typically intravascular for most of their length and heat transfer and dissipation from the leads into the blood may prevent dangerous levels of lead heating to be reached or maintained for the intravascular segments of pacemaker leads. However, this remains to be evaluated.

For certain segments of these leads, it is theoretically possible that sufficient power deposition or heating may be induced within these leads (i.e., those unconnected to a pulse generator) to result in local tissue injury or burn during an MR procedure. An *ex vivo* study conducted by Achenbach et al. substantiates this contention, whereby temperature increases of up to 63.1 degrees C were recorded at the tips of pacemaker electrodes during MR imaging performed in phantoms. An investigation by Shellock et al. (2005) further substantiated that excessive temperatures can occur for unconnected cardiac pacing leads.

A case report by Masaki et al. described an iatrogenic second-degree burn caused by a catheter (percutaneous transluminal coronary angioplasty or PTCA) encased by tubular, braided stainless steel. The presence of this PTCA catheter caused a superficial burn of the abdomen during an MRI procedure performed at 1.5-Tesla and further illustrates the potential risks associated with MRI examinations and cardiovascular catheters that are made from conducting, metallic materials.

Because of possible deleterious and unpredictable effects, patients referred for MR procedures with cardiovascular catheters and accessories that have internally or externally-positioned conductive wires or similar components should not undergo MR procedures because of the possible associated risks, unless MR-safety testing information demonstrates otherwise. Further support of this recommendation is based on the fact that inappropriate use of monitoring devices during MR procedures is often the cause of patient injuries. For example, burns have resulted in the MR environment in association with the use of devices that utilize conductive wires.

[MR healthcare professionals are advised to contact the respective manufacturer in order to obtain the latest safety information to ensure patient safety relative to the use of an MR procedure.]

REFERENCES

Achenbach S, Moshage W, Diem B, Bieberle T, Schibgilla V, Bachmann K. Effects of magnetic resonance imaging on cardiac pacemakers and electrodes. Am Heart J 1997;134:467-473

Dempsey MF, Condon B, Hadley DM. Investigation of the factors responsible for burns during MRI. J Magn Reson Imaging 2001;13:627-631.

ECRI, Health devices alert. A new MRI complication? May 27, 1988.

Masaki F, Shuhei Y, Riko K, Yohjiro M. Iatrogenic second-degree burn caused by a catheter encased tubular braid of stainless steel during MRI. Burns. 2007 Sep 13; [Epub ahead of print]

Shellock FG. Magnetic Resonance Procedures: Health Effects and Safety. CRC Press, LLC, Boca Raton, FL, 2001.

Shellock FG, Kanal E. Magnetic Resonance: Bioeffects, Safety, and Patient Management. Second Edition, Lippincott-Raven Press, New York, 1996.

Shellock FG, Shellock VJ. Cardiovascular catheters and accessories: *Ex vivo* testing of ferromagnetism, heating, and artifacts associated with MRI. J Magn Reson Imaging 1998;8:1338-1342.

Shellock FG, Valencerina S, Fischer L. MRI-related heating of pacemaker at 1.5- and 3-Tesla: Evaluation with and without pulse generator attached to leads. Circulation 112;Supplement II:561, 2005.

Carotid Artery Vascular Clamps

To date, each carotid artery vascular clamp tested in association with a 1.5-Tesla MR system displayed positive magnetic field interactions. However, only the Poppen-Blaylock carotid artery vascular clamp is considered contraindicated for patients undergoing MR procedures due to the existence of substantial ferromagnetism. The other carotid artery clamps were considered safe for patients exposed to MR systems because they were deemed "weakly" ferromagnetic. With the exception of the Poppen-Blaylock clamp, patients with the other carotid artery vascular clamps that have been evaluated for magnetic field interactions have been imaged by MR systems with static magnetic fields up to 1.5-Tesla without experiencing discomfort or neurological sequelae.

REFERENCES

Shellock FG. Magnetic Resonance Procedures: Health Effects and Safety. CRC Press, LLC, Boca Raton, FL, 2001.

Shellock FG, Kanal E. Magnetic Resonance: Bioeffects, Safety, and Patient Management. Second Edition, Lippincott-Raven Press, New York, 1996.

Teitelbaum GP, Lin MCW, Watanabe AT, et al. Ferromagnetism and MR imaging: safety of carotid vascular clamps. AJNR Am J Neuroradiol 1990;11:267-272.

Celsius Control System

The **Celsius Control System** (INNERCOOL Therapies, San Diego, CA) provides physicians with a state-of-the-art, endovascular technology that can safely and rapidly lower the patient body temperature, precisely maintain a chosen target temperature and rewarm patients to normothermic levels.

Medical research suggests there are a number of potential clinical applications for the Celsius Control System such as inducing mild hypothermia in surgery, stroke and heart attack or for temperature control in surgical and critical care procedures.

The Celsius Control System consists of an endovascular catheter, console and proprietary disposables. The distal portion of the catheter incorporates a flexible Temperature Control Element (TCE) that is cooled or warmed with saline solution circulated in a closed-loop manner from the console. When placed in the inferior vena cava, the TCE exchanges thermal energy directly with the blood, resulting in cooling or warming of the downstream organs and body. The Celsius Control System does not infuse fluid into the patient, nor is blood circulated outside of the body.

INNERCOOL Therapies received FDA clearance in January 2003 for the Celsius Control System to induce, maintain and reverse mild hypothermia in neurosurgical patients in surgery and recovery/intensive care. Subsequent indications for the CCS have also been obtained in fever control and cardiac surgery.

Clinical experience with the Celsius Control System has shown average cool down rates of 5.0 - 6.0 degrees C/hr, target temperature control of ±0.1 degrees C and average rewarm rates of 2.0 - 3.0 degrees C/hr.

Celsius Control System

The Celsius Control System consists of a disposable endovascular heat transfer catheter, administration cassette, and a console. The distal portion of the catheter (10.7 Fr. and 14 Fr.) has a flexible, metallic temperature control element (TCE) that is cooled or warmed by sterile saline circulated within it from the Celsius Control Console. The administration cassette connects the catheter to the console, maintaining the sterility of the saline conduit. The TCE does not expand inside the body so the outer diameter of the TCE will remain consistent throughout the entire cooling/warming procedure unlike balloon based cooling systems which expand to outer diameters of 24 Fr.-47 Fr. during use.

The TCE has a proprietary surface of alternating helices that induces mixing and significantly enhances heat transfer directly with the blood flowing in the inferior vena cava. In addition, the use of a flexible metal heat exchanger, further optimizes heat transfer due to the high thermal conductivity of metal. The flexibility of the TCE is achieved through uniquely designed segmented bellows joints. The catheter can also be placed in an operating room or ICU setting without the need for continuous fluoroscopy.

The TCE and catheter are coated with the Applause heparin coating from Surmodics, Inc. The Applause coating is covalently bonded to the surface of Innercool catheters through a proprietary PhotoLink process. Covalent bonding insures a more durable, active heparin coating compared to the short-lived nature of ionically bound heparin coatings. The Applause coating has demonstrated that over 80% of the heparin activity remains after 28-days of saline incubation.

Accutrol Catheter

INNERCOOL Therapies' Accutrol catheter contains an integrated temperature sensor, which can accurately determine the patient's core body temperature within 0.1°C of pulmonary artery temperature. The proprietary, novel Accutrol software control algorithm provides automated body temperature control. The Accutrol system eliminates the need to place bladder or rectal probes, which can be slow to react to actual decreases in core body temperature, may be uncomfortable to the patient and time-consuming to place.

Temperature control at target temperature is very tight and allows for gradual rewarming times, which can be programmed from 3 to 24 hours. The Accutrol catheter is beneficial in the critical care environment where gradual rewarming may be warranted.

Standard catheter

The Standard catheter incorporates the same design features as the Accutrol catheter including performance attributes. However, an external core temperature feedback probe is required for operation

MAGNETIC RESONANCE IMAGING (MRI)

The Celsius Control Catheter is "MR Conditional" according to the American Society for Testing and Materials (ASTM) International, Designation: F2503-05. Standard Practice for Marking Medical Devices and Other Items for Safety in the Magnetic Resonance Environment.

ASTM International, 2005. The Celsius Control Catheter demonstrates no known hazards when a "head-only" MRI procedure is performed according to the conditions stated in this labeling.

It is important to read and understand this document in its entirety before conducting a head-only MRI (magnetic resonance imaging) procedure on a patient with an indwelling Celsius Control Catheter. Failure to strictly adhere to these guidelines may result in serious injury to the patient. This information applies to the following INNERCOOL Therapies products:

Catalog No.
11-10-65-1 Celsius Control Standard Catheter 10.7 Fr.
11-14-65-1 Celsius Control Standard Catheter 14 Fr.
11-10-65-2 Celsius Control Accutrol Catheter 10.7 Fr.
11-14-65-2 Celsius Control Accutrol Catheter 14 Fr

Warnings
-Disconnect Celsius Control Catheter from the Celsius Control Console completely prior to entering the MRI environment. Failure to do so may result in serious injury to the patient. It is not possible to continue therapy with the system during an MRI procedure.

-This labeling information applies to "head-only" MRI procedures conducted using a 1.5- Tesla transmit/receive RF head coil or a transmit RF body/receive-only head coil, *ONLY*.

<u>**MRI examinations of other parts of the body is strictly prohibited with the Celsius Control Catheter** *in situ*.</u>

-Testing has not been performed using other MR systems operating at other static magnetic field strengths (i.e., 1.5-Tesla, <u>*only*</u>) and, therefore, other scanners should not be used to perform an MRI examination on a patient who has an indwelling Celsius Control Catheter.

-The Celsius Control Catheter must be properly positioned per the directions for use with the catheter introduced through the femoral vein of either the left or right groin of the patient and advanced into the IVC such that the catheter is parallel to the bore of the MR system. Do not perform the MRI examination with the Celsius Control Catheter placed in any other configuration. Failure to follow this guideline may result in serious injury to the patient.

-Using the transmit/receive RF head coil, do not exceed an MR system reported whole body averaged specific absorption rate (SAR) greater than 0.4-W/Kg.

-Using the transmit RF body coil/receive-only head coil, do not exceed an MR system reported whole body averaged SAR of greater than 3.5-W/Kg.

Overview

The Celsius Control Catheter has undergone extensive *in vitro* testing to demonstrate that, by following specific guidelines, it is safe to perform a head-only MRI procedure on a patient with this device in a 1.5-Tesla MR system, ONLY. Variability among MR systems, differences in how scanners estimate or calculate specific absorption rates (SAR) cannot be simulated comprehensively using in vitro techniques. This document outlines recommended guidelines and specific conditions under which the Celsius Control Catheter has been shown to pose minimal risk to a patient undergoing a head only MRI procedure. Deviation from these guidelines may increase the potential for serious harm to the patient. MRI conditions utilizing MR systems with higher or lower static magnetic fields have not been assessed for the Celsius Control Catheter and, as such, must be avoided to ensure patient safety. The user of this information assumes full responsibility for the consequences of conducting a MRI examination on a patient with an indwelling Celsius Control Catheter.

Magnetic Field Interactions

Translation Attraction and Torque. Magnetic materials contained within an implanted or indwelling device may experience translational or rotational forces when brought into the static magnetic field of a MRI system. The Celsius Control Catheter contains relatively minor magnetic materials. In vitro testing demonstrated that the Celsius Control Catheter is not substantially affected by translational attraction and torque related to exposure to a 1.5 Tesla MR system.

MRI-Related Heating

Under certain conditions, RF fields generated by MRI can induce substantial currents in metallic components contained within medical device products. This may rapidly produce significant heating of a device. Failure to follow the recommendations contained in this communication may result in the generation of thermal lesions and serious patient harm. In vitro testing demonstrated that the Celsius Control Catheter is not substantially affected by the RF fields related to exposure to a 1.5 Tesla MR system under the conditions used for testing.

MRI Artifacts

The presence of the Celsius Control Catheter will cause moderate artifacts on the MR image depending on the pulse sequence parameters used for MRI. However, the artifacts are confined to the position of the

Celsius Control Catheter and, as such, will not affect the diagnostic use of MR imaging for head only MRI examinations.

Procedure

In addition to standard safety procedures for MRI, the following precautions must be followed specific to the Celsius Control Catheter:

1) Inform the patient of the potential risks of undergoing a MRI procedure with the Celsius Control Catheter.

2) Disconnect all cables and patient monitoring devices attached to the Celsius Control Catheter prior to transporting the patient into the MRI environment.

3) The MRI procedure must be performed using a 1.5-Tesla MR system, *only*.

4) MRI examinations must be performed to image the ***head only.*** Use only the following types of radio frequency (RF) coils for the MRI procedure:
   a) Transmit/receive RF head coil
   b) Transmit body RF coil/receive-only head coil.

5) Using the transmit/receive RF head coil, do not exceed an MR system reported SAR of 0.4-W/kg. Using the transmit RF body coil/receive-only RF head coil, do not exceed an MR system reported SAR of 3.5-W/kg.

6) It is important to place the Celsius Control Catheter in a specific geometry to minimize the potential for excessive heating during the MRI procedure. The Celsius Control Catheter must be properly positioned as per the directions for use with the catheter introduced through the femoral vein of either the left or right groin of the patient and advanced into the IVC such that the catheter is parallel to the bore of the MR system. Do not perform the MRI examination with the Celsius Control Catheter placed in any other configuration. Failure to follow this guideline may result in serious injury to the patient.

7) Ensure that the proper patient weight is used for the SAR calculations. Verify that the MRI system has appropriately calculated and updated the SAR value after all parameter changes have been made.

8) A knowledgeable MRI expert (e.g., MRI physicist, MRI-trained radiologist, etc.) must verify that all set-up steps and settings have been properly implemented and checked prior to performing the head only MRI procedure.

9) Verify that all proposed MRI examination parameters and conditions for the Celsius Control Catheter comply with the instructions

described herein. If they do not comply, do not perform the head only MRI procedure.

10) Provide the patient with a means by which he/she can alert the MR system operator during the MRI procedure if any discomfort or unusual sensations should occur.

11) Monitor the patient continuously during the head only MRI examination and be prepared respond or to terminate the MRI procedure immediately in the event of a complaint.

12) Determine if the patient has any other implants or conditions that would prohibit or contraindicate a head only MRI examination. Do not conduct a head only MRI examination if any conditions or implanted devices that would prohibit or contraindicate a MRI are present.

[MR healthcare professionals are advised to contact the manufacturer to ensure that the latest safety information is obtained and carefully followed in order to ensure patient safety relative to the use of an MR procedure.]

REFERENCE

http://www.innercool.com/

Cerebrospinal Fluid (CSF) Shunt Valves

Hydrocephalus is the accumulation of cerebrospinal fluid in the brain, resulting from increased production, or more commonly, pathway obstruction or decreased absorption of the fluid. Cerebrospinal fluid (CSF) shunts have been used for decades for the treatment of hydrocephalus. A CSF shunt involves establishing an accessory pathway for the movement of CSF in order to bypass an obstruction of the natural pathways.

The shunt is positioned to enable the CSF to be drained from the cerebral ventricles or sub-arachnoid spaces into another absorption site (e.g., the right atrium of the heart or the peritoneal cavity) through a system of small catheters. A regulatory device, such as a valve, may be inserted into the pathway of the catheters. In general, the valve keeps the CSF flowing away from the brain and moderates the pressure or flow rate. Some valves are fixed pressure valves (i.e., monopressure valves) and others have adjustable settings. The drainage system using catheters and valves enables the excess CSF within the brain to be evacuated and, thereby, the pressure within the cranium to be reduced.

There are many different types of CSF shunt valves and associated accessories used for treatment of hydrocephalus. In general, for shunt valves that utilize magnetic components, highly specific safety guidelines must be followed in order to perform MRI procedures safely in patients with these devices.

CODMAN HAKIM Programmable Valves

Description. The CODMAN HAKIM Programmable Valve (CSF shunt valve, Codman, a Johnson & Johnson Company, Raynham, MA) includes a valve mechanism that incorporates a flat 316L stainless steel spring in which the calibration is accomplished by a combination between a pillar and a micro-adjustable telescoping fulcrum. The valve chassis is made of titanium. The ball and cone are manufactured from synthetic ruby. Intraventricular pressure is maintained at a constant level by the ball and cone valve seat design.

The pressure setting of the spring in the inlet valve unit is noninvasively adjusted by the use of an external programmer, which activates the stepper motor within the valve housing. The programmer transmits a codified magnetic signal to the motor allowing eighteen pressure settings, ranging from 30 mm to 200 mm H_2O (294 to 1960 Pa) in 10 mm (98 Pa) increments. These are operating pressures of the valve unit and have been determined with a flow rate of 15–25 ml H_2O per hour.

The valve is classified by its working pressure with a specified flow rate and not by the opening and closing pressures. The pressure that a valve sustains with a given flow is the parameter that reflects the working pressure of the valve once it is implanted. Before shipment, each valve is calibrated with special equipment: Duplication of these test procedures cannot be accomplished in the operating room.

Indications. The CODMAN HAKIM Programmable Valves are implantable devices that provide constant intraventricular pressure and drainage of CSF for the management of hydrocephalus.

Programmable Valve Configurations

- In-line with SIPHONGUARD Device
- In-line
- Right Angle with SIPHONGUARD Device
- Right Angle
- Cylindrical with Prechamber
- Cylindrical
- Micro with RICKHAM® Reservoir
- Micro

CODMAN HAKIM In-line and Right Angle Valves include a programmable valve with a low profile and flat bottom, and an in-line or right angle integral reservoir with or without SIPHONGUARD.

CODMAN HAKIM Cylindrical Valves include a programmable valve, a pumping chamber, and an outlet valve available with or without a prechamber.

CODMAN HAKIM Micro Valves include a programmable valve with or without an integral RICKHAM reservoir.

WARNINGS. Subjecting the valve to strong magnetic fields may change the setting of the valve.

- The use of Magnetic Resonance (MR) systems up to 3-Tesla will not damage the valve mechanism, but may change the setting of the valve. Confirm the valve setting after an MRI procedure.
- Common magnets greater than 80 gauss, such as household magnets, loudspeaker magnets, and language lab headphone magnets, may affect the valve setting when placed close to the valve.
- Magnetic fields generated from microwaves, high-tension wires, electric motors, transformers, etc., do not affect the valve setting.

Read the *MRI Information* before performing an MRI procedure on a patient implanted with the programmable valve.

MRI Information

The CODMAN HAKIM Programmable Valve (CSF shunt valve, Codman, a Johnson & Johnson Company, Raynham, MA) is "MR Conditional" according to ASTM F 2503. The valve demonstrates no known hazards when an MRI is performed under the following conditions:

- MRI can be performed at any time after implantation
- Use an MR system with a static magnetic field of 3 T or less
- Use an MR System with a spatial gradient of 720 gauss/cm or less
- Limit the exposure to RF energy to a whole-body-averaged specific absorption rate (SAR) of 3 W/kg for 15 minutes
- Verify the valve setting after the MRI procedure (see *Programming the Valve*)

In non-clinical testing, the valve produced a temperature rise of 0.4-degrees C at a maximum whole-body-averaged specific absorption rate (SAR) of 3-W/kg for 15 minutes of MR scanning in a 3-T Excite General Electric MR scanner.

MR image quality may be compromised if the area of interest is relatively close to the device. Distortion may be seen at the boundaries of the artifact. Therefore, optimization of the MR imaging parameters may be necessary.

The following table provides a comparison between the signal void and imaging pulse sequence at 3-Tesla:

Signal Void	Pulse Sequence	Imaging plane
1,590-mm^2	T1-weighted, spin echo	Parallel

1,022-mm^2	T1-weighted, spin echo	Perpendicular
2,439-mm^2	Gradient echo	Parallel
2,404-mm^2	Gradient echo	Perpendicular

Delta Shunt Assembly

The Delta Shunt Assembly (Medtronic Neurosurgery, Goleta, CA) combines the Delta valve with an integral, open-end, radiopaque peritoneal catheter. All Delta shunt assemblies incorporate the same product features as the Delta valves. These include injectable reservoir domes, occluders for selective flushing, and a completely non-metallic design. The valves are fabricated of dissimilar materials - polypropylene and silicone elastomer - reducing the chance of valve sticking and deformation. The normally closed Delta chamber mechanism minimizes over-drainage by utilizing the principles of hydrodynamic leverage. Because of the non-metallic design, the Delta shunt is safe for patients undergoing MRI procedures.

POLARIS Adjustable Pressure Valve

The POLARIS Adjustable Pressure Valve (Sophysa USA, Inc., Crown Point, IN) has magnets made of Samarium-Cobalt, which are specially treated to preserve permanent magnetization, even after repeated exposure to MRI at 3-Tesla. The principle of the POLARIS Adjustable Pressure Valve is based on the variation in pressure exerted on a ball by a semicircular spring at different points along its curvature. The flat semicircular calibrated spring determines an operating pressure. Because of the unique design of the POLARIS Adjustable Pressure Valve, it is considered to be acceptable for patients undergoing MRI procedures at 3-Tesla or less.

Although the magnetic self-locking system for the POLARIS Adjustable Pressure Valve is designed to be insensitive to magnetic fields associated with exposure to MRI, it is recommended that the following procedure be performed when a patient undergoes an MRI examination:

1) Confirm the position of the rotor before entering the MR system room, using the locating instrument and the reading/adjustment instrument.
2) Perform the MRI examination.
3) Check the position of the rotor (i.e., the setting) as soon as the patient leaves the MR system room.

4) If the position of the rotor has changed, reset it to its original position using the reading/adjustment instrument following the described procedure.

proGAV Programmable Valve

The programmable valve, proGAV (Aesculap, Inc., Center Valley, PA), has magnetic components used for the programming mechanism. This device recently underwent evaluations relative to the use of a 3-Tesla MR system (i.e., tested for magnetic field interactions, heating, artifacts, and functional alterations). In consideration of the results of these tests, in order to take proper precautions to ensure patient safety, the following guidelines are recommended for scanning a patient with this device:

1) A patient with the programmable valve, proGAV, may undergo MRI at 3-T or less immediately after implantation.
2) Prior to MRI, the programmable valve setting should be determined by appropriate personnel using proper equipment.
3) The exposure to RF energy should be limited to a whole body averaged SAR of 2.1-W/kg for 15-min.
4) After MRI, the proGAV programmable valve setting should be determined and re-set, as needed.

Pulsar Valve

The Pulsar Valve (Sophysa USA, Inc., Costa Mesa, CA) for CSF drainage is a monopressure valve. Its principal is based on the play of a silicone membrane, calibrated in low, medium, or high pressure, ensuring a proximal regulation of CSF flow through the shunt system. The Pulsar Valve is safe for patients undergoing MRI procedures.

Sophy Mini Monopressure Valve

The Sophy Mini Monopressure Valve (Sophysa USA, Inc., Costa Mesa, CA) for CSF drainage has a ball-in-cone mechanism. This device is safe for patients undergoing MRI procedures.

Strata, Strata II, and Strata NSC Programmable CSF Shunt Valves

MRI Information

The Strata, Strata NSC, and Strata II Programmable CSF shunt valves (Medtronic Neurosurgery, Goleta, CA) are Magnetic Resonance Conditional (MR conditional) in accordance with ASTM F2503. MRI systems of up to 3.0-Tesla may be used any time after implantation and will not damage the Strata, Strata NSC, or Strata II valve mechanisms, but can change the performance level setting. The performance level setting should always be checked before and after MRI exposure. The results of the tests performed to assess magnetic field interactions, artifacts, and heating, indicated the presence of the valves evaluated should present no substantial risk to a patient undergoing an MRI procedure using the following conditions:

- Static magnetic field of 3.0 Tesla or less
- Spatial Gradient of 720 Gauss/cm or less
- Radio Frequency (RF) Fields with an average Specific Absorption Rate (SAR) of 3 W/kg for 15 minutes. Using the GE 3T Excite HD Magnetic Resonance Imaging System, the valve experienced a maximum temperature change of 0.4°C over a 15 minute exposure period. The table below provides maximum signal voids (artifact sizes) for standard imaging pulse sequences at 3 Tesla per ASTM F2119.

Signal Void	Pulse Sequence	Imaging plane
35.16-cm^2	T1-weighted, spin echo	Parallel
33.03-cm^2	T1-weighted, spin echo	Perpendicular
75.91-cm^2	Gradient echo	Parallel
66.55-cm^2	Gradient echo	Perpendicular

Adjustment Kits

Do **NOT** take the Adjustment Tool into an MRI facility as these magnets could potentially be a safety hazard to the patient and/or user. Proximity to MRI suite may impede the mechanism in the Indicator Tool due to the field strength of an MRI magnet. Move out of the vicinity prior to attempting to verify a valve setting.

SOPHY Adjustable Pressure Valve

The principle of the SOPHY Adjustable Pressure Valve (Sophysa USA, Inc., Costa Mesa, CA) resides in the variation in pressure exerted on a ball by a semi-circular spring at various points along its circumference. The spring is attached to a magnetic rotor whose position can be noninvasively altered using an adjustment magnet. A series of indentations allows a variety of positions to be selected, each position representing a different pressure setting. The valve's ball-in-cone mechanism maintains the selected pressure constant without significant drift.

Because a magnetic component is associated with this device, special MR safety precautions exist for scanning patients with the SOPHY Adjustable Pressure Valve, as follows:

- The pressure settings should always be checked in case of shock on the implantation site.
- Changing pressure settings must only be performed by a neurosurgeon.
- The patient must be advised that carrying his Patient Identification Card is important and necessary for the follow-up of the clinical conditions.
- Patients undergoing MRI exposure should be advised that they might feel a small yet harmless effect due to MRI.
- The pressure settings should always be checked before and after MRI exposure, or after strong magnetic field exposure.
- The patient must be advised that in the case of implantation on the skull vibrations due to CSF flow may be perceived.
- Patients with implanted valve systems must be kept under close observation for symptoms of shunt failure.

[MR healthcare professionals are advised to contact the respective manufacturer in order to obtain the latest safety information to ensure patient safety relative to the use of an MR procedure.]

REFERENCES

Anderson RCE, Walker ML, Viner JM, Kestle JRW. Adjustment and malfunction of a programmable valve after exposure to toy magnets. J Neurosurg (Pediatrics) 2004;101:222-225.

Codman, a Johnson and Johnson Company, http://www.codman.com

Fransen P. Transcutaneous pressure-adjustable valves and magnetic resonance imaging: an ex vivo examination of the Codman-Medos programmable valve and the Sophy adjustable pressure valve. Neurosurgery 1998;42:430.

Fransen P, Dooms G, Thauvoy C. Safety of the adjustable pressure ventricular valve in magnetic resonance imaging: problems and solutions. Neuroradiology 1992;34:508-509.

Inoue T, Kuzu Y, Ogasawara K, Ogawa A. Effect of 3-Tesla magnetic resonance imaging on various pressure programmable shunt valves. J Neurosurg 2005;103(2 Suppl):163-5.

Lindner D, Preul C, Trantakis C, Moeller H, Meixensberger J. Effect of 3-T MRI on the function of shunt valves--evaluation of Paedi GAV, Dual Switch and proGAV. Eur J Radiol 2005;56:56-9.

Ludemann W, Rosahl SK, Kaminsky J, Samii M. Reliability of a new adjustable shunt device without the need for readjustment following 3-Tesla MRI. Childs Nerv Syst 2005;21:227-229.

Medtronic Neurosurgery, Goleta, CA; Cerebral Spinal Fluid Shunt Valves and Accessories, http://www.medtronic.com/neurosurgery/shunts.html

Miwa K, Kondo H, Sakai N. Pressure changes observed in Codman-Medos programmable valves following magnetic exposure and filliping. Childs Nerv Syst 2001;17:150-153.

Ortler M, Kostron H, Felber S. Transcutaneous pressure-adjustable valves and magnetic resonance imaging: an ex vivo examination of the Codman-Medos programmable valve and the Sophy adjustable pressure valve. Neurosurgery 1997;40:1050-1057.

Schneider T, Knauff U, Nitsch J, Firsching R. Electromagnetic field hazards involving adjustable shunt valves in hydrocephalus. J Neurosurg 2002;96:331-334.

Shellock FG. MR safety and Cerebral Spinal Fluid Shunt (CSF) Valves. Signals, No. 51, Issue 4, pp. 10, 2004.

Shellock FG, Habibi R, Knebel J. Programmable CSF shunt valve: *In vitro* assessment of MRI safety at 3-Tesla. American Journal of Neuroradiology, 2006;27:661-665.

Shellock FG, Wilson SF, Mauge CP. Magnetically-programmable shunt valve: MRI at 3-Tesla. Magnetic Resonance Imaging 2007;25:1116-21.

Sophysa USA, Inc., Cerebral Spinal Fluid Shunt Valves and Accessories, http://www.sophysa.com

Zemack G, Romner B. Seven years of clinical experience with the programmable Codman Hakim valve: a retrospective study of 583 patients. J Neurosurg 2000;92:941-8.

Cochlear Implants

Cochlear implants are electronically-activated devices. Consequently, an MR procedure may be contraindicated for a patient with this type of implant because of the possibility of injuring the patient and/or altering or damaging the function of the device. In general, individuals with cochlear implants should be prevented from entering the MR environment unless specific guidelines exist to ensure safety for these devices.

Investigations have been conducted to determine if there are situations and specific conditions for a patient with a cochlear implant to safely undergo an MR procedure. These studies have resulted in highly specific guidelines that must be followed in order to safely perform MR examinations in patients with certain cochlear implants. Notably, some cochlear implants require the use of a 0.2-Tesla or 0.3-Tesla MR system, *only,* as part of the guidelines. In other cases, the magnet associated with the cochlear implant may require removal prior to the MRI examination and the replacement following the scan. Additional MRI concerns include possible demagnetization of the internal magnet associated with the cochlear implant be exposure to the powerful static magnetic field of the MR system, as well as the substantial artifacts that exist if this magnet remains in place during an MRI examination. See specific information below.

Hires 90K Implant and MRI (Advanced Bionics, Sylmar, CA)*

INFORMATION FOR MRI HEALTHCARE WORKERS

The HiRes 90K implant, with the internal magnet removed, has been tested with 1.5-Tesla/64-MHz and 0.3-Tesla/12-MHz MRI systems. MRI is contraindicated except under the circumstances described below.

Do not allow patients with a HiRes 90K cochlear implant to be in the area of an MRI system unless the following conditions have been met:
-The internal magnet must be surgically removed and replaced with the Magnet Insert Dummy before the patient undergoes an MRI procedure.
-The external sound processor and headpiece are removed before entering a room where an MRI scanner is located.
-MRI parameters should be selected to ensure a Specific Absorption Rate

(SAR) of less than 1.0 W/kg in the head region.
-Continuous verbal and visual monitoring of the patient should be performed throughout the MRI procedure.

Image shadowing may extend as far as 7-cm squared area from the implant, resulting in loss of diagnostic information in the implant vicinity. The extent of the shadowing may be minimized by adjusting the signal parameters.

For additional information regarding the use of MRI with the HiRes 90K implant, please contact Advanced Bionics Technical Support.

Information for Patients

What is Magnetic Resonance Imaging? Magnetic resonance imaging (MRI) is a technique for taking remarkably clear and detailed pictures of internal organs and tissues using radio waves and a strong magnetic field.

When might a person be referred for an MRI? MRI is a sensitive exam for brain tumors, strokes, and certain chronic disorders of the nervous system such as multiple sclerosis. In addition, MRI might be recommended as a means of documenting disease of the cardiovascular system, pituitary gland, eye or inner ear.

Is the cochlear implant safe with MRI? Only after the magnet has been removed. As referrals for MRI are increasing, it is comforting to know that your implant is safe with this imaging technique. But you must be sure to have the magnet removed first.

The United States Food and Drug Administration (FDA) cleared the HiResolution Bionic Ear System's HiRes 90K implant for Magnetic Resonance Imaging (MRI) at 0.3-Tesla and 1.5-Tesla with the internal magnet removed.

The magnetic and electrical properties of an MRI machine can potentially cause harm to a patient with a cochlear implant and damage the device. Therefore a patient with a cochlear implant should not be near an MRI machine, whether or not in use, unless the following conditions have been met:
-Internal magnet has been removed
-External processor and headpiece have been removed

A cochlear implant recipient should always consult with their implant surgeon before any imaging is performed, regardless of the imaging technique.

If an MRI is needed, what are the steps required to remove the magnet of the cochlear implant? Removing the magnet is a quick and easy procedure typically performed under local anesthesia. Your surgeon will shave a small area of hair directly over the implant. A small incision will be made exposing the implant. The magnet is gently removed and replaced with a sterilized insert. The incision is then closed. You may experience some swelling and slight discomfort following the procedure.

Will I be able to wear my processor after the magnet is removed? Once the incision has healed, you will be able to wear your processor. You should check with your implant center before resuming device use. Your audiologist will assist you in coupling the headpiece to the implant. Typically, a small hair clip is attached to hold the headpiece in place over the implant.

Can the magnet be replaced after an MRI? Yes, your surgeon can replace the magnet after an MRI is completed, provided that further MRI evaluations are not anticipated. Under local anesthesia, your surgeon will shave the hair over the implant and make a small incision. The sterilized insert is removed and replaced with a new sterilized magnet ordered from Advanced Bionics.

If necessary, can the HiResolution Bionic Ear System's HiRes 90K be implanted without the magnet? Yes, your surgeon can elect to remove the magnet from the HiRes 90K before the device is implanted. In this case, the surgeon will order the sterilized insert with the device and replace the magnet with the sterilized insert at the time of surgery.

What recommendations should be provided to the radiologist/technologist when an MRI is ordered for a cochlear implant recipient? Your implant center can provide the MRI technologist or radiologist with the HiResolution Bionic Ear System's HiRes 90K package insert. Further instructions are provided when the implant center orders the sterilized insert or replacement magnet from Advanced Bionics that can be forwarded to the MRI technologist as well.

Are other imaging techniques available? How is MRI different? There are many imaging techniques used today including x-rays, computed tomography (CT) scans, positron emission tomography (PET) scans, and ultrasound. MRI requires specialized equipment and expertise and allows evaluation of some body structures that may not be as visible with other imaging methods. Your medical team will discuss these options with you and determine which technique is optimal for your healthcare needs.

What do we need to do if we want to replace the magnet after the MRI? Provided additional MRIs are not anticipated, the center can order a sterilized "replacement magnet" CI-1412 from Advanced Bionics'

Customer Service. The replacement magnet will come with a surgical insert title "MRI for HiRes 90k implant" which provides detailed surgical instructions.

The Insert Dummy and Replacement Magnets are ordered SEPARATELY.

Can we implant the HiRes 90K without the magnet to begin with? Yes, order the Insert Dummy with the device. The surgical insert titled "MRI for HiRes 90K implant" that accompanies the insert dummy includes detailed surgical instructions for removing the magnet prior to implantation.

What specific recommendations can we provide the MRI technologist? The HiRes 90K implant is FDA approved for PRI testing at 0.3-Tesla and 1.5-Tesla with the magnet removed. The external hardware must also be removed before the patient enters the MRI testing room/suite. The center can provide the technologist with the "MRI for HiRes 90K implant" surgical insert that accompanies the insert dummy or replacement magnet.

[*Information provided with permission from Advanced Bionics, Sylmar, CA]

[MR healthcare professionals are advised to contact the manufacturer to ensure that the latest safety information is obtained and carefully followed in order to ensure patient safety relative to the use of an MR procedure.]

PULSAR COCHLEAR IMPLANT, PULSARCI[100] COCHLEAR IMPLANT, MED-EL CORPORATION

The Pulsar Cochlear Implant, PULSARCI[100] Cochlear Implant, MED-EL Corporation, Durham, NC) has the following information stated with regard to using MR imaging in patients with this device:

MRI Safe - Without Magnet Removal

Many cochlear implant users will require an MRI (Magnetic Resonance Imaging) scan at some point in their lifetime, so MRI compatibility is an important consideration when selecting a cochlear implant. MED-EL is the only cochlear implant manufacturer to offer MRI safety without surgical removal of the internal magnet. At MED-EL, we recognize the importance of providing access to critical medical treatment, including MRI, without disruption to your life or your hearing.

PULSARCI[100] is MRI safe at 0.2-Tesla

- No need for surgery to remove and replace the internal magnet
- No incision or swelling to heal after an MRI scan
- No recovery time to affect implant use or performance

- No additional risk to the patient
- No significant impact on MRI image quality
- No limitations on daily activities following an MRI scan
- No risk of magnet displacement

[MR healthcare professionals are advised to contact the manufacturer to ensure that the latest safety information is obtained and carefully followed in order to ensure patient safety relative to the use of an MR procedure.]

Nucleus 24 Series, Cochlear Implant (Cochlear Corporation)

Magnetic Resonance Imaging (MRI)
The Nucleus 24 cochlear implant and some Nucleus 22 cochlear implants have a removable magnet and specific design characteristics to enable it to withstand MRI up to 1.5 tesla, but not higher.

For patients with a Nucleus 22 cochlear implant without a removable magnet, MRI is contraindicated.

The Nucleus 24 cochlear implant has a removable magnet and specific design characteristics to enable it to withstand MRI up to 1.5 Tesla static field, a 64 MHz RF pulsed field, and pulsed gradient fields up to 20 Tesla/ sec. If the cochlear implant's magnet is in place, it must be removed surgically before the patient undergoes a MRI procedure.

Magnetic Resonance Imaging (MRI) is contraindicated except under the circumstances described below. Patients with a cochlear implant should not enter a room where a MRI scanner is located except under the following special circumstances. The patient must remove the speech processor and headset before entering a room where a MRI scanner is located.

If the implant's magnet is still in place, the implant may move, causing pain and/or tissue damage if the recipient is exposed to MRI. Once the magnet is surgically removed, the metal in the cochlear implant will affect the quality of the MRI, but no damage to the implant will occur. Image shadowing may extend as far as 6-cm from the implant, thereby resulting in loss of diagnostic information in the vicinity of the implant.

The MRI static field exerts a small force on the implant, even without the magnet. Without the magnet, the maximum force is less than the normal weight of the implant. This may be perceptible during the MRI procedure but is not harmful.

If there is doubt that the patient has a cochlear implant with a removable magnet, the physician should use an x-ray to check the radiopaque lettering on the implant. There are three platinum letters printed on each implant. If the middle letter is a "C", "H", "J", "L", "P", "T", "2", "5" or "7" the implant has a removable magnet. Once the magnet has been removed, MRI can be performed.

Removing the Magnet
(when the patient needs a single MRI)

If an implant user develops a condition likely to require a single MRI examination, the magnet must be surgically removed. Surgery is usually performed under local anesthetic in a minor procedure room. A local injection of lidoocaine with 1:100,000 or 1:200,000 Epinephrine is used. The area over the magnet is shaved and the area is prepared for the incision. A curved incision is made posterior to the implant. The surgeon cuts through any fibrous growth around the implant to expose the magnet.

If a retaining suture runs across the magnet, the surgeon may bend the suture to expose the magnet. A dry sterile dressing is applied over the wound and the patient is taken for MRI examination. The recess may remain empty, with sterility maintained for a period of up to four hours. After the examination, a sterile magnet is replaced and the wound closed. A sterile dressing is applied overnight.

Magnet Removal
(when it is anticipated that the patient will need repeated MRIs in the future)

If it is anticipated that a patient will need repeated MRIs in the future, the surgeon may elect to remove the magnet on a more long-term basis. If it is known prior to implantation that the patient will need repeated MRIs in the future, the surgeon may elect to remove the magnet from the implant prior to implantation.

In these cases, the magnet may be removed and replaced with a non-magnetic titanium plug. The plug prevents the growth of fibrous tissue into the recess, which could make the future placement of a magnet difficult.

If the device has not yet been implanted, the magnet should be removed under sterile conditions. The cochlear implant is removed from its sterile packaging and placed on a flat stable surface with the magnet's star symbol facing upward. The protective tubing should not be removed from the electrode array until implantation. Using an elevator, the lip of the silicone recess may be gently lifted in order to shell the magnet out of the recess. When removing the magnet, the pressure applied to the antenna of the implant should be minimized. If the device is already implanted, a similar method should be used to shell out the magnet while leaving the device in-situ. The sterile non-magnetic plug may then be inserted into the recess.

Replacing the Magnet

The magnet is replaced when there is no further need for MRI examinations. After exposure of the magnet recess, an elevator may be used to lift the lip of the recess and position the magnet. A sterile magnet should be inserted with the star symbol (denoting polarity) facing up. The wound is closed and a sterile dressing is applied.

Note to MR Healthcare Professionals: Different MRI guidelines exist for different countries. As such, use the appropriate information for your country. Visit www.Cochlear.com to obtain the proper information.

[MR healthcare professionals are advised to contact the respective manufacturer in order to obtain the latest safety information to ensure patient safety relative to the use of an MR procedure.]

REFERENCES

Chou H-K, McDougall JA, Can KW. Absence of radiofrequency heating from auditory implants during magnetic resonance imaging. Bioelectromagnetics 1995;16:307-316.

Deneuve S, Loundon N, et al. Cochlear implant magnet displacement during magnetic resonance imaging. Otol Neurotol. 2008;29:789-190.

Gubbels SP, McMenomey SO. Safety study of the Cochlear Nucleus 24 device with internal magnet in the 1.5 Tesla magnetic resonance imaging scanner. Laryngoscope. 2006;116:865-71.

Heller JW, et al. Evaluation of MRI compatibility of the modified nucleus multi-channel auditory brainstem and cochlear implants. Am J Otol 1996;17:724-729.

http://www.advancedbionics.comhttp://www.Cochlear.com

http://www.MEDEL.com

Majdani O, Rau TS, Gotz F, et al. Artifacts caused by cochlear implants with non-removable magnets in 3T MRI: phantom and cadaveric studies. Eur Arch Otorhinolaryngol. 2009. [Epub ahead of print]

Majdani O, Leinung M, Rau T, et al. Demagnetization of cochlear implants and temperature changes in 3.0T MRI environment. Otolaryngol Head Neck Surg. 2008;139:833-9.

Ouayoun M, et al. Nuclear magnetic resonance and cochlear implant. Ann Otolaryngol Chir Cervicofac 1997;114:65-70.

Shellock FG. Magnetic Resonance Procedures: Health Effects and Safety. CRC Press, LLC, Boca Raton, FL, 2001.

Teissl C, Kremser C, Hochmair ES, Hochmair-Desoyer IJ. Cochlear implants: *in vitro* investigation of electromagnetic interference at MR imaging-compatibility and safety aspects. Radiology 1998;208:700-708.

Teissl C, Kremser C, Hochmair ES, Hochmair-Desoyer IJ. Magnetic resonance imaging and cochlear implants: compatibility and safety aspects. J Magn Reson Imaging 1999;9:26-38.

Coils, Stents, Filters, and Grafts

Coils, stents, filters and vascular grafts have been evaluated relative to the use of MR systems. Several of these demonstrated magnetic field interactions in association with scanners. Fortunately, the devices that exhibited positive magnetic field interactions typically become incorporated securely in tissue within six weeks after implantation due to ingrowth and other mechanisms. Therefore, for most coils, filters, stents and grafts that have been tested, it is unlikely that these implants would become moved or dislodged as a result of exposure to MR systems operating at 1.5-Tesla or less. Additionally, many of these items have now been evaluated at 3-Tesla (see below). MRI-related heating may also be of concern for certain configurations or shapes for coils, stents, filters and vascular grafts.

Many of these implants are made from nonferromagnetic materials, such as the LGM IVC filter (Vena Tech) used for caval interruption and the Wallstent biliary endoprosthesis [Schneider (USA), Inc.] used for treatment of biliary obstruction. As such, these implants are acceptable for patients undergoing MR procedures relative to the use of the particular field strength utilized in *ex vivo* testing (for specific information, see **The List**). Notably, it is unnecessary to wait an extended period of time after surgery to perform an MR procedure in a patient with a "passive" metallic implant that is made from a nonmagnetic material (see **Guidelines for the Management of the Post-Operative Patient Referred for a Magnetic Resonance Procedure**). In fact, there are reports in the peer-reviewed literature that describe placement of vascular stents using MR-guidance at 1.5-Tesla and 3-Tesla. The only exception may be if there are concerns associated with MRI-related heating.

Patients with the specific coils, stents, filters and vascular grafts indicated in **The List** have had procedures using MR systems operating at static magnetic field strengths of 3-Tesla or less without reported injuries or other problems. Despite the past track record of safety, MRI facilities should never have a "general" policy to scan patients with these implants if the acceptable MRI conditions are unknown or if there is no specific MRI labeling information available. One of the reasons for this is that new coils, stents, filters and vascular grafts are developed on an ongoing basis. Additionally, to date, not all such devices have undergone comprehensive MRI testing, including with respect to the 3-Tesla MRI environment.

A study by Taal et al. supports the fact that not all stents are safe for patients undergoing MR procedures. This investigation was performed to evaluate potential problems for four different types of stents: the Ultraflex (titanium alloy), the covered Wallstent (Nitinol), the Gianturco stent (Cook), and the modified Gianturco stent (Song) - the last two are made from stainless steel. Taal et al. reported "an appreciable attraction force and torque" found for both types of Gianturco stents. In particular, "the Gianturco (Cook) stent pulled toward the head with a force of 7 g…however, it is uncertain whether this is a potential risk for dislodgment." In consideration of these results the investigators advised, "…specific information on the type of stent is necessary before a magnetic resonance imaging examination is planned."

MRI at 3-Tesla and Coils, Stents, Filters and Vascular Grafts. Different coils, stents, filters and vascular grafts have been evaluated at 3-Tesla. Of these implants, two displayed magnetic field interactions that exceeded the American Society for Testing and Materials (ASTM) International guideline for safety (i.e., the deflection angles were greater than 45 degrees). However, similar to other comparable implants, tissue ingrowth and other mechanims are sufficient to prevent them from posing a substantial risk to a patient or individual in the 3-Tesla MR environment. Thus, these issues warrant further consideration.

MRI at 3-Tesla: Bare Metal and Drug Eluting Coronary Stents. Patients with coronary artery disease are often treated by percutaneous transluminal coronary angioplasty (PTCA). Re-narrowing at the angioplasty site, or restenosis, occurs in as many as 50% of patients following PTCA. Therefore, after coronary artery intervention, either a bare metal or drug eluting stent is placed in an effort to prevent restenosis. There is considerable attention focused on the use of drug eluting stents to prevent coronary artery restenosis that tends to occur in a substantial number of patients following stenting with "bare" devices. Studies have reported that drug eluting stents reduce the incidence of target vessel failure compared to uncoated metallic stents. As such, drug eluting stents are now used on a widespread basis in patients with coronary artery disease.

MRI information has been obtained for many bare metal and drug eluting coronary artery stents, which have been reported to be acceptable for patients undergoing MR procedures at 3-Tesla or less (i.e., based on assessments of magnetic field interactions and MRI-related heating). Of note is that, for most of these coronary artery stents, patients with these implants may undergo MRI procedures immediately after placement. Please refer to **The List** for specific information.

REFERENCES

Ahmed S, Shellock FG. Magnetic resonance imaging safety: implications for cardiovascular patients. Journal of Cardiovascular Magnetic Resonance 2001;3:171-181.

Bueker A, et al. Real-time MR fluoroscopy for MR-guided iliac artery stent placement. J Magn Reson Imaging 2000;12:616-622.

Hennemeyer CT, Wicklow K, Feinberg DA, Derdeyn CP. In vitro evaluation of platinum Guglielmi detachable coils at 3-T with a porcine model: safety issues and artifacts. Radiology 2001;219:732-737.

Hiramoto JS, Reilly LM, Schneider DB, et al. Long-term outcome and reintervention after endovascular abdominal aortic aneurysm repair using the Zenith stent graft. J Vasc Surg. 2007;45:461-452

Hug J, et al. Coronary arterial stents: safety and artifacts during MR imaging. Radiology 2000;216:781-787.

Girard MJ, et al. Wallstent metallic biliary endoprosthesis: MR imaging characteristics. Radiology 1992;184:874-876.

Green SR, Gianchandani YB. Wireless magnetoelastic monitoring of biliary stents. Journal of Microelectromechanical Systems. 2009;18:64-78.

Kaya MG, et al. Long-term clinical effects of magnetic resonance imaging in patients with coronary artery stent implantation. Coron Artery Dis. 2009; 20:138-42.

Kiproff PM, et al. Magnetic resonance characteristics of the LGM vena cava filter: technical note. Cardiovasc Intervent Radiol 1991;14:254-255.

Leibman CE, Messersmith RN, Levin DN, et al. MR imaging of inferior vena caval filter: safety and artifacts. AJR Am J Roentgenol 1988;150:1174-1176.

Manke C, Nitz WR, Djavidani B, et al. MR imaging-guided stent placement in iliac arterial stenoses: A feasibility study. Radiology 2001;219:527-534.

Marshall MW, Teitelbaum GP, Kim HS, et al. Ferromagnetism and magnetic resonance artifacts of platinum embolization microcoils. Cardiovasc Intervent Radiol 1991;14:163-166.

Nehra A, Moran CJ, Cross DT, Derdeyn CP. MR safety and imaging of Neuroform Stents at 3-T. Am J Neuroradiol 2004;25:1476-1478.

Patel M, Albert TSE, Kandzari DE, et al. Acute myocardial infarction: safety of cardiac MR imaging after percutaneous revascularization with stents. Radiology 2006;674-680.

Porto I, Selvanayagam J, Ashar V, Neubauer S, Banning AP. Safety of magnetic resonance imaging one to three days after bare metal and drug-eluting stent implantation. Am J Cardiol 2005;96:366-8.

Rutledge JM, Vick GW, Mullins CE, Grifka RG. Safety of magnetic resonance immediately following Palmaz stent implant: a report of three cases. Catheter Cardiovasc Interv 2001;53:519-523.

Shellock FG. MR Safety at 3-Tesla: Bare Metal and Drug Eluting Coronary Artery Stents. Signals No. 53, Issue 2, pp. 26-27, 2005.

Shellock FG. Biomedical implants and devices: assessment of magnetic field interactions with a 3.0-Tesla MR system. J Magn Reson Imaging 2002;16:721-732.

Shellock FG. Magnetic Resonance Procedures: Health Effects and Safety. CRC Press, LLC, Boca Raton, FL, 2001.

Shellock FG, Detrick MS, Brant-Zawadski M. MR-compatibility of the Guglielmi detachable coils. Radiology 1997;203:568-570.

Shellock FG. Forder J. Drug eluting coronary stent: *In vitro* evaluation of magnetic resonance safety at 3-Tesla. Journal of Cardiovascular Magnetic Resonance 2005;7:415-419.

Shellock FG, Gounis M, Wakhloo A. Detachable coil for cerebral aneurysms: *In vitro* evaluation of magnet field interactions, heating, and artifacts at 3-Tesla. American Journal of Neuroradiology 2005;26:363-366.

Shellock FG, Morisoli S, Kanal E. MR procedures and biomedical implants, materials, and devices: 1993 update. Radiology 1993;189:587-599.

Shellock FG, Shellock VJ. Stents: Evaluation of MRI safety. Am J Roentgenol 1999;173:543-546.

Sommer T, et al. High field MR imaging: magnetic field interactions of aneurysm clips, coronary artery stents and iliac artery stents with a 3.0 Tesla MR system. Rofo Fortschr Geb Rontgenstr Neuen Bildgeb Verfahr 2004;176:731-8.

Spuentrup E, et al. Magnetic resonance-guided coronary artery stent placement in a swine model. Circulation 2002;105:874-879.

Taal BG, Muller SH, Boot H, Koop W. Potential risks and artifacts of magnetic resonance imaging of self-expandable esophageal stents. Gastrointestinal Endoscopy 1997;46:424-429.

Teitelbaum GP, Bradley WG, Klein BD. MR imaging artifacts, ferromagnetism, and magnetic torque of intravascular filters, stents, and coils. Radiology 1988;166:657-664.

Teitelbaum GP, Lin MCW, Watanabe AT, et al. Ferromagnetism and MR imaging: safety of cartoid vascular clamps. AJNR Am J Neuroradiol 1990;11:267-272.

Teitelbaum GP, Ortega HV, Vinitski S, et al. Low artifact intravascular devices: MR imaging evaluation. Radiology 1988;168:713-719.

Teitelbaum GP, Raney M, Carvlin MJ, et al. Evaluation of ferromagnetism and magnetic resonance imaging artifacts of the Strecker tantalum vascular stent. Cardiovasc Intervent Radiol 1989;12:125-127.

Watanabe AT, Teitelbaum GP, Gomes AS, et al. MR imaging of the bird's nest filter. Radiology 1990;177:578-579.

Cranial Flap Fixation Clamps and Similar Devices

After performing a craniotomy, bone flaps are typically fixed with wire, suture material, or small plates and screws. Problems related to cranial bone flap fixation after craniotomy are more common with the trend for performing smaller craniotomies that are frequently utilized for minimally invasive surgical procedures. The use of small plates and screws for fixation of cranial bone flaps has improved the overall attachment process and end result. However, this technique requires a considerable amount of time and expense compared to using wire and suture techniques.

Because of the various problems with bone flap fixation, a special metallic implant system, named the Craniofix (Aesculap, Inc., Central Valley, PA) was developed for fixation of cranial bone flaps after craniotomy. MR tests conducted to assess magnetic field interaction, heating, and artifacts indicated that the clamps used for the cranial bone flap fixation system present no risk to the patient in the MR environment of MR systems operating at 1.5-Tesla or less. Furthermore, the quality of the diagnostic MR images was acceptable, particularly for conventional spin echo or fast spin echo pulse sequences. Other devices used for similar applications have also been evaluated MR related issues.

MRI at 3-Tesla and Cranial Fixation Implants and Devices. Several different cranial or burr hole fixation implants and devices made from titanium or titanium alloy have been tested at 3-Tesla. These were found to be acceptable for patients undergoing MR procedures.

CranioFix Titanium Clamps (Information dated 11/11/09 - Aesculap Inc., Center Valley, PA) are indicated for the fixation of cranial bone flaps after a craniotomy. They are manufactured from a titanium alloy (Ti_6Al_4V) which is non-ferromagnetic and may be safely exposed to MRI. All CranioFix Titanium Clamps (FF099T, FF100T, FF101T, FF490T, FF491T, and FF492T) have been tested and proven MR-safe per ASTM-2052-02* up to 3.0 Tesla.

For additional information, please refer to the following publications:

(1) Shellock, F.G. (2009). Reference manual for MR safety, implants, and devices. Los Angeles: Biomedical Research Publishing Group.

(2) Shellock, F.G. (2002). Biomedical implants and devices: Assessment of magnetic field interactions with a 3.0 Tesla MR system. JMRI, 16, 721-732

*These Aesculap devices were cleared by FDA as "MR-Safe" per ASTM-2052-02. Due to a change in definition within this standard, F 2503-2005-08, these devices are now termed as "MR Conditional" by ASTM. The FDA has not mandated a revision to our labeling because the device material and performance have not changed.

REFERENCES

Shellock FG. Biomedical implants and devices: assessment of magnetic field interactions with a 3.0-Tesla MR system. J Magn Reson Imaging 2002;16:721-732.

Shellock FG. Magnetic Resonance Procedures: Health Effects and Safety. CRC Press, LLC, Boca Raton, FL, 2001.

Shellock FG, Shellock VJ. Evaluation of cranial flap fixation clamps for compatibility with MR imaging. Radiology 1998;207:822-825.

Dental Implants, Devices, and Materials

Many of the dental implants, devices, materials, and objects evaluated for ferromagnetic qualities exhibited measurable deflection forces (e.g., brace bands, brace wires, etc.) but only the ones with magnetically-activated components present potential problems for patients during MR procedures (also, see **Magnetically-Activated Implants and Devices**). The issues that exist for magnetically-activated dental implants include possible demagnetization of the magnetic components and the substantial artifacts that these magnets produce on MR imaging.

Dental implants, devices, and materials made from ferromagnetic materials tend to be held in place with sufficient counter-forces to prevent them from causing problems related to movement or dislodgment during in association with MR systems operating 3-Tesla or less.

REFERENCES

Gegauff A, Laurell KA, Thavendrarajah A, et al. A potential MRI hazard: forces on dental magnet keepers. J Oral Rehabil 1990;17:403-410.

Hubalkova H, La Serna P, Linetskiy I, Dostalova T. Dental alloys and magnetic resonance imaging. Int Dent J. 2006;56:135-41.

Lissac MI, Metrop D, Brugigrad, et al. Dental materials and magnetic resonance imaging. Invest Radiol 1991;26:40-45.

New PFJ, Rosen BR, Brady TJ, et al. Potential hazards and artifacts of ferromagnetic and nonferromagnetic surgical and dental materials and devices in nuclear magnetic resonance imaging. Radiology 1983;147:139-148.

Shellock FG. *Ex vivo* assessment of deflection forces and artifacts associated with high-field strength MRI of "mini-magnet" dental prostheses. Magn Reson Imaging 1989;7 (Suppl 1):38.

Shellock FG. Magnetic Resonance Procedures: Health Effects and Safety. CRC Press, LLC, Boca Raton, FL, 2001.

Shellock FG, Crues JV. High-field strength MR imaging and metallic biomedical implants: an *ex vivo* evaluation of deflection forces. Am J Roentgenol 1988;151:389-392.

Diaphragms

A contraceptive diaphragm may have a metallic ring that maintains it in position during use. Thus, certain contraceptive diaphragms display positive magnetic field interactions in association with exposure to MR systems and, because of the metallic component, substantial artifacts may also be found. MR examinations have been performed in patients with these devices without complaints or adverse sensations related to movement. Furthermore, there is no danger of heating for a contraceptive diaphragm during an MR procedure under conditions currently recommended by the United States Food and Drug Administration. Therefore, the presence of a diaphragm is not a contraindication for a patient undergoing an MR examination using an MR system operating at 3-Tesla or less. Regardless of the afore-mentioned information, it is best to remove a contraceptive diaphragm prior to an MRI examination.

REFERENCES

Shellock FG. Magnetic Resonance Procedures: Health Effects and Safety. CRC Press, LLC, Boca Raton, FL, 2001.

Shellock FG, Kanal E. Magnetic Resonance: Bioeffects, Safety, and Patient Management. Second Edition, Lippincott-Raven Press, New York, 1996.

Dressings Containing Silver and MRI Procedures

Clarification: Antimicrobial Dressings Containing Silver Aren't Necessarily Hazardous during MR Scans*

[*ECRI Institute. Antimicrobial dressings containing silver may cause pain and burns during MR scans [Hazard Report and clarification]. Health Devices 2007 Jul;36(7):232-3 and 2008 Feb; 37(2):60-2. Copyright 2007, 2008 ECRI Institute. Reprinted with permission.]

In our July 2007 issue, we published a Hazard Report titled "Antimicrobial Dressings Containing Silver May Cause Pain and Burns during MR Scans" in which we reported on a patient who suffered pain during a magnetic resonance (MR) scan. The patient was wearing dressings containing silver, which acts as an antimicrobial agent. We discussed the possibility that the silver in the dressings might have been heated by the radio-frequency (RF) energy that is present during any MR scan.

Our report on this incident has given some readers the impression that patients wearing dressings containing silver should never undergo MR scans. That is not the case. We are publishing this update to further explain the issue and clarify our recommendations. In particular, we want to make the following points clear:

First, the fact that a patient is wearing silver-containing dressings should not keep the patient from having an MR examination.

Second, the reason that some silver-containing dressings are contraindicated by the dressing manufacturer for use during MR scans is because they could produce artifacts and distortions in the MR image, not because of any risk they might pose to the patient (although such risk cannot be conclusively ruled out).

Third, the exact cause of the patient's pain in the reported incident was never determined; the silver-containing dressings are only one of the possible causes.

DISCUSSION

Our position on silver-containing dressings in MR scans. We believe that the presence of antimicrobial dressings containing silver should not disqualify a patient from undergoing an MR scan. We do advise, whenever feasible, that such dressings be removed before a scan and that the wound be washed with water to remove as many traces of silver as possible. The reason for doing so is to minimize any detrimental effects the silver might have on the quality of the image. If it isn't feasible to remove the dressings, we believe the scan should still be carried out.

However, clinicians should be aware that there may be a risk, albeit remote, that the silver in the dressing— some of which will have been absorbed into the wound and its exudate—could become heated by the RF energy present during the scan (see Possible Causes of Pain, below). As in any MR procedure, the patient should be monitored closely, and any report of unusual pain or heating should be promptly addressed, as described in our Recommendations.

Note that the dressings are only likely to be a concern if the dressed area will be included in the scanned area. If, for example, a head scan is being performed and there are silver-containing dressings on the patient's foot, there is probably no reason the dressings need to be disturbed.

Possible causes of pain.

In the reported incident, the patient was an amputee whose stump was being scanned. The stump had been covered with silver-containing dressings. During the MR acquisition, the patient experienced significant pain, and the scan was aborted.

A week later, the study was continued, after the dressing had been removed and the wound lightly washed with water at the advice of the dressing manufacturer. However, the patient still experienced significant pain, and the reporting hospital noted that the amputation stump retained a silvery sheen despite the washing. It was suspected that the MR energy had interacted with the silver. But no further testing was undertaken to verify that suspicion.

Silver is not ferromagnetic, so the patient's pain could not have been caused by any magnetic effects of the MR field on the silver. As discussed above, though, MR scans create RF energy, which can induce electrical currents within electrical conductors. These currents can cause heating and lead to patient burns. This has been previously reported by Wagle and Smith (2000) and Franiel et al. (2006). However, empirical testing with implants and devices shows that excessive heating only occurs for those that have an elongated shape forming a closed loop of a certain diameter (Dempsey and Condon 2001). In the case that we reported, it is conceivable that the silver formed a large conducting loop around the wound; but the large amount of silver that would be needed makes this unlikely. Also, although the patient felt a burning sensation, there were no visible signs of a burn. So the evidence is far from conclusive.

RECOMMENDATIONS

Until further empirical testing is done to establish the required conditions, if any, necessary to produce a heating effect, the following revised recommendations should be followed:

1)   Alert MR healthcare workers that some silver-containing antimicrobial dressings are contraindicated for MR exams in order to avoid artifacts. Therefore, if contraindicated dressings are close to the region being scanned or within the transmit RF coil, they should be removed if possible. However, a patient wearing such a dressing should not be prevented from having an MR procedure.

2)   In some cases, it may be possible to reapply the same dressing to the patient after the scan. Whether this can be done depends in part on the amount of exudates on the dressing. The decision to reapply a dressing must be made by qualified staff.

3)   As with any MR procedure, the patient should be carefully monitored and instructed to immediately report any unusual pain or heating. All such cases should be investigated immediately. If it is not possible to determine the cause of the pain and alleviate the problem (e.g., by applying a cold compress), then the procedure should be abandoned.

4)   Report any similar occurrences of patient pain or burns to the dressing manufacturer and to ECRI Institute. Full details of the procedure should be recorded, including the field strength, coil used, and scan parameters.

REFERENCES

Dempsey MF, Condon B. Thermal injuries associated with MRI. Clin Radiol. 2001 Jun;56:457-65

Franiel T, Schmidt S, Klingebiel R. First-degree burns on MRI due to nonferrous tattoos. AJR Am J Roentgenol. 2006;187(5):W556

Tope WD, Shellock FG. Magnetic resonance imaging and permanent cosmetics (tattoos): survey of complications and adverse events. J Magn Reson Imaging. 2002;15:180-4.

Wagle WA, Smith M. Tattoo-induced skin burn during MR imaging. AJR Am J Roentgenol. 2000;174:1795.

Wagner M, Lanfermann H, Zanella F. MR-induced burn-reaction in a female patient with "permanent make-up" Rofo. 2006;178:728-30.

Yuh WT, Fisher DJ, Shields RK, Ehrhardt JC, Shellock FG. Phantom limb pain induced in amputee by strong magnetic fields. J Magn Reson Imaging. 1992;2:221-3.

Dressings Containing Silver and MRI Procedures: Aquacel AG

Aquacel Ag (ConvaTec, Skillman, New Jersey) is a dressing that contains ionic silver, which combines the antibacterial action of silver with a barrier dressing that utilizes Hydrofiber technology (E.R. Squibb & Sons, LLC, New Brunswick, NJ) to absorb large amounts of wound exudate without requiring frequent dressing changes.

Nyenhuis and Duan (2009) evaluated MRI issues for this dressing at 1.5- and 3-Tesla. Based on the findings, the Aquacel Ag wound dressing impregnated with ionic silver was reported to be "MR safe" (an item that poses no known hazards in all MRI environments), particularly since it exhibited magnetic and electric properties to human tissues. Therefore, Aquacel Ag dressing may be left in place in a patient undergoing an MRI procedure at 3-Tesla or less.

REFERENCE

Nyenhuis J, Duan L. An evaluation of MRI safety and compatibility of a silver-impregnated antimicrobial wound dressing. J Am Coll Radiol. 2009;6:500-5.

ECG Electrodes

Using only electrocardiograph (ECG) electrodes tested specifically with regard to the MRI environment is strongly recommended to ensure patient safety and proper recording of the electrocardiogram. Tests should include an evaluation of magnetic field interactions, MRI-related heating, and characterization of artifacts. Various ECG electrodes have been specially developed for use during MR procedures to protect the patient from potentially hazardous conditions and to minimize MRI-related artifacts. **The List** provides a compilation of ECG electrodes that have been evaluated for MR-safety using MR systems operating with static magnetic fields up to 1.5-Tesla. Some have been assessed at 3-Tesla, as well. Importantly, these electrodes should be used according to the guidelines provided by the manufacturers of the ECG monitoring devices.

REFERENCES

Shellock FG. MRI and ECG electrodes. Signals, No. 29, Issue 1, pp. 10-14, 1999.

Shellock FG. Magnetic Resonance Procedures: Health Effects and Safety. CRC Press, LLC, Boca Raton, FL, 2001.

Epidural Pump, ambIT Epidural Pump

ambIT Epidural Pump, Model 22028

The ambIT Trialing Drug Infusion Pump/ambIT external epidural pump (Medtronic, Inc.,   Sorensen Medical, Inc.) is used to infuse medication and/or fluids into patients primarily for pain management. Routes of delivery are generally intravenous, epidural and/or regional.

MRI Information
Warnings
Safety hazards such as under infusion may be associated with external radio frequency interference (RFI) or electromagnetic radiation. Typical equipment which may generate such radiation include x-ray machines, MRI equipment, and any other non-shielded electrical equipment.

REFERENCE

http://www.medtronic.com/

Essure Device

The Essure Device (Conceptus, San Carlos, CA) is a metallic implant developed for permanent female contraception. The presence of this implant is intended to alter the function and architecture of the fallopian tube, resulting in permanent contraception. The Essure Device is composed of 316L stainless steel, platinum, iridium, nickel-titanium alloy, silver solder, and polyethylene terephthalate (PET) fibers.

The MRI assessment of this device involved testing for magnetic field interactions (1.5-Tesla), heating, induced electrical currents, and artifacts using previously described techniques. There were no magnetic field interactions, the highest temperature changes were $\leq +0.6°C$, and the induced electrical currents were minimal. Furthermore, artifacts should not create a substantial problem for diagnostic MR imaging unless the area of interest is in the exact same position as where this implant is located. Thus, the findings indicated that it is acceptable for a patient with the Essure Device to undergo an MR procedure at 1.5-Tesla or less.

MRI at 3-Tesla and the Essure Device. The Essure Device has been evaluated (i.e., tested for magnetic field interactions and MRI-related heating) at 3-Tesla and found to be acceptable for patients undergoing MR procedures at this field strength.

REFERENCES

Shellock FG. Biomedical implants and devices: assessment of magnetic field interactions with a 3.0-Tesla MR system. J Magn Reson Imaging 2002;16:721-732.

Shellock FG. New metallic implant used for permanent female contraception: evaluation of MR safety. Am J Roentgenol 2002;178:1513-1516.

External Fixation Devices

Most orthopedic implants and materials do not pose problems for patients undergoing MR procedures. However, because of the length of the implant or the formation of a conductive loop, MR examinations may be hazardous for certain orthopedic implants, namely external fixation systems.

External fixation systems comprise specially designed frames, clamps, rods, rod-to-rod couplings, pins, posts, fasteners, wire fixations, fixation bolts, washers, nuts, hinges, sockets, connecting bars, screws and other components used in orthopedic and reconstructive surgery. Indications for external fixation systems are varied and include the following treatment applications:

- Open and closed fracture fixation;
- Pseudoarthroses of long bones (both congenital and acquired);
- Limb lengthening by metaphyseal or epiphyseal distraction;
- Correction of bony or soft tissue defects; and
- Correction of bony or soft tissue deformities.

The assessment of MRIissues for external fixation systems is especially challenging because of the myriad of possible components (many of which are made from conductive materials) and configurations used for these devices. The primary concern is MRI-related heating which is dependent on the particular aspects of the external fixation system. Importantly, the specific MRI conditions (strength of the static magnetic field, RF frequency, type of RF transmit coil, pulse sequence, body part imaged, position of the fixation device relative to the transmit RF coil, etc.) directly impact the safety aspects of scanning patients with external fixation systems.

For example, Luechinger et al. used MRI to study "large orthopedic external fixation clamps and related components". Forces induced by a 3-Tesla MR scanner were compiled for newly designed nonmagnetic clamps and older clamps that contained ferromagnetic components. Heating trials were performed in 1.5- and 3-Tesla MR systems for two assembled external fixation frames. Forces of the newly designed clamps were more than a factor 2 lower as the gravitational force on the device whereas, magnetic forces on the older devices showed over 10 times the force induced by earth acceleration of gravity. No torque effects could be found for the newly designed clamps.

Temperatures recorded at the tips of Schanz screws in the 1.5-Tesla MR system showed a rise of 0.7 degrees C for a pelvic frame and of 2.1 degrees C for a diamond knee bridge frame when normalized to a specific absorption rate (SAR) of 2 W/kg. The normalized temperature increases in the 3-Tesla MR system were 0.9 degrees C for the pelvic frame and 1.1 degrees C for the knee bridge frame. Large external fixation frames assembled with the newly designed clamps (390 Series Clamps), carbon fiber reinforced rods, and implant quality 316L stainless steel Schanz screws met acceptable safety guidelines when tested at 3-Tesla. Notably, this information pertains to the specific configuration of the fixation device that underwent testing, relative to the MRI conditions that were used.

To ensure patient safety, guidelines must be applied on a case-by-case basis. Therefore, MR healthcare professionals are referred to product labeling approved by the U.S. Food and Drug Administration for a given external fixation system. Importantly, this information may only apply to a particular configuration for the external fixation device.

Vibration Associated With MR Procedures. Graf et al. reported that torque acting on metallic implants or instruments due to eddy-current induction in associated with MR imaging can be considerable. Larger implants (such as fixation devices) made from conducting materials are especially affected. Gradient switching was shown to produce fast alternating torque. Significant vibrations at off-center positions of the metal parts may explain why some patients with metallic implants may report feeling sensations of "heating" during MR examinations.

[MR healthcare professionals are advised to contact the respective manufacturer in order to obtain the latest safety information to ensure patient safety relative to the use of an MR procedure.]

REFERENCE

Graf H, Lauer UA, Schick F. Eddy-current induction in extended metallic parts as a source of considerable torsional moment. Journal of Magnetic Resonance Imaging 2006;23:585-590.

Luechinger R, Boesiger P, Disegi JA. Safety evaluation of large external fixation clamps and frames in a magnetic resonance environment. J Biomed Mater Res B Appl Biomater. 2007;82:17-22.

Shellock FG. External Fixation Devices and MRI Safety. Signals, No. 56, Issue 1, pp. 15, 2006.

Foley Catheters With and Without Temperature Sensors

Most Foley catheters utilized to drain the bladder have no or few metallic components. Accordingly, these devices are acceptable for patients undergoing MR procedures. However, certain Foley catheters have sensors to measure the temperature of the urine in the bladder, which is an appropriate means of determining "deep" body or core temperature. This type of Foley catheter typically has a thermistor or thermocouple located on or near the tip of the device and a wire that runs the length of the catheter to a connector that plugs into a temperature monitor. Sometimes an additional external cable is also used. A Foley catheter with a temperature sensor should never be connected to an external cable and/or the temperature monitor because this equipment has not been shown to be safe for patients undergoing MR examinations.

Several Foley catheters with temperature sensors have been evaluated in the MR environment by determining magnetic field interactions, artifacts, and heating. In general, the findings of this assessment indicated that it would be safe to perform MR procedures in patients with certain Foley catheters with temperature sensors as long as specific recommendations are followed.

Similar to other devices with conductive components, the position of the wire of a Foley catheter with a temperature sensor has an important effect on the amount of heating that develops during an MR procedure. Therefore, to prevent excessive heating associated with an MR procedure, a Foley catheter with a temperature sensor must be positioned in a straight configuration (without a loop) down the center of the MR system and away from transmit RF coil. The metal connector must not touch the patient. Additional recommendations for the specific Foley catheters with temperature sensors that have undergone MRI testing include, the following:

1) If the Foley catheter with a temperature sensor has a removable connector cable or extension, it should be disconnected prior to the MR procedure.
2) Remove all electrically conductive material from the bore of the MR system that is not required for the procedure (i.e., unused surface coils, cables, etc.).

3) Keep electrically conductive material that must remain in the bore of the MR system from directly contacting the patient by placing insulation or space between the conductive material and the patient.
4) Position the Foley catheter with a temperature sensor in a straight configuration down the center of the MR system table to prevent cross points, coils, and loops.
5) Ensure that the connector does not touch the patient.
6) MR imaging should be performed using MR systems shown to be acceptable and safe for patients (e.g., operating at a specific static magnetic field and frequency, 1.5-Tesla/64-MHz, or other tested field strength/frequency level).
7) Follow the **Instructions for Use** for a given Foley catheter with a temperature sensor with regard to the MR system whole body averaged specific absorption rate.
8) Monitor the patient continuously using a verbal means (e.g., intercom). If the patient reports any unusual sensation, discontinue the MR procedure immediately. Notably, MRI procedures should not be performed in patients that are unable to communicate (e.g., sedated, anesthetized, etc.).

Specific labeling instructions for a given Foley catheter with temperature sensor must be carefully followed. Importantly, not all Foley catheters with temperature sensors are acceptable for patients undergoing MR procedures.

An example of specific instructions for a Foley catheter with temperature sensor that has FDA approved MRI labeling is, as follows:

Foley Catheter with Temperature Sensor, Bardex Latex-Free Temperature-Sensing 400-Series Foley Catheter (C. R. Bard, Inc., Covington, GA)

MRI Safety Instructions

Warning: This product should never be connected to the temperature monitor or connected to a cable during an MRI procedure. Failure to follow this guideline may result in serious injury to the patient. Refer to *Instructions for Use*. It is important to closely follow these specific conditions that have been determined to permit the examination to be conducted safely. Any deviation may result in a serious injury to the patient.

Non-clinical testing demonstrated that these Foley catheters with temperature sensors are MR Conditional. A patient with one of these devices can be scanned safely immediately after placement under the following conditions:

- Static magnetic field of 3-Tesla or less with regard to magnetic field interactions.
- Spatial gradient magnetic field of 720-Gauss/cm or less with regard to magnetic field interactions.
- Maximum MR system reported, whole-body-averaged specific absorption rate (SAR) of 3.5-W/kg at 1.5-Tesla or 3-W/kg at 3-Tesla for 15 minutes of scanning (i.e., per pulse sequence).

Importantly, the MRI procedure should be performed using an MR system operating at a static magnetic field strength of 1.5-Tesla or 3-Tesla, ONLY. The safe use of an MR system operating at lower or higher field strength for a patient with a Foley catheter with temperature sensor has not been determined.

Special Instructions: The position of the wire of the Foley Catheter with Temperature Sensor has an important effect on the amount of heating that may develop during an MRI procedure. Accordingly, the Foley catheter with temperature sensor must be positioned in a straight configuration down the center of the patient table (i.e., down the center of the MR system without any loop) to prevent possible excessive heating associated with an MRI procedure.

Additional safety instructions include the following:

(1) The Foley catheter with temperature sensor should not be connected to the temperature monitoring equipment during the MRI procedure.

(2) If the Foley catheter with temperature sensor has a removable catheter connector cable, it should be disconnected prior to the MRI procedure.

(3) Remove all electrically conductive material from the bore of the MR system that is not required for the procedure (i.e., unused surface coils, cables, etc.).

(4) Keep electrically conductive material that must remain in the bore of the MR system from directly contacting the patient by placing thermal and/or electrical insulation (including air) between the conductive material and the patient.

(5) Position the Foley catheter with a temperature sensor in a straight configuration down the center of the patient table to prevent cross points and conductive coils or loops.

(6) The wire and connector of the Foley catheter with temperature sensor should not be in contact with the patient during the MRI procedure. Position the device, accordingly.

(7) MR imaging should be performed using an MR system with static magnetic strength of 1.5-Tesla or 3-Tesla, ONLY.

(8) At 1.5-Tesla, the MR system reported whole body averaged SAR should not exceed 3.5- W/kg for 15-min. of scanning.

(9) At 3-Tesla, the MR system reported whole body averaged SAR should not exceed 3-W/kg for 15-min of scanning.

In addition to the above, the **Guidelines to Prevent Excessive Heating and Burns Associated with Magnetic Resonance Procedures** should be considered and implemented, as needed.

[MR healthcare professionals are advised to contact the respective manufacturer in order to obtain the latest safety information to ensure patient safety relative to the use of an MR procedure.]

REFERENCES

Dempsey MF, Condon B, Hadley DM. Investigation of the factors responsible for burns during MRI. J Magn Reson Imaging 2001;13:627-631.

http://www.bardmedical.com/

Shellock FG. Magnetic Resonance Procedures: Health Effects and Safety. CRC Press, LLC, Boca Raton, FL, 2001.

Shellock FG, Kanal E. Magnetic Resonance: Bioeffects, Safety, and Patient Management. Second Edition, Lippincott-Raven Press, New York, 1996.

FREEHAND Implantable Functional Neurostimulator System (FNS)

The FREEHAND Implantable Functional Neurostimulator System (FNS)(NeuroControl, Cleveland, OH) is a radiofrequency (RF) powered motor control neuroprosthesis that consists of both implanted and external components. It utilizes low levels of electrical current to stimulate the peripheral nerves that innervate muscles in the forearm and hand providing functional hand grasp patterns. The NeuroControl FREEHAND System consists of the following subsystems:

- The **Implanted Components** include the Implantable Receiver-Stimulator, Epimysial and Intramuscular Electrodes, and Connectors (sleeves and springs).
- The **External Components** include the External Controller, Transmit Coil, Shoulder Position Sensor, Battery Charger, and Remote On/Off Switch.
- The **Programming System** consists of the Pre-configured Personal Computer loaded with the Programming Interface Software, the Interface Module, and a Serial Cable.
- The **Surgical Implementation Components** include the **Electrode Positioning Kit** (the Surgical Stimulator, Epimysial Probe, Anode Plate, and Clip Lead) and
- The **Intramuscular Electrode Insertion Tool Kit** (the Intramuscular Probe and the Cannula). The Intramuscular Electrode is preloaded in the Lead Carrier with Carrier Cover.

The NeuroControl FREEHAND System is intended to improve a patient's ability to grasp, hold, and release objects. It is indicated for use in patients who:

- are tetraplegic due to C5 or C6 level spinal cord injury (ASIA Classification)
- have adequate functional range of motion of the upper extremity
- have intact lower motor neuron innervation of the forearm and hand musculature and
- are skeletally mature

WARNINGS

The NeuroControl FREEHAND System may only be prescribed, implanted, or adjusted by clinicians who have been trained and certified in its implementation and use.

- **Monopolar Electrosurgical Instruments** should not be used on the implanted upper extremity. These tools could damage the Implantable Receiver-Stimulator. Bipolar electrosurgical instruments can be used safely in coagulating mode.
- **Electrostatic Discharge (ESD)** may damage the FREEHAND Implantable Receiver-Stimulator during intraoperative handling. Handle only as instructed in the Clinician's Manual.
- **Neuromuscular Blocking Agents** (long-acting) should not be administered during implantation surgery. These agents render nerves unresponsive to electrical stimulation and may compromise the proper installation of the device.

PRECAUTIONS

- **Surface Stimulation**: Electrical surface stimulation (muscle stimulator, EMG, or TENS) should be used with caution on or near the implanted upper extremity as it may damage the system. Contact NeuroControl prior to applying surface stimulation.
- **X-rays, mammography, ultrasound**: X-ray imaging (e.g., CT or mammography), and ultrasound have not been reported to affect the function of the Implantable Receiver-Stimulator or Epimysial Electrodes. However, the implantable components may obscure the view of other anatomic structures.
- **MRI**: Testing of the FREEHAND System in a 1.5-Tesla scanner exposed to a whole body averaged Specific Absorption Rate (SAR) of 1.1 W/kg for a 30 minute duration resulted in localized temperature rises no more than 2.7 degrees C in a gelled saline filled phantom (without blood flow) and translational force less than that of a 3-gram mass and torque of 0.063 N-cm (significantly less than produced by the weight of the device). A patient with a FREEHAND System may undergo an MR procedure using a shielded or unshielded MR system with a static magnetic field of 1.5-Tesla only. The implantable components may obscure the view of other nearby anatomic structures. Artifact size is dependent on a variety of factors including the type of pulse sequence used for imaging (e.g. larger for gradient echo pulse sequences and smaller for spin echo and fast spin echo pulse sequences), the direction of the

frequency encoding, and the size of the field of view used for imaging. The use of non-standard scanning modes to minimize image artifact or improve visibility should be applied with caution and with the Specific Absorption Rate (SAR) not to exceed an average of 1.1 W/kg and gradient magnetic fields no greater than 20 Tesla/sec. The use of Transmit Coils other than the scanner's Body Coil or a Head Coil is prohibited. Testing of the function of each electrode should be conducted prior to MRI scanning to ensure that no leads are broken. Do not expose patients to MRI if any lead is broken or if integrity cannot be established as excessive heating may result in a broken lead. The external components of the FREEHAND System must be removed prior to MRI scanning. Patients must be continuously observed during the MR procedure and instructed to report any unusual sensations (e.g., warming, burning, or neuromuscular stimulation). Scanning must be discontinued immediately if any unusual sensation occurs. Contact NeuroControl Corporation for additional information.

- **Antibiotic prophylaxis:** Standard antibiotic prophylaxis for patients with an implant should be utilized to protect the patient when invasive procedures (e.g., oral surgery) are performed.
- **Ultrasound**: Therapeutic ultrasound should not be performed over the area of the Implantable Receiver-Stimulator or Epimysial Electrodes as it may damage the system.
- **Diathermy**: Therapeutic diathermy should not be used in patients with the NeuroControl FREEHAND System as it may damage the system.
- **Therapeutic Radiation**: The electronic components in the FREEHAND System may be damaged by therapeutic ionizing radiation. The damage that occurs may not be immediately detectable. Any changes in sensation or muscle contraction should be reported to the physician. If the changes are painful or uncomfortable the patient should stop using the FREEHAND System pending review by the clinician.
- **Invasive Procedures**: To avoid unintentional damage to implanted components, invasive procedures such as drawing blood or administering an intravenous infusion should be avoided on the implanted arm or in the area of the Implantable Receiver-Stimulator or near sites of the Epimysial Electrodes.
- **Serum CPK levels**: Exercise and muscle activity are known to cause changes in certain blood enzymes measured by standard laboratory and clinical tests, such as serum CPK. Exercise,

whether volitional or induced by electrical stimulation, may produce elevated serum CPK levels. If a FREEHAND System patient has elevated CPK, fractionation is indicated to differentiate between CK-MM from skeletal muscle and CK-MB from cardiac muscle that could be the result of cardiac injury.

- **Drug Interactions**: Muscle inhibitors and muscle relaxants may affect the strength of muscle contraction achieved using the FREEHAND System. It is recommended that these medications be stabilized prior to implementing the FREEHAND System so that muscle response to electrical stimulation can be accurately evaluated.

- **Electrostatic Discharge (ESD)** exposure can cause loss of current amplitude programmability which also produces stimulus current amplitude higher than default. This does not result in any increased safety concerns from stimulation, has not caused compromise in hand function, and device operation will remain stable in this mode of operation. If a patient indicates that an increase in grasp strength is suddenly observed, this malfunction mode should be considered and evaluated. Changes in hand grasp can be managed by reprogramming grasp patterns, usually lowering stimulus pulse widths.

- **Pacemaker Warning Areas**: Patients should avoid areas posted with a warning to persons who have an implanted pacemaker. Contact NeuroControl Corporation for additional information.

- **Studies have not been conducted** on the use of the NeuroControl FREEHAND System in patients with the following conditions:

- children who are skeletally immature (usually males < 16 years, females < 15 years)

- prior history of a major chronic systemic infection or other illness that would increase the risk of surgery

- poorly controlled autonomic dysreflexia

- seizures and balance disorders

- pregnancy

Risks and benefits in patients with any of these conditions should be carefully evaluated before using the FREEHAND System.

- **Safety critical tasks:** Patients should be advised to avoid performing tasks which may be critical to their safety, e.g., controlling an automobile (throttle or brake), handling an object that could injure the patient (scald or burn), etc.

- The patient should be advised to avoid the use of a compression cuff for measuring blood pressures on the arm in which the FREEHAND System is implanted.

- **Post-operatively**, the patient should be advised to regularly check the condition of his or her skin across the hand, across the volar and dorsal aspects of the forearm, and across the chest where the FREEHAND System Receiver-Stimulator, leads and Electrodes are located for signs of redness, swelling, or breakdown. If skin breakdown becomes apparent, patients should contact their clinician immediately. The clinician should treat the infection, taking into consideration the extra risk presented by the presence of the implanted materials.

- **Keep it dry**: The user should avoid getting the external components, cables, and attachments of the FREEHAND System wet.

- The patient and caregiver should be advised to **inspect the cables and connectors** regularly for fraying or damage and replace components when necessary.

[Excerpted with permission from the Package Insert, FREEHAND System, NeuroControl Corporation, Cleveland, OH]

[MR healthcare professionals are advised to contact the respective manufacturer in order to obtain the latest safety information to ensure patient safety relative to the use of an MR procedure.]

Glaucoma Drainage Implants (Shunt Tubes)

A glaucoma drainage implant or device, also known as a shunt tube, is implanted to maintain an artificial drainage pathway to control intraocular pressure for patients with glaucoma. Intraocular pressure is lowered when aqueous humor flows from inside the eye through the tube into the space between the plate that rests on the scleral surface and surrounding fibrous capsule. The implantation of a glaucoma drainage device is used to treat glaucoma that is refractory to medical and standard surgical therapy. These are usually cases where standard drainage procedures have failed or have a poor prognosis including failed trabeculectomy, juvenile glaucoma, neovascular glaucoma and glaucoma secondary to uveitis, traumatic glaucoma, cataract with glaucoma and high risk cases of primary glaucoma.

Importantly, for certain glaucoma drainage implants, radiographic findings may suggest the diagnosis of an orbital foreign body if the ophthalmic history is unknown, as reported by Ceballos and Parrish. In this case report, a patient was denied an MRI examination for fear of dislodging an apparent "metallic foreign body." In fact, the patient had a Baerveldt glaucoma drainage implant, which was mistakenly identified as an orbital metallic object based on its radiographic characteristics (i.e., due to the presence of barium-impregnated silicone).

At least one glaucoma drainage implant, the Ex-PRESS miniature glaucoma shunt (Optonol Ltd., Neve Ilan, Israel) is made from 316L stainless steel which, according to De Feo et al., may affect MRI examinations of the optic nerve. Geffen et al. reported that the Ex-PRESS glaucoma shunt is acceptable for patients undergoing MRI at 3-Tesla or less.

Many other glaucoma drainage implants are made from nonmetallic materials and are safe for patients undergoing MRI procedures. Commonly used devices that do not contain metal include, the following:

- Baerveldt glaucoma drainage implant (Pharmacia Co., Kalamazoo, MI)
- Krupin-Denver eye valve to disc implant (E. Benson Hood Laboratories, Pembroke, MA)

- Ahmed glaucoma valve (New World Medical, Rancho Cucamonga, CA)
- Molteno drainage device (Molteno Ophthalmic Ltd., Dunedin, New Zealand)
- Joseph valve (Valve Implants Limited, Hertford, England)

REFERENCES

Ceballos EM, Parrish RK. Plain film imaging of Baerveldt glaucoma drainage implants. American Journal of Neuroradiology 2002;23;935-937.

Dahan E, Carmichael TR. Implantation of a miniature glaucoma device under a scleral flap. J Glaucoma 2005;14:98-102.

De Feo F, Roccatagliata L, Bonzano L, et al. Magnetic resonance imaging in patients implanted with Ex-PRESS stainless steel glaucoma drainage microdevice. Am J Ophthalmol. 2009;147:907-11.

Geffen N, Trope GE, et al. Is the Ex-PRESS Glaucoma Shunt Magnetic Resonance Imaging Safe? J Glaucoma. 2009 Aug 5. [Epub ahead of print]

Hong CH, Arosemena A, Zurakowski D, Ayyala RS. Glaucoma drainage devices: a systematic literature review and current controversies. Surv Ophthalmol 2005;50:48-60.

Jeon TY, Kim HJ, Kim ST, Chung TY, Kee C. MR imaging features of giant reservoir formation in the orbit: an unusual complication of Ahmed glaucoma valve implantation. AJNR Am J Neuroradiol. 2007;28:1565-1566.

Sidoti PA, Baerveldt G. Glaucoma drainage implants. Curr Opin Ophthalmol 1994;5:85-98.

Traverso CE, De Feo F, Messas-Kaplan A, Denis P, Levartovsky S, Sellem E, Badalà F, Zagorski Z, Bron A, Belkin M. Long term effect on IOP of a stainless steel glaucoma drainage implant (Ex-PRESS) in combined surgery with phacoemulsification. British Journal of Ophthalmology 2005;89:425-429.

Guidewires

Advances in interventional MR procedures have resulted in the need for guidewires that are acceptable for endovascular therapy, drainage procedures, and other similar applications. Conventional guidewires are made from stainless steel or Nitinol, materials known to be conductive. Accordingly, radiofrequency fields used for MR procedures may induce substantial currents in guidewires, leading to excessive temperature increases and potential injuries.

Liu et al. studied the theoretical and experimental aspects of the RF heating resonance phenomenon of an endovascular guidewire. A Nitinol-based guidewire (Terumo, Tokyo, Japan) was inserted into a vessel phantom and imaged using 1.5- and 0.2-Tesla MR systems with continuous temperature monitoring at the guidewire tip. The guidwire was deployed in the phantom in a "straight" manner. The heating effects due to different experimental conditions were examined. A model was developed for the resonant current and the associated electric field produced by the guidewire acting as an antenna. Temperature increases of up to 17 degrees C were measured while imaging the guidewire at an off-center position in the 1.5-Tesla MR system. Power absorption produced by the resonating wire decreased as the repetition time was increased. No temperature rise was measured during MRI performed using the 0.2-Tesla MR system. Thus, considering the potential utility of low-field, open MR systems for MR-guided endovascular interventions, it is important to be aware of the safety of such applications for metallic guidewires and the potential hazards associated with using a guidewire with MR systems operating at other static magnetic field strengths, including 3-Tesla.

An investigation conducted by Konings et al. examined the radiofrequency (RF) heating of an endovascular guidewire frequently used in interventional MR procedures. A Terumo guidewire was partly immersed in an oblong saline bath to simulate an endovascular intervention. The temperature rise of the guidewire tip during MR imaging was measured using a Luxtron fluoroptic thermometry system. Starting from a baseline level of 26 degrees C, the tip of the guidewire reached temperatures up to 74 degrees C after 30 seconds of scanning using a 1.5-Tesla MR system. Touching the guidewire produced a skin burn.

The excessive heating of a linear conductor, like the guidewire that underwent evaluation, could only be explained by resonating RF waves. According to Konings et al., the capricious dependencies of this resonance phenomenon have severe consequences for safety guidelines of interventional MR procedures involving guidewires.

Recent advances in guidewire designs reporte by Kocaturk et al. and Kramer et al. have yielded guidewires that appear to be more acceptable for interventional MRI procedures with respect to both safety and visualization aspects.

REFERENCES

Buecker A. Safety of MRI-guided vascular interventions. Minim Invasive Ther Allied Technol. 2006;15:65-70.

Kocaturk O, et al. Whole shaft visibility and mechanical performance for active MR catheters using copper-nitinol braided polymer tubes. J Cardiovasc Magn Reson. 2009;11:29.

Konings MK, Bartels LW, Smits HJ, Bakker CJ. Heating around intravascular guidewires by resonating RF waves. J Magn Reson Imaging 2000;12:79-85.

Kramer NA, et al. Preclinical evaluation of a novel fiber compound MR guidewire in vivo. Invest Radiol. 2009;44:390-7.

Lin C-Y, Farahani K, Lu DSK, Shellock FG. Safety of MRI-guided endovascular guidewire applications. Proceedings of the International Society of Magnetic Resonance Imaging, 1999;7:1015.

Shellock FG. Magnetic Resonance Procedures: Health Effects and Safety. CRC Press, LLC, Boca Raton, FL, 2001.

Shellock FG. Radiofrequency-induced heating during MR procedures: A review. Journal of Magnetic Resonance Imaging. 2000;12: 30-36.

Halo Vests and Cervical Fixation Devices

Halo vests and cervical fixation devices may be constructed from a combination of metallic components and other materials. Although some commercially available halo vests and cervical fixation devices are composed entirely of nonferromagnetic metals, there may be hazards due to excessive MRI-related heating that can be generated because of the conductive nature of the metallic components. Additionally, there is a potential for the patient's tissue to be involved in part of a current loop, such that excessive heating and burn injury may occur. The currents generated within a ring or conductive loop is of additional concern because eddy current induction can cause image degradation. Adjusting the phase encoding direction of the pulse sequence so that it is parallel to the axis of the halo vest may reduce artifacts associated with eddy currents during MR imaging.

Serious injuries have occurred in patients with halo vests and cervical fixation devices that have undergone MR procedures. For example, Kim et al. (2003) described a case of a patient that underwent MRI at 1.5-Tesla wearing a titanium halo vest system (the name, model and manufacturer of this device were not provided). After the MR procedure, substantial burns were evident on the scalp of the right two posterior pins. According to the report, "the stoic patient had clearly perceived significant burning pain during MR imaging, but did not notify the technicians."

Fortunately, certain halo vests and cervical fixation devices have been designed to specifically be acceptable for patients undergoing MR procedures at 1.5-Tesla and 3-Tesla (see **The List**).

Vibration Effects. A study was conducted to evaluate the possible heating of halo vests and cervical fixation devices during MR imaging performed at 1.5-Tesla MR system using a variety of pulse sequences. The data indicated that no substantial heating was detected for the specific devices tested. Of interest is that there appeared to be subtle motions of the halo ring associated with a magnetization transfer contrast (MTC) pulse sequence, as shown by recordings obtained using a motion sensitive, laser-Doppler flow monitor.

Apparently, the imaging parameters used for the MTC pulse sequence produced sufficient vibration of the halo ring to create the sensation of heating. Patients may interpret these rapid vibrations as a "heating" sensation. This is likely to occur when the vibration frequency is at a level that stimulates nerve receptors located in the subcutaneous region, which detect sensations of pain and temperature changes.

The aforementioned is a hypothesis based on the available experimental data and requires further investigation to substantiate this theory. However, additional support for this premise comes from a report by Hartwell and Shellock. In this case, a halo ring and vest (removed from a patient who complained of severe "burning" in a front skull pin during MR imaging) was evaluated for heating and other potential problems associated with MR imaging. This work was performed in conjunction with the neurosurgeon who applied the device to the patient. The halo ring and vest were connected similar to the manner used on the patient. A fluid-filled Plexiglas phantom was placed within the vest. The device was then placed in a 1.5-Tesla MR system and imaging was performed using the same parameters that were associated with the "burning" sensation experienced by the patient. The neurosurgeon remained inside of the MR system to visually observe the cervical fixation device and to maintain physical contact (i.e., touching the skull pins and other components) during the MR procedure.

No perceivable temperature change was noted for the metallic components during MR imaging. However, these components (e.g., halo ring, vertical supports, vest bolts, etc.) vibrated substantially during MR imaging. Furthermore, when the skull pins were held firmly during the scan, there was a "drilling" sensation, which could be interpreted as a "burning" effect. Nevertheless, the skull pins remained cool to the touch throughout the MR procedure. Recent work conducted at 3-Tesla likewise supports the fact that substantial vibration occurs in cervical fixation devices (Unpublished observations, F.G. Shellock, 2009).

Graf et al. reported that torque acting on metallic implants or instruments due to eddy-current induction in associated with MR imaging can be considerable. Larger implants (such as fixation devices) made from well-conducting materials are especially affected. Gradient switching was shown to produce fast alternating torque. Significant vibrations at off-center positions of the metal parts may explain why some patients with metallic implants sometimes report feeling heating sensations during MR examinations.

In consideration of the above, it is inadvisable to permit patients with certain cervical fixation devices to undergo MR procedures using an

MTC pulse sequence until this problem can be further characterized to avoid unwanted patient responses, regardless of the lack of safety concern related to excessive heating. Other comparable pulse sequences should likewise be avoided when performing MR imaging of patients with halo vests and cervical fixation devices until the precise cause of this problem is determined and fully characterized. Additionally, all instructions for use and patient application information provided by halo vest and cervical fixation device manufacturers should be carefully followed.

MRI at 3-Tesla and Cervical Fixation Devices. To date, several cervical fixation devices have undergone MRI testing at 3-Tesla. MRI information for these devices are, as follows:

'LiL Angel Pediatric Halo System with Jerome Halo Vest and Resolve Glass-composite Halo Ring and Resolve Ceramic-tipped Skull Pins

'LiL Angel Pediatric Halo System with Resolve Halo Vest and Resolve Glass-composite Halo Ring and Resolve Ceramic-tipped Skull Pins

Resolve Halo System with Jerome Halo Vest and Resolve Glass-composite Halo Ring and Resolve Ceramic-tipped Skull Pins

Resolve Halo System with Resolve Halo Vest and Resolve Glass-composite Halo Ring and Resolve Ceramic-tipped Skull Pins (Each above product from OSSUR Reykjavik, Iceland and OSSUR AMERICAS, Aliso Viejo, CA)

Non-clinical testing has demonstrated that each product indicated above used as a cervical fixation or cervical traction device or system is MR Conditional. A patient with this system may undergo MRI safely under the following conditions:

- Static magnetic field of 3-Tesla or less
- Maximum spatial gradient magnetic field of 720 Gauss/cm or less
- Maximum MR system reported, specific absorption rate (SAR) of 3.0 W/kg for 15 minutes of scanning

In non-clinical testing, this system produced maximum temperature changes of 0.6 degrees C or less at a maximum MR system reported, specific absorption rate (SAR) of 3.0 W/kg for 15 minutes of MRI using a 3-Tesla MR system (Excite, Software G3.0-052B, General Electric Healthcare, Milwaukee, WI). MR image quality may be compromised if the area of interest is in the exact same area or relatively close to the position of the Skull Pins. Therefore, it may be necessary to optimize MR imaging parameters for the presence of these metallic objects.

Important Note: All of the materials used for the above products included metals with very low magnetic susceptibility (e.g., commercially pure titanium, Titanium alloy, Aluminum, etc.) or are nonmetallic and nonconductors. Accordingly, little or no substantial magnetic field interactions are present for these products in association with the 3-Tesla MR system.

PMT Halo System with Carbon Graphite Open Back Ring and Titanium Skull Pin (PMT Corporation, Chanhassen, MN)

Non-clinical testing has demonstrated that the PMT Halo System with Carbon Graphite Open Back Ring and Titanium Skull Pins used as a cervical fixation or cervical traction device or system is MR Conditional. A patient with this system may undergo MRI safely under the following conditions:

- Static magnetic field of 3-Tesla and 1.5-Tesla only.
- Maximum spatial gradient magnetic field of 720 Gauss/cm or less
- Maximum MR system reported, specific absorption rate (SAR) of 3.0 W/kg for 15 minutes of scanning

In non-clinical testing, this system produced maximum temperature changes of 0.5 degrees C or less at a maximum MR system reported, specific absorption rate (SAR) of 3.0 W/kg for 15 minutes of MRI using a 3-Tesla MR system (Excite, Software G3.0-052B, General Electric Healthcare, Milwaukee, WI). MR image quality may be compromised if the area of interest is in the exact same area or relatively close to the position of the Titanium Skull Pins. Therefore, it may be necessary to optimize MR imaging parameters for the presence of these metallic objects.

Important Note: All of the materials used for the above products included metals with very low magnetic susceptibility (e.g., commercially pure titanium, Titanium alloy, Aluminum, etc.) or are nonmetallic and nonconductors. Accordingly, little or no substantial magnetic field interactions are present for these products in association with the 3-Tesla MR system.

Bremer Halo Crown System with Bremer Air Flo Vest and Titanium Skull Pins (DePuy Spine Inc., Raynham, MA)

Non-clinical testing has demonstrated that the Bremer Halo Crown System with Bremer Air Flo Vest and Titanium Skull Pins used as a cervical fixation or cervical traction device or system is MR Conditional. A patient with this system may undergo MRI safely under the following conditions:

- Static magnetic field of 3-Tesla or less
- Maximum spatial gradient magnetic field of 720 Gauss/cm or less
- Maximum MR system reported, specific absorption rate (SAR) of 3.0 W/kg for 15 minutes of scanning

In non-clinical testing, this system produced maximum temperature changes of 0.6 degrees C or less at a maximum MR system reported, specific absorption rate (SAR) of 3.0 W/kg for 15 minutes of MRI using a 3-Tesla MR system (Excite, Software G3.0-052B, General Electric Healthcare, Milwaukee, WI). MR -image quality may be compromised if the area of interest is in the exact same area or relatively close to the position of the Titanium Skull Pins. Therefore, it may be necessary to optimize MR imaging parameters for the presence of these metallic objects.

Important Note: All of the materials used for the above products included metals with very low magnetic susceptibility (e.g., commercially pure titanium, Titanium alloy, Aluminum, etc.) or are nonmetallic and nonconductors. Accordingly, little or no substantial magnetic field interactions are present for these products in association with the 3-Tesla MR system.

Bremer 3D Halo Crown System with Bremer Air Flo Vest and Titanium Skull Pins (DePuy Spine Inc., Raynham, MA)

Non-clinical testing has demonstrated that the Bremer 3D Halo Crown System with Bremer Air Flo Vest and Titanium Skull Pins used as a cervical fixation or cervical traction device or system is MR Conditional. A patient with this system may undergo MRI safely under the following conditions:

- Static magnetic field of 3-Tesla or less
- Maximum spatial gradient magnetic field of 720 Gauss/cm or less
- Maximum MR system reported, specific absorption rate (SAR) of 3.0 W/kg for 15 minutes of scanning

In non-clinical testing, this system produced maximum temperature changes of 0.6 degrees C or less at a maximum MR system reported, specific absorption rate (SAR) of 3.0 W/kg for 15 minutes of MRI using a 3-Tesla MR system (Excite, General Electric). MR image quality may be compromised if the area of interest is in the exact same area or relatively close to the position of the Titanium Skull Pins. Therefore, it may be necessary to optimize MR imaging parameters for the presence of these metallic objects.

Important Note: All of the materials used for the above products included metals with very low magnetic susceptibility (e.g., commercially pure titanium, Titanium alloy, Aluminum, etc.) or are nonmetallic and nonconductors. Accordingly, little or no substantial magnetic field interactions are present for these products in association with the 3-Tesla MR system.

[MR healthcare professionals are advised to contact the respective manufacturer in order to obtain the latest safety information to ensure patient safety relative to the use of an MR procedure.]

REFERENCES

Ballock RT, Hajed PC, Byrne TP, et al. The quality of magnetic resonance imaging, as affected by the composition of the halo orthosis. J Bone Joint Surg 1989;71-A:431-434.

Clayman DA, Murakami ME, Vines FS. Compatibility of cervical spine braces with MR imaging. A study of nine nonferrous devices. AJNR Am J Neuroradiol 1990;11:385-390.

Diaz F, Tweardy L, Shellock FG. Cervical fixation devices: MRI issues at 3-Tesla. Spine (in press)

Graf H, Lauer UA, Schick F. Eddy-current induction in extended metallic parts as a source of considerable torsional moment. Journal of Magnetic Resonance Imaging 2006;23:585-590.

Hartwell CG, Shellock FG. MRI of cervical fixation devices: Sensation of heating caused by vibration of metallic components. J Magn Reson Imaging 1997;7:771.

Hua J, Fox RA. Magnetic resonance imaging of patients wearing a surgical traction halo. J Magn Reson Imaging 1996;:1:264-267.

Kim LJ, Sonntag VK, Hott JT, Nemeth JA, Klopfenstein JD, Tweardy L. Scalp burns from halo pins following magnetic resonance imaging. Case Report. Journal of Neurosurgery 2003;99:186.

Malko JA, Hoffman JC, Jarrett PJ. Eddy-current-induced artifacts caused by an "MR-compatible" halo device. Radiology 1989;173:563-564.

Shellock FG. MR imaging and cervical fixation devices: assessment of ferromagnetism, heating, and artifacts. Magn Reson Imaging 1996;14:1093-1098.

Shellock FG. Magnetic Resonance Procedures: Health Effects and Safety. CRC Press, LLC, Boca Raton, FL, 2001.

Shellock FG, Slimp G. Halo vest for cervical spine fixation during MR imaging. AJR Am J Roentgenol 1990;154:631-632.

Hearing Aids and Other Hearing Systems

External hearing aids are included in the category of electronically-activated devices that may be found in patients referred for MR procedures. Exposure to the magnetic fields used for MR examinations can easily damage these devices. Therefore, a patient or other individual with an external hearing aid must not enter the MR environment. Fortunately, to prevent damage, an external hearing aid can be readily identified and removed from the patient or individual prior to permitting entrance to the MR system room.

Other hearing devices may have external components as well as pieces that are surgically implanted. Hearing devices with external and internal components may be especially problematic for patients and individuals in the MR environment. Accordingly, patients and individuals with these particular hearing devices may not be allowed into the MR environment because of the risk of damaging the components. The manufacturers of these devices should be contacted for current MRI information.

(For information on other hearing systems, refer to the sections: **Baha, Bone Conduction Implant**, **Cochlear Implants**, and **InSound XT Series and Lyric Hearing Device**).

[MR healthcare professionals are advised to contact the respective manufacturer in order to obtain the latest safety information to ensure patient safety relative to the use of an MR procedure.]

REFERENCES

Shellock FG. Magnetic Resonance Procedures: Health Effects and Safety. CRC Press, LLC, Boca Raton, FL, 2001.

Shellock FG, Kanal E. Magnetic Resonance: Bioeffects, Safety, and Patient Management. Second Edition, Lippincott-Raven Press, New York, 1996.

Heart Valve Prostheses and Annuloplasty Rings

Many heart valve prostheses and annuloplasty rings have been evaluated for MR issues, especially with regard to the presence of magnetic field interactions associated with exposure to MR systems operating at field strengths of as high as 4.7-Tesla. Of these, the majority displayed measurable yet relatively minor magnetic field interactions. That is, because the actual attractive forces exerted on the heart valve prostheses and annuloplasty rings were minimal compared to the force exerted by the beating heart (i.e., approximately 7.2-N), an MR procedure is not considered to be hazardous for a patient that has any heart valve prosthesis or annuloplasty ring tested relative to the field strength of the magnet (i.e., MR system) used for the evaluation. Importantly, this recommendation includes the Starr-Edwards Model Pre-6000 heart valve prosthesis previously suggested to be a potential risk for a patient undergoing an MR examination.

With respect to clinical MR procedures, there has been no report of a patient incident or injury related to the presence of a heart valve prosthesis or annuloplasty ring. However, it should be noted that not all heart valve prostheses have been evaluated and at least one prototype exists that has magnetic components.

A study by Edwards et al. examined the effects of aging on cardiac tissue strength and its ability to withstand forces associated with a 4.7-T magnet. The goal of this research was to determine the forces required to cause partial or total detachment of a heart valve prosthesis in patients with age-related degenerative diseases exposed to MRI. Edwards et al. concluded that specific age-related degenerative cardiac diseases stiffen and strengthen tissue, resulting in significant forces required to pull a suture through valve annulus tissue. Importantly, these forces are substantially greater than those magnetically induced at 4.7-T. Accordingly, patients with degenerative valvular diseases are unlikely to be at risk during exposure to static magnetic fields less than or equal to 4.7-T.

Heart Valve Prostheses and the Lenz Effect. Condon and Hadley reported the theoretical possibility of a previously unconsidered electromagnetic interaction with heart valves that contain metallic disks or leaflets. Basically, any metal (i.e., not just ferromagnetic material) moving through a magnetic field will develop another magnetic field that opposes the primary magnetic field. This phenomenon is referred to as the "Lenz effect". In theory, "resistive pressure" may develop with the potential to inhibit both the opening and closing aspects of the mechanical heart valve prosthesis. The Lenz effect is proportional to the strength of the static magnetic field. Accordingly, there may be problems for patients with heart valves that have metal leaflets undergoing MR procedures using MR systems operating at static magnetic fields greater than 1.5-Tesla. However, this phenomenon has not been observed in association with MR procedures.

MRI at 3-Tesla and Heart Valve Prostheses and Annuloplasty Rings. Findings obtained at 3-Tesla for various heart valve prostheses and annuloplasty rings that underwent testing indicated that certain implants exhibit relatively minor magnetic field interactions. Similar to heart valve prostheses and annuloplasty rings tested at 1.5-Tesla, because the actual attractive forces exerted on these implants are deemed minimal compared to the force exerted by the beating heart, MR procedures at 3-Tesla are not considered to be hazardous for patients or individuals that have these devices. To date, for the heart valves that have been tested, MRI-related heating has not been shown to reach substantial levels.

REFERENCES

Ahmed S, Shellock FG. Magnetic resonance imaging safety: implications for cardiovascular patients. Journal of Cardiovascular Magnetic Resonance 2001;3:171-181.

Condon B, Hadley DM. Potential MR hazard to patients with metallic heart valves: the Lenz effect. Journal of Magnetic Resonance Imaging 2000;12:171-176.

Edwards, M-B, Taylor KM, Shellock FG. Prosthetic heart valves: evaluation of magnetic field interactions, heating, and artifacts at 1.5-Tesla. Journal of Magnetic Resonance Imaging. 2000;12:363-369.

Edwards MB, Draper ER, Hand JW, Taylor KM, Young IR. Mechanical testing of human cardiac tissue: some implications for MRI safety. J Cardiovasc Magn Reson. 2005;7:835-40

Frank H, Buxbaum P, Huber L, et al. *In vitro* behavior of mechanical heart valves in 1.5-T superconducting magnet. Eur J Radiol 1992;2:555-558.

Hassler M, Le Bas JF, Wolf JE, et al. Effects of magnetic fields used in MRI on 15 prosthetic heart valves. J Radiol 1986;67:661-666.

Medtronic Heart Valves, Medtronic, Inc., Minneapolis, MN, Permission to publish 3-Tesla MR testing information for Medtronic Heart Valves provided by Kathryn M. Bayer, Senior Technical Consultant, Medtronic Heart Valves, Technical Service.

Pruefer D, et al. In vitro investigation of prosthetic heart valves in magnetic resonance imaging: evaluation of potential hazards. J Heart Valve Disease 2001;10:410-414.

Randall PA, Kohman LJ, Scalzetti EM, et al. Magnetic resonance imaging of prosthetic cardiac valves *in vitro* and *in vivo*. Am J Cardiol 1988;62:973-976.

Shellock FG. Magnetic Resonance Procedures: Health Effects and Safety. CRC Press, LLC, Boca Raton, FL, 2001.

Shellock FG. Biomedical implants and devices: assessment of magnetic field interactions with a 3.0-Tesla MR system. J Magn Reson Imaging 2002;16:721-732.

Shellock FG. Prosthetic heart valves and annuloplasty rings: assessment of magnetic field interactions, heating, and artifacts at 1.5-Tesla. Journal of Cardiovascular Magnetic Resonance 2001;3:159-169.

Shellock FG, Morisoli SM. *Ex vivo* evaluation of ferromagnetism, heating, and artifacts for heart valve prostheses exposed to a 1.5-Tesla MR system. J Magn Reson Imaging 1994;4:756-758.

Shellock FG, Shellock VJ. MRI Safety of cardiovascular implants: evaluation of ferromagnetism, heating, and artifacts. Radiology 2000;214:P19H.

Soulen RL. Magnetic resonance imaging of prosthetic heart valves [Letter]. Radiology 1986;158:279.

Soulen RL, Budinger TF, Higgins CB. Magnetic resonance imaging of prosthetic heart valves. Radiology 1985;154:705-707.

Hemostatic Clips, Other Clips, Fasteners, and Staples

Various hemostatic vascular clips, other types of clips, fasteners, and staples evaluated for magnetic field interactions were not attracted by static magnetic fields of MR systems operating at 3-Tesla or less. These implants were made from nonferromagnetic materials such as tantalum, commercially pure titanium, and nonferromagnetic forms of stainless steel. Additionally, some forms of ligating, hemostatic, or other types of clips are made from biodegradable materials. Therefore, patients that have the implants made from nonmagnetic or "weakly" magnetic materials listed in **The List** are not at risk for injury during MR procedures. Importantly, for the devices that have been tested, there has never been a report of an injury to a patient in association with a hemostatic vascular clip, other type of clip, fastener, or staple in the MR environment. Patients with nonferromagnetic versions of these implants may undergo MR procedures immediately after they are placed.

Vascular grafts frequently have clips or fasteners applied that may present problems for MR imaging because of the associated artifacts. Weishaupt et al. evaluated the artifact size on three-dimensional MR angiograms as well as the MR safety for 18 different commercially available hemostatic and ligating clips. All of the clips were safe at 1.5-Tesla insofar as there was no heating or magnetic field interactions measured for these implants.

Specific MRI-related labeling statements for certain hemostatic clips that require further attention during the pre-MRI screening procedure are, as follows:

Resolution Clip. The Resolution Clip (Boston Scientific Corporation) is indicated for placement within the gastrointestinal tract for the purpose of endoscopic marking or hemostasis. Currently, the Resolution Clip is labeled, as follows: "Do not perform MRI procedures on patients who have had clips placed within their gastrointestinal tract, as this could be harmful to patients."

Long Clip, HX-600-090L. The Long Clip HX-600-090L (Olympus Medical Systems Corporation) is indicated for placement within the gastrointestinal tract for the purpose of endoscopic marking, hemostasis, or closure of GI tract luminal perforations within 20-mm as a supplementary method. Currently, the Long Clip HX-600-090L is labeled, as follows: "Do not perform MRI procedures on patients who have clips placed within their gastrointestinal tracts. This could be harmful to the patient."

Additional information: Olympus endoscopic clips have been shown to remain in the patient an average of 9.4 days, but retention is based on a variety of factors and may result in a longer retention period. Prior to MRI, the physician should confirm there are no residual clips in the GI tract. The following techniques may be used for confirmation:

(1) View the lesion under radiologic imaging. Olympus clip fixing devices are radiopaque. By using x-ray, the physician can determine if any residual clips are in the gastrointestinal tract. If no clips are evident under radiologic imaging, MRI may be accomplished.

(2) Endoscopically examine the lesion. If no clips remain at the lesion, MRI may be accomplished.

QuickClip2, HX-201LR-135 & HX-201UR-135. The QuickClip2, HX-201LR-135 & HX-201UR-135 (Olympus Medical Systems Corporation) are indicated for placement within the gastrointestinal tract for the purpose of endoscopic marking, hemostasis, or closure of GI tract luminal perforations within 20-mm as a supplementary method. Currently, the QuickClip2 (HX-201LR-135 & HX-201UR-135) is labeled, as follows: "Do not perform MRI procedures on patients who have clips placed within their gastrointestinal tracts. This could be harmful to the patient."

Additional information: Olympus endoscopic clips have been shown to remain in the patient an average of 9.4 days, but retention is based on a variety of factors and may result in a longer retention period. Prior to MRI, the physician should confirm there are no residual clips in the GI tract. The following techniques may be used for confirmation:

(1) View the lesion under radiologic imaging. Olympus clip fixing devices are radiopaque. By using x-ray, the physician can determine if any residual clips are in the gastrointestinal tract. If no clips are evident under radiologic imaging, MRI may be accomplished.

(2) Endoscopically examine the lesion. If no clips remain at the lesion, MRI may be accomplished.

QuickClip2 Long, HX-201LR-135L & HX-201UR-135L. The QuickClip2 Long, HX-201LR-135L & HX-201UR-135L (Olympus Medical Systems Corporation) are indicated for placement within the gastrointestinal tract for the purpose of endoscopic marking, hemostasis, or closure of GI tract luminal perforations within 20-mm as a supplementary method. Currently, the QuickClip2 Long (HX-201LR-135L & HX-201UR-135L) is labeled, as follows: "Do not perform MRI procedures on patients who have clips placed within their gastrointestinal tracts. This could be harmful to the patient."

Additional information: Olympus endoscopic clips have been shown to remain in the patient an average of 9.4 days, but retention is based on a variety of factors and may result in a longer retention period. Prior to MRI, the physician should confirm there are no residual clips in the GI tract. The following techniques may be used for confirmation:

(1) View the lesion under radiologic imaging. Olympus clip fixing devices are radiopaque. By using x-ray, the physician can determine if any residual clips are in the gastrointestinal tract. If no clips are evident under radiologic imaging, MRI may be accomplished.

(2) Endoscopically examine the lesion. If no clips remain at the lesion, MRI may be accomplished.

TriClip Endoscopic Clipping Device. An investigation by Gill et al. involving excised tissue exposed to 1.5-Tesla MR system, reported that the TriClip (TriClip Endoscopic Clipping Device, Wilson-Cook Medical Inc., Winston-Salem, NC) demonstrated "detachment from gastric tissue". Therefore, the TriClip should be considered unsafe for MRI.

MRI at 3-Tesla and Hemostatic Clips, Other Clips, Fasteners, and Staples. At 3-Tesla, a variety of hemostatic clips, other clips, fasteners, and staples have been evaluated for MR safety. In general, these devices do not present an additional risk to patients undergoing MR procedures. Please refer to **The List** for specific information.

REFERENCES

Brown MA, Carden JA, Coleman RE, et al. Magnetic field effects on surgical ligation clips. Magn Reson Imaging 1987;5:443-453.

Barrafato D, Henkelman RM. Magnetic resonance imaging and surgical clips. Can J Surg 1984;27:509-512.

Gill KR, Pooley RA, Wallace MB. Magnetic resonance imaging compatibility of endoclips. Gastrointest Endosc. 2009;70:532-6

Raju GS. Endoclips for GI endoscopy. Gastrointestinal Endoscopy 2004; 59:267-279.

Resolution Clip information, http://www.bostonscientific.com/templatedata/imports/collateral/Endoscopy/prospec_resolution_01_us.pdf

Shellock FG. Hemostatic Clips and MRI Procedures: Some Safe…Some May Not Be. Signals No. 66, pp. 20-21, 2008.

Shellock FG. Magnetic Resonance Procedures: Health Effects and Safety. CRC Press, LLC, Boca Raton, FL, 2001.

Shellock FG. MR imaging of metallic implants and materials: a compilation of the literature. Am J Roentgenol 1988;151:811-814.

Shellock FG. Biomedical implants and devices: assessment of magnetic field interactions with a 3.0-Tesla MR system. J Magn Reson Imaging 2002;16:721-732.

Shellock FG, Crues JV. High-field strength MR imaging and metallic biomedical implants: an *ex vivo* evaluation of deflection forces. AJR Am J Roentgenol 1988;151:389-392.

Shellock FG, Morisoli S, Kanal E. MR procedures and biomedical implants, materials, and devices: 1993 update. Radiology 1993;189:587-599.

Shellock FG, Swengros-Curtis J. MR imaging and biomedical implants, materials, and devices: an updated review. Radiology 1991;180:541-550.

Weishaupt D, Quick HH, Nanz D, Schmidt M, Cassina PC, Debatin JF. Ligating clips for three-dimensional MR angiography at 1.5-T: *in vitro* evaluation. Radiology 2000;214:902-907.

InSound XT Series and Lyric Hearing Device

MRI Information

For the **InSound XT Series** and **Lyric Hearing Device** (InSound Medical, Newark, CA), each hearing system must be removed prior to an MRI procedure. Furthermore, these devices are not allowed in the MR system room. Each device may be self-removed if an MRI examination is required.

[MR healthcare professionals are advised to contact the manufacturer to ensure that the latest safety information is obtained and carefully followed in order to ensure patient safety relative to the use of an MR procedure.]

REFERENCE

http://www.insoundmedical.com/

Insulin Pumps

Insulin Pumps (Animas Corporation, a Johnson and Johnson Company). This MRI information pertains to the following insulin pumps from Animas Corporation, a Johnson and Johnson Company:

-Animas 2020 Insulin Pump

-IR Animas 1200

-IR 1000 Insulin Pump

-IR 1100 Insulin Pump

-IR 1200 Insulin Pump

Each insulin pump indicated above should not be exposed to very strong electromagnetic fields, such as MRIs, RF welders or magnets used to pick up automobiles. Very strong magnetic fields, such as that associated with MRI, can "magnetize" the portion of the insulin pump's motor that regulates insulin delivery and, thus, damage this device.

For the patient: If you plan to undergo an MRI, remove the insulin pump beforehand and keep it outside of the MR system room during the procedure.

If the pump is accidentally allowed into the MR system room, disconnect the pump immediately and contact Animas Pump Support for important instructions.

For the Healthcare Professional: DO NOT bring the insulin pump into the MR system at any time. If the pump is accidentally allowed into the MR system room, disconnect the pump immediately and contact Animas Pump Support for important instructions.

[MR healthcare professionals are advised to contact the manufacturer to ensure that the latest safety information is obtained and carefully followed in order to ensure patient safety relative to the use of an MR procedure.]

Cozmo Pump, Infusion Pump

According to the User Manual for the Cozmo Pump (Deltec, Inc., St. Paul, MN), which is a device used to administer insulin, the following is stated regarding Magnetic Resonance Imaging (MRI):

"Caution: Avoid strong electromagnetic fields, like those present with Magnetic Resonance Imaging (MRI) and direct x-ray, as they can affect

how the pump works. If you cannot avoid them, you must take the pump off."

[MR healthcare professionals are advised to contact the respective manufacturer in order to obtain the latest safety information to ensure patient safety relative to the use of an MR procedure.]

Medtronic MiniMed 2007 Implantable Insulin Pump System (Medtronic Minimed, Northridge, CA)

The Medtronic MiniMed 2007 Implantable Insulin Pump System (Medtronic Minimed, Northridge, CA) may offer treatment advantages for diabetes patients who have difficulty maintaining consistent glycemic control. Patients that have not responded well to intensive insulin therapy, including multiple daily insulin injections or continuous subcutaneous insulin infusion using an external pump, may be primary candidates for the Medtronic MiniMed 2007 System. The Medtronic MiniMed 2007 System delivers insulin into the peritoneal cavity in short, frequent bursts or "pulses", similar to how pancreatic beta cells secrete insulin.

Medtronic MiniMed 2007 Implantable Insulin Pump System and MRI.

The Medtronic MiniMed 2007 Implantable Insulin Pump is designed to withstand common electrostatic and electromagnetic interference but must be removed prior to undergoing an MR procedure. Any magnetic field exceeding 600 gauss will interfere with the proper functioning of the pump for as long as the pump remains in that field. Fields much higher than that, such as those emitted by an MR system, may cause irreparable damage to the pump.

By comparison, infusion sets (MMT-11X, MMT-31X, MMT-32X, MMT-37X, MMT-39X) used with this device contain no metallic components and are safe to be used and can remain attached to the patient during an MR procedure. The only exceptions would be Polyfin infusion sets. Polyfin infusion sets (MMT-106 AND MMT-107, MMT-16X, MMT-30X, MMT-36X) have a surgical steel needle that remains in the subcutaneous tissue. These infusion sets should be removed prior to any MR procedure. **[Reprinted with permission from Medtronic, Minimed]**

MiniMed Paradigm REAL-Time Insulin Pump and Continuous Glucose Monitoring System (522 and 722 Insulin Pumps; Medtronic Minimed, Northridge, CA)

MRI Information for Patients
Magnetic fields

Do **not** use pump cases that have a magnetic clasp.

Do **not** expose your insulin pump to MRI equipment or other devices that generate very strong magnetic fields.

The magnetic fields in the immediate vicinity of these devices can damage the part of the pump's motor that regulates insulin delivery, possibly resulting in over-delivery and severe hypoglycemia.

Your pump must be removed and kept outside the room during magnetic resonance imaging (MRI) procedures.

If your pump is inadvertently exposed to a strong magnetic field, discontinue use and contact your local help line or representative for further assistance.

The insulin pump, transmitter, and sensor must be removed prior to entering the MRI environment.

[Reprinted with permission from Medtronic, Minimed]

[MR healthcare professionals are advised to contact the respective manufacturer in order to obtain the latest safety information to ensure patient safety relative to the use of an MR procedure.]

REFERENCES

http://www.animascorp.com
http://www.animascorp.com/products/pr_userguide.shtml
http://www.cozmore.com
http://www.minimed.com

Intrauterine Contraceptive Devices and Other Devices

Intrauterine contraceptive devices (IUD) may be made from nonmetallic materials (e.g., plastic) or a combination of nonmetallic and metallic materials. Copper is typically the metal used in an IUD, however, stainless steel or other metals may also be utilized. The "Copper T" and "Copper 7" both have a fine copper coil wound around a portion of the IUD. Testing conducted to determine the MR-safety aspects of copper IUDs indicated that these objects are safe for patients in the MR environment using MR systems operating at 1.5-Tesla or less. This includes the Multiload Cu375, the Nova T (containing copper and silver), and the Gyne T IUDs. An artifact may be seen for the metallic component of the IUD, however, the extent of this artifact is relatively small because of the low magnetic susceptibility of copper.

Zieman M and Kanal E reported 3-Tesla MRI *in vitro* test results for the Copper T 380A IUD. No significant deflection, torque, heating or artifact was found. Thus, this IUD is acceptable for patients undergoing MRI at 3-Tesla or less.

Importantly, stainless steel IUDs exist and, to date, these devices have not undergone testing to determine if they are acceptable for patients in association with MR procedures.

The Mirena intrauterine system (IUS) is a hormone-releasing device that contains levonorgestrel to prevent pregnancy (Berlex Laboratories, Wayne, NJ). This T-shaped device is made entirely from nonmetallic materials that include polyethylene, barium sulfate (i.e., which makes it radiopaque), and silicone. Therefore, the Mirena is safe for patients undergoing MR procedures using MR systems operating at all static magnetic field strengths.

The Implanon implant (Etonogestrel) is a single-rod, nonmetallic, subdermal device that offers women up to three years of contraceptive protection. This implant is acceptable for patients undergoing MR procedures at all static magnetic field strengths.

REFERENCES

Hess T, Stepanow B, Knopp MV. Safety of intrauterine contraceptive devices during MR imaging. Eur Radiol 1996;6:66-68.

http://www.implanon.com/

Kido A, et al. Intrauterine devices and uterine peristalsis: evaluation with MRI. Magn Reson Imaging. 2008;26:54-8.

Mark AS, Hricak H. Intrauterine contraceptive devices: MR imaging. Radiology 1987;162:311-314.

Mirena (levonorgestrel-releasing intrauterine system (IUS), Product Insert information, Berlex Laboratories, Wayne, NJ

Shellock FG. Magnetic Resonance Procedures: Health Effects and Safety. CRC Press, LLC, Boca Raton, FL, 2001.

Westerway SC, Picker R, Christie J. Implanon implant detection with ultrasound and magnetic resonance imaging. Aust NZ Obstet Gynaecol 2003;43:346-350.

Zhuang LQ, Yang BY. Comparison of clinical effects of stainless steel IUDs with and without copper. Shengzhi Yu biun. 1984;4:48-50.

Zieman M, Kanal E. Copper T 380A IUD and magnetic resonance imaging. Contraception. 2007;75:93-5.

IsoMed Implantable Constant-Flow Infusion Pump

IsoMed: All models beginning with 8472
Medtronic, Inc., Minneapolis, MN

Reference: IsoMed Technical Manual (220666-001)

Exposure of IsoMed pumps to Magnetic Resonance Imaging (MRI) fields of 1.5 T (Tesla) has demonstrated no impact on pump performance and a limited effect on the quality of the diagnostic information.

Testing on the IsoMed pump has established the following with regard to MRI safety and diagnostic issues.

Implant Heating During MRI Scans

Specific Absorption Rate (SAR): Presence of the pump can potentially cause a two-fold increase of the local temperature rise in tissues near the pump. During a 20-minute pulse sequence in a 1.5 T (Tesla) GE Signa Scanner with a whole-body average SAR of 1 W/kg, a temperature rise of 1 degree Celsius in a static phantom was observed near the pump implanted in the "abdomen" of the phantom. The temperature rise in a static phantom represents a worst case for physiological temperature rise and the 20-minute scan time is representative of a typical imaging session. Implanting the pump in other locations may result in higher temperature rises in tissues near the pump.

In the unlikely event that the patient experiences uncomfortable warmth near the pump, the MRI scan should be stopped and the scan parameters adjusted to reduce the SAR to comfortable levels.

Peripheral Nerve Stimulation

Time-Varying Gradient Magnetic Fields: Presence of the pump may potentially cause a two-fold increase of the induced electric field in tissues near the pump. With the pump implanted in the abdomen, using pulse sequences that have dB/dt up to 20 T/s, the measured induced electric field near the pump is below the threshold necessary to cause stimulation.

In the unlikely event that the patient reports stimulation during the scan, the proper procedure is the same as for patients without implants — stop the MRI scan and adjust the scan parameters to reduce the potential for nerve stimulation.

Static Magnetic Field

For magnetic fields up to 1.5 T, the magnetic force and torque on the IsoMed pump will be less than the force and torque due to gravity.

In the unlikely event that the patient reports a slight tugging sensation at the pump implant site, an elastic garment or wrap may be used to prevent the pump from moving and reduce the sensation the patient may experience.

Image Distortion

The IsoMed pump will cause image dropout on MRI images in the region surrounding the pump. The extent of image artifact depends on the pulse sequence chosen with gradient echo sequences generally causing the most image dropout. Spin echo sequences will cause image dropout in a region approximately 50% larger than the pump itself, about 12 cm across, but with little image distortion or artifact beyond that region.

Minimizing Image Distortion

MRI image artifact may be minimized by careful choice of pulse sequence parameters and location of the angle and location of the imaging plane. However, the reduction in image distortion obtained by adjustment of pulse sequence parameters will usually be at a cost in signal-to-noise ratio. These general principles should be followed:

- use imaging sequences with stronger gradients for both slice and read encoding directions. Employ higher bandwidth for both RF pulse and data sampling.
- choose an orientation for read-out axis that minimizes the appearance of in-plane distortion.
- use spin echo (SE) or gradient echo (GE) MRI imaging sequences with a relatively high data sampling bandwidth.
- use shorter echo time (TE) for gradient echo technique, whenever possible.
- be aware that the actual imaging slice shape can be curved in space due to the presence of the field disturbance of the pump (as stated above).

- identify the location of the implant in the patient and when possible, orient all imaging slices away from the implanted pump.

[MR healthcare professionals are advised to contact the respective manufacturer in order to obtain the latest safety information to ensure patient safety relative to the use of an MR procedure.]

REFERENCE

Medtronic Neurological Technical Services Department, Tech Note. MRI Guidelines for Neurological Products, Issue No. NTN 04-03 Rev 2, July, 2005, Important Note: Before scanning a patient with this implant or device, obtain the latest MRI safety information by contacting Medtronic, Neurological Technical Services Department (800) 707-0933 or visit www.Medtronic.com

Licox CC1.P1 Oxygen and Temperature Probe, Brain Tissue Oxygen Monitoring System

Licox CC1.P1 Oxygen and Temperature Probe, Brain Tissue Oxygen Monitoring System (Integra NeuroSciences, Plainsboro, NJ)

MRI SAFETY OF THE LICOX IT2 COMPLETE BRAIN TUNNELING PROBE KIT INCLUDING THE MODEL CC1.P1 OXYGEN AND TEMPERATURE PROBE AND MODEL VK5.2 PARENTERAL PROBE GUIDE AT 1.5 TESLA

It is important to read and understand this document in its entirety before conducting an MRI (magnetic resonance imaging) procedure on a patient with an implanted Licox CC1.P1 Oxygen and Temperature Probe. Failure to strictly adhere to these guidelines may result in serious injury to the patient.

This information applies to the following Integra products:

- Model IT2 Complete Brain Tunneling Probe Kit, consisting of
- Model CC1.P1 Oxygen and Temperature Probe
- Model VK5.2 Parenteral Probe Guide

WARNINGS

- These guidelines apply to MRI procedures conducted using a 1.5 Tesla MR System, ONLY.
- Testing has not been performed on other MR Systems and therefore should not be used.
- Use only normal operating mode. Do not perform MR scans in the 1st level or higher level control mode.
- Disconnect all cables and patient monitoring devices from the Licox CC1.P1 probe prior to entering the MRI environment. Failure to do so may result in serious injury to the patient. It is not possible to monitor brain oxygen tension during MRI procedures using this device.

- The position or orientation of the Licox CC1.P1 catheter and VK5.2 Parenteral Probe Guide does not impact their MRI safety characteristics.

DO NOT EXCEED AN RF (RADIO FREQUENCY) WHOLE BODY AVERAGED SAR (SPECIFIC ABSORPTION RATE) OF 1.0 W/Kg IN THE HEAD OR BODY DURING THE MRI PROCEDURE.

OVERVIEW

The Licox IT2 Complete Brain Tunneling Probe Kit including the CC1.P1 Oxygen and Temperature Probe and VK5.2 Parenteral Probe Guide were subjected to MRI testing, which included radio frequency induced heating, magnetically induced displacement force and torque to demonstrate that these components were considered "MR Conditional" as defined in ASTM F2503, Standard Practice for Marking Medical Devices and Other Items for Safety in the Magnetic Resonance Environment using a 1.5-Tesla MR system, ONLY. Testing has not been performed on other MR Systems and therefore should not be used.

This document outlines recommended guidelines and specific conditions under which the Licox IT2 Complete Brain Tunneling Probe Kit has been shown to pose minimal risk to a patient undergoing an MRI procedure.

Deviation from these guidelines may increase the potential for serious harm to the patient. MRI conditions utilizing MR systems with higher or lower static magnetic fields have not been assessed for the Licox IT2 Complete Brain Tunneling Probe Kit and, as such, must be avoided to ensure patient safety.

MRI – LICOX IT2 INTERACTIONS

MRI INDUCED HEATING

Under certain conditions, RF fields generated by MRI can induce substantial currents in metallic components contained within medical device products. This may rapidly produce significant heating of a device. Failure to follow the recommendations contained in this communication may result in the generation of thermal lesions and serious patient harm.

MAGNETIC FIELD INTERACTIONS -

Magnetic materials contained within an implanted device may experience translational attraction or rotational forces when brought into the static magnetic field of an MR system. The Licox CC1.P1 Probe contains magnetic material and has been shown in safety testing to not be substantially affected by translational attraction and torque related to exposure to a 1.5 Tesla static magnetic field of an MR system.

IMAGE ARTIFACTS -

The presence of the Licox CC1.P1 Probe will cause minor artifacts on the MR image. It is up to the discretion of the interpreting physician to determine if the location of the sensor is in the area of imaging interest and whether it will adversely affect the quality of the diagnostic information required from the MRI procedure.

The Licox CC1.P1 connector will cause substantial artifacts and distortion on the MR image. As such, position the connector away from the anatomy of interest during the MRI procedure.

PROCEDURE -

In addition to standard safety procedures for MRI, the following precautions must be followed specific to the Licox IT2 product:

1) Inform the patient of the potential risks of undergoing an MRI procedure with this device. Disconnect all cables and patient monitoring devices attached to the Licox IT2 prior to transporting the patient into the MRI environment.
2) Use only the following types of radio frequency (RF) coils for the MRI procedure:
    a) Transmit/receive RF body coil
    b) Transmit body coil/receive-only head coil
    c) Transmit/receive head coil
    d) Transmit/receive lower extremity coil - for imaging of lower extremities only, not for imaging the head of patients.
3) Set MRI parameters to the lowest usable whole body averaged SAR level. **THIS MUST NOT EXCEED A WHOLE BODY AVERAGED SAR OF 1.0 W/kg IN THE HEAD OR BODY** to minimize the risk of excessive heating of device components.
4) Verify that the MR system has appropriately calculated and updated the SAR value after all parameter changes have been made. Ensure that the proper patient weight is used for the SAR calculations.
5) For head scans using the transmit body coil the local SAR must be less than 2.0-W/kg.
6) A knowledgeable MRI expert (e.g., MRI physicist, MRI-trained radiologist) must verify that all set-up steps and settings have been properly implemented and checked prior to performing the MRI procedure.
7) If conscious and alert, provide the patient with a means of alerting the MRI system operator of unusual sensations. Instruct the patient to

watch for sensations such as overheating or shock. Terminate the MRI procedure immediately if so notified by the patient.

8) Monitor the patient continuously during the MRI examination and be prepared to stop and respond in the event of an emergency.

[MR healthcare professionals are advised to contact the respective manufacturer in order to obtain the latest safety information to ensure patient safety relative to the use of an MR procedure.]

REFERENCES

www.integra-ls.com

Licox MR Safety Fact Sheet: Licox IT2 Complete Brain Oxygen and Temperature Tunneling Probe Kit - 5/06 (Integra NeuroSciences, Plainsboro, NJ)

http://www.integra-ls.com/products/?product=48; click on MRI Safety to the right or go directly to http://www.integrals.com/pdfs/MRI_Safety.pdf

Magnetically-Activated Implants and Devices

Various types of implants and devices incorporate magnets as a means of activating the implant. The magnet may be used to retain the implant in place (e.g., certain prosthetic devices), to guide a ferromagnetic object into a specific position, to permit the functional aspects of the implant, to change the operation of the implant (e.g., adjustable pressure valves), or to program the device. Because there is a high likelihood of perturbing the function, demagnetizing, or displacing these implants, MR procedures typically should not be performed in patients with these implants or devices. However, in some cases, patients with magnetically-activated implants and devices may undergo MR procedures as long as certain precautions are followed (for example, see section entitled **Cerebrospinal Fluid (CSF) Shunt Valves and Accessories**).

Implants and devices that use magnets (e.g., certain types of dental implants, magnetic sphincters, magnetic stoma plugs, magnetic ocular implants, otologic implants, and other prosthetic devices) may be damaged by exposure to MR systems which, in turn, may necessitate surgery to replace or reposition them. For example, Schneider et al. reported that an MR examination is capable of demagnetizing the permanent magnet associated with an otologic implant (i.e., the Audiant magnet). Obviously, this has important implications for patients undergoing MR procedures.

Whenever possible, and if this can be done without risk to the patient, a magnetically-activated implant or device (e.g., an externally applied prosthesis or magnetic stoma plug) should be removed from the patient prior to the MR procedure. This will permit the examination to be performed safely. Knowledge of the specific aspects of the magnetically-activated implant or device is essential to recognize potential problems and to guarantee that an MR procedure may be performed safely on the patient.

Extrusion of an eye socket magnetic implant in a patient imaged with a 0.5-Tesla MR system has been described. This type of magnetic prosthesis is used in a patient after enucleation. A removable eye prosthesis adheres with a magnet of opposite polarity to a permanent implant sutured to the rectus muscles and conjunctiva by magnetic attraction through the conjunctiva. This "magnetic linkage" is intended to permit the eye prosthesis to move in a coordinated fashion with that of eye movement. In the reported incident, the static magnetic field of the MR system produced sufficient attraction of the ferromagnetic portion of the prosthesis to cause injury to the patient.

Certain dental prosthetic appliances utilize magnetic forces to retain the implant in place. The magnet may be contained within the prosthesis and attached to a ferromagnetic post implanted in the mandible or the magnetic component may be the implanted component. Therefore, whether or not an MR procedure may be performed without problems depends on the configuration of the magnetically-active dental implant.

REFERENCES

Gaston A, Marsault C, Lacaze A, et al. External magnetic guidance of endovascular catheters with a superconducting magnet: preliminary trials. J Neuroradiol 1988;15:137-147.

Grady MS, Howard MA, Molloy JA, et al. Nonlinear magnetic stereotaxis: three dimensional *in vivo* remote magnetic manipulation of a small object in canine brain. Med Phys 1990;17:405-415.

Majdani O, Leinung M, Rau T, et al. Demagnetization of cochlear implants and temperature changes in 3.0T MRI environment. Otolaryngol Head Neck Surg. 2008;139:833-9.

Ranney DF, Huffaker HH. Magnetic microspheres for the targeted controlled release of drugs and diagnostic agents. Ann NY Acad Sci 1987;507:104-119.

Schneider ML, Walker GB, Dormer KJ. Effects of magnetic resonance imaging on implantable permanent magnets. Am J Otol 1995;16:687-689.

Shellock FG. Magnetic Resonance Procedures: Health Effects and Safety. CRC Press, LLC, Boca Raton, FL, 2001.

Shellock FG. Ex vivo assessment of deflection forces and artifacts associated with high-field strength MRI of "mini-magnet" dental prostheses. Magn Reson Imaging 1989;7 (Suppl 1):38.

Young DB, Pawlak AM. An electromagnetically controllable heart valve suitable for chronic implantation. ASAIO Trans 1990;36:M421-M425.

Yuh WTC, Hanigan MT, et al. Extrusion of an eye socket magnetic implant after MR imaging examination: potential hazard to a patient with eye prosthesis. J Magn Reson Imaging 1991;1:711-713.

Miscellaneous Implants and Devices

Many miscellaneous implants, materials, devices, and objects have been tested with regard to MR procedures and the MR environment. For example, various types of firearms have been evaluated in the MR environment. These firearms exhibited strong ferromagnetism. In fact, two of the six firearms that underwent testing discharged in a reproducible manner while in the MR system room. Obviously, firearms should remain outside of the MR environment to prevent problems or possible injuries.

MR-guided biopsy, therapeutic, and minimally invasive surgical procedures are important clinical applications that are performed on conventional, open-architecture, or "double-donut" MR systems specially designed for this work. These procedures present challenges for the instruments and devices that are needed to support these interventions. Metallic surgical instruments and other devices potentially pose hazards (e.g., "missile" effects) or other problems (i.e., image artifacts and distortion that can obscure the area of interest) that must be addressed to apply MR-guided techniques effectively. Various manufacturers have used "weakly" ferromagnetic, nonferromagnetic or nonmetallic materials to make special instruments for interventional MR procedures.

Other medical products and devices have been developed with metallic components that are either entirely nonferromagnetic (e.g., stereotactic head-frame, Compass International, Inc., Rochester, MN) or made from metals that have a low magnetic susceptibility (e.g., titanium, non-magnetic types of stainless steel, etc.) that are acceptable for use in the MR environment.

MRI at 3-Tesla and Miscellaneous Implants and Devices. Many implants and devices have been tested in association with 3-Tesla MR systems. Refer to **The List** to determine information about specific miscellaneous implants and devices assessed at 3-Tesla.

REFERENCES

Go KG, Kamman RL, Mooyaart EL. Interaction of metallic neurosurgical implants with magnetic resonance imaging at 1.5-Tesla as a cause of image distortion and of hazardous movement of the implant. Clin Neurosurg 1989;91:109-115.

Kanal E, Shaibani A. Firearm safety in the MR imaging environment. Radiology 1994;193:875-876.

Lufkin R, Jordan S, Lylyck P, et al. MR imaging with topographic EEG electrodes in place. AJNR Am J Neuroradiol 1988;9:953-954.

Planert J, Modler H, Vosshenrich R. Measurements of magnetism-forces and torque moments affecting medical instruments, implants, and foreign objects during magnetic resonance imaging at all degrees of freedom. Medical Physics 1996;23:851-856.

Shellock FG. Biomedical implants and devices: assessment of magnetic field interactions with a 3.0-Tesla MR system. J Magn Reson Imaging 2002;16:721-732.

Shellock FG. MR-compatibility of an endoscope designed for use in interventional MR procedures. AJR Am J Roentgenol 1998;71:1297-1300.

Shellock FG. Magnetic Resonance Procedures: Health Effects and Safety. CRC Press, LLC, Boca Raton, FL, 2001.

Shellock FG. MR safety update 2002: Implants and devices. J Magn Reson Imaging 2002;16:485-496.

Shellock FG. Metallic neurosurgical implants: assessment of magnetic field interactions, heating, and artifacts at 1.5-Tesla. Radiology 2001;218:611.

Shellock FG. Surgical instruments for interventional MRI procedures: assessment of MR safety. J Magn Reson Imaging 2001;13:152-157.

Shellock FG, Shellock VJ. Ceramic surgical instruments: evaluation of MR-compatibility at 1.5-Tesla. J Magn Reson Imaging 1996;6:954-956.

Shellock FG, Shellock VJ. Evaluation of MR compatibility of 38 bioimplants and devices. Radiology 1995;197:174.

To SYC, Lufkin RB, Chiu L. MR-compatible winged infusion set. Comput Med Imag Graph 1989;13:469-472.

Zhang J, Wilson CL, Levesque MF, Behnke EJ, Lufkin RB. Temperature changes in nickel-chromium intracranial depth electrodes during MR scanning. AJNR Am J Neuroradiol 1993;14:497-500.

Neurostimulation Systems: General Information

The incidence of patients receiving implanted neurostimulation or neuromodulation systems for treatment of neurological disorders and other conditions is increasing. Because of the inherent design and intended function of neurostimulation systems, the electromagnetic fields used for MR procedures may produce a variety of problems with these devices. For example, altered function of a neurostimulation system that results from exposure to the electromagnetic fields of an MR system may cause discomfort, pain, or injury to the patient. MRI-related heating has been reported to create the greatest concern for many different devices used for neuromodulation. Importantly, the exact criteria for the particular neurostimulation system with regard to the implantable pulse generator (PG), leads, electrodes, and operational aspects of the device and the MR system conditions must be defined by comprehensive testing and carefully followed to ensure patient safety.

[MR healthcare professionals are advised to contact the respective manufacturer in order to obtain the latest safety information to ensure patient safety relative to the use of an MR procedure.]

REFERENCES

Baker K, Nyenhuis JA, Hridlicka G, Rezai AR, Tkach JA, Sharan A, Shellock FG. Neurostimulator implants: assessment of magnetic field interactions associated with 1.5- and 3.0-Tesla MR systems. Journal of Magnetic Resonance Imaging 2005;21:72-77.

Baker KB, Tkach JA, Nyenhuis JA, Phillips M, Shellock FG, Gonzalez-Martinez J, Rezai AR. Evaluation of specific absorption rate as a dosimeter of MRI-Related implant heating. Journal of Magnetic Resonance Imaging 2004;20:315-320.

Baker KB, Tkach J, Hall JD, Nyenhuis JA, Shellock FG, Rezai AR. Reduction of MRI-related heating in deep brain stimulation leads using a lead management system. Neurosurgery 2005;57:392-397.

Baker KB, Tkach JA, Phillips MD, Rezai AR. Variability in RF-induced heating of a deep brain stimulation implant across MR systems. J Magn Reson Imaging 2006;24:1236-42.

Bhidayasiri R, Bronstein JM, Sinha S, Krahl SE, Ahn S, Behnke EJ, Cohen MS, Frysinger R, Shellock FG. Bilateral neurostimulation systems used for deep brain stimulation: *In vitro* study of MRI-related heating at 1.5-Tesla and implications for clinical imaging of the brain. Magnetic Resonance Imaging 2005;23:549-555.

Chhabra V, Sung E, et al. Safety of magnetic resonance imaging of deep brain stimulator systems: a serial imaging and clinical retrospective study. J Neurosurg. 2009 Aug 14. [Epub ahead of print]

De Andres J, Valia JC, et al. Magnetic resonance imaging in patients with spinal neurostimulation systems. Anesthesiology. 2007;106:779-86.

Dormont D, Cornu P, Pidoux B, Bonnet AM, Biondi A, Oppenheim C, Hasboun D, Damier P, et al. Chronic thalamic stimulation with three-dimensional MR stereotactic guidance. AJNR Am J Neuroradiol 1997;18:1093-1097.

Elkelini MS, Hassouna MM. Safety of MRI at 1.5-Tesla in patients with implanted sacral nerve neurostimulator. Eur Urol. 2006 Aug;50(2):311-6.

Finelli DA, Rezai AR, Ruggieri P, Tkach J, Nyenhuis J, Hridlicka G, Sharan A, Stypulkowski PH, Shellock FG. MR-related heating of deep brain stimulation electrodes: an *in vitro* study of clinical imaging sequences. AJNR Am J Neuroradiol 2002;23:1795-1802.

Georgi A-C, Stippich C, Tronnier VM, Heiland S. Active deep brain stimulation during MRI: a feasibility study. Magn Reson in Medicine 2003;51:380-388.

Gleason CA, Kaula NF, Hricak H, et al. The effect of magnetic resonance imagers on implanted neurostimulators. Pacing Clin Electrophysiol 1992;15:81-94.

Henderson J, Tkach J, Phillips M, Baker K, Shellock FG, Rezai A. Permanent neurological deficit related to magnetic resonance imaging in a patient with implanted deep brain stimulation electrodes for Parkinson's disease: Case report. Neurosurgery 2005;57:E1063.

Kovacs N, Nagy F, Kover F, et al. Implanted deep brain stimulator and 1.0-Tesla magnetic resonance imaging. J Magn Reson Imaging. 2006;24:1409-12.

Larson PS, Richardson RM, Starr PA, Martin AJ. Magnetic resonance imaging of implanted deep brain stimulators: experience in a large series. Stereotact Funct Neurosurg. 2008;86:92-100.

Liem LA, van Dongen VC. Magnetic resonance imaging and spinal cord stimulation systems. Pain 1997;70:95-97.

Mogilner AY, Rezai AR. Brain stimulation: history, current clinical application, and future prospects. Acta Neurochir Suppl. 2003;87:115-120.

Mohsin SA, Sheikh NM, Saeed U. MRI-induced heating of deep brain stimulation leads. Phys Med Biol. 2008;53:5745-56.

Phillips MD, Baker KB, Lowe MJ, et al. Parkinson disease: pattern of functional MR imaging activation during deep brain stimulation of subthalamic nucleus--initial experience. Radiology. 2006;239:209-16.

Rezai AR, et al. Thalamic stimulation and functional magnetic resonance imaging: localization of cortical and subcortical activation with implanted electrodes. J Neurosurg 1999;90;583-590.

Rezai AR, Baker K, Tkach J, Phillips M, Hrdlicka G, Sharan A, Nyenhuis J, Ruggieri P, Henderson J, Shellock FG. Is magnetic resonance imaging safe for patients with neurostimulation systems used for deep brain stimulation (DBS)? Neurosurgery 2005;57:1056-1062.

Rezai AR, Finelli D, Ruggieri P, Tkach J, Nyenhuis JA, Shellock FG. Neurostimulators: Potential for excessive heating of deep brain stimulation electrodes during MR imaging. Journal of Magnetic Resonance Imaging 2001;14:488-489.

Rezai AR, Finelli D, Nyenhuis JA, Hrdlick G, Tkach J, Ruggieri P, Stypulkowski PH, Sharan A, Shellock FG. Neurostimulator for deep brain stimulation: Ex vivo evaluation of MRI-related heating at 1.5-Tesla. Journal of Magnetic Resonance Imaging 2002;15:241-250.

Rezai AR, Phillips M, Baker K, Sharan AD, Nyenhuis J, Tkach J, Henderson J, Shellock FG. Neurostimulation system used for deep brain stimulation (DBS): MR safety issues and implications of failing to follow guidelines. Investigative Radiology 2004;39:300-303.

Rise MT. Instrumentation for neuromodulation. Archives Of Medical Research 2000;31:237-247.

Shellock FG. MRI Safety and Neuromodulation Systems.In: NEUROMODULATION Krames ES, Peckham PH, Rezai, AR, Editors. Academic Press/Elsevier, New York, 2009.

Shellock FG. Magnetic Resonance Procedures: Health Effects and Safety. CRC Press, LLC, Boca Raton, FL, 2001.

Shellock FG. MR imaging and electronically-activated devices. Radiology. 219:294-295, 2001.

Shellock FG. MR safety update 2002: Implants and devices. Journal of Magnetic Resonance Imaging 2002;16:485-496.

Shellock FG. Begnaud J, Inman DM. VNS Therapy System: *In vitro* evaluation of MRI-related heating and function at 1.5- and 3-Tesla. Neuromodulation 2006;9:204-213.

Shellock FG, Cosendai G, Park S-M, Nyenhuis JA. Implantable microstimulator: magnetic resonance safety at 1.5-Tesla. Investigative Radiology 2004;39:591-594.

Smith CD, Kildishev AV, Nyenhuis JA, Foster KS, Bourland JD, Interactions of MRI magnetic fields with elongated medical implants. J Appl Physics 2000; 87:6188-6190.

Smith CD, Nyenhuis JA, Kildishev AV. Chapter 16. Health effects of induced electrical currents: Implications for implants. In: Magnetic resonance: health effects and safety, FG Shellock, Editor, CRC Press, Boca Raton, FL, 2001; pp. 393-413.

Spiegel J, et al. Transient dystonia following magnetic resonance imaging in a patient with deep brain stimulation electrodes for the treatment of Parkinson disease. J Neurosurgery 2003;99:772-774.

Tagliati M, Jankovic J, et al. and the National Parkinson Foundation DBS Working Group. Safety of MRI in patients with implanted deep brain stimulation devices. Neuroimage. 2009;47 Suppl 2:T53-7.

Tronnier VM, Stauber A, Hahnel S, Sarem-Aslani A. Magnetic resonance imaging with implanted neurostimulation systems: an in vitro and in vivo study. Neurosurgery 1999;44:118-25.

Utti RJ, Tsuboi Y, et al, Wharen RE. Magnetic resonance imaging and deep brain stimulation. Neurosurgery 2002;51:1423-1431.

Zonenshayn M, Mogilner AY, Rezai AR. Neurostimulation and functional brain stimulation. Neurological Research 2000;22;318-325.

Neurostimulation Systems: Deep Brain Stimulation

The Effects of Magnetic Resonance Imaging (MRI) on Deep Brain Stimulation System (Activa) for Movement Disorders
Medtronic Inc., Minneapolis, MN

Models:

Kinetra: 7428
Soletra: 7426
Itrel II: 7424
Activa PC Deep Brain Neurostimulator (Model 37601)
Activa RC Deep Brain Neurostimulator (Model 37612)

MRI and Activa Therapy

Introduction

It is important to read this section in its entirety before conducting an MRI examination on a patient with any implanted Activa System component.

Due to the number and variability of parameters that affect MRI compatibility, the safety of patients or continued functioning of Activa Systems exposed to MRI cannot be absolutely ensured. MRI systems generate powerful electromagnetic fields that can produce a number of interactions with implanted components of the Activa neurostimulation system. Some of these interactions, especially heating, are potentially hazardous and can lead to serious injury or death. However, with appropriate control measures, particularly with respect to the selection of MRI parameters and RF coils, it is generally possible to safely perform an MRI head scan on an Activa patient. In addition, Activa System components can affect the MRI image, potentially impacting the diagnostic use of this modality. The following information describes the potential interactions and control measures that should be taken to minimize the risks from these interactions.

Contraindication: Implantation of an Activa Brain Stimulation System is contraindicated for patients who will be exposed to Magnetic Resonance Imaging (MRI) using a full body transmit radio-frequency (RF) coil, a receive-only head coil, or a head transmit coil that extends over the chest area. Performing MRI with this equipment can cause tissue lesions from component heating, especially at the lead electrodes, resulting in serious and permanent injury including coma, paralysis, or death.

Warnings:

- Do not conduct an MRI examination on a patient with any implanted Activa System component until you read and fully understand all the information in this section. Failure to follow all warnings and guidelines related to MRI can result in serious and permanent injury including coma, paralysis, or death.

- In-vitro testing has shown that exposure of the Activa neurostimulator system to MRI at parameters other than those described in this guideline can induce significant heating at the lead electrodes or at breaks in the lead. Excessive heating may occur even if the lead and/or extension are the only part of the Activa System that is implanted. Excessive heating can result in serious and permanent injury including coma, paralysis, or death.

- MRI examinations of patients with an implanted Activa System should only be done if absolutely needed and then only if these guidelines are followed. MRI should not be considered for Activa patients if other potentially safer diagnostic methods such as CT, X-ray, ultrasound, or other methods will provide adequate diagnostic information.

- A responsible individual with expert knowledge about MRI, such as an MRI radiologist or MRI physicist, must assure all procedures in this guidelines are followed and that the MRI scan parameters, especially RF specific absorption rate (SAR) and gradient dB/dt parameters, comply with the recommended settings, both for the pre-scan (tuning) and during the actual MRI examination. The responsible individual must verify that parameters entered into the MRI system meet the guidelines in this section.

- Do not conduct an MRI examination if the patient has any other implants or limiting factors that would prohibit or contraindicate an MRI examination.

Cautions:

- The neurostimulator, especially those without filtered feedthroughs such as the Itrel II Model 7424, may be reset or potentially damaged when subjected to an MRI examination. If reset, the neurostimulator must be reprogrammed. If damaged, the neurostimulator must be replaced.

- MRI images may be severely distorted or image target areas can be completely blocked from view near the implanted Activa System components, especially near the neurostimulator. If the MRI targeted image area is near the neurostimulator, it may be necessary to move the neurostimulator to obtain an image, or use alternate imaging techniques. Do not remove the neurostimulator and leave the lead system implanted as this can result in higher than expected lead heating.

- Carefully weigh any decision to perform magnetic resonance imaging (MRI) examinations on patients who require the neurostimulator to control tremor. Image quality during MRI examinations may be reduced, because the tremor may return when the neurostimulator is turned off.

- If possible, do not sedate the patient so that the patient can provide feedback of any problems during the examination.

- Monitor the patient during the MRI examination. Verify that the patient is feeling normal and is responsive between each individual scan sequence of the MRI examination. Discontinue the MRI immediately if the patient becomes unresponsive to questions or experiences any heating, pain, shocking sensations/uncomfortable stimulation, or unusual sensations.

Note: The MRI guidelines provided here may significantly extend the MRI examination time or prevent some types of MRI examinations from being conducted on Activa patients.

General Information on MRI

An MRI system produces three types of electromagnetic fields that may interact with implanted neurostimulation systems. All three of these fields are necessary to produce an MRI image. Each of these fields can also produce specific but different types of interactions with implanted neurostimulator systems. These fields include:

- **Static Magnetic Field.** This is a steady state non-varying magnetic field that is normally always ON, even when no scan is underway. In a 1.5 Tesla MRI system, the static magnetic field is approximately 30,000 times greater than the magnetic field of the earth.

- **Gradient Magnetic Field.** This is a low-frequency pulsed magnetic field that is only present during a scan. The gradient magnetic field can induce voltages onto the lead system that may result in unintended stimulation or functional interactions with the neurostimulator.

- **RF Field.** This is a pulsed radio frequency (RF) field that is only present during a scan. It can be produced by a variety of transmission RF coils such as a whole body transmit coil or an extremity coil such as a transmit/receive head coil. Only a transmit/receive head coil should be used as the other RF coils can expose more of the lead system to RF energy, thereby increasing the risk of excessive heating and thermal lesions possibly resulting in coma, paralysis, or death.

MRI Interactions with Implanted Activa Systems

MRI/neurostimulation system interactions are various, and the risk to the patient can range from minimal to severe. These interactions include the following:

Heating – The MRI RF field induces voltages onto the lead system that can produce significant heating effects at the lead electrode-tissue interface or at the location of any breaks in the neurostimulator lead system. Component heating from the MRI RF field is the most serious risk from MRI exposure. Failure to follow these MRI recommendations can result in thermal lesions possibly resulting in coma, paralysis, or death.

Magnetic Field Interactions – Magnetic field interactions such as force and torque effects are produced by the static magnetic field. Any magnetic material will be attracted to the static magnetic field of the MRI. The force and torque effects may produce movement of the neurostimulator that can be uncomfortable to the patient, open a recent incision, or both. Activa System components are designed with minimal magnetic materials.

Induced Stimulation – Gradient magnetic fields may induce voltages onto the lead system that may cause unintended stimulation. The voltage of the induced stimulation pulses is proportional to the time rate of change (dB/dt) of the gradient pulses, the effective loop area created by the neurostimulator lead system, and the location of the lead system with respect to the gradient coils of the MRI.

Effects on Neurostimulator Function – The static, gradient, and RF fields of the MRI may affect the neurostimulator operation and programming. The static magnetic field may cause the neurostimulator to turn ON or OFF if the neurostimulator uses a magnetically controlled switch that allows the patient to control stimulation by the application of a handheld magnet. Additionally, the MRI RF, static, and gradient fields may temporarily affect or disable other functions, such as telemetry or stimulation pulses. Parameters will need to be reprogrammed if the MRI causes a POR (Power On Reset) of the neurostimulator.

Image Artifacts and Distortion – The neurostimulation system components, particularly the neurostimulator, can cause significant imaging artifacts and/or distortion of the MRI image, particularly if the neurostimulator components contain magnetic material. The neurostimulator can cause the MRI image to be completely blocked from view (i.e., signal loss or signal "void") or severely distorted within several inches of the neurostimulator.

MRI Procedure

Scope

These MRI/neurostimulator exposure guidelines apply to Activa Systems comprising combinations of the following components:

- Neurostimulator Models: Itrel II 7424, Soletra 7426, Kinetra 7428
- Lead Extension Models: 7495, 7482
- Lead Models: DBS 3387, 3389

Supervision

A responsible individual such as an MRI radiologist or MRI physicist must assure these procedures are followed. If the MRI is operated by an MRI technician, it is strongly recommended the responsible individual verifies that the MRI recommendations are followed.

Preparation

Do the following prior to performing an MRI examination on an Activa patient:

1) Inform the patient of the risks of undergoing an MRI.
2) Check if the patient has any other implants or conditions that would prohibit or contraindicate an MRI examination. Do not conduct an MRI examination if any are found.

3) Verify that all proposed MRI examination parameters comply with the "MRI Operation Settings" on Table 2. If not, the parameters must be modified to meet these requirements. If this cannot be done, do not perform an MRI.

4) If the patient has implanted leads but does not have an implanted neurostimulator, perform the following steps:

- Wrap the external portion of the leads/percutaneous extensions with insulating material.
- Keep the external portion of the leads/percutaneous extensions out of contact with the patient.
- Keep the external leads/percutaneous extensions straight, with no loops, and running down the center of the head coil.

5) If the patient has an implanted neurostimulator, perform the following steps:

- Review the neurostimulator with a clinician programmer and print out a copy of the programmed parameters for reference.
- Test for possible open circuits by measuring impedance and battery current on all electrodes in unipolar mode (see Table 1). If an open circuit is suspected, obtain an x-ray to identify whether the open circuit is caused by a broken lead wire. If a broken lead wire is found, do not perform an MRI.

Warning: An MRI procedure should not be performed in a patient with an Activa System that has a broken lead wire because higher than normal heating may occur at the break or the lead electrodes which can cause thermal lesions. These lesions may result in coma, paralysis, or death.

Table 1. Measurement Values Indicating Possible Open Circuits

Neurostimulator	Impedance	Battery Current
Itrel II Model 7424	>2000	<10 µA
Soletra Model 7426	>2000	<10 µA
Kinetra Model 7428	>4000	<15 µA

- If the Activa System is functioning properly and no broken lead wires are found, program the neurostimulator to the settings provided in Table 2.

Table 2. Recommended Neurostimulator Settings for MRI

Parameter	Setting
Stimulation output	OFF (all programs)

Stimulation mode	Bipolar (all programs)
Amplitude	0 Volts (all programs)
Magnetic (reed) switch	Disabled (Kinetra Model 7428 only)
Other parameters	Do not change

MRI Operation Settings

Prior to the MRI examination, a responsible individual such as an MRI radiologist or MRI physicist must assure the examination will be conducted according to the following MRI requirements. If standard MRI pulse sequences will be used, they must meet these requirements. If they do not, the pulse parameters must be adjusted so that they comply with these requirements:

Warning: In-vitro testing has shown that exposure of the Activa System to MRI under conditions other than described in this guideline can induce excessive heating at the lead electrodes or at breaks in the lead to cause lesions. These lesions may result in coma, paralysis, or death.

- Use only a 1.5 Tesla horizontal bore MRI (do not use open sided or other field strength MRI systems).
- Use only a transmit/receive head coil.

Contraindication: Implantation of an Activa Brain Stimulation System is contraindicated for patients who will be exposed to Magnetic Resonance Imaging (MRI) using a full body transmit radio-frequency (RF) coil, a receive-only head coil, or a head transmit coil that extends over the chest area. Performing MRI with this equipment can cause tissue lesions from component heating, especially at the lead electrodes, resulting in serious and permanent injury including coma, paralysis, or death.

- Enter the correct patient weight into the MRI console to assure the head SAR is estimated correctly.
- Use MRI examination parameters that limit the head SAR to 1/10 (0.1) W/kg or less for all RF pulse sequences.

Warnings

- Ensure the SAR value is the value for head SAR. Some MRI systems may only display SAR, whole body SAR, or local body SAR. Make sure the value being limited to 1/10 (0.1) W/kg is for head SAR. Excessive heating may occur if the wrong SAR value is used.
- If MRI parameters must be manually adjusted after the initial automatic MRI prescan, do not make any adjustments that will

increase the SAR value. Some MRI machines may not automatically update the displayed SAR value if manual adjustments are made. This may lead to higher than expected temperature increases in the Activa System, particularly at the lead electrodes.

- Limit the gradient dB/dt field to 20 Tesla/second or less.

Note: The recommendations provided are based on in-vitro testing and should result in a safe MRI examination of a patient with an implanted Medtronic Activa System. However, due to the many variables that affect safety, Medtronic cannot absolutely ensure safety or that the neurostimulator will not be damaged. The user of this information assumes full responsibility for the consequences of conducting an MRI examination on a patient with an implanted Activa System.

Prior to the MRI Examination

Prior to the scan examination, the responsible individual must verify the MRI examination parameters comply with these guidelines.

- Patients with implanted Activa Systems should be informed of the risks of undergoing an MRI.
- If possible, do not use sedation so the patient can inform the MRI operator of any heating, discomfort, or other problems.
- Instruct the patient to immediately inform the MRI operator if any discomfort, stimulation, shocking, or heating occurs during the examination.

During the MRI Examination

- Monitor the patient both visually and audibly. Check the patient between each imaging sequence. Discontinue the MRI examination immediately if the patient is unable to respond to questions or reports any problems.
- Conduct the examination using only the MRI pulse sequence that the MRI radiologist or physicist has confirmed meets the MRI requirements above.

Post MRI Examination Review

- Verify that the patient is feeling normal.
- Verify that the neurostimulator is functional.
- Reprogram the neurostimulator to pre-MRI settings.

[MR healthcare professionals are advised to contact the respective manufacturer in order to obtain the latest safety information to ensure patient safety relative to the use of an MR procedure.]

REFERENCES

http://www.medtronic.com/

Neurostimulation System: Enterra Therapy, Gastric Electrical Stimulation (GES)

The **Enterra Therapy, Gastric Electrical Stimulation (GES) System** (Medtronic, Inc., Minneapolis, MN), is a neurostimulation system indicated for treatment of patients with chronic, intractable (drug refractory) nausea and vomiting secondary to gastroparesis of diabetic or idiopathic etiology. Gastroparesis is a stomach disorder in which food moves through the stomach more slowly than normal. In some patients, this condition results in severe, chronic nausea and vomiting that cannot be adequately controlled by available drugs. These patients have difficulty eating and may require some form of tube feeding to ensure adequate nutrition. Enterra Therapy uses mild electrical pulses to stimulate the stomach. This electrical stimulation helps to control the symptoms associated with gastroparesis, including nausea and vomiting.

Enterra Therapy has been used successfully in people for several years. Worldwide clinical trials have been conducted in patients with severe symptoms of nausea and vomiting associated with gastroparesis. The results (Medtronic FDA Application H990014) showed that the therapy successfully reduced symptoms of nausea and vomiting in patients for whom drug treatments did not work. Patients also experienced improvements in other upper GI symptoms, solid food intake, and a reduction in hypoglycemic attacks, as well as significant improvements in health related quality of life.

Enterra Models: 7425G, 3116

Patients with an implanted device should not be exposed to the electromagnetic fields produced by magnetic resonance imaging (MRI). Use of MRI may potentially result in system failure or dislodgment, heating, or induced voltages in the neurostimulator and/or lead. An induced voltage through the neurostimulator or lead may cause uncomfortable, "jolting," or "shocking," levels of stimulation.

Clinicians should carefully weigh the decision to use MRI in patients with an implanted neurostimulation system, and note the following:

- Magnetic and radio-frequency (RF) fields produced by MRI may change the neurostimulator settings, activate the device, and injure the patient.
- Patients treated with MRI should be closely monitored and programmed parameters verified upon cessation of MRI.

[MR healthcare professionals are advised to contact the respective manufacturer in order to obtain the latest safety information to ensure patient safety relative to the use of an MR procedure.]

REFERENCE

http://www.medtronic.com/

Neurostimulation System: InterStim Therapy - Sacral Nerve Stimulation (SNS) for Urinary Control

InterStim Therapy - Sacral Nerve Stimulation (SNS) for Urinary Control (Medtronic, Inc., Minneapolis, MN) is a treatment for urinary urge incontinence, non-obstructive urinary retention, and significant symptoms of urgency-frequency in patients who have failed or could not tolerate more conservative treatments. In properly selected patients, InterStim Therapy can be dramatically successful in reducing or eliminating symptoms. The implantable InterStim System uses mild electrical stimulation of the sacral nerve that influences the behavior of the bladder, sphincter, and pelvic floor muscles.

This information on MRI pertains to the following Medtronic Neuromodulation products:
InterStim: Model number 3023
InterStim II: Model number 3058

Magnetic resonance imaging (MRI) – MRI is not recommended for a patient who has any implanted component of a neurostimulation system. Exposing a patient with an implanted neurostimulation system or component to MRI may potentially injure the patient or damage the neurostimulator. Clinicians should carefully weigh the decision to use MRI in patients with an implanted neurostimulation system, and note the following:

Induced electrical currents from the MRI to the neurostimulation system or component may cause heating, especially at the lead electrode site, resulting in tissue damage. Induced electrical currents may also stimulate or shock the patient.

Note: This warning applies even if only a lead or extension is implanted.

Factors that increase the risks of heating and patient injury include, but are not limited to, the following:

- High MRI Specific Absorption Rate (SAR) Radio Frequency (RF) power levels.
- MRI RF transmit coil that is near or extends over the implanted lead.
- Implanted leads with small surface area electrodes.
- Short distances between lead electrodes and tissue that is sensitive to heat.
- An MRI may permanently damage the neurostimulator, requiring it be removed or replaced.
- An MRI may affect the normal operation of the neurostimulator. An MRI can also reset the neurostimulator to power-on-reset values requiring reprogramming by a trained InterStim clinician.
- The neurostimulator can move within the implant pocket and align with the MRI field, resulting in discomfort or reopening of a recent implant incision.

In addition, the image details from MRI may be degraded, distorted, or blocked from view by the implanted neurostimulation system.

Patients treated with MRI should be closely monitored and programmed parameters verified upon cessation of MRI.

[MR healthcare professionals are advised to contact the respective manufacturer in order to obtain the latest safety information to ensure patient safety relative to the use of an MR procedure.]

REFERENCE

http://www.medtronic.com/

Neurostimulation Systems: Spinal Cord Stimulation

St. Jude Medical

Genesis, GenesisXP, GenesisRC, Eon, Eon C, Eon Mini, and Renew

The Genesis, GenesisXP, GenesisRC, Eon, EonC, Eon Mini, and Renewneuromodulation devices (St. Jude Medical)) used for spinal cord stimulation are indicated as aids in the management of chronic intractable pain of the trunk and/or limbs including unilateral or bilateral pain associated with any of the following: failed back surgery syndrome, intractable low back and leg pain, as well as for the treatment of other conditions.

MRI Information

The labeling information for these afore-mentioned products states: "**Warnings/Precautions:** Diathermy therapy, cardioverter defibrillators, magnetic resonance imaging (MRI), explosive or flammable gases, theft detectors and metal screening devices, lead movement, operation of machinery and equipment, postural changes, pediatric use, pregnancy, and case damage. Patients who are poor surgical risks, with multiple illnesses, or with active general infections should not be implanted."

REFERENCE

http://sjmneuropro.com

Neurostimulation Systems: Spinal Cord Stimulation

Medtronic, Inc

PrimeAdvanced Spinal Cord Neurostimulator (PrimeAdvanced, Model 37702)
RestoreAdvanced Spinal Cord Neurostimulator (RestoreAdvanced, Model 37713)
RestoreUltra Spinal Cord Neurostimulator (RestoreUltra, Model 37712)

Models:

Itrel 3: 7425
Restore: 37711
Synergy: 7427
SynergyPlus: 7479
Synergy Versitrel: 7427V
SynergyCompact: 7479B

Medtronic, Minneapolis, MN

MRI and Neurostimulation Therapy for Chronic Pain

Medtronic recommends that you do not conduct an MRI examination of any part of the body on a patient using a radio-frequency (RF) transmit body coil. If all of the instructions stated in this section are followed, MRI examinations of the head only using an RF transmit/receive head coil may be safely performed.

It is important to read this information in its entirety before conducting an MRI examination on a patient with any implanted component of a Medtronic neurostimulation system for chronic pain. These instructions do not apply to other implantable products or other devices, products, or items.

Contact Medtronic if you have any questions.www.Medtronic.com

Due to the number and variability of parameters that affect MRI compatibility, the safety of patients or continued functioning of neurostimulation systems exposed to MRI cannot be absolutely ensured. MRI systems generate powerful electromagnetic fields that can produce a number of interactions with implanted components of the neurostimulation system. Some of these interactions, especially heating, are potentially hazardous and can lead to serious injury or death. However, when all instructions stated in this section are followed, MRI examinations of the head only may be safely performed. In addition, neurostimulation system components can affect the MRI image, potentially impacting the diagnostic use of this modality. The following information describes the potential interactions and control measures that should be taken to minimize the risks from these interactions.

The instructions in this section describe how to conduct a head-only MRI examination of a patient with a neurostimulation system implanted for chronic pain, using a transmit/receive head coil of a 1.5-Tesla horizontal bore MRI. MRI examinations of any other part of the body are not recommended, as these require the use of the MRI RF transmit body coil, which may produce hazardous temperatures at the location of the implanted lead electrodes.

Warnings

MRI RF transmit body coil – Medtronic recommends that you do not conduct an MRI examination using an RF transmit body coil on a patient with any implanted neurostimulation system component because the interaction of the MRI with the neurostimulation system may lead to serious injury or death. See the section "Risks associated with MRI examination".

MRI transmit/receive head coil – An MRI examination of the head only (no other part of the body) can be conducted safely using an RF transmit/receive head coil when all instructions in this section are followed.

Limitations

- MRI should not be considered for patients with neurostimulation systems if other potentially safer diagnostic methods such as CT x-ray, ultrasound, or others will provide adequate diagnostic information.
- These instructions apply only to Medtronic neurostimulation therapies for chronic pain for approved indications.

- The instructions in this section apply to all Medtronic fully implantable neurostimulators, leads, and extensions used for chronic pain therapy.

Note: The instructions contained in this section are not applicable to MRI examinations of patients with radiofrequency (RF) neurostimulators. Medtronic recommends physicians not prescribe MRI for a patient who has an implanted Itrel 3 Model 7425 Neurostimulator. The Itrel 3 Neurostimulator is highly susceptible to reset or damage when subjected to an MRI examination. If reset, the neurostimulator must be reprogrammed. If damaged, the neurostimulator must be replaced. The Itrel 3 Neurostimulator has an increased risk of induced electrical current, which may stimulate or shock the patient.

Contact Medtronic for information about newer models or any updates.

- The RF transmit/receive head coil must not cover any implanted system component.
- If the patient has any other implants or products that prohibit or contraindicate an MRI examination, follow the instructions from the manufacturer. The instructions in this section apply only to the Medtronic products listed above.
- Do not conduct an MRI examination if the patient's neurostimulation system has a broken lead wire, because higher than normal heating may occur at the break or lead electrodes. Excessive heating can cause tissue damage and result in severe injury or death.
- Physicians should not prescribe MRI for patients undergoing trial neurostimulation and having systems that are not fully implanted.

If the MRI targeted image area is near the neurostimulator, it may be necessary to move the neurostimulator to obtain an image, or use alternate imaging techniques. MRI images may be severely distorted or image target areas can be completely blocked from view near the implanted neurostimulation system components, especially near the neurostimulator.

- Do not remove the neurostimulator and leave the lead system implanted as this can result in higher than expected lead heating. Excessive heating can cause tissue damage and result in severe injury or death.

Risks associated with MRI examination – Exposing a patient with an implanted neurostimulation system or component to MRI may potentially injure the patient or damage the neurostimulator. The known potential risks are as follows:

- Induced electrical currents from the MRI to the neurostimulation system or component may cause heating, especially at the lead-electrode site, resulting in tissue damage. Induced electrical currents may also stimulate or shock the patient.

Note: This warning applies even if only a lead or extension is implanted.

Factors that increase the risks of heating and patient injury include, but are not limited to, the following:

- High MRI specific absorption rate (SAR) RF power levels
- Low impedance leads or extensions (Medtronic product names or model numbers designated by a "Z," an "LZ," or "low impedance")
- MRI RF transmit/receive coil that is near or extends over the implanted lead system
- Implanted lead systems with small surface area electrodes
- Short distances between lead electrodes and heat-sensitive tissue
- Exposure to gradients exceeding a dB/dt limit of 20 Tesla per second may result in overstimulation or shocking, particularly for unipolar-capable devices.
- MRI may permanently damage the neurostimulator, requiring explant or replacement.
- MRI may affect the operation of the neurostimulator. The MRI may also reset the parameters to power-on-reset settings, requiring reprogramming with the clinician programmer. The Itrel 3 Model 7425 Neurostimulator is highly susceptible to reset or damage when subjected to an MRI examination. If reset, the neurostimulator must be reprogrammed. If damaged, the neurostimulator must be replaced. An Itrel 3 neurostimulator also might exhibit unpredictable behavior if subjected to an MRI examination.

The neurostimulator may move within the implant pocket and align itself with the MRI field, which may cause patient discomfort or a recent neurostimulator implant incision to open.

Cautions

Patient interaction during MRI – If possible, do not sedate the patient so that the patient can provide feedback of any problems during the examination.

Monitor the patient during the MRI examination. Verify that the patient is feeling normal and is responsive between each individual scan sequence of the MRI examination. Discontinue the MRI immediately if the patient becomes unresponsive to questions or experiences any heating, pain, shocking sensations/ uncomfortable stimulation, or unusual sensations.

MRI procedure using an RF transmit/receive head coil

Supervision

If all of the instructions stated in this section are followed, MRI examinations of the head using an RF transmit/receive head coil may be safely performed.

Prior to the MRI examination, an individual with the proper knowledge of MRI equipment such as an MRI radiologist or MRI physicist must ensure the MRI examination will be conducted according to the information outlined in this section.

Note: Due to the additional requirements in these instructions, MRI examination time maybe significantly extended.

MRI exposure requirements

Prior to an MRI examination, determine whether the patient has multiple active medical device implants (such as deep-brain stimulation systems, implantable cardiac defibrillators, and others). The most restrictive MRI exposure requirements must be used if the patient has multiple active medical device implants. Contact the appropriate manufacturers of the devices if you have questions.

If the following requirements cannot be met, do not proceed with the MRI examination.

- Use only an RF transmit/receive head coil.*
- Use only a 1.5-Tesla horizontal bore MRI (do not use open sided or other field strength MRI systems).
- Enter the correct patient weight into the MRI console to ensure the head SAR is estimated correctly. The MRI scan sequences must meet the following requirements. If they do not, the pulse parameters must be adjusted so that they comply with these requirements.

- Use MRI examination parameters that limit the head SAR to 1.5 W/kg or less for all RF pulse sequences.
- Limit the gradient dB/dt field to 20 Tesla per second or less.

*Important: If you are unsure if your MRI has RF transmit/receive head coil capability or if it displays "head SAR", check with your MRI manufacturer.

Note: The requirements provided are based on *in-vitro* testing and should result in a safe MRI examination of a patient with an implanted Medtronic neurostimulation system when all instructions in this section are followed. However, due to the many variables that affect safety, the safety of patients or continued functionality of neurostimulator systems exposed to MRI cannot be absolutely ensured. The user of this information assumes full responsibility for the consequences of conducting an MRI examination on a patient with an implanted neurostimulation system.

Preparation for the MRI examination

Do the following prior to performing an MRI examination on a patient with an implanted neurostimulation component:

1) Inform the patient of all of the risks of undergoing an MRI examination as stated in this section.
2) If possible, do not use sedation so the patient can inform the MRI operator of any heating, discomfort, or other problems.
3) Instruct the patient to immediately inform the MRI operator if any discomfort, stimulation, shocking, or heating occurs during the examination.
4) Determine if the patient has any other implants or conditions that would prohibit or contraindicate an MRI examination. If you are unclear what implants may be present, perform an x-ray to determine implant type and location. Do not conduct an MRI examination if any conditions or implants that would prohibit or contraindicate an MRI are present.
5) Verify that all proposed MRI examination parameters comply with the "MRI exposure requirements" (see above). If not, the parameters must be modified to meet these requirements. If parameters cannot be modified, do not perform an MRI.
6) If the patient has implanted leads but does not have an implanted neurostimulator, perform the following steps:

- Wrap the external portion of the leads/percutaneous extensions with insulating material, such as dry gauze.
- Keep the external portion of the leads/percutaneous extensions out of contact with the patient.
- Keep the external leads/percutaneous extensions straight, with no loops, and running down the center of the head coil.

7) If the patient has an implanted neurostimulator, perform the following steps:

- Review the neurostimulator with a clinician programmer and print out a copy of the programmed parameters for reference.
- Test for possible open circuits by measuring impedance on all electrodes. An impedance measurement greater than 4000 for Synergy Plus, Synergy Compact, Synergy Versitrel, Synergy, or Itrel 3 indicates a possible open circuit. An impedance measurement greater than 3600 for Restore indicates a possible open circuit.
- If an open circuit is suspected, obtain an x-ray to identify whether the open circuit is caused by a broken lead wire. If a broken lead wire is found, do not perform an MRI examination.

Warning: Do not conduct an MRI examination if the patient's neurostimulation system has a broken lead wire, because higher than normal heating may occur at the break or lead electrodes. Excessive heating can cause thermal lesions and result in severe injury or death.

8) If the system is functioning properly and no broken lead wires are found, program the neurostimulator to the settings provided in Table 1.

Table 1. Recommended neurostimulator settings for MRI examinations

Parameter	Setting
Stimulation output	OFF (all programs)
Stimulation mode	Bipolar (all programs)
Amplitude	0 Volts (all programs)
Magnetic (reed) switch	Disabled (Itrel 3 Model 7425 only)
Other parameters	Do not change

During the MRI examination

- Monitor the patient both visually and audibly. Check the patient between each imaging sequence. Discontinue the MRI examination immediately if the patient is unable to respond to questions or reports any problems.

- Conduct the examination using only the MRI pulse sequence that the MRI radiologist or physicist has confirmed meets the "MRI exposure requirements" outlined in this section.

Post-MRI examination review

- Verify that the patient feels normal.
- Verify that the neurostimulator is functional.
- Reprogram the neurostimulator to pre-MRI settings.

Models:
Mattrix: 3272, 3271

Reference: Pain Therapy IFP (221351-001)

Medtronic recommends physicians **not** prescribe an MRI for a patient who has any implanted component of a [Mattrix] system. Exposing a patient with a [Mattrix] system or component to an MRI may potentially injure the patient and/or damage the receiver. The known potential risks are as follows:

- Induced electrical currents from the MRI to the [Mattrix] system or component may cause heating, especially at the lead electrode site, resulting in tissue damage. Induced electrical currents may also stimulate or shock the patient.

Note: This warning applies even if only a lead or extension is implanted.

Heating risks are affected by a number of factors involving the MRI equipment and the implanted [Mattrix] system. Factors that increase the risks of heating and patient injury include, but are not limited to, the following:

- High MRI Specific Absorption Rate (SAR) Radio Frequency (RF) power levels
- Low impedance leads or extensions (Medtronic product names or model numbers designated by a "Z," an "LZ," or "low impedance")
- MRI RF transmit coil that is near or extends over the implanted lead system
- Implanted lead systems with small surface area electrodes

- Short separation distances between lead electrodes and thermally sensitive tissue
- An MRI may permanently damage the receiver, which may require explant or possible replacement.
- An MRI may affect the functional operation of the receiver
- The receiver may move within the implant pocket and align itself with the MRI field, which may cause patient discomfort or a recent receiver implant incision to open.

In addition, the image details from MRI may be degraded, distorted, or blocked from view by the implanted [Mattrix] system.

[MR healthcare professionals are advised to contact the respective manufacturer in order to obtain the latest safety information to ensure patient safety relative to the use of an MR procedure.]

REFERENCE

http://www.medtronic.com/

Neurostimulation System: Vagus Nerve Stimulation

Vagus Nerve Stimulation, Vagal Nerve Stimulator, VNS Therapy, NeuroCybernetic Prosthesis (NCP) System

(Cyberonics, Inc., Houston, TX)

Current MRI information for the Vagal Nerve Stimulator, VNS Therapy, NeuroCybernetic Prosthesis (NCP) System (Cyberonics, Inc., Houston, TX) may be found by visiting http://www.cyberonics.com/ and http://www.vnstherapy.com/.

Important Note: Highly specific conditions must be followed in orer to safety perform MRI in patients with the Vagal Nerve Stimulator, VNS Therapy, NeuroCybernetic Prosthesis (NCP) System.

MAGNETIC RESONANCE IMAGING (MRI)

Caution: Magnetic resonance imaging (MRI) should not be performed with a magnetic resonance body coil in the transmit mode. The heat induced in the Lead by an MRI body scan can cause injury.

If an MRI should be done, use only a transmit and receive type of head coil. Magnetic and RF fields produced by MRI may change the Pulse Generator settings (change to reset parameters) or activate the device. Stimulation has been shown to cause the adverse events reported in the "Adverse Events" section in the indication-specific parts of the multi-part physician manuals. MRI compatibility was demonstrated using a 1.5T General Electric Signa Imager with a Model 100 Pulse Generator and 300 Lead only. Model 101, 102, 102R, 103, and 104 Pulse Generators are functionally equivalent to the Model 100. Model 302, 303, and 304 Leads are functionally equivalent to the Model 300. Testing on this imager as performed on a phantom* indicated that the following Pulse Generator and MRI procedures can be used safely without adverse events:

- Pulse Generator output programmed to 0 mA for the MRI procedure, and afterward, retested by performing the System Diagnostics (Lead Test) and reprogrammed to the original settings

- Head coil type: transmit and receive only

- Static magnetic field strength: less than or equal to 2.0 tesla

- Specific absorption rate (SAR): less than 1.3 W/kg for a 154.5-lb (70-kg) patient

- Time-varying intensity: less than 10 tesla/sec

Use caution when other MRI systems are used, since adverse events may occur because of different magnetic field distributions. Consider other imaging modalities when appropriate.

Caution: Procedures in which the RF is transmitted by a body coil should not be done on a patient who has the VNS Therapy System. Thus, protocols must not be used that utilize local coils that are RF-receive only, with RF-transmit performed by the body coil. Note that some RF head coils are receive-only, and that most other local coils, such as knee and spinal coils, are also RF receive-only. **These coils must not be used in patients with the VNS Therapy System.**

(*) A phantom is a material resembling a body in mass, composition, and dimensions that is used to measure absorption of radiation.

[MR healthcare professionals are advised to contact the respective manufacturer in order to obtain the latest safety information to ensure patient safety relative to the use of an MR procedure.]

REFERENCES

http://www.cyberonics.com/

http://www.vnstherapy.com/

http://www.vnstherapy.com/epilepsy/hcp/manuals/default.aspx

Ocular Implants, Lens Implants, and Devices

Of the different ocular implants, lens implants, and devices tested in the MR environment, the Fatio eyelid spring, the retinal tack made from martensitic (i.e., ferromagnetic) stainless steel (Western European), the Troutman magnetic ocular implant, and the Unitek round wire eyelid spring demonstrated positive magnetic field interactions in association with exposure to 1.5-Tesla MR systems. By comparison, many of the lens implants pose no hazard to the patient during an MRI procedure since they do not contain metallic materials (see **The List**). ·

A patient with a Fatio eyelid spring or round wire eyelid spring may experience discomfort but would probably not be injured as a result of exposure to an MR system. In fact, patients have undergone MR procedures with eyelid wires after having a protective plastic covering placed around the globe along with a firmly applied eye patch as a precaution.

The retinal tack made from martensitic stainless steel and Troutman magnetic ocular implant may injure a patient undergoing an MR procedure, although no such case has ever been reported.

[For additional information pertaining to ocular related prostheses, see **Glaucoma Drainage Implants (Shunt Tubes)**, **Magnetically-Activated Implants and Devices**, and **Scleral Buckle (Scleral Buckling Procedure**.]

REFERENCES

Albert DW, Olson KR, Parel JM, et al. Magnetic resonance imaging and retinal tacks. Arch Ophthalmol 1990;108:320-321.

de Keizer RJ, Te Strake L. Intraocular lens implants (pseudophakoi) and steelwire sutures: a contraindication for MRI? Doc Ophthalmol 1984;61:281-284.

Joondeph BC, Peyman GA, Mafee MF, et al. Magnetic resonance imaging and retinal tacks [Letter]. Arch Ophthalmol 1987;105:1479-1480.

Marra S, Leonetti JP, Konior RJ, Raslan W. Effect of magnetic resonance imaging on implantable eyelid weights. Ann Otol Rhinol Laryngol 1995;104:448-452.

Roberts CW, Haik BG, Cahill P. Magnetic resonance imaging of metal loop intraocular lenses. Arch Ophthalmol 1990;108:320-321.

Seiff SR, Vestel KP, Truwit CL. Eyelid palpebral springs in patients undergoing magnetic resonance imaging: an area of possible concern [Letter]. Arch Ophthalmol 1991;109:319.

Shellock FG. Magnetic Resonance Procedures: Health Effects and Safety. CRC Press, LLC, Boca Raton, FL, 2001.

Shellock FG, Kanal E. Magnetic Resonance: Bioeffects, Safety, and Patient Management. Second Edition, Lippincott-Raven Press, New York, 1996.

Shellock FG, Myers SM, Schatz CJ. Ex vivo evaluation of ferromagnetism determined for metallic scleral "buckles" exposed to a 1.5-T MR scanner. Radiology 1992;185:288-289.

Orthopedic Implants, Materials, and Devices

Most of the orthopedic implants, materials, and devices evaluated in the MR environment are made from nonferromagnetic materials and, therefore, are safe for patients undergoing MR procedures. However, in certain instances, due to the length or formation of a conductive loop, MRI-related heating may be a problem for some orthopedic implants, especially external fixation systems, (see below).

The Perfix interference screw used for reconstruction of the anterior cruciate ligament has been found to be highly ferromagnetic. Because this interference screw is firmly imbedded in bone for its specific application, it is held in place with sufficient retentive forces to prevent movement or dislodgment. Patients with Perfix interference screws have safely undergone MR procedures using MR systems operating at 1.5-Tesla.

The presence of the Perfix interference screw causes extensive image distortion during MR imaging of the knee. Therefore, interference screws made from materials with low magnetic susceptibility should be used for reconstruction of the anterior cruciate ligament if MR imaging is to be utilized for subsequent evaluation of the knee.

Patients with the MR safe or MR conditional orthopedic implants, materials, and devices indicated in **The List** have undergone MR procedures using MR systems operating at static magnetic fields up to 3-Tesla without incident.

External Fixation Systems. External fixation systems comprise specially designed frames, clamps, rods, rod-to-rod couplings, pins, posts, fasteners, wire fixations, fixation bolts, washers, nuts, hinges, sockets, connecting bars, screws and other components used in orthopedic and reconstructive surgery. Indications for external fixation systems are varied and include the following treatment applications:

- Open and closed fracture fixation;
- Pseudoarthroses of long bones (both congenital and acquired);
- Limb lengthening by metaphyseal or epiphyseal distraction;
- Correction of bony or soft tissue defects; and
- Correction of bony or soft tissue deformities.

The assessment of MRI issues for external fixation systems is particularly challenging because of the myriad of possible components (many of which are made from conductive materials) and configurations used for these devices. The primary concern is MRI-related heating which is dependent on particular aspects of the external fixation system. Importantly, the MRI conditions (field strength, RF field, RF transmit coil, pulse sequence, body part imaged, etc.) used greatly impacts the safety aspects of scanning patients with external fixation systems.

To ensure patient safety, guidelines are typically applied on a case by case basis and, therefore, MR users are referred to product labeling approved by the U.S. Food and Drug Administration for a given external fixation system. Notably, the acceptable MRI conditions typically apply to the specific configuration(s) used in the evaluation of a given fixation device, ONLY. Other configurations may be unsafe.

Vibration Associated With MR Procedures. Graf et al. reported that torque acting on metallic implants or instruments due to eddy-current induction in associated with MR imaging can be considerable. Larger implants (such as fixation devices) made from well-conducting materials are especially affected. Gradient switching was shown to produce fast alternating torque. Significant vibrations at off-center positions of the metal parts may explain why some patients with metallic implants sometimes report feeling heating sensations during MR examinations.

MRI at 3-Tesla and Orthopedic Implants, Materials, and Devices. A variety of orthopedic implants have been evaluated for magnetic field interactions at 3-Tesla (see **The List**). All of these are considered to be safe based on findings for deflection angles, torque, and the intended *in vivo* uses of these devices. For some orthopedic implants, MRI-related heating was evaluated, as needed, and is a concern for certain devices, especially external fixation systems.

[MR healthcare professionals are advised to contact the respective manufacturer in order to obtain the latest safety information to ensure patient safety relative to the use of an MR procedure.]

REFERENCES

Graf H, Steidle G, Martirosian P, Lauer UA, Schick F. Metal artifacts caused by gradient switching. Magnetic Resonance in Medicine 2005;54;231-234.

Luechinger R, Boesiger P, Disegi JA. Safety evaluation of large external fixation clamps and frames in a magnetic resonance environment. J Biomed Mater Res B Appl Biomater. 2007;82:17-22.

Lyons CJ, Betz RR, Mesgarzadeh M, et al. The effect of magnetic resonance imaging on metal spine implants. Spine 1989;14:670-672.

McComb C, Allan D, Condon B. Evaluation of the translational and rotational forces acting on a highly ferromagnetic orthopedic spinal implant in magnetic resonance imaging. J Magn Reson Imaging. 2009;29:449-53.

Mechlin M, Thickman D, Kressel HY, et al. Magnetic resonance imaging of postoperative patients with metallic implants. AJR Am J Roentgenol 1984;143:1281-1284.

Mesgarzadeh M, Revesz G, Bonakdarpour A, et al. The effect on medical metal implants by magnetic fields of magnetic resonance imaging. Skeletal Radiol 1985;14:205-206.

Shellock FG. Magnetic Resonance Procedures: Health Effects and Safety. CRC Press, LLC, Boca Raton, FL, 2001.

Shellock FG. Biomedical implants and devices: assessment of magnetic field interactions with a 3.0-Tesla MR system. J Magn Reson Imaging 2002;16:721-732.

Shellock FG, Crues JV. High-field-strength MR imaging and metallic bioimplants: an *in vitro* evaluation of deflection forces and temperature changes induced in large prostheses [Abstract]. Radiology 1987;165:150.

Shellock FG, Kanal E. Magnetic Resonance: Bioeffects, Safety, and Patient Management. Second Edition, Lippincott-Raven Press, New York, 1996.

Shellock FG, Mink JH, Curtin S, et al. MRI and orthopedic implants used for anterior cruciate ligament reconstruction: assessment of ferromagnetism and artifacts. J Magn Reson Imaging 1992;2:225-228.

Shellock FG, Morisoli S, Kanal E. MR procedures and biomedical implants, materials, and devices: 1993 update. Radiology 1993;189:587-599.Stradiotti P, et al. Metal-related artifacts in instrumented spine. Techniques for reducing artifacts in CT and MRI: state of the art. Eur Spine J. 2009;18 Suppl 1:102-8.

Yang CW, Liu L, et al. Magnetic resonance imaging of artificial lumbar disks: safety and metal artifacts. Chin Med J (Engl). 2009;20;122:911-6.

Otologic Implants

Of the otologic implants evaluated for the presence of magnetic field interactions (note: MRI-related heating is not considered to be an issue for these relatively small implants), the McGee stapedectomy piston prosthesis, made from platinum and chromium-nickel alloy stainless steel, is ferromagnetic. The manufacturer has recalled this otologic implant. Patients who received this device have been issued warnings to avoid MR procedures. The specific item and lot numbers of the McGee implants recalled and considered to be a contraindication for MR procedures are as follows (Personal Communication, Winston Geer, Smith & Nephew Richards Inc., Barlett, TN, 1995):

Item No.	Lot Number
14-0330	1W91100, 4UO9690
14-0331	4U09700
14-0332	1W91110, 4U58540, 4U86300
14-0333	4U09710, 1W34390, 2WR4073
14-0334	4U09720, 1W34390, 2WR4073
14-0335	1W34400, 4U09730
14-0336	3U18350, 3U50470, 4UR2889
14-0337	3U18370, 4UR2889
14-0338	3U18390, 4U02900, 4UR1453
14-0339	3U18400, 3U50500
14-0340	3U18410, 3U50500
14-0341	3U41200, 4UR2889

MRI at 3-Tesla and Otologic Implants. Many otologic implants have been evaluated for magnetic field interactions at 3-Tesla (see **The List**). In consideration of the relatively small sizes of these items, MRI-related heating is not a concern at 3-Tesla. For the ones tested, all are considered to be acceptable for patients based on findings for deflection angles, torque, and the intended *in vivo* uses of these specific devices.

For example, MRI testing at 3-Tesla was conducted on the following product from Micromedics, Inc:

Stainless Steel Vent Tube & Stainless Steel Wire

Because of the size of the metallic mass associated with this particular product, the MRI test findings (MR Conditional 6, 3-Tesla or less) apply to all of the products listed below (Micromedics, Inc., Eagan, MN):

VT-0205-, Fluoroplastic with stainless steel wire
VT-0702-, Silicone with stainless steel wire
VT-1402-, Stainless Steel with stainless steel wire
VT-1412-, Titanium with stainless steel wire
VT-1505-, Polyethylene with stainless steel wire

REFERENCES

Applebaum EL, Valvassori GE. Effects of magnetic resonance imaging fields on stapedectomy prostheses. Arch Otolaryngol 1985;11:820-821.

Applebaum EL, Valvassori GE. Further studies on the effects of magnetic resonance fields on middle ear implants. Ann Otol Rhinol Laryngol 1990;99:801-804.

Bauknecht HC, et al. Behaviour of titanium middle ear implants at 1.5 and 3 Tesla field strength in magnetic resonance imaging. Laryngorhinootologie. 2009;88:236-40.

Fritsch MH. MRI scanners and the stapes prosthesis. Otol Neurotol 2007;28:733-8.

Fritsch MH, Mosier KM. MRI compatibility issues in otology. Curr Opin Otolaryngol Head Neck Surg. 2007;15:335-340.

Fritsch MH, Gutt JJ. Ferromagnetic movements of middle ear implants and stapes prostheses in a 3-T magnetic resonance field. Otol Neurotol. 2005;26:225-230.

Leon JA, Gabriele OF. Middle ear prothesis: significance in magnetic resonance imaging. Magn Reson Imaging 1987;5:405-406.

Martin AD, Driscoll CL, Wood CP, Felmlee JP. Safety evaluation of titanium middle ear prostheses at 3.0 Tesla. Otolaryngol Head Neck Surg 2005;132:537-42.

Nogueira M, Shellock FG. Otologic bioimplants: Ex vivo assessment of ferromagnetism and artifacts at 1.5-Tesla. AJR Am J Roentgenol 1995;163:1472-1473.

Shellock FG. Magnetic Resonance Procedures: Health Effects and Safety. CRC Press, LLC, Boca Raton, FL, 2001.

Shellock FG, Morisoli S, Kanal E. MR procedures and biomedical implants, materials, and devices: 1993 update. Radiology 1993;189:587-599.

White DW. Interaction between magnetic fields and metallic ossicular prostheses. Am J Otol 1987;8:290-292.

Wild DC, Head K, Hall DA. Safe magnetic resonance scanning of patients with metallic middle ear implants. Clin Otolaryngol. 2006;31:508-510.

Oxygen Tanks and Gas Cylinders

According to Chaljub et al., accidents related to ferromagnetic oxygen tanks and other gas cylinders that can become projectiles might be increasing. In fact, missile-related accidents for these objects as well as other items have resulted in at least one fatality, several injuries, damage to MR systems, and down-time (i.e., loss of revenue) for many MRI centers.

Therefore, MRI facilities must implement a policy for safe administration of oxygen to patients undergoing MR procedures. In lieu of utilizing pipes to directly deliver gases to patients, the use of non-magnetic (usually aluminum) gas cylinders is one means of preventing "missile effect" hazards in the MR environment. Non-magnetic oxygen tanks and cylinders for other gases are commercially available from various vendors.

MRI centers should have a sufficient number of nonmagnetic oxygen tanks and strict policies to prevent emergency staff members from introducing ferromagnetic objects into the MR environment. Notably, some hospital-based MR centers have nonmagnetic oxygen tanks used throughout their buildings to prevent projectile accidents.

Nonmagnetic tanks must be prominently labeled and/or color-coded to avoid confusion with magnetic cylinders. Furthermore, all healthcare workers that work in the MR environment must be informed regarding the fact that only nonmagnetic oxygen and other gas cylinders are allowed into the MR system room.

Nonmagnetic/weakly magnetic (i.e., MR conditional) oxygen regulators, flow meters, cylinder carts, cylinder stands, cylinder holders for wheelchairs, and suction devices are also commercially available to provide safe respiratory support and management of patients in the MR environment and for transfer to and from the MRI facility.

REFERENCES

Chaljub G, et al. Projectile cylinder accidents resulting from the presence of ferromagnetic nitrous oxide or oxygen tanks in the MR suite. American Journal of Roentgenology 2001;177:27-30.

Colletti PM. Size "H" oxygen cylinder: accidental MR projectile at 1.5-Tesla. Journal of Magnetic Resonance Imaging 2004;19:141-143.

ECRI. Patient Death Illustrates the Importance of Adhering to Safety Precautions in Magnetic Resonance Environments. ECRI, Plymouth Meeting, PA, Aug. 6, 2001.

Jolesz FA, et al. Compatible instrumentation for intraoperative MRI: expanding resources. Journal of Magnetic Resonance Imaging, 1998;8:8-11.

Keeler EK, et al. Accessory equipment considerations with respect to MRI compatibility. Journal of Magnetic Resonance Imaging, 1998;8:12-18.

Shellock FG. Magnetic Resonance Procedures: Health Effects and Safety. CRC Press, Boca Raton, FL, 2001.

Palatal System Implant Assembly

The Palatal System Implant Assembly (Pavad Medical, Inc., Fremont, CA) is designed to treat sleep disordered breathing.

MRI Information

The Palatal System Implant Assembly was determined to be MR-conditional according to the terminology specified in the ASTM International, Designation: F2503-05. Standard Practice for Marking Medical Devices and Other Items for Safety in the Magnetic Resonance Environment.

Non-clinical testing demonstrated that the Palatal System Implant Assembly is MR Conditional. A patient with this implant can be scanned safely immediately after placement under the following conditions:

- Static magnetic field of 1.5-Tesla
- Maximum spatial gradient magnetic field of 250-Gauss/cm
- Maximum MR system reported whole-body-averaged specific absorption rate (SAR) of 3.5-W/kg for 15 minutes of scanning.

In non-clinical testing, the Palatal System Implant Assembly produced a temperature rise of 0.8 °C at a maximum MR system-reported whole body averaged specific absorption rate (SAR) of 3.5-W/kg for 15-minutes of MR scanning in a 1.5-Tesla MR system using a transmit/receive body coil (1.5-Tesla, Magnetom, Software Numaris/4, Version Syngo MR 2002B DHHS, Siemens Medical Solutions, Malvern, PA).

MR image quality may be compromised if the area of interest is in the exact same area or relatively close to the position of the Palatal System Implant Assembly. Therefore, optimization of MR imaging parameters to compensate for the presence of this implant may be necessary. The following chart provides artifact information for the Palatal System Implant Assembly in relation to different pulse sequences at 1.5-Tesla:

Pulse sequence	Signal Void
T1-weighted spin echo, long axis orientation	2.7-cm^2
T1-weighted spin echo, short axis orientation	2.7-cm^2
Gradient echo, long axis orientation	8.8-cm^2
Gradient echo, short axis orientation	9.6-cm^2

MRI Procedures and Function of the Palatal System Implant Assembly

The effects of MRI procedures on the functional aspects of Palatal System Implant Assembly devices were assessed. In-vitro testing was performed on a phantom with six Palatal System Implant Assembly devices placed in various orientations relative to the MR system. MRI was conducted using 1.5-Tesla/64 MHz MR system (transmit/receive RF body coil) to perform 8 different MR imaging pulse sequences, as follows: T1-weighted spin echo, T1-weighted fast spin echo, T2-weighted spin echo, T2- weighted fast spin echo, three dimensional fast gradient echo, turbo/fast gradient echo, turbo/fast spoiled gradient echo, echo planar imaging.

The findings indicated that there was no apparent damage or alteration in the function of the Palatal System Implant Assembly. Thus, the Palatal System Implant Assembly was demonstrated to maintain full functionality after exposure to the MRI conditions indicated above.

Additional guidelines for the Palatal System Implant Assembly include:

- Do not use MR systems other than 1.5 Tesla MR systems.
- Continuously monitor the patients using visual and audio means (i.e., intercom system) throughout the MR procedure
- Instruct the patient to alert the MR system operator of any unusual sensations or problems so the MR system operator can terminate the MRI procedure, if needed.
- Provide the patient with a means to alert the MR system operator of any unusual sensations or problems that may be experienced during the MRI procedure.

Patent Ductus Arteriosus (PDA) Occluders, Atrial Septal Defect (ASD) Occluders, Ventricular Septal Defect (VSD) Occluders, and Patent Foramen Ovale (PFO) Closure Devices

Cardiac occluders and closure devices are implants used to treat patients with patient ductus arteriosus (PDA), atrial septal defect (ASD), ventricular septal defect (VSD), or patent foramen ovale (PFO) heart conditions. For implants that have been evaluated relative to the use of 1.5-T MR systems, as long as the proper size occluder or closure device is used, the amount of retention provided by the folded-back, hinged arms of the device is sufficient to keep it in place, acutely. Eventually, tissue growth covers the cardiac occluder or closure device and facilitates retention.

Certain metallic PDA, ASD, VSD occluders and PFO closure devices tested for magnetic qualities were made from either 304V stainless steel or MP35N. Occluders made from 304V stainless steel were found to be "weakly" ferromagnetic, whereas those made from MP35N were nonferromagnetic in association with a 1.5-Tesla MR system.

Patients with cardiac occluders made from MP35N (i.e., a nonferromagnetic alloy) may undergo MR procedures at 1.5-Tesla or less any time after placement of these implants. However, patients with cardiac occluders made from 304V stainless steel (i.e., a "weakly ferromagnetic" material) are advised to wait a minimum of six weeks after placement of these devices before undergoing MR procedures. This wait period permits tissue ingrowth to provide additional retentive forces for the occluders made from weakly ferromagnetic materials.

If there is any question about the integrity of the retention aspects of a metallic cardiac occluder made from a ferromagnetic material, the patient or individual should not be allowed into the MR environment or to undergo an MR procedure.

MRI at 3-Tesla and PDA, ASD, VSD Occluders and PFO Closure Devices. Various PDA, ASD, VSD occluders and PFO closure devices have been evaluated at 3-Tesla (see **The List**). All of these are considered to be acceptable based on findings for deflection angles, torque, MRI-related heating and the intended *in vivo* uses of these specific devices.

REFERENCES

Shellock FG, Morisoli SM. Ex vivo evaluation of ferromagnetism and artifacts for cardiac occluders exposed to a 1.5-Tesla MR system. J Magn Reson Imaging 1994;4:213-215.

Shellock FG. Magnetic Resonance Procedures: Health Effects and Safety. CRC Press, LLC, Boca Raton, FL, 2001.

Shellock FG, Valencerina S. Septal repair implants: evaluation of MRI safety at 3-Tesla. Magnetic Resonance Imaging 2005;23:1021-1025.

Pellets and Bullets

The majority of pellets and bullets tested in the MR environment were found to be composed of nonferromagnetic materials. Ammunition that proved to be ferromagnetic tended to be manufactured in foreign countries and/or used for military applications. Shrapnel typically contains steel and, therefore, presents a potential hazard for patients undergoing MR procedures.

Because pellets, bullets, and shrapnel are frequently contaminated with ferromagnetic materials, the risk versus benefit of performing an MR procedure should be carefully considered. Additional consideration must be given to whether the metallic object is located near or in a vital anatomic structure, with the assumption that the object is likely to be ferromagnetic and can potentially move.

In an effort to reduce lead poisoning in "puddling" type ducks, the federal government requires many of the eastern United States to use steel shotgun pellets instead of lead. The presence of steel shotgun pellets presents a potential hazard to patients undergoing MR procedures and causes substantial imaging artifacts at the immediate position of these metallic objects.

In one case, a small metallic BB located in a subcutaneous site caused painful symptoms in a patient exposed to an MR system, although no serious injury occurred. In consideration of this information, MR healthcare professionals should exercise caution when deciding to perform MR procedures in patients with pellets, bullets, shrapnel or other similar ballistic objects.

Smugar et al. conducted an investigation to determine whether neurological problems developed in patients with intraspinal bullets or bullet fragments in association with MR imaging performed at 1.5-Tesla. Patients were queried during scanning for symptoms of discomfort, pain, or changes in neurological status. Additionally, detailed neurological examinations were performed prior to MRI, post MRI, and at the patients' discharge. Based on these findings, Smugar et al. concluded that patients with complete spinal cord injury may undergo MR imaging if they have intraspinal bullets or fragments without concern for affects on their physical or neurological status. Thus, metallic fragments in the spinal canals of paralyzed patients are believed to represent only a relative contraindication to MR procedures.

REFERENCES

Shellock FG. Magnetic Resonance Procedures: Health Effects and Safety. CRC Press, LLC, Boca Raton, FL, 2001.

Shellock FG, Kanal E. Magnetic Resonance: Bioeffects, Safety, and Patient Management. Second Edition, Lippincott-Raven Press, New York, 1996.

Smugar SS, Schweitzer ME, Hume E. MRI in patients with intraspinal bullets. J Magn Reson Imaging 1999;9:151-153.

Teitelbaum GP. Metallic ballistic fragments: MR imaging safety and artifacts [Letter]. Radiology 1990;177:883.

Teitelbaum GP, Yee CA, Van Horn DD, et al. Metallic ballistic fragments: MR imaging safety and artifacts. Radiology 1990;175:855-859.

Penile Implants

Several types of penile implants and prostheses have been evaluated in the MR environment. Of these, two (i.e., the Duraphase and Omniphase models) demonstrated substantial ferromagnetic qualities when exposed to a 1.5-Tesla MR system. Fortunately, it is unlikely for a penile implant to severely injure a patient undergoing an MR procedure because of the degree of magnetic field interactions associated with a 1.5-Tesla MR system. This is especially true when one considers the manner in which this device is utilized. Nevertheless, it would undoubtedly be uncomfortable for a patient with a ferromagnetic penile implant to undergo an MR examination. For this reason, subjecting a patient with the Duraphase or Omniphase penile implant to the MR environment or an MR procedure is inadvisable.

MRI at 3-Tesla and Penile Implants. Several different penile implants have been tested in association with 3-Tesla MR systems. Findings for these specific penile implants indicated that they either exhibited no magnetic field interactions or relatively minor or "weak" magnetic field interactions. Accordingly, these specific penile implants are considered acceptable for patients undergoing MR procedures using MR systems operating at 3-Tesla or less (see **The List**).

REFERENCES

Shellock FG. Magnetic Resonance Procedures: Health Effects and Safety. CRC Press, LLC, Boca Raton, FL, 2001.

Shellock FG, Crues JV, Sacks SA. High-field magnetic resonance imaging of penile prostheses: *in vitro* evaluation of deflection forces and imaging artifacts [Abstract]. In: Book of Abstracts, Society of Magnetic Resonance in Medicine. Berkeley, CA: Society of Magnetic Resonance in Medicine, 1987;3:915.

Shellock FG, Kanal E. Magnetic Resonance: Bioeffects, Safety, and Patient Management. Second Edition, Lippincott-Raven Press, New York, 1996.

Pessaries

A pessary is a small medical device that is inserted into the vagina or rectum and held in place by the pelvic floor musculature. In some instances, a pessary may contain metal to permit forming it into a shape to facilitate proper retention. Typically, the pessary is a firm ring or similar structure that presses against the wall of the vagina and urethra to help decrease urinary leakage or other condition. Indications for the pessary include pelvic support defects, such as uterine prolapse and vaginal prolapse, as well as stress urinary incontinence.

MRI Information. A wide variety of pessary styles exist, including those made entirely from nonmetallic, nonconducting materials (e.g., plastic, silicone, or latex) as well as those that have metallic components. Obviously, pessaries made from nonmetallic, nonconducting materials pose no problems for patients undergoing MRI. However, pessaries that have metallic components cause substantial artifacts and may pose risks to patients undergoing MR examinations. Notably, to date, there are no reports of injuries or other issues related to performing MRI in patients with these devices.

REFERENCES

Brubacker L. The vaginal pessary. In: Friedman AJ, ed. American Urogynecologic Society Quarterly Report 1991;9(3).

Davila GW. Vaginal prolapse: management with nonsurgical techniques. Postgrad Med 1996;99: 171-6,181,184-5.

Deger RB, Menzin AW, Mikuta JJ. The vaginal pessary: past and present. Postgrad Obstet Gynecol 1993;13:1-8.

Komesu YM, et al. Restoration of continence by pessaries: magnetic resonance imaging assessment of mechanism of action. Am J Obstet Gynecol. 2008;198:563.e1-6.

Miller DS. Contemporary use of the pessary. In: Sciarra JJ, ed. Gynecology and obstetrics. Revised 1997 ed. Philadelphia: Lippencott-Raven, 1997:1-12.

Zeitlin MP, Lebherz TB. Pessaries in the geriatric patient. J Am Geriatr Soc 1992;40:635-9.

PillCam Capsule Endoscopy Device

The PillCam (M2A, PillCam SB, PillCam ESO, PillCam ESO2) Capsule Endoscopy Device (Given Imaging Inc., Norcross, GA) is an ingestible device for use in the gastrointestinal tract. Peristalsis moves the PillCam Capsule smoothly and painlessly throughout the gastrointestinal tract, transmitting color video images as it passes. The procedure allows patients to continue daily activities during the endoscopic examination. The PillCam Capsule Endoscopy Device is a first-line tool in the detection of abnormalities of the small bowel.

The PillCam Capsule Endoscopy Device has been utilized to diagnose diseases of the small intestine including Crohn's Disease, celiac disease and other malabsorption disorders, benign and malignant tumors of the small intestine, vascular disorders and medication related small bowel injuries.

MRI Information

The User Manual for the PillCam Capsule Endoscopy Device states:

"Undergoing an MRI while the capsule is inside the patient's body may result in serious damage to his/her intestinal tract or abdominal cavity. If the patient did not positively verify the excretion of the PillCam Capsule from his/her body, he/she should contact the physician for evaluation and possible abdominal X-ray before undergoing an MRI examination."

[Reprinted with permission from Given Imaging Inc., Norcross, GA]

REFERENCE

www.givenimaging.com

RF BION Microstimulator

Surgically implanted neurostimulators and electrodes may be utilized to provide functional electrical stimulation of the affected site. However, these devices may be associated with considerable surgical morbidity and expense. As such, there has been an on-going effort to develop technology that combines the reliability of using an implanted device with a low morbidity and low cost procedure. This effort has yielded a miniaturized, implantable device designed for functional electrical stimulation.

In 1988, Heetderks first demonstrated the feasibility of using a millimeter-sized, neural prosthetic implant. Over the years, this so-called "microstimulator" evolved to its present form. The microstimulator now exists as a relatively small, wireless, digitally controlled stimulator that is implanted using a minimally invasive procedure to provide electrical pulses to a muscle or nerve. This device receives power and command signals by inductive coupling from an externally worn coil that generates a radiofrequency magnetic field. The microstimulator is currently undergoing clinical trials to assess its therapeutic effect on a variety of neurological disorders including urinary incontinence, shoulder subluxation, drop foot, ventilator-dependant respiratory deficiencies, and sleep apnea.

RF BION Microstimulator. The implantable RF BION Microstimulator (Alfred E. Mann Foundation for Scientific Research, Valencia, CA and Advanced Bionics Corporation, Valencia, CA) is a wireless device designed for functional electrical stimulation of the peripheral nervous system. This hermetically-sealed implant is a small, lightweight, cylindrical-shaped device (length, 16.6-mm; diameter-2.4 mm; mass, 0.265-g) made of a ceramic tube closed on each end by titanium caps and contains components made from titanium, gold, copper, ferrite, platinum, iridium, silicon, zirconium, and tantalum. The active electrodes are welded on each end cap: an iridium disk on the cathodal side and a platinum-iridium eyelet on the anodal side.

The microstimulator receives power and digital commands via a 2-MHz radiofrequency magnetic field link generated from an external coil that is worn by the patient. The RF Bion Microstimulator produces asymmetric, biphasic, capacitively coupled constant-current pulses. Stimulation circuitry and a receiving multi-turn loop antenna are contained within the microstimulator. The antenna is wound around two pieces of ferrite, cut from a cylinder of radius 0.74-mm. Because of the small size of this microstimulator, it may be implanted through a specially designed, trocar-based 12- or 14-gauge implant tool or via a small surgical opening for placement near a nerve or at the motor unit of a muscle. A suture passed through one of the end caps allows the microstimulator to be maintained acutely in a properly implanted position.

MRI and the RF BION Microstimulator

Safety information for the use of a magnetic resonance imaging (MRI) procedure (i.e., imaging, angiography, functional imaging, spectroscopy, etc.) in a patient with the RF BION Microstimulator is highly specific to the type of MR system and conditions used to determine safety criteria for this implant. Safety information for MR procedures described herein pertains to the use of MR systems operating with static magnetic fields of 1.5-Tesla, gradient magnetic fields of 20-Tesla/second or less, and a whole body averaged specific absorption rate (SAR) of 2.0 W/kg or less for 15-minutes of imaging.

Warning: The effects on the RF BION Microstimulator of performing MRI procedures using other MR systems and other conditions have not been determined.

The following information describes testing that was performed on the effect of magnetic resonance imaging (MRI) procedures on an implanted RF BION Microstimulator.

MR procedures MUST ONLY be performed according to the following information:

Magnetic Field Interactions. Magnetic field interactions (translational attraction and torque) were assessed for the RF BION Microstimulator in association with exposure to a 1.5-Tesla MR system. The RF BION Microstimulator displays relatively moderate magnetic field interactions. [The deflection angle measured for the RF BION Microstimulator was 58 degrees. Thus, the magnetic force is 1.6 times the gravitational force (0.42 g). The maximal magnetic torque was calculated to be equal to 3.9 times the "gravity torque", the product of the implant's length and weight. Therefore, torque can be viewed as a force equivalent to 0.98 g acting on one end of the RF BION Microstimulator with the other end fixed.] Because of the presence of the ferrite material (mass of 32 mg), the intended *in vivo* use of this implant must be considered.

Notably, tissue encapsulation around the RF BION Microstimulator is a major factor that will retain this implant *in situ*. *In vivo* research demonstrated that counter-forces provided by encapsulation (i.e., fibrous tissue) that occurs 2 to 3 weeks after implantation will prevent the RF BION Microstimulator from being moved or dislodged in association with the exposure to a 1.5-Tesla MR system. Therefore, considering that the mass of the RF BION Microstimulator is relatively small (0.25 g), and this implant does not contain any sharp ends, magnetic field interactions associated with exposure to a 1.5-Tesla MR system will not move or dislodge this implant after a conservative post-op waiting period of 6 to 8 weeks.

Interactions with Time-Varying Magnetic Fields. The potential interactions of the RF BION Microstimulator with magnetic resonance imaging (MRI)-related time-varying magnetic fields (gradient and RF) were theoretically and experimentally investigated with respect to a 1.5-Tesla/64-MHz MR system.

Effects of Radiofrequency Fields. Based on theoretical analysis and *in vitro* experiments, the presence of the RF BION Microstimulator in a patient undergoing an MRI procedure at a whole-body-averaged specific absorption rate (SAR) of 2-W/kg for 15-min. will not result in a substantial increase in temperature. Therefore, a patient with the RF BION Microstimulator is not at increased risk with respect to MRI-related heating of this implant under the conditions used for this assessment.

Effects of Gradient Fields. The electric field in the body induced by the MRI pulsed gradient magnetic fields may exceed 5 V/m. Given the size and shape of the RF BION Microstimulator, this field intensity induces minimal voltage (95 mV) along the length of the implant. Importantly, concentration of the gradient currents will be no greater than that resulting from the concentration rising from bones surrounded by tissue. Therefore, no physiological impact is expected by the interaction between the RF BION Microstimulator with the gradient currents in the tissue of a patient with this implant undergoing an MR procedure at 1.5-Tesla/64 MHz. Accordingly, a patient with the RF BION Microstimulator may safely be exposed to the gradient magnetic fields (dB/dt) at levels that are currently allowed for 1.5-Tesla MR systems operating with conventional pulse sequences and standard accessories (e.g., surface RF coils).

Warning: Unconventional or non-standard MR techniques have not been assessed for the RF BION Microstimulator and, therefore, must be avoided.

MRI Procedures and Function of the RF BION Microstimulator. The effects of MRI procedures on the functional aspects of the RF BION System were assessed. *In vitro* testing was performed on a phantom with nine RF BION devices placed in various orientations relative to the MR system.

MR imaging was conducted using 1.5-Tesla/64-MHz MR system (transmit/receive RF body coil) to perform 15 different MR imaging pulse sequences, as follows: (1) T1-weighted, spin echo pulse sequence, (2) T1-weighted, fast spin echo pulse sequence, (3) T2-weighted, spin echo pulse sequence, (4) T2-weighted, fast spin echo pulse sequence, (5) Gradient echo, two dimensional pulse sequence, (6) Gradient echo, three dimensional pulse sequence, (7) Fast gradient echo, two dimensional pulse sequence, (8) Fast gradient echo, three dimensional pulse sequence, (9) Fast spoiled gradient echo, two dimensional pulse, sequence, (10) Fast spoiled gradient echo, three dimensional pulse sequence, (11) T1-weighted, spin echo pulse sequence with high whole-body averaged specific absorption rate (1.1 W/kg), (12) T1-weighted, fast spin echo pulse sequence with high whole-body averaged specific absorption rate (1.1 W/kg), (13) T2-weighted, spin echo pulse sequence with high whole body averaged specific absorption rate (1.1 W/kg), (14) T2-weighted, fast spin echo pulse sequence with high whole-body averaged specific absorption rate (1.1 W/kg), and (15) Gradient echo, three dimensional pulse sequence with magnetization transfer contrast with high whole-body averaged specific absorption rate (1.1 W/kg)

The findings indicated that there was no apparent damage or alteration in the functional aspects of the RF BION Microstimulators. Thus, the RF BION Microstimulator was demonstrated to maintain full functionality after exposure to the MR imaging conditions indicated above.

Warning: The effect of using any other MR imaging pulse sequence or procedure on the RF BION Microstimulator is unknown.

Additional MRI Safety Guidelines for the RF BION Microstimulator

- DO NOT use MR systems other than 1.5 Tesla MR systems.
- Continuously monitor the patient using visual and audio means (i.e., intercom system) throughout the MR procedure.
- Instruct the patient to alert the MR system operator of any unusual sensations or problems so the MR system operator can terminate the MRI procedure, if needed.
- Provide the patient with a means to alert the MR system operator of any unusual sensations or problems that may be experienced during the MR procedure.

Post-MRI Procedure Recommendations for the RF BION Microstimulator. After undergoing an MRI procedure, the RF BION Microstimulator should be checked to ensure that it is working properly. To do so, stimulation threshold measurements should be obtained and compared to pre-MRI procedure threshold levels.

[For additional information about this product, including safety guidelines, contact the Alfred E. Mann Foundation, Valencia, CA; http://www.aemf.org and Advanced Bionics Corporation, Sylmar, CA; http://www.advancedbionics.com/]

[MR healthcare professionals are advised to contact the respective manufacturer in order to obtain the latest safety information to ensure patient safety relative to the use of an MR procedure.]

REFERENCES

Arcos, I, Davis R, Fey K, Mishler D, Sanderson D, Tanacs C, Vogel MJ, Wolf R, Zilberman Y, Schulman J. Second-generation microstimulator. Artificial Organs 2002;26:228-231.

Cameron T, Loeb GE, Peck RA, Schulman JH, Strojnik P, Troyk PR. Micromodular implants to provide electrical stimulation of paralyzed muscles and limbs. IEEE Trans Biomed Eng 1997; 44:781-90.

Heetderks, WJ. RF powering of millimeter- and submillimeter-sized neural prosthetic implants. IEEE Trans Biomed Eng 1988;35:323-327.

Loeb GE, Peck RA, Moore WH, Hood K. BION system for distributed neural prosthetic interfaces. Med Eng Phys. 2001;23:9-18.

Shellock FG, Cosendai G, Park S-M, Nyenhuis JA. Implantable microstimulator: magnetic resonancesafety at 1.5-Tesla. Investigative Radiology 2004;39:591-594.

Walter JS, Riedy L, King W, Wheeler JS, Najafi K, Anderson CL, Gudausky TM, Dokmeci M. Short-term bladder-wall response to implantation of microstimulators. J Spinal Cord Med. 1997;20:319-23.

Zealear DL, Garren KC, Rodriguez RJ, Reyes JH, Huang S, Dokmeci MR, Najafi K. The biocompatibility, integrity, and positional stability of an injectable microstimulator for reanimation of the paralyzed larynx. IEEE Trans Biomed Eng. 2001;48:890-7.

Reveal Plus Insertable Loop Recorder

The 9526 Reveal Plus Insertable Loop Recorder (ILR, Medtronic, Inc., Minneapolis, MN) is an implantable, single-use, programmable device containing two surface electrodes for continuous recording of the patient's subcutaneous electrocardiogram. This device is used to record the electrocardiogram subcutaneously and is indicated for patients who experience transient symptoms that may suggest a cardiac arrhythmia and patients with clinical syndromes or situations at increased risk of cardiac arrhythmias.

MRI S and the Reveal Plus Insertable Loop Recorder

The Reveal Plus Insertable Loop Recorder contains no lead wires or large loops of electrically conductive material. The electromagnetic fields produced during magnetic resonance imaging may adversely affect the data stored by the Reveal Plus Insertable Loop Recorder. Therefore, consideration must be given to interrogating the Reveal Plus Insertable Loop Recorder in order to save the data that could become corrupted or erased. Accordingly, careful planning in conjunction with the physician responsible for the patient's Reveal Plus Insertable Loop Recorder is necessary.

Also, since this device contains ferromagnetic components, strong magnetic fields associated with the MR system may apply a mechanical force on the Reveal Plus Insertable Loop Recorder. Accordingly, the patient may feel slight movement of this device. While this does not represent a safety hazard, the patient must be informed of this possibility to avoid undue concern.

Additional information may be found in the Reveal Plus 9526 Insertable Loop Recorder System Product Information Manual, as follows:

- For information on how to interrogate and save data, refer to "How to Interrogate the ILR" and " How to Save To Disk," both in Chapter 3.
- For information on resetting collection data/parameters, refer to "Clearing Memory Without Changing Gain and Sensitivity Settings" in Chapter 2.

- For testing patient triggered storage integrity, refer to "Storing an Event in a Clinical Setting" in Chapter 2.

[Information provided with permission, Medtronic, Inc., Minneapolis, MN]

[MR healthcare professionals are advised to contact the respective manufacturer in order to obtain the latest safety information to ensure patient safety relative to the use of an MR procedure.]

REFERENCES

Gimbel JR, Wilkoff BL. Artefact mimicking tachycardia during magnetic resonance imaging in a patient with an implantable loop recorder. Heart. 2003;89:e10

Gimbel JR. Magnetic resonance imaging of implantable cardiac rhythm devices at 3.0 Tesla. Pacing Clin Electrophysiol. 2008;31:795-801.

http://www.medtronic.com/physician/reveal/mri.html

Krahn A., Klein G, Yee R., Norris C. Final results from a pilot study with an implantable loop recorder to determine the etiology of syncope in patients with negative non-invasive and invasive testing. American Journal of Cardiology 82:117-119, 1998.

Reveal Syncope Validation Project (RSVP) Clinical Summary. Medtronic data on file.

Shellock FG, et al. Cardiac pacemakers, ICDs, and loop recorder: Evaluation of translational attraction using conventional ("long-bore") and "short-bore" MR systems at 1.5- and 3-Tesla. Journal of Cardiovascular Magnetic Resonance 2003;5:387-397.

Shellock FG. MR Safety and the Reveal Insertable Loop Recorder. Signals, No. 49, Issue 3, pp. 8, 2004.

Wong JA, Yee R, Gula LJ, et al. Feasibility of magnetic resonance imaging in patients with an implantable loop recorder. Pacing Clin Electrophysiol. 2008;31:333-7.

Reveal DX 9528 and Reveal XT 9529, Insertable Cardiac Monitors

Reveal DX Model 9528 Insertable Cardiac Monitor (Medtronic, Inc., Minneapolis, MN)

The Reveal DX Model 9528 Insertable Cardiac Monitor is a small, leadless device that is typically implanted under the skin, in the chest. Two electrodes on the body of the device continuously monitor the patient's subcutaneous ECG. The device memory can store up to 22.5 min. of ECG recordings from patient-activated episodes and up to 27 min. of ECG recordings from automatically detected arrhythmias.

MRI Conditions For Use

MR Conditional – The Reveal XT has been demonstrated to pose no known hazards in a specified MR environment with the conditions of use specified in this section. Non-clinical testing has demonstrated that the Reveal XT is safe for use in the MRI environment when used according to the instructions provided in this section. The Reveal XT can be safely scanned in patients under the following conditions:

• Closed bore, cylindrical magnet with static magnetic field must be 1.5 T or 3.0 T.

• Whole body gradient systems with gradient slew rate specification must be ≤200 T/m/s.

• Whole body Specific Absorption Rate (SAR) as reported by the MRI equipment must be ≤2.0 W/kg; head SAR as reported by the MRI equipment must be ≤3.2 W/kg.

• The uninterrupted duration of active scanning (when radio frequency (RF) and gradients are on) over the chest during MRI must not exceed 30 min. If additional chest scans beyond 30 min are necessary, a waiting period of at least 10 min is required.

In non-clinical testing, the device produced a temperature rise of less than 4 °C (7.2 °F). A maximum whole body average SAR was used for a 30 min scanning period. In the 1.5 T device (manufacturer Philips, model Intera, software version 2.1.3.2, Field strength B1 of 4.5 µT), the maximum SAR level of 4.0 W/kg was used, which was displayed on the

MRI scanner console. In the 3 T device (manufacturer Philips, model Achieva, software version 2.1.3.2, Field strength B1 of 1.6 µT) a maximum SAR level of 0.9 W/kg was used, which was displayed on the MRI scanner console.

Reveal DX Model 9528 Insertable Cardiac Monitor (Medtronic, Inc., Minneapolis, MN)

The Reveal DX Model 9528 Insertable Cardiac Monitor is a small, leadless device that is typically implanted under the skin, in the chest. Two electrodes on the body of the device continuously monitor the patient's subcutaneous ECG. The device memory can store up to 22.5 min. of ECG recordings from patient-activated episodes and up to 27 min. of ECG recordings from automatically detected arrhythmias.

MRI Conditions For Use

MR Conditional – The Reveal DX has been demonstrated to pose no known hazards in a specified MR environment with the conditions of use specified in this section. Non-clinical testing has demonstrated that the Reveal DX is safe for use in the MRI environment when used according to the instructions provided in this section. The Reveal DX can be safely scanned in patients under the following conditions:

• Closed bore, cylindrical magnet with static magnetic field must be 1.5 T or 3.0 T.

• Whole body gradient systems with gradient slew rate specification must be $\leq$200 T/m/s.

• Whole body Specific Absorption Rate (SAR) as reported by the MRI equipment must be $\leq$2.0 W/kg; head SAR as reported by the MRI equipment must be $\leq$3.2 W/kg.

• The uninterrupted duration of active scanning (when radio frequency (RF) and gradients are on) over the chest during MRI must not exceed 30 min. If additional chest scans beyond 30 min are necessary, a waiting period of at least 10 min is required.

In non-clinical testing, the device produced a temperature rise of less than 4 °C (7.2 °F). A maximum whole body average SAR was used for a 30 min scanning period. In the 1.5 T device (manufacturer Philips, model Intera, software version 2.1.3.2, Field strength B1 of 4.5 µT), the maximum SAR level of 4.0 W/kg was used, which was displayed on the MRI scanner console. In the 3 T device (manufacturer Philips, model Achieva, software version 2.1.3.2, Field strength B1 of 1.6 µT) a maximum SAR level of 0.9 W/kg was used, which was displayed on the

MRI scanner console.

[Information provided with permission, Medtronic, Inc., Minneapolis, MN]

[MR healthcare professionals are advised to contact the respective manufacturer in order to obtain the latest safety information to ensure patient safety relative to the use of an MR procedure.]

REFERENCE

http://www.medtronic.com

St. Jude Medical (SJM) Confirm, Implantable Cardiac Monitor

St. Jude Medical (SJM) Confirm, Model DM2100

Implantable Cardiac Monitor, St. Jude Medical, Sylmar, CA

The St. Jude Medical (SJM) Confirm Implantable Cardiac Monitor (ICM) (St. Jude Medical, Sylmar, CA) is designed to monitor and store ECG data and to communicate with the St. Jude Medical, Merlin Patient Care System and the SJM Confirm external patient activator. The SJM Confirm ICM is an implantable patient-activated and automatically-activated monitoring system that records subcutaneous ECG and is indicated in the following cases:

- Patients with clinical syndromes or situations at increased risk of cardiac arrhythmias
- Patients who experience transient symptoms that may suggest a cardiac arrhythmia

MRI Information

MRI for patients with implanted devices has been contraindicated by MRI manufacturers. Clinicians should carefully weigh the decision to use MRI in patients with implanted devices. MRI may cause device malfunction or injury to the patient.

[MR healthcare professionals are advised to contact the respective manufacturer in order to obtain the latest safety information to ensure patient safety relative to the use of an MR procedure.]

REFERENCE

User's Manual, SJM Confirm, Model DM2100, Implantable Cardiac Monitor, St. Jude Medical, Sylmar, CA

SAM Sling

The SAM Sling (SAM Medical Products, Newport, OR) is a force-controlled circumferential pelvic belt designed to provide safe and effective reduction and stabilization of open-book pelvic fractures. Pelvic ring fractures are devastating injuries, accompanied by extensive internal bleeding that can often be fatal. Since the mid-nineteenth century, the standard first-aid protocol has been to wrap a bedsheet or belt around the victim's hips, cinch it tight, and hope for the best. It's a technique that works, even for the worst type of pelvic fractures, known as open-book fractures because the pelvic ring has sprung open, like the pages of a book. Compression "closes the book," reduces pain, slows bleeding, and promotes clot formation as the patient is transported to an emergency department.

The problem with bed sheets and belts is that they're an extremely inexact methodology. Not only is there no control over how tightly the sheet is cinched, but until development began on the SAM Sling, nobody knew how tightly it should be cinched or exactly where on the body it should be placed. Imagine how it would be if the only way to measure blood pressure was with un-calibrated instruments, each of which was different. With pelvic ring fractures, too much compression force shifts the broken ends of bones and causes additional damage—too little allows bleeding to continue.

In 2002, researchers at a leading hospital determined that the optimum safe pressure for closing unstable open-book fractures falls in a range centered on approximately 150 Newtons, or 33 pounds. That allowed the creation of the SAM Sling's patented "autostop" buckle, which has spring-loaded prongs that lock the buckle in place when the right amount of force is applied. Not only is there no guesswork needed, the autostop buckle simply won't allow the belt to be over-tightened.

Important Warnings

MRI Information

Based on in vitro testing, the SAM Sling will not present a hazard or risk to a patient undergoing an MRI procedure using an MR system operating at 3-Tesla or less. The SAM Sling contains ferromagnetic springs in the buckle. Therefore, it is important to ensure that the SAM Sling is firmly applied to the patient prior to entry into the MRI environment (as stated in the labeling for this device). Accordingly, there will be no hazard or risk to a patient undergoing an MRI procedure. The SAM Sling should not be removed from the patient while in the MR system room.

- This product is not recommended for use on children.

REFERENCE

SAM Medical Products, http://www.sammedical.com

Scleral Buckle
(Scleral Buckling Procedure)

The application of a scleral buckle (note, this is a procedure not an implant) or "scleral buckling" is a surgical technique used to repair retinal detachments and was first used experimentally by ophthalmic surgeons in 1937. By the early 1960's, scleral buckling became the method of choice when the development of new materials, particularly silicone, offered surgeons better opportunities to improve patient care.

The buckling element is usually left in place permanently. The element pushes in, or "buckles," the sclera toward the middle of the eye. This buckling effect on the sclera relieves the traction on the retina, allowing the retinal tear to settle against the wall of the eye. The buckle effect may cover only the area behind the detachment, or it may encircle the eyeball like a ring. The buckle holds the retina against the sclera until scarring seals the tear and prevents fluid leakage, which could cause further retinal detachment. Scleral buckles come in many shapes and sizes. The encircling band is usually a thin silicone band sewn around the circumference of the sclera of the eye. In rare instances, a metallic clip may be used. Some clips may pose a risk to patients undergoing MRI procedures.

Tantalum Clips
Tantalum clips were found to be less bulky than sutures, allowing the surgeon to adjust the tension of the circling band for the scleral buckle. These clips did not cause tissue reaction and did not harbor infection. Because tantalum is a nonmagnetic metal, Tantalum clips are considered to be acceptable for patients undergoing MRI procedures.

REFERENCES

Bakshandeh H, Shellock FG, Schatz CJ, Morisoli SM. Metallic clips used for scleral buckling: ex vivo evaluation of ferromagnetism at 1.5 T. J Magn Reson Imaging. 1993;3:559.

Lincoff H. Radial buckling in the repair of retinal detachment. Int Ophthalmol Clin. 1976;16:127-34.

Michels RG. Scleral buckling methods for rhegmatogenous retinal detachment. Retina. 1986;6:1-49.

Sleuth Implantable ECG Monitoring System

The Sleuth Implantable ECG Monitoring System (Sleuth and Sleuth AT, Models 2010 and 2020, Transoma Medical, St. Paul, MN) is an implantable, patient- and automatically-activated cardiac monitoring system that records subcutaneous electrocardiogram (ECG) and is indicated for patients with clinical syndromes or situations at increased risk of cardiac arrhythmias and patients who experience transient symptoms that may suggest a cardiac arrhythmia.

MRI INFORMATION

MR Conditional: 1.5-T MRI

NOTE: The monitoring system does not need to be adjusted during MR scanning. However, MR scanning may cause electromagnetic interference that may cause the system to record ECG events. MR scanning may also interfere with the quality of the ECG signal. Therefore, ECG data acquired during an MR scan may be inaccurate or unusable.

The Sleuth IMD (Models 2010 and 2020) was determined to be MR conditional based on information provided in the following document: American Society for Testing and Materials (ASTM) International, Designation: F2503-05. Standard Practice for Marking Medical Devices and Other Items for Safety in the Magnetic Resonance Environment. ASTM International, 100 Barr Harbor Drive, PO Box C700, West Conshohocken, Pennsylvania, 2005.

Non-clinical testing has demonstrated the Sleuth IMD is MR conditional. It can be scanned safely under:

- static magnetic field of 1.5-Tesla
- spatial gradient magnetic field of 250 Gauss/cm
- maximum MR system reported whole-body-averaged specific absorption rate (SAR) of 3.5 W/kg for 15 minutes of scanning

In non-clinical testing in a phantom, the device produced a temperature rise of less than or equal to 1.3 degrees C at a maximum whole-body-averaged specific absorption rate (SAR) of 3.5 W/kg for 15 minutes of

MR scanning in a 1.5-Tesla MR system (Magnetom, Siemens Medical Solutions, Malvern, PA, Software Numaris/4, Version Syngo MR 2002B DHHS Active-shielded, horizontal field scanner).

The maximum whole body averaged specific absorption rate (SAR) reported was measured by the MR system. MR image quality may be compromised if the area of interest is in the same area or relatively close to the position of the Sleuth IMD. The table below provides maximum signal voids (artifact size) for the standard imaging pulse sequences at 1.5 Tesla per ASTM F2119:

Signal Void	Pulse Sequence	Imaging Plane
115 cm^2	T1-weighted spin echo	Parallel
68 cm^2	T1-weighted spin echo	Perpendicular
162 cm^2	Gradient echo	Parallel
280 cm^2	Gradient echo	Perpendicular

The effect of performing MRI procedures using higher static magnetic field or higher levels of RF energy on a patient with the IMD has not been determined. MRI healthcare professionals are advised to contact Transoma Medical to ensure that the latest safety information is obtained and carefully followed to ensure patient safety relative to the use of an MR procedure.

Note: Magnetic forces may act on the housing of the implanted IMD and result in a tugging sensation that patients may feel. This force does not pose a safety hazard, but to mitigate patient alarm, patients should be made aware of the possibility of such a sensation.

[*The information for the Sleuth was reprinted with permission by Transoma Medical, St. Paul, MN, http://transomamedical.com]

[MR healthcare professionals are advised to contact the manufacturer to ensure that the latest safety information is obtained and carefully followed in order to ensure patient safety relative to the use of an MR procedure.]

REFERENCE

http://transoma.com/

Surgical Instruments and Devices

Interventional magnetic resonance (MR) techniques have evolved into clinically viable surgical and therapeutic applications. This has resulted in the development and performance of innovative procedures that include percutaneous biopsy (e.g., breast, bone, brain, abdominal, etc.), endoscopic surgery of the abdomen, spine, and sinuses, open brain surgery, and MR-guided monitoring of thermal therapies (i.e., laser-induced, RF-induced, and cryomediated procedures).

Surgical instruments and devices are an important necessity for interventional MR. Besides the typical MR safety concerns, there are possible hazards in the interventional MR environment related to the surgical instruments and devices that must be addressed to ensure the safety of healthcare practitioners and patients. Many of the conventional instruments and devices are made from metallic materials that can create substantial problems in association with interventional MR.

The interventional MR safety issues that exist for surgical instruments and devices include unwanted movement caused by magnetic field interactions (e.g., the "missile effect", translational attraction, torque), issues related to eddy currents, and heat generated by RF power deposition. Furthermore, the operational aspects of various instruments may be adversely impacted by the electromagnetic fields used for MR imaging. Artifacts associated with the use of a surgical instrument or device can be particularly problematic if in the imaging area of interest during its intended use. To address these problems, various surgical instruments and devices have been developed that do not present an additional risk or problem to the patient or MR healthcare practitioner in the interventional MR environment.

REFERENCES

Hinks RS, Bronskill MJ, Kucharczyk W, Bernstein M, Collick BD, Henkelman RM. MR systems for image-guided therapy. J Magn Reson Imaging 1998;8:19-25.

Jolesz FA. Interventional and intraoperative MRI: a general overview of the field. J Magn Reson Imaging 1998;3-7.

Jolesz FA. Image-guided procedures and the operating room of the future. Radiology 1997; 204:601-612.

Jolesz FA, et al. Compatible instrumentation for intraoperative MRI: expanding resources. J Magn Reson Imaging 1998;8:8-11.

Shellock FG. Compatibility of an endoscope designed for use in interventional MR imaging procedures. AJR Amer J Roentgenol 1998;171:1297-1300.

Shellock FG. Metallic surgical instruments for interventional MRI procedures: evaluation of MR safety. J Magn Reson Imaging 2001;13:152-157.

Shellock FG. MRI safety of instruments designed for interventional MRI: assessment of ferromagnetism, heating, and artifacts. Workshop on New Insights into Safety and Compatibility Issues Affecting In Vivo MR, Syllabus, International Society of Magnetic Resonance in Medicine, Berkeley, 1998; pp. 39.

Shellock FG, Shellock VJ. Ceramic surgical instruments: Evaluation of MR-compatibility at 1.5 Tesla. J Magn Reson Imaging 1996;6:954-956.

Sutures

Sutures are made from a variety of materials, including those that are nonmetallic and metallic. Various sutures with the needles removed have been testing at 1.5- and 3-Tesla. For the thirteen different sutures evaluated at 1.5-Tesla, all were shown to be acceptable for patients.

MRI at 3-Tesla and Sutures. At 3-Tesla, most of the sutures evaluated displayed no magnetic field interactions, while two (Flexon suture and Steel suture, United States Surgical, North Haven, CT) showed minor deflection angles and torque. For these two sutures, the *in situ* application of these materials provides sufficient counter-forces to prevent movement or dislodgment. Therefore, in consideration of the intended *in vivo* use of these materials, all of the sutures with the needles removed tested to date are regarded to be acceptable at 3-Tesla.

REFERENCES

American Society for Testing and Materials (ASTM) Designation: F 2052. Standard test method for measurement of magnetically induced displacement force on passive implants in the magnetic resonance environment. In: Annual Book of ASTM Standards, Section 13, Medical Devices and Services, Volume 13.01 Medical Devices; Emergency Medical Services. West Conshohocken, PA, 2002, pp. 1576-1580.

Shellock FG. Biomedical implants and devices: assessment of magnetic field interactions with a 3.0-Tesla MR system. J Magn Reson Imaging J Magn Reson Imaging 2002;16:721-732.

SynchroMed, SynchroMed EL, and SynchroMed II Drug Infusion Systems

The Effects of Magnetic Resonance Imaging (MRI) on Medtronic Drug Infusion Systems

For SynchroMed pump models 8615, 8616, 8617 and 8618 please refer to the MRI Information for the SynchroMed EL Pump.

Before any medical procedure is begun, patients must always inform any health care personnel that they have an implanted drug infusion system and share this information about MRI with them.

MRI Information for the SynchroMed EL Pump

Models: **SynchroMed EL**: All models beginning with 8626, 8627
Reference: SynchroMed IsoMed Information for Prescribers Manual

Introduction

SynchroMed EL pump performance has not been established for greater than 3.0 Tesla (T) horizontal, closed-bore MRI scanners. SynchroMed EL pump performance has not been established using other types of MRI scanners such as open-sided or standing MRI.

Temporary motor stall and stall recover

The magnetic field of the MRI scanner will temporarily stop the rotor of the SynchroMed EL pump motor and suspend drug infusion for the duration of the MRI exposure. The pump should resume normal operation upon termination of MRI exposure; however, there is the potential for an extended delay in pump recovery after exiting the MRI magnetic field because exposure to the MRI magnetic field may cause the motor gears within the pump to bind temporarily without permanent damage. This is caused by the potential for backward rotation of the pump rotor magnet when it aligns with the MRI magnetic field. This temporary binding may delay the return of proper infusion after the pump is removed from the MRI magnetic field. While extended delays in pump recovery are unlikely, reports have indicated that there is the potential for a two to twenty-four hour delay in return to proper drug infusion after completion of an MRI scan.

Warning: Patients receiving intrathecal baclofen therapy (e.g. Lioresal Intrathecal) are at higher risk for adverse events, as baclofen withdrawal can lead to a life threatening condition if not treated promptly and effectively. For complete product information, refer to the Lioresal Intrathecal (baclofen injection) Package Insert. For information on other drugs, please refer to the product labeling for the drug being administered.

Potential for permanent motor stall

90 degrees alignment of an implanted pump with the z axis of 1.5 T and 3.0 T horizontal, closed-bore magnetic resonance imaging (MRI) scanners can cause MRI-induced demagnetization of the internal pump motor magnets, which can result in permanent, nonrecoverable stoppage of the pump. This is due to the orientation of the pump with respect to the magnetic field of a horizontal, closed-bore MRI system. SynchroMed EL pump performance has not been established using other types of MRI scanners such as open-sided or standing MRI.

Note: If the pump face is oriented at 90 degrees to the z-axis, the refill port would be facing towards the patient's feet or head.

Preparation for the MRI examination

Prior to MRI, the physician should ensure the pump is not oriented 90 degrees with respect to the z-axis of the MRI scanner. The physician should also determine if the patient implanted with a SynchroMed EL pump can safely be deprived of drug delivery. If the patient cannot be safely deprived of drug delivery, alternative delivery methods for the drug can be used during the time required for the MRI scan. If there is concern that depriving the patient of drug delivery may be unsafe for the patient during the MRI procedure, medical supervision should be provided while the MRI is conducted.

Note: Prior to the MRI scan, confirm that the pump program settings are documented in case reprogramming is required after the scan.

Post-MRI examination review

Upon completion of the MRI scan, or shortly thereafter, the SynchroMed EL pump must be interrogated using the clinician programmer in order to confirm that electromagnetic interference from the MRI has not affected the pump status. If interrogation using the clinician programmer shows that a "Pump Memory Error" occurred, the physician must reprogram the pump in order for proper drug infusion to resume. A Pump Memory Error Alarm (double tone) will accompany a Pump Memory Error. If this occurs, notify:

- -US only: Medtronic Technical Services at 1-800-707-0933.

The SynchroMed EL pump does not detect or alarm for motor stalls. A physician should confirm a SynchroMed EL pump has resumed proper drug infusion after an MRI by performing a pump roller study. If a pump roller study cannot be performed, patients must be closely monitored for return of underlying symptoms to confirm the pump has resumed proper drug infusion after an MRI. The duration of monitoring depends on the drug and the delivery rate. Consult the patient's providing physician for likely time period for return of symptoms in the event of a pump stoppage.

Additional safety and diagnostic issues

Testing on the SynchroMed EL pump has established the following with regard to other MRI safety and diagnostic issues:

Tissue heating adjacent to implant during MRI scans

Specific absorption rate (SAR) — Presence of the pump can potentially cause an increase of the local temperature in tissues near the pump. During a 20-minute pulse sequence in a 1.5 T GE Signa scanner with a whole-body average SAR of 1 W/kg, a temperature increase of 1 degrees C in a static phantom was observed near the pump implanted in the "abdomen" of the phantom. The 20-minute scan time is representative of a typical imaging session. Implanting the pump more lateral to the midline of the abdomen may result in greater temperature increases in tissues near the pump.

Testing in a 3.0 T GE Signa scanner using transmit-receive RF body coil (at an MR system reported whole body averaged SAR of 3.0 W/kg and a spatial peak SAR of 5.9 W/kg) resulted in maximum heating of 1.7 degrees C for the SynchroMed EL pump.

In the unlikely event that the patient experiences uncomfortable warmth near the pump, the MRI scan should be stopped and the scan parameters adjusted to reduce the SAR to comfortable levels.

Peripheral nerve stimulation during MRI scans

Time-varying gradient magnetic fields — Presence of the pump may potentially cause a two-fold increase of the induced electric field in tissues near the pump. With the pump implanted in the abdomen, using pulse sequences that have dB/dt up to 20 T/s, the measured induced electric field near the pump is below the threshold necessary to cause stimulation.

In the unlikely event that the patient reports stimulation during the scan, the proper procedure is the same as for patients without implants—stop the MRI scan and adjust the scan parameters to reduce the potential for nerve stimulation.

Static magnetic field

For magnetic fields up to 3.0 T, the magnetic force and torque on the pump will be less than the force and torque due to gravity. The patient may experience a slight tugging sensation at the pump implant site. An elastic garment or wrap will prevent the pump from moving and reduce the sensation the patient may experience.

Image distortion

The pump contains ferromagnetic components that will cause image distortion and image dropout in areas around the pump. The severity of image artifact is dependent on the MR pulse sequence used. For spin echo pulse sequences, the area of significant image artifact may be 20-25 cm across. Images of the head or lower extremities should be largely unaffected.

Minimizing image distortion — Careful choice of pulse sequence parameters and location of the angle and location of the imaging plane may minimize MR image artifact; however, the reduction in image distortion obtained by adjustment of pulse sequence parameters will usually be at a cost in signal-to-noise ratio. The following general principles should be followed:

- Use imaging sequences with stronger gradients for both slice and read encoding directions. Employ higher bandwidth for both radio-frequency pulse and data sampling.
- Choose an orientation for read-out axis that minimizes the appearance of in-plane distortion.
- Use spin echo or gradient echo MR imaging sequences with a relatively high data sampling bandwidth.

- Use shorter echo time for gradient echo technique, whenever possible.

- Be aware that the actual imaging slice shape can be curved in space due to the presence of the field disturbance of the pump (as stated above).

- Identify the location of the implant in the patient, and when possible, orient all imaging slices away from the implanted pump.

MRI Information for SynchroMed II Pump

Models: **SynchroMed II**: All models beginning with 8637
Reference: SynchroMed IsoMed Information for Prescribers Manual

Introduction

SynchroMed II pump performance has not been established for greater than 3.0 Tesla (T) horizontal, closed-bore MRI scanners. SynchroMed II pump performance has not been established using other types of MRI scanners such as open-sided or standing MRI.

Temporary motor stall and stall recovery

The magnetic field of the MRI scanner will temporarily stop the rotor of the SynchroMed II pump motor and suspend drug infusion for the duration of the MRI exposure. The pump should resume normal operation upon termination of MRI exposure; however, there is the potential for an extended delay in pump recovery after exiting the MRI magnetic field because exposure to the MRI magnetic field may cause the motor gears within the pump to bind temporarily without permanent damage. This is caused by the potential for backward rotation of the pump rotor magnet when it aligns with the MRI magnetic field. This temporary binding may delay the return of proper infusion after the pump is removed from the MRI magnetic field. While extended delays in pump recovery are unlikely, reports have indicated that there is the potential for a two to twenty-four hour delay in return to proper drug infusion after completion of an MRI scan.

Warning: Patients receiving intrathecal baclofen therapy (e.g. Lioresal Intrathecal) are at higher risk for adverse events, as baclofen withdrawal can lead to a life threatening condition if not treated promptly and effectively. For complete product information, refer to the Lioresal Intrathecal (baclofen injection) Package Insert.

For information on other drugs, please refer to the product labeling for the drug being administered.

Time required for stall and recovery detection

The SynchroMed II pump detects motor stall and motor stall recovery. Medtronic does not recommend programming the SynchroMed II pump to "stopped pump mode" prior to an MRI because of the possibility of an increased delay in the detection of an extended motor stall. Motor stall events are recorded in the pump event log and can be reviewed using the clinician programmer. A motor stall will also cause the pump alarm to sound (two tone alarm). The slower the programmed delivery rate, the longer it may take for the stall detection algorithm to log motor stall and motor stall recovery. For pumps programmed to deliver at least 0.048 ml/day, the motor stall detection (with audible alarm) should occur within 20 minutes of exposure to the MRI magnetic field. Stall recovery detection should occur within 20 minutes of exiting the MRI magnetic field. The detection of a motor stall and detection of motor stall recovery may each take up to 90 minutes if the pump is programmed to minimum rate mode (0.006 ml/day).

Potential for delay in logging motor stall events

In some cases, electromagnetic interference (EMI) from an MRI scan can interfere with normal event logging. If this occurs, it may cause the pump to switch into the telemetry mode. 'Telemetry mode' is a special state in which the pump is able to communicate with the clinician programmer. While in this state, the pump infuses normally; however, some error logging and the audible alarm for motor stall are suspended. If the pump switches into telemetry mode due to EMI, the pump resumes drug delivery after leaving the MRI magnetic field; however, pump motor stall and motor stall recovery detection function is not active until the post-MRI pump interrogation ends telemetry mode (refer to "Post-MRI examination review"). Due to this issue, if the interrogation is not performed upon completion of the MRI scan or shortly thereafter, review of the pump logs may indicate that the pump ceased drug delivery for an extended period of time, when in fact it had recovered normally. In this scenario, you may receive an erroneous "stopped pump period may exceed tube set" error message.

Note: In some cases, the SynchroMed II pump event log may not register motor stall recovery until after the pump has been interrogated a second time due to the effect of electromagnetic interference on the pump.

Potential for permanent motor stall

90 degrees alignment of an implanted pump with the z axis of 1.5 T and 3.0 T horizontal, closed-bore magnetic resonance imaging (MRI) scanners can cause MRI-induced demagnetization of the internal pump motor magnets, which can result in permanent, nonrecoverable stoppage of the pump. This is due to the orientation of the pump with respect to the magnetic field of a horizontal, closed-bore MRI system. SynchroMed II pump performance has not been established using other types of MRI scanners such as open-sided or standing MRI.

Note: If the pump face is oriented at 90 degrees to the z-axis, the refill port would be facing towards the patient's feet or head.

Preparation for the MRI examination

Prior to MRI, the physician should ensure the pump is not oriented 90 degrees with respect to the z axis of the MRI scanner. The physician should also determine if the patient implanted with a SynchroMed II pump can safely be deprived of drug delivery. If the patient cannot be safely deprived of drug delivery, alternative delivery methods for the drug can be used during the time required for the MRI scan. If there is concern that depriving the patient of drug delivery may be unsafe for the patient during the MRI procedure, medical supervision should be provided while the MRI is conducted.

Post-MRI examination review

Upon completion of the MRI scan, or shortly thereafter, the physician must confirm that therapy has properly resumed by interrogating the SynchroMed II pump with the clinician programmer. For pumps programmed to deliver at least 0.048 ml/day, the detection of the motor stall should occur within 20 minutes of MRI exposure.

Detection of the motor stall: Recovery and recording of the recovery in the pump event log will typically occur within 20 minutes of the removal of the pump from the MRI magnetic field.

Note: Both the detection of the motor stall and detection of the motor stall recovery may each take up to 90 minutes if the pump is programmed to minimum rate mode (0.006 ml/day). In the unlikely event that electromagnetic interference from the MRI scan causes a change to "safe state", the pump will automatically switch to minimum rate mode (infusion at 0.006 ml/day). The pump must be reprogrammed in order for proper infusion to resume.

The following pump interrogation guidelines should be used to determine whether the pump has resumed proper function (refer to the SynchroMed II Programming Guide for information about how to interrogate the pump and view event logs).

1) At least 20 minutes after completing MRI exposure, interrogate the pump using the clinician programmer and select the check box to download event logs. If the event log states "Motor Stall Occurred" and "Motor Stall Recovery Occurred", normal function of the pump has returned.

2) If event log **does not** show stall and recovery, wait 20 minutes after the initial interrogation, re-interrogate the pump using the clinician programmer, and review the event logs again. (This will address the potential for event logging delays due to electromagnetic interference from the MRI magnetic field.)

If the event log states "Motor Stall Occurred" and **does not** state "Motor Stall Recovery Occurred", there is a potential for an extended motor stall due to temporary gear binding. Contact:

- US only: Medtronic Technical Services at 1-800-707-0933.
- In all other cases, the pump has resumed its normal operation.

Additional safety and diagnostic issues

Testing on the SynchroMed II pump has established the following with regard to other MRI safety and diagnostic issues:

Tissue heating adjacent to implant during MRI scans

Specific absorption rate (SAR) — Presence of the pump can potentially cause an increase of the local temperature in tissues near the pump. During a 20-minute pulse sequence in a 1.5 T GE Signa scanner with a whole-body average SAR of 1 W/kg, a temperature increase of 1 degrees C in a static phantom was observed near the pump implanted in the "abdomen" of the phantom. The 20-minute scan time is representative of a typical imaging session. Implanting the pump more lateral to the midline of the abdomen may result in greater temperature increases in tissues near the pump. Testing in a 3.0 T GE Signa scanner using transmit-receive RF body coil (at an MR system reported whole body averaged SAR of 3.0 W/kg and a spatial peak SAR of 5.9 W/kg) resulted in maximum heating of 2.7 degrees C for the SynchroMed II pump.

- In the unlikely event that the patient experiences uncomfortable warmth near the pump, the MRI scan should be stopped and the scan parameters adjusted to reduce the SAR to comfortable levels.

Peripheral nerve stimulation during MRI scans

Time-varying gradient magnetic fields — Presence of the pump may potentially cause a two-fold increase of the induced electric field in tissues near the pump. With the pump implanted in the abdomen, using pulse sequences that have dB/dt up to 20 T/s, the measured induced electric field near the pump is below the threshold necessary to cause stimulation. In the unlikely event that the patient reports stimulation during the scan, the proper procedure is the same as for patients without implants—stop the MRI scan and adjust the scan parameters to reduce the potential for nerve stimulation.

Static magnetic field

For magnetic fields up to 3.0 T, the magnetic force and torque on the pump will be less than the force and torque due to gravity. The patient may experience a slight tugging sensation at the pump implant site. An elastic garment or wrap will prevent the pump from moving and reduce the sensation the patient may experience.

Image distortion

The pump contains ferromagnetic components that will cause image distortion and image dropout in areas around the pump. The severity of image artifact is dependent on the MR pulse sequence used. For spin echo pulse sequences, the area of significant image artifact may be 20-25 cm across. Images of the head or lower extremities should be largely unaffected.

Minimizing image distortion — Careful choice of pulse sequence parameters and location of the angle and location of the imaging plane may minimize MR image artifact; however, the reduction in image distortion obtained by adjustment of pulse sequence parameters will usually be at a cost in signal-to-noise ratio. The following general principles should be followed:

- Use imaging sequences with stronger gradients for both slice and read encoding directions. Employ higher bandwidth for both radio-frequency pulse and data sampling.
- Choose an orientation for read-out axis that minimizes the appearance of in-plane distortion.

- Use spin echo or gradient echo MR imaging sequences with a relatively high data sampling bandwidth.
- Use shorter echo time for gradient echo technique, whenever possible.
- Be aware that the actual imaging slice shape can be curved in space due to the presence of the field disturbance of the pump (as stated above).
- Identify the location of the implant in the patient, and when possible, orient all imaging slices away from the implanted pump.

[MR healthcare professionals are advised to contact the respective manufacturer in order to obtain the latest safety information to ensure patient safety relative to the use of an MR procedure.]

REFERENCES

http://www.medtronic.com

http://professional.medtronic.com/landingpage/index.htm

TheraSeed Radioactive Seed Implant

The TheraSeed radioactive seed implant (Theragenics Corporation, Buford, GA) is used to deliver low-level radiation to the prostate to treat cancer. The TheraSeed radioactive seed is a relatively small implant comprised of a titanium tube with two graphite pellets and a lead marker inside. The outside dimensions of tube are approximately length 0.177" in length with a diameter of 0.032".

Palladium-103 is the isotope contained in the TheraSeed implant. Because the radiation is so low and the seeds are placed so precisely, virtually all the radiation is absorbed by the prostate. Treatments with the TheraSeed implant may involve placement in the prostate of from 80 to 120 of these devices. These "seeds" are implanted with "spacers" between them and placed according to treatment plans, so that they do not contact one another during their intended "*in vivo*" use.

Magnetic resonance tests (magnetic field interactions, heating, induced currents, and artifacts) conducted on the TheraSeed revealed that this implant is acceptable for patients undergoing MR procedures at 3-Tesla or less.

REFERENCE

http://www.theraseed.com/

Transdermal Medication Patches and Other Drug Delivery Patches

A transdermal patch allows continuous and prolonged drug delivery that may be more effective and safer than oral medication. In addition, patches offer the potential to deliver medications that would otherwise require injections. Future advances in technology will expand the utilization of drug patches. For example, researchers are currently working on various technologies to force larger molecules through the skin. These so-called "active patches" may permit the delivery of insulin to diabetics, as well as the administration of red-cell stimulating erythropoietin for treatment of anemia patients without injections.

Several anecdotal reports have indicated that transdermal medication patches that contain aluminum foil or other similar metallic component may cause excessive heating or a burn in a patient undergoing an MR procedure. For example, a Deponit (nitroglycerin transdermal delivery system) patch that contains an aluminum foil component, was worn by a patient during MR imaging. This patient received a second-degree burn during the examination that was performed using conventional pulse sequences and standard imaging procedures (Personal communication, Robert E. Mucha, Schwarz Pharma, Milwaukee, WI; 1995). This injury was likely due to MRI-related heating of the metallic foil associated with this transdermal patch.

The U.S. Food and Drug Administration is aware of at least two other adverse events in which patients wearing nicotine transdermal patches during MRI examinations experienced burns. In one case, the patient was wearing a nicotine (Habitrol) transdermal patch. When the patient was removed from the scanner at the completion of the MRI procedure, he stated that his arm was "burning". Upon examination, his upper left arm appeared to be mildly erythematous and there was a small blister where the patch was located. In another case, a patient underwent a short (less than 40 seconds) MRI examination of the lumbar spine while wearing a nicotine transdermal patch. Later, the patient complained of burn lines on his upper arms that were associated with this patch.

In consideration of the above, a patient wearing a transdermal patch that has a metallic component must be identified prior to undergoing an MR procedure. The patient's physician should be contacted to determine if it is possible to temporarily remove the medication patch to prevent excessive heating and burns. After the MR examination, a new patch should be applied following the directions of the prescribing physician (Personal communication, Robert E. Mucha, Schwarz Pharma, Milwaukee, WI; 1995). Importantly, this procedure should be conducted in consultation with the physician responsible for prescribing the transdermal patch or otherwise responsible for the management of the patient.

The Institute for Safe Medical Practices has stated that medication patches such as ANDRODERM, TRANSDERM-NITRO, DEPONIT, NICODERM, NICOTROL, CATAPRES-TTS, and possibly others should be removed prior to an MR examination. In addition, other patches to be aware of include the nicotine patch marketed as Habitrol and its "private label" equivalents and Scopolamine\Hyoscine HydroBromide, marketed as TransDerm Scop (Personal Communication, 05/19/04, Crispin C. Fernandez, M.D. Medical Affairs, Novartis Consumer Health, Inc. Parsippany, NJ).

Notably, not all transdermal medication patches contain a metallic component and, therefore, these patches do not need to be removed from the patient for the MRI examination.

ActiPatch

ActiPatch (BioElectronics, Frederick, MD) is a medical, drug-free device that delivers pulsed electromagnetic frequency therapies to accelerate healing of soft tissue injuries. The ActiPatch has an embedded battery-operated microchip that delivers continuous pulsed therapy to reduce pain and swelling.

MRI and the ActiPatch. The ActiPatch must be removed prior to performing an MRI procedure to prevent possible damage to this device and the potential risk of excessive heating.

REFERENCES

http://www.bioelectronicscorp.com/

Institute for Safe Medical Practices, Medication Safety Alert! Burns in MRI patients wearing transdermal patches. Vol. 9, Issue 7, April 8, 2004. http://www.ismp.org/msaarticles/burnsprint.htm

Kanal E, Barkovich AJ, Bell C, et al. ACR guidance document for safe MR practices: 2007. AJR Am J Roentgenol. 2007;188:1447-1474.

Kuehn BM. FDA warning: remove drug patches before MRI to prevent burns to skin. JAMA. 2009;301:1328.

FDA Public Health Advisory: Risk of Burns during MRI Scans from Transdermal Drug Patches with Metallic Backings
[Reprinted with permission.]

The FDA has been made aware of information about certain transdermal patches (medicated patches applied to the skin) that contain aluminum or other metals in the backing of the patches. Patches that contain metal can overheat during an MRI scan and cause skin burns in the immediate area of the patch.

Transdermal patches slowly deliver medicines through the skin. Some patches contain metal in the layer of the patch that is not in contact with the skin (the backing). The metal in the backing of these patches may not be visible. The labeling for most of the medicated patches that contain metal in the backing provides a warning to patients about the risk of burns if the patch is not removed before an MRI scan. However, not all transdermal patches that contain metal have this warning for patients in the labeling.

The FDA is in the process of reviewing the labeling and composition of all medicated patches to ensure that those made with materials containing metal provide a warning about the risk of burns to patients who wear the patches during an MRI scan.

Until this review is complete, FDA recommends that healthcare professionals referring patients to have an MRI scan identify those patients who are wearing a patch before the patients have the MRI scan. The healthcare professional should advise these patients about the procedures for removing and disposing of the patch before the MRI scan, and replacing the patch after the MRI scan. MRI facilities should follow published safe practice recommendations concerning patients who are wearing patches (1, 2).

Until this safety issue is resolved, FDA recommends that patients who use medicated patches (including nicotine patches) do the following:

- Tell the doctor referring you for an MRI scan that you are using a patch and why you are using it (such as, for pain, smoking cessation, hormones)
- Ask your doctor for guidance about removing and disposing of the patch before having an MRI scan and replacing it after the procedure.
- Tell the MRI facility that you are using a patch. You should do this when making your appointment and during the health history questions you are asked when you arrive for your appointment.

The FDA urges health care professionals and patients to report possible cases of skin burns while wearing patches during an MRI to the FDA through the MedWatch program by phone (1-800-FDA-1088) or by the Internet at http://www.fda.gov/medwatch/index.html.

(1) Kanal, et. al, "ACR Guidance Document for Safe MR Practices: 2007," AJR 2007; 188:1–27.

(2) Guidelines for Screening Patients For MR Procedures and Individuals for the MR Environment, Institute for Magnetic Resonance Safety, Education, and Research, www.imrser.org, 2009.

FDA Update: (03/09/2009)

FDA has evaluated the composition of available patches to determine which of them contain metal components and to assure that this information is included in their labeling. Based on current information from this evaluation, FDA is working with the manufacturers of the following patches to update the labeling to include adequate warnings to patients about the risk of burns to the skin if the patch is worn during an MRI scan. It should be noted that some of the drugs listed may have a generic equivalent and more than one size and strength of patch. FDA will update this posting as information becomes available.

Proprietary Name Generic/Established Name

Catapres TTS / Clonidine
Neupro / Rotigotine
Lidopel / Lidocaine HCl and epinephrine
Synera / Lidocaine/Tetracaine
Transderm-Scop / Scopolamine
Prostep / Nicotine transdermal system
Habitrol / Nicotine transdermal system
Nicotrol TD / Nicotine transdermal system
Androderm / Testosterone transdermal system
Fentanyl / Fentanyl
Salonpas Power Plus / Methyl Salicylate/Menthol

Vascular Access Ports, Infusion Pumps*, and Catheters

Vascular access ports, infusion pumps, and catheters are implants and devices commonly used to provide long-term vascular administration of chemotherapeutic agents, antibiotics, analgesics and other medications (also, see information pertaining to the **AccuRx Constant Flow Implantable Pump, Ambulatory Infusion Pumps, Insulin Pumps,** the **IsoMed Implantable Constant-Flow Infusion Pump**, and the **SynchroMed, SynchroMED EL,** and **SynchroMed II Drug Infusion Systems**). Vascular access ports are usually implanted in a subcutaneous pocket over the upper chest wall with the catheters inserted in the jugular, subclavian, or cephalic vein.

Vascular access ports have a variety of similar features (e.g., a reservoir, central septum, and catheter) and may be constructed from different materials including stainless steel, titanium, silicone, and plastic. Because of the widespread use of vascular access ports and associated catheters and the high probability that patients with these devices may require MR procedures, it has been important to determine the MR safety aspects of these implants.

Three of the implantable vascular access ports and catheters evaluated for safety with MR procedures showed measurable magnetic field interactions during exposure to the MR systems (typically 1.5-Tesla) used for testing, but the interactions were minor relative to the *in vivo* applications of these implants. Therefore, an MR procedure is acceptable when using an MR system operating at 1.5-Tesla or less in a patient that has one of the vascular access ports or catheters shown in **The List**.

With respect to MR imaging and artifacts, in general, vascular access ports that will produce the least amount of artifact are made entirely from nonmetallic materials. The ones that produce the largest artifacts are composed of metal(s) or have metal in an unusual shape (e.g., the OmegaPort Access Devices).

Even vascular access ports made entirely from nonmetallic materials are seen on the MR images because they contain silicone. The septum portion vascular access ports is typically made from silicone. Using MR imaging, the Larmor precessional frequency of fat is close to that of silicone (i.e.,

100 Hz at 1.5-T). Therefore, silicone used in the construction of a vascular access port may be observed on MR images with varying degrees of signal intensity depending on the pulse sequence that is used.

If a radiologist did not know that this type of vascular access port was present in a patient, the MR signal produced by the silicone component of the device could be considered an abnormality, or at the very least, present a confusing image. For example, this may cause a diagnostic problem in a patient evaluated for a rupture of a silicone breast implant, because silicone from the vascular access port may be misread as an "extracapsular silicone implant rupture."

MRI at 3-Tesla and Vascular Access Ports and Catheters. For the vascular access ports assessed for magnetic field interactions at 3-Tesla, these did not exhibit substantial magnetic field interactions and, therefore, will not move or dislodge in this MR environment. For the accessories, some showed measurable magnetic field interactions (see **The List**). However, during the *intended use* of these accessories, it is unlikely that they will present a problem in the 3-Tesla MR environment considering that the simple application of a small piece of adhesive tape or other appropriate means of retention effectively counterbalances the magnetic qualities of these devices (Unpublished Observations, F.G. Shellock).

REFERENCES

American Society for Testing and Materials (ASTM) Designation: F 2052. Standard test method for measurement of magnetically induced displacement force on passive implants in the magnetic resonance environment. In: Annual Book of ASTM Standards, Section 13, Medical Devices and Services, Volume 13.01 Medical Devices; Emergency Medical Services. West Conshohocken, PA, 2002, pp. 1576-1580.

Shellock FG. Magnetic Resonance Procedures: Health Effects and Safety. CRC Press, LLC, Boca Raton, FL, 2001.

Shellock FG. Biomedical implants and devices: assessment of magnetic field interactions with a 3.0-Tesla MR system. J Magn Reson Imaging J Magn Reson Imaging 2002;16:721-732.

Shellock FG, Nogueira M, Morisoli S. MR imaging and vascular access ports: *ex vivo* evaluation of ferromagnetism, heating, and artifacts at 1.5-T. J Magn Reson Imaging 1995;4:481-484.

Shellock FG, Shellock VJ. Vascular access ports and catheters tested for ferromagnetism, heating, and artifacts associated with MR imaging. Magn Reson Imaging 1996;14:443-447.

VeriChip Microtransponder

The VeriChip Microtransponder is a miniaturized, implantable radio frequency identification device (RFID). The Microtransponder is a passive device that contains an electronic circuit, which is activated externally by a low-power electro-magnetic field emitted by a battery powered scanner. The Microtransponder is implanted subcutaneously.

With regard to MRI procedures, the labeling for this device states: Patients with the VeriChip Microtransponder may safely undergo MRI diagnostics, in up to 7-Tesla cylindrical systems. See section below.

INSTRUCTIONS FOR PATIENTS UNDERGOING MRI

- The patient should be monitored continuously throughout the MRI procedure using visual and audio means (e.g., intercom system).
- Instruct the patient to alert the MR system operator of any unusual sensations or problems so that, if necessary, the MR system operator can immediately terminate the procedure.
- Provide the patient with a means to alert the MR system operator of any unusual sensations or problems.
- Do not perform MRI if the patient is sedated, anesthetized, confused or otherwise unable to communicate with the MR system operator.

REFERENCE

http://www.verichipcorp.com

VOCARE Bladder System, Implantable Functional Neuromuscular Stimulation

The NeuroControl VOCARE Bladder System is a radiofrequency (RF) powered motor control neuroprosthesis or neurostimulation system that consists of both implanted and external components. The VOCARE Bladder System delivers low levels of electrical stimulation to a spinal cord injured patient's intact sacral spinal nerve roots to elicit functional contraction of the muscles innervated by them. The NeuroControl VOCARE Bladder System consists of the following subsystems:

- The **Implanted Components** include the Implantable Receiver-Stimulator and Extradural Electrodes.
- The **External Components** include the External Controller, External Transmitter, External Cable, Transmitter Tester, Battery Charger and Power Cord.
- The **Surgical Components** include the Surgical Stimulator, Intradural Surgical Probe, Extradural Surgical Probe, Surgical Test Cable, and Silicone Adhesive.

The NeuroControl VOCARE Bladder System is indicated for the treatment of patients who have clinically complete spinal cord lesions (ASIA Classification) with intact parasympathetic innervation of the bladder and are skeletally mature and neurologically stable, to provide urination on demand and to reduce post-void residual volumes of urine. Secondary intended use is to aid in bowel evacuation.

CONTRAINDICATIONS

The NeuroControl VOCARE Bladder System is contraindicated for patients with the following characteristics:

- Poor or inadequate bladder reflexes
- Active or recurrent pressure ulcers
- Active sepsis
- Implanted cardiac pacemaker

WARNINGS

The NeuroControl VOCARE Bladder System may only be prescribed, implanted, or adjusted by clinicians who have been trained and certified in its implementation and use.

PRECAUTIONS

- **X-rays, Diagnostic Ultrasound**: X-ray imaging, and diagnostic ultrasound have not been reported to affect the function of the Implantable Receiver-Stimulator or Extradural Electrodes. However, the implantable components may obscure the view of other anatomic structures.

- **MRI**: Testing of the VOCARE Bladder System in a 1.5-Tesla scanner with a maximum spatial gradient of 450 gauss/cm or less, exposed to an average Specific Absorption Rate (SAR) of 1.1 W/kg, for a 30 minute duration resulted in localized temperature rises up to 5.5 degrees C in a gel phantom (without blood flow) and translational force less than that of a 12 gram mass and torque of 0.47 N-cm (less than that produced by the weight of the device). A patient with a VOCARE Bladder System may undergo an MR procedure using a shielded or unshielded MR system with a static magnetic field of 1.5-Tesla only and a maximum spatial gradient of 450 gauss/cm or less. The implantable components may obscure the view of other nearby anatomic structures. Artifact size is dependent on variety of factors including the type of pulse sequence used for imaging (e.g. larger for gradient echo pulse sequences and smaller for spin echo and fast spin echo pulse sequences), the direction of the frequency encoding, and the size of the field of view used for imaging. The use of non-standard scanning modes to minimize image artifact or improve visibility should be applied with caution and with the Specific Absorption Rate (SAR) not to exceed an average of 1.1 W/kg and gradient magnetic fields no greater than 20 Tesla/sec. The use of Transmit RF Coils other than the scanner's Body RF Coil or a Head RF Coil is prohibited. Testing of the function of each electrode should be conducted prior to MRI scanning to ensure no leads are broken. Do not expose patients to MRI if any lead is broken or if integrity cannot be established as excessive heating may result in a broken lead. Patients should be advised to empty their bladder or bowel prior to MRI scanning as a precaution. The external components of the VOCARE Bladder System must be removed prior to MRI scanning. Patients must be continuously observed during the MRI procedure and instructed to report any unusual sensations (e.g., warming, burning, or neuromuscular stimulation). Scanning must be discontinued immediately if any unusual sensation occurs. Contact NeuroControl Corporation for additional information.

- **Therapeutic Ultrasound, Therapeutic Diathermy, and Microwave Therapy**: Therapeutic ultrasound, therapeutic diathermy, and microwave therapy should not be performed over the area of the Implantable Receiver-Stimulator or Extradural Electrodes as it may damage the VOCARE Bladder System.

- **Electrocautery:** Do not touch the Implantable Components of the VOCARE Bladder System with electrocautery instruments. Do not use electrocautery within 1 cm of the metal electrode contacts.

- **Antibiotic Prophylaxis:** Standard antibiotic prophylaxis for patients with an implant should be utilized to protect the patient when invasive procedures (e.g., oral surgery) are performed.

- **Drug Interactions**: Anticholinergic medications, or other medications which reduce the contraction of smooth muscle, may reduce the strength of bladder contraction achieved using the VOCARE Bladder System. Anticholinergic medications should be discontinued at least three days prior to evaluating patients for the VOCARE Bladder System and prior to implantation surgery so that bladder reflexes and response to electrical stimulation can be accurately evaluated. In addition, long-acting neuromuscular blocking agents must not be used during surgery.

- **Prior procedures** (such as bladder neck surgery or bladder augmentation) or conditions (such as severe urethral damage, stricture, or erosion) may affect patient suitability for the VOCARE Bladder System or clinical outcome. Patients with bladder augmentation may not be candidates for this procedure unless they can still achieve appropriate bladder pressures through reflex contractions. Patients should be thoroughly evaluated and counseled regarding the effect of any prior procedures or conditions.

- **Post-operative incontinence** may occur following posterior rhizotomy, which is typically performed in conjunction with implantation of the VOCARE Bladder System. While rhizotomy generally abolishes reflex incontinence, some patients may still experience stress incontinence. Patients should be evaluated for open bladder neck pre-operatively and counseled regarding the factors that may increase the risk of stress incontinence.

- **Bowel motility** may be affected by the rhizotomy procedure and by use of the VOCARE Bladder System. Patients should be advised that the rhizotomy may decrease the response to suppositories and digital stimulation of the rectum. Conversely, use of the VOCARE Bladder System may increase bowel motility. Patients may need to adjust the frequency and/or method of their bowel management routine postoperatively.

- The **rhizotomy** procedure typically performed in conjunction with implantation of the VOCARE Bladder System may cause loss of erectile function and ejaculation in men who had these responses before surgery.

- **Spinal instability** may result from the laminectomies required during implantation and rhizotomy surgery. Patients should be evaluated carefully for added risk factors, such as significant osteoporosis or scoliosis.

- **Studies have not been conducted** on the use of the NeuroControl VOCARE Bladder System in pregnant women.

- **Post-operatively**, the patient should be advised to check the condition of his or her skin over the VOCARE Bladder System Receiver-Stimulator and leads daily for signs of redness, swelling, or breakdown. If skin breakdown becomes apparent, patients should contact their clinician immediately. The clinician should treat the infection aggressively, taking into consideration the extra risk presented by the presence of the implanted materials.

- **Unintended Stimulation:** While there have been no reports of VOCARE Bladder System activation or malfunction due to electromagnetic interference (such as from retail anti-theft detectors, airport metal detectors, or other electronic devices) testing has not been conducted to rule out the possibility of this occurring. Patients should be advised to notify their clinician if they experience **unintended** stimulation when the VOCARE Bladder System is **not** in use. If possible, patients should note when and where the stimulation occurred.

- **Keep it dry**: The user should avoid getting the external components, cables, and attachments of the VOCARE Bladder System wet.

- The patient and caregiver should be advised to **inspect the external cables and connectors** daily for fraying or damage and replace components when necessary.

- To avoid possible interference, patients with electric wheelchairs should be advised to **turn off their wheelchair controller** prior to turning on the VOCARE Bladder System External Controller.

- **External Defibrillation:** The effect of external defibrillation on the VOCARE Bladder System is unknown.

- Patients should be advised to turn off the VOCARE Bladder System External Controller when not in use. **The External Transmitter can become hot** if the VOCARE Bladder System is left on for extended periods of time.

[Excerpted with permission from VOCARE Bladder System Implantable Functional Neuromuscular Stimulator, NeuroControl Corporation, Valley View, OH]

[MR healthcare professionals are advised to contact the respective manufacturer in order to obtain the latest safety information to ensure patient safety relative to the use of an MR procedure.]

The List – Information and Terminology

The List contains information for thousands of implants, devices, materials, and other products. The objects in **The List** are divided into general categories to facilitate access and review of pertinent information.

To properly utilize **The List**, particular attention must be given to the information indicated for the highest static magnetic **Field Strength** used for testing and the **Status** information indicated for a given **Object** (*Note:* These specific terms correspond to the column headings for information compiled in **The List**). In addition, for certain objects (e.g., those designated as *Conditional 5*), it will be necessary to refer to specific recommendations or guidelines in **SECTION II** of this textbook or to contact the manufacturer or the implant or device for the latest MRI information, particularly if the implant/device in question is electronically-activated or otherwise an "active" implant. Frequently, specific MRI information is best found at the implant/device company's website. See **Appendix III** for a list of company websites.

The relevant terminology for **The List** is, as follows:

Object: This is the implant, device, material, or product that underwent evaluation relative to an MR procedure or the MR environment. Information is also provided for the material(s) used to make the object and the manufacturer of the object, if known. The term "SS" refers to stainless steel. Note that there are magnetic and nonmagnetic forms of stainless steel.

Status: This information pertains to the results of the tests conducted for the object. Testing typically included an assessment of magnetic field interactions (i.e., deflection and/or torque) and MRI-related heating, as needed. In some cases, medical products were assessed for induced electrical currents and the impact of an MR procedure or the MR environment on the functional aspects of the object.

Information for each object has been specifically categorized using a **Status** designation, which indicates the object to be **Safe, Conditional, or Unsafe**, as follows (***IMPORTANT NOTE***: See the section entitled *Terminology Applied to Implants and Devices):

Safe – The object is considered to be safe for the patient undergoing an MR procedure or an individual in the MR environment, with special reference to the highest static magnetic field strength that was used for the MR safety test. The object has undergone testing to demonstrate that it is safe or it is made from material(s) considered to be safe with regard to the MR environment (e.g., plastic, silicone, glass, etc.) or an MR procedure. Refer to additional information for the particular object indicated in the text of **SECTION II** of this textbook (see **Table of Contents**).

Terminology from the American Society for Testing and Materials (ASTM) International and utilized by the Food and Drug Administration refers to <u>MR safe</u> as an item that poses no known hazards in all MRI environments. Using the current terminology, MR safe items include non-conducting, non-metallic, non-magnetic items such as a plastic Petri dish.

Conditional – The object may or may not be safe for the patient undergoing an MR procedure or an individual in the MR environment, depending on the specific conditions that are present.

Current terminology from the American Society for Testing and Materials (ASTM) International and utilized by the Food and Drug Administration refers to <u>MR conditional</u> as an item that has been demonstrated to pose no known hazards in a specified MRI environment with specified conditions of use. Field conditions that define the MRI environment include static magnetic field strength, spatial gradient, dB/dt (time varying magnetic fields), radio frequency (RF) fields, and specific absorption rate (SAR). Additional conditions, including specific configurations of the item (e.g., the routing of leads used for a neurostimulation system), may be required.

The MR conditional information has been sub-categorized to indicate specific recommendations for the particular object, as follows:

Conditional 1 – The object is acceptable for the patient or individual in the MR environment, despite the fact that it showed positive findings for magnetic field interactions during testing. Notably, the object is considered to be "weakly" ferromagnetic, *only*.

In general, the object is safe because the magnetic field interactions were characterized as "mild" or "weak" relative to the *in vivo* forces or counter-forces present for the object. For example, certain prosthetic heart valve prostheses and annuloplasty rings showed measurable magnetic field interactions during exposure to the MR systems used for testing, but the magnetic field interactions were less than the forces exerted on the implants by the beating heart.

Additionally, there may be substantial "retentive" or counter-forces provided by the presence of sutures or other means of fixation (e.g., screws, cement, etc.), tissue ingrowth, scarring, or granulation that serve to prevent the object from presenting a risk or hazard to the patient undergoing an MR procedure or an individual in the MR environment.

For a device or product that is used for an MR-guided procedure (e.g., laryngoscope, endoscope, etc.), there may be minor magnetic field interactions in association with the MR system. Eddy currents may also be present. However, the device or product is considered to be acceptable if it is used in its "intended" manner, as specified by the manufacturer. Special attention should be given to the strength of the static magnetic field used for testing the device or product. Functional or operational aspects may need to be considered. Additionally, specific recommendations for the use of the device or product in the MR environment or during an MR procedure (i.e., typically presented in the Product Insert or Instructions for Use) should be followed carefully. See also Conditional 7 information below.

Conditional 2 – These particular "weakly" ferromagnetic coils, filters, stents, clips, cardiac occluders, or other implants typically become firmly incorporated into the tissue six weeks following placement. Therefore, it is unlikely that these objects will be moved or dislodged by interactions with the magnetic fields of MR systems operating at the static magnetic field strength used for testing. Furthermore, to date, there has been no report of an injury to a patient or individual in association with an MR procedure for these coils, stents, filters, cardiac occluders or other similar implants designated as "Conditional 2".

Of note is that if the implant is made from a nonmagnetic material (e.g., Phynox, Elgiloy, titanium, titanium alloy, MP35N, Nitinol, etc.), it is _not_ necessary to wait a minimum of six weeks before performing and MR procedure using an MR system operating at 1.5-Tesla or less (in some cases, this may also apply to 3-Tesla MR systems).

Special Note: If there is any concern regarding the integrity of the implant or the integrity of the tissue with regard to its ability to

retain the object in place during an MR procedure or during exposure to the MR environment, the patient or individual should not be allowed into the MR environment.

Conditional 3 – Certain transdermal patches with metallic foil (e.g., Deponit, nitroglycerin transdermal delivery system) or other metallic components, although not attracted to an MR system, have been reported to heat excessively during MR procedures. This excessive heating may produce discomfort or burn a patient or individual wearing a transdermal patch with a metallic component. Therefore, it is recommended that the patch be removed prior to the MR procedure. A new patch should be applied immediately after the examination. This procedure should only be done in consultation with the patient's or individual's personal physician responsible for prescribing the transdermal medication patch.

Conditional 4 - This halo vest or cervical fixation device may have ferromagnetic component parts, however, the magnetic field interactions have not been determined. Nevertheless, there has been no report of patient injury in association with the presence of this device in the MR environment at the static magnetic field strength used for MR safety testing. Issues may still be present with regard to MRI-related heating. As such, guidelines provided in the Product Insert or Instructions for Use for a given halo vest or cervical fixation device should be carefully followed. Halo vests and cervical fixation devices made from conducting metals may heat excessively during an MR procedure, resulting in serious patient injury. Contact the manufacturer for further information. Also, refer to recent information for cervical fixation devices, as several have now been evaluated at 3-Tesla.

Conditional 5 - This object is acceptable for a patient undergoing an MR procedure or an individual in the MR environment *only* if specific guidelines or recommendations are followed (see specific information for a given object in **SECTION II** and contact the manufacturer for further information). Please refer to the specific criteria for performing the MR procedure by reviewing the information for the object in this textbook. Consult the manufacturer of the particular device for the latest safety information. Frequently, this information is best found at the company's website. *A list of biomedical company websites is shown in **Appendix III**.*

Conditional 6 - This implant/device was determined to be MR-conditional according to the terminology specified in the American Society for Testing and Materials (ASTM) International,

Designation: F2503-05. Standard Practice for Marking Medical Devices and Other Items for Safety in the Magnetic Resonance Environment.

Non-clinical testing demonstrated that the implant/device is MR Conditional. A patient with this implant/device can be scanned safely immediately after placement under the following conditions:

- Static magnetic field of 3-Tesla or less
- Maximum spatial gradient magnetic field of 720-Gauss/cm or less
- Maximum MR system reported whole-body-averaged specific absorption rate (SAR) of 3-W/kg for 15 minutes of scanning.

In non-clinical testing, the implant/device produced a temperature rise of less than or equal to 3.0 degrees C at a maximum MR system-reported whole body averaged specific absorption rate (SAR) of 3-W/kg for 15-minutes of MR scanning in a 3-Tesla MR system using a transmit/receive body coil (Excite, Software G3.0-052B, General Electric Healthcare, Milwaukee, WI).

MR image quality may be compromised if the area of interest is in the exact same area or relatively close to the position of the implant/device. Therefore, optimization of MR imaging parameters to compensate for the presence of this implant/device may be necessary.

Attention: Contact the manufacturer of this implant/device for further information, as needed.

Conditional 7 - *Important Note:* This device is not intended for use during the operation of an MR system for an MR procedure. That is, this device should not be inside of the bore of the MR system, exposing this device to the time-varying and RF fields activated during an MR procedure.

Attention: Contact the manufacturer of this implant/device for further information.

Conditional 8 – Note: This information pertains to an implant/device that has MRI labeling at 1.5-Tesla and 3-Tesla. In some cases, it may pertain to a single and two-overlapped version of a stent. Contact the manufacturer for additional MRI information, as needed.

The implant/device was determined to be MR-conditional according to the terminology specified in the American Society for Testing and

Materials (ASTM) International, Designation: F2503-05. Standard Practice for Marking Medical Devices and Other Items for Safety in the Magnetic Resonance Environment.

Non-clinical testing demonstrated that the implant/device is MR Conditional. A patient with this implant/device can be scanned safely immediately after placement under the following conditions:

For magnetic field interactions,

-Static magnetic field of 3-Tesla or less

-Maximum spatial gradient magnetic field of 720-Gauss/cm or less

MRI-Related Heating

In non-clinical testing, the implant/device produced the following temperature rises during MRI performed for 15-min in 1.5-Tesla (1.5-Tesla/64-MHz, Magnetom, Siemens Medical Solutions, Malvern, PA. Software Numaris/4, Version Syngo MR 2002B DHHS) and 3-Tesla (3-Tesla/128-MHz, Excite, Software G3.0-052B, General Electric Healthcare, Milwaukee, WI) MR systems, using MR system reported, whole body averaged SAR of 3-W/kg or less, as follows:

Highest temperature change	*MRI Condition*
Less than or equal to 3.0 degrees C	1.5-T/64-MHz
Less than or equal to 3.0 degrees C	3-T/128-MHz

Artifact Information

MR image quality may be compromised if the area of interest is in the exact same area or relatively close to the position of the implant/device. Therefore, optimization of MR imaging parameters to compensate for the presence of this implant/device may be necessary.

Attention: Contact the manufacturer of this implant/device for further information.

Terminology from the American Society for Testing and Materials (ASTM) International and utilized by the Food and Drug Administration refers to <u>MR Unsafe</u> as an item that is known to pose hazards in all MRI environments. MR Unsafe items include magnetic items such as a pair of ferromagnetic scissors.

Unsafe 1 – The object is considered to pose a potential or realistic risk or hazard to a patient or individual in the MR environment primarily as the result of movement or dislodgment of the object. Other hazards may also exist. Therefore, in general, the presence of this object is considered to be a contraindication for an MR procedure and/or for an individual to enter the MR environment. Note that the "default" static magnetic field strength for an unsafe implant or device is 1.5-Tesla.

Unsafe 2 – This object displays only minor magnetic field interactions which, in consideration of the *in vivo* application of this object, is unlikely to pose a hazard or risk in association with movement or dislodgment. Nevertheless, the presence of this object is considered to be a contraindication for an MR procedure or for an individual in the MR environment. Potential risks of performing an MR procedure in a patient or individual with this object are related to possible induced currents, excessive heating, or other potentially hazardous conditions. Therefore, it is inadvisable to perform an MR procedure in a patient or individual with this object.

For example, although certain cardiovascular catheters and accessories typically do not exhibit magnetic field interactions, there are other mechanisms whereby these devices may pose a hazard to the patient or individual or in the MR environment (e.g., excessive MRI-related heating).

The Swan-Ganz thermodilution catheter (and other similar catheters) displays no attraction to the MR system. However, there has been a report of a Swan-Ganz catheter that "melted" in a patient during an MR procedure. Therefore, the presence of this cardiovascular catheter and any other similar device is considered to be a contraindication for a patient undergoing an MR procedure.

Field Strength – This is the highest strength of the static magnetic field of the MR system that was used for safety testing of the object. In most cases, a 1.5-Tesla MR system was used for testing. However, there are some objects that were tested at field strengths lower (e.g., 0.15-Tesla) or higher (e.g., 3-Tesla) than 1.5-Tesla. *Note that the "default" field strength for an unsafe implant or device is 1.5-Tesla.*

There are MR systems with static magnetic field strengths that exceed 3.0-Tesla (i.e., as high as 8-Tesla or 9.4-Tesla). Some objects have been assessed to determine the relative amount of magnetic field interactions in association with these very high-field-strength MR systems.

Important Note: An object that exhibits only "mild" or "weak" magnetic field interactions in association with exposure to a 1.5-Tesla MR system may be attracted with sufficient force by a higher field strength scanner (e.g., 3-Tesla), potentially posing a risk to a patient or individual. Therefore, careful consideration must be given to each object relative to the static magnetic field strength of the MR system used for testing as well as the conditions that are present for the patient or individual under consideration prior to exposure to the MR environment. Furthermore, for implants and devices that have an elongated shape or form a loop of a certain diameter, MRI-related heating may be of concern. Please refer to **3-Tesla MR Safety Information for Implants and Devices** in this textbook for additional guidance and recommendations.

Reference – This is the peer-reviewed publication or other documentation used for the MRI safety information indicated for a particular object.

*Terminology Applied to Implants and Devices

IMPORTANT NOTE: See the section in this textbook entitled, **Terminology Applied to Implants and Devices,** in order to be familiar with the proper terms used for MRI labeling.

Also, for a comprehensive explanation, see Shellock FG, Woods TO, Crues JV. MRI labeling information for implants and devices: Explanation of terminology. Radiology 2009;253:26-30 (available as a PDF file on *www.IMRSER.org*)

Use of Terminology

The current MRI labeling terminology is intended to help elucidate matters related to biomedical implants and devices to ensure the safe use of MRI technology. Notably, this terminology (i.e., MR safe, MR conditional, and MR unsafe) has not been applied *retrospectively* to implants and devices that previously received U.S. Food and Drug Administration (FDA) approved labeling using the terms "MR safe" or "MR compatible" (i.e., this applies to those objects tested prior to December, 2005). Accordingly, this should be understood to avoid undue confusion regarding the matter of MRI-related labeling for "older" vs. "newer" implants, or those that have undergone retesting.

REFERENCES

American Society for Testing and Materials (ASTM) International, Designation: F2503-05. Standard Practice for Marking Medical Devices and Other Items for Safety in the Magnetic Resonance Environment. ASTM International, West Conshohocken, PA, 2005.

Shellock FG, Woods TO, Crues JV. MRI labeling information for implants and devices: Explanation of terminology. Radiology 2009;253:26-30.

Woods TO. Standards for medical devices in MRI: present and future. J Magn Reson Imaging. 2007;26:1186-9.

Woods TO. Guidance for Industry and FDA Staff - Establishing Safety and Compatibility of Passive Implants in the Magnetic Resonance (MR) Environment. Document issued on: August 21, 2008; http://www.fda.gov/cdrh/osel/guidance/1685.html

Object	Status	Field Strength (T)	Reference

Aneurysm Clips

Object	Status	Field Strength (T)	Reference
Aesculap AVM clip *curved, Phynox,* *Aesculap Inc., Center Valley, PA*	Safe	1.5, 3	
Aesculap AVM clip *straight, Phynox,* *Aesculap Inc., Center Valley, PA*	Safe	1.5, 3	
Codman AVM Micro Clip *Codman & Shurtleff, Inc.,* *a Johnson & Johnson Company,* *http://www.codman.com/DePuy/index.html*	Conditional 6	3	116
Codman Slim-Line Aneurysm Clip *Codman & Shurtleff, Inc.,* *a Johnson & Johnson Company,* *http://www.codman.com/DePuy/index.html*	Conditional 6	3	116
Codman Slim-Line Aneurysm Clip Graft *Codman & Shurtleff, Inc.,* *a Johnson & Johnson Company,* *http://www.codman.com/DePuy/index.html*	Conditional 6	3	116
Codman Slim-Line Mini Aneurysm Clip *Codman & Shurtleff, Inc.,* *a Johnson & Johnson Company,* *http://www.codman.com/DePuy/index.html*	Conditional 6	3	116
Codman Slim-Line Temporary Vessel Aneurysm Clip *Codman & Shurtleff, Inc.,* *a Johnson & Johnson Company,* *http://www.codman.com/DePuy/index.html*	Conditional 6	3	116
Downs Multi-Positional *Aneurysm Clip, 17-7PH*	Unsafe 1	1.39	1
Drake (DR 14, DR 21) *Aneurysm Clip,* *Edward Weck, Triangle Park, NJ*	Unsafe 1	1.39	1
Drake (DR 16) *Aneurysm Clip,* *Edward Weck, Triangle Park, NJ*	Unsafe 1	0.147	1
Drake Aneurysm Clip *301 SS,* *Edward Weck, Triangle Park, NJ*	Unsafe 1	1.5	2
Heifetz Aneurysm Clip *17-7PH,* *Edward Weck, Triangle Park, NJ*	Unsafe 1	1.89	4

Object	Status	Field Strength (T)	Reference
Heifetz Aneurysm Clip *Elgiloy,* *Edward Weck, Triangle Park, NJ*	Safe	1.89	2
Housepian Aneurysm Clip	Unsafe 1	0.147	1
Kapp Aneurysm Clip *405 SS, V. Mueller*	Unsafe 1	1.89	2
Kapp, Curved Aneurysm Clip *404 SS, V. Mueller*	Unsafe 1	1.39	1
Kapp, Straight Aneurysm Clip *404 SS, V. Mueller*	Unsafe 1	1.39	1
L-Aneurysm Clip System *Titanium,* *Peter Lazic GmbH, http://www.lazic.de*	Safe	3	
Mayfield Aneurysm Clip *301 SS,* *Codman, Randolf, MA*	Unsafe 1	1.5	3
Mayfield Aneurysm Clip *304 SS,* *Codman, Randolf, MA*	Unsafe 1	1.89	5
McFadden Aneurysm Clip *301 SS,* *Codman, Randolf, MA*	Unsafe 1	1.5	2
McFadden Vari-Angle, Aneurysm Clip *micro clip, fenestrated, 9-mm straight blade, MP35N,* *Codman,* *Johnson & Johnson Professional, Inc., Raynham, MA*	Safe	1.5	
McFadden Vari-Angle, Aneurysm Clip *micro clip, 9-mm straight blade, MP35N,* *Codman,* *Johnson & Johnson Professional, Inc., Raynham, MA*	Safe	1.5	
Olivercrona *Aneurysm Clip*	Safe	1.39	1
Perneczky Aneurysm Clip *curved, 20-mm,* *Zeppelin Chirurgische Instrumente, Germany*	Safe	1.5	
Perneczky Aneurysm Clip *curved, 9-mm,* *Zeppelin Chirurgische Instrumente, Germany*	Safe	1.5	
Perneczky Aneurysm Clip *straight, 2-mm blade, SS alloy,* *Zeppelin Chirugishe Instrumente, Pullach, Germany*	Safe	1.5, 3	82
Perneczky Aneurysm Clip *straight, 3-mm,* *Zeppelin Chirurgische Instumente, Germany*	Safe	1.5	

Object	Status	Field Strength (T)	Reference
Perneczky Aneurysm Clip *straight, 6-mm blade, SS alloy,* *Zeppelin Chirugishe Instrumente, Pullach, Germany*	Safe	1.5, 3	82
Perneczky Aneurysm Clip *straight, 7-mm blade, SS alloy,* *Zeppelin Chirugishe Instrumente, Pullach, Germany*	Safe	1.5, 3	82
Perneczky Aneurysm Clip *straight, 9-mm,* *Zeppelin Chirurgische Instrumente, Germany*	Safe	1.5	
Pivot Aneurysm Clip *17-7PH*	Unsafe 1	1.89	5
R. Spetzler Titanium Aneurysm Clip *for Permanent Occlusion, 5-mm Fenestrated Bayonet,* *11-mm blade length (M-9248), Ti6Al4V (Titanium alloy),* *Allegiance Healthcare Corporation,* *V. Mueller Neuro/Spine, San Carlos, CA*	Safe	1.5, 3	
R. Spetzler Titanium Aneurysm Clip *for Permanent Occlusion, 5-mm Fenestrated Straight,* *12-mm blade length (M-9227), Ti6Al4V (Titanium alloy),* *Allegiance Healthcare Corporation,* *V. Mueller Neuro/Spine, San Carlos, CA*	Safe	1.5, 3	
R. Spetzler Titanium Aneurysm Clip *for Permanent Occlusion, Mini 40 degree Side,* *5-mm blade length (M-9450), Ti6Al4V (Titanium alloy),* *Allegiance Healthcare Corporation,* *V. Mueller Neuro/Spine, San Carlos, CA*	Safe	1.5, 3	
R. Spetzler Titanium Aneurysm Clip *for Permanent Occlusion, Standard Bayonet,* *12-mm blade length (M-9152), Ti6Al4V (Titanium alloy),* *Allegiance Healthcare Corporation,* *V. Mueller Neuro/Spine, San Carlos, CA*	Safe	1.5, 3	
R. Spetzler Titanium Aneurysm Clip *for Permanent Occlusion, Standard Straight,* *15-mm blade length (M-9113), Ti6Al4V (Titanium alloy),* *Allegiance Healthcare Corporation,* *V. Mueller Neuro/Spine, San Carlos, CA*	Safe	1.5, 3	
Scoville Aneurysm Clip *EN58J,* *Downs Surgical, Inc., Decatur, GA*	Safe	1.89	2
Slim-Line Aneurysm Clip *Fenestrated Straight, 4-mm opening, 6-mm blade, MP35N,* *Codman, Codman & Shurtleff, Inc.,* *Johnson and Johnson Company, Raynham, MA*	Safe	1.5, 3	

Object	Status	Field Strength (T)	Reference
Spetzler Pure Titanium Aneurysm Clip *Model C-2200, straight, 5-mm blade, C.P. Titanium,* *NMT Neurosciences, Duluth, Georgia*	Safe	1.5, 3	82
Spetzler Pure Titanium Aneurysm Clip *Model C-2203, straight, 11-mm blade, C.P. Titanium,* *NMT Neurosciences, Duluth, Georgia*	Safe	1.5, 3	82
Spetzler Pure Titanium Aneurysm Clip *Model C-2212, curved, 7-mm blade, C.P. Titanium,* *NMT Neurosciences, Duluth, Georgia*	Safe	1.5, 3	82
Spetzler Pure Titanium Aneurysm Clip *Model C-2214, curved, 11-mm blade, C.P. Titanium,* *NMT Neurosciences, Duluth, Georgia*	Safe	1.5, 3	82
Spetzler Pure Titanium Aneurysm Clip *Model C-2224, straight,* *11-mm/3.5-mm fenestrated blade, C.P. Titanium,* *NMT Neurosciences, Duluth, Georgia*	Safe	1.5, 3	82
Spetzler Pure Titanium Aneurysm Clip *Model C-2526, straight,* *11-mm blade, C.P. Titanium,* *NMT Neurosciences, Duluth, Georgia*	Safe	1.5, 3	82
Spetzler Pure Titanium Aneurysm Clip *straight, 9-mm blade,* *C. P. Titanium, Elekta Instruments, Atlanta, GA*	Safe	1.5, 3	82
Spetzler Titanium Aneurysm Clip *straight, 13-mm blade, double turn, C.P. Titanium,* *Elekta Instruments, Inc., Atlanta, GA*	Safe	1.5	68
Spetzler Titanium Aneurysm Clip *straight, 13-mm blade, single turn, C.P. Titanium,* *Elekta Instruments, Inc., Atlanta, GA*	Safe	1.5, 3	68, 82
Spetzler Titanium Aneurysm Clip *straight, 9-mm blade, double turn, C.P. Titanium,* *Elekta Instruments, Inc., Atlanta, GA*	Safe	1.5	68
Spetzler Titanium Aneurysm Clip *straight, 9-mm blade, single turn, C.P. Titanium,* *Elekta Instruments, Inc., Atlanta, GA*	Safe	1.5, 3	68, 82
Stevens Aneurysm Clip *silver alloy*	Safe	0.15	6
Sugita Aneurysm Clip *Elgiloy, Downs Surgical, Inc., Decatur, GA*	Safe	1.89	2
Sugita Aneurysm Clip *Fenestrated large, bent, 7.5-mm, Elgiloy,* *Mizuho America, Inc., Beverly, MA*	Safe	1.5, 3	82

Object	Status	Field Strength (T)	Reference
Sugita Titanium Aneurysm Clip *mini temporary, angled, 5-mm blade, Titanium alloy,* *Mizuho America, Inc., Beverly, MA*	Safe	1.5	
Sugita Titanium Aneurysm Clip *mini temporary, straight large, 6-mm blade, Titanium alloy,* *Mizuho America, Beverly, MA*	Safe	1.5	
Sugita Titanium Aneurysm Clip *mini temporary, straight slim, 6-mm blade, Titanium alloy,* *Mizuho America, Beverly, MA*	Safe	1.5	
Sugita Titanium Aneurysm Clip *mini, angled, 5-mm blade, Titanium alloy,* *Mizuho America, Inc., Beverly, MA*	Safe	1.5	
Sugita Titanium Aneurysm Clip *mini, angled, 7-mm blade, Titanium alloy,* *Mizuho America, Inc., Beverly, MA*	Safe	1.5	
Sugita Titanium Aneurysm Clip *mini, bayonet, 5-mm blade, Titanium alloy,* *Mizuho America, Inc., Beverly, MA*	Safe	1.5	
Sugita Titanium Aneurysm Clip *mini, curved slim, 5.2-mm blade, Titanium alloy,* *Mizuho America, Inc., Beverly, MA*	Safe	1.5	
Sugita Titanium Aneurysm Clip *mini, curved slim, 6.7-mm blade, Titanium alloy,* *Mizuho America, Inc., Beverly, MA*	Safe	1.5	
Sugita Titanium Aneurysm Clip *mini, curved slim, 8.2-mm blade, Titanium alloy,* *Mizuho America, Inc., Beverly, MA*	Safe	1.5	
Sugita Titanium Aneurysm Clip *mini, curved, 4.5-mm blade, Titanium alloy,* *Mizuho America, Inc., Beverly, MA*	Safe	1.5	
Sugita Titanium Aneurysm Clip *mini, curved, 5.5-mm blade, Titanium alloy,* *Mizuho America, Inc., Beverly, MA*	Safe	1.5	
Sugita Titanium Aneurysm Clip *mini, curved, 5-mm blade, Titanium alloy,* *Mizuho America, Inc., Beverly, MA*	Safe	1.5	
Sugita Titanium Aneurysm Clip *mini, side curved, 7-mm blade, Titanium alloy,* *Mizuho America, Inc., Beverly, MA*	Safe	1.5	
Sugita Titanium Aneurysm Clip *mini, straight large, 6-mm blade, Titanium alloy,* *Mizuho America, Inc., Beverly, MA*	Safe	1.5	

Object	Status	Field Strength (T)	Reference
Sugita Titanium Aneurysm Clip *mini, straight slim, 4-mm blade, Titanium alloy,* *Mizuho America, Inc., Beverly, MA*	Safe	1.5	
Sugita Titanium Aneurysm Clip *mini, straight slim, 6-mm blade, Titanium alloy,* *Mizuho America, Inc., Beverly, MA*	Safe	1.5	
Sugita Titanium Aneurysm Clip *mini, straight small, 4-mm blade, Titanium alloy,* *Mizuho America, Inc., Beverly, MA*	Safe	1.5	
Sugita Titanium Aneurysm Clip *standard, 1/4 curved, 11-mm blade, Titanium alloy,* *Mizuho America, Inc., Beverly, MA*	Safe	1.5	
Sugita Titanium Aneurysm Clip *standard, 1/4 curved, large, 8.6-mm blade, Titanium alloy,* *Mizuho America, Beverly, MA*	Safe	1.5	
Sugita Titanium Aneurysm Clip *standard, 1/4 curved, small, 7.6-mm blade, Titanium alloy,* *Mizuho America, Beverly, MA*	Safe	1.5	
Sugita Titanium Aneurysm Clip *standard, 45 degree curved, large, 10-mm blade,* *Titanium alloy,* *Mizuho America, Inc., Beverly, MA*	Safe	1.5	
Sugita Titanium Aneurysm Clip *standard, 45 degree curved, medium, 7.5-mm blade,* *Titanium alloy,* *Mizuho America, Beverly, MA*	Safe	1.5	
Sugita Titanium Aneurysm Clip *standard, 45 degree curved, small, 5-mm blade,* *Titanium alloy,* *Mizuho America, Inc., Beverly, MA*	Safe	1.5	
Sugita Titanium Aneurysm Clip *standard, angled, 12-mm blade, Titanium alloy,* *Mizuho America, Inc., Beverly, MA*	Safe	1.5	
Sugita Titanium Aneurysm Clip *standard, angled, 8-mm blade, Titanium alloy,* *Mizuho America, Inc., Beverly, MA*	Safe	1.5	
Sugita Titanium Aneurysm Clip *standard, bayonet large, 12-mm blade, Titanium alloy,* *Mizuho America, Inc., Beverly, MA*	Safe	1.5	
Sugita Titanium Aneurysm Clip *standard, bayonet small, 10-mm blade, Titanium alloy,* *Mizuho America, Inc., Beverly, MA*	Safe	1.5	
Sugita Titanium Aneurysm Clip *standard, bayonet, 7-mm blade, Titanium alloy,* *Mizuho America, Inc., Beverly, MA*	Safe	1.5	

Object	Status	Field Strength (T)	Reference
Sugita Titanium Aneurysm Clip *standard, curved (155 g), 9-mm blade, Titanium alloy,* *Mizuho America, Inc., Beverly, MA*	Safe	1.5	
Sugita Titanium Aneurysm Clip *standard, curved (160 g), 9-mm blade, Titanium alloy,* *Mizuho America, Inc., Beverly, MA*	Safe	1.5	
Sugita Titanium Aneurysm Clip *standard, for Permanent Occlusion, 45 degree angled,* *19-mm, serrated blade, Titanium alloy,* *Mizuho America, Inc., Beverly, MA*	Safe	1.5, 3	82
Sugita Titanium Aneurysm Clip *standard, J-angled, large, 9-mm blade, Titanium alloy,* *Mizuho America, Inc., Beverly, MA*	Safe	1.5	
Sugita Titanium Aneurysm Clip *standard, J-angled, medium, 7.5-mm blade, Titanium alloy,* *Mizuho America, Beverly, MA*	Safe	1.5	
Sugita Titanium Aneurysm Clip *standard, J-angled, small, 6-mm blade, Titanium alloy,* *Mizuho America, Inc., Beverly, MA*	Safe	1.5	
Sugita Titanium Aneurysm Clip *standard, L-angled, large, 10-mm blade, Titanium alloy,* *Mizuho America, Inc., Beverly, MA*	Safe	1.5	
Sugita Titanium Aneurysm Clip *standard, L-angled, medium, 7.5-mm blade, Titanium alloy,* *Mizuho America, Beverly, MA*	Safe	1.5	
Sugita Titanium Aneurysm Clip *standard, L-angled, small, 5-mm blade, Titanium alloy,* *Mizuho America, Inc., Beverly, MA*	Safe	1.5	
Sugita Titanium Aneurysm Clip *standard, L-curved, large, 10-mm blade, Titanium alloy,* *Mizuho America, Inc., Beverly, MA*	Safe	1.5	
Sugita Titanium Aneurysm Clip *standard, L-curved, small, 7.5-mm blade, Titanium alloy,* *Mizuho America, Inc., Beverly, MA*	Safe	1.5	
Sugita Titanium Aneurysm Clip *standard, side angled, 12-mm blade, Titanium alloy,* *Mizuho America, Inc., Beverly, MA*	Safe	1.5	
Sugita Titanium Aneurysm Clip *standard, side angled, 8-mm blade, Titanium alloy,* *Mizuho America, Inc., Beverly, MA*	Safe	1.5	
Sugita Titanium Aneurysm Clip *standard, side curved bayonet, 8.5-mm blade, Titanium alloy,* *Mizuho America, Beverly, MA*	Safe	1.5	

Object	Status	Field Strength (T)	Reference
Sugita Titanium Aneurysm Clip *standard, side curved, 9-mm blade, Titanium alloy,* *Mizuho America, Inc., Beverly, MA*	Safe	1.5	
Sugita Titanium Aneurysm Clip *standard, slight curved bayonet, 12-mm blade, Titanium alloy,* *Mizuho America, Beverly, MA*	Safe	1.5	
Sugita Titanium Aneurysm Clip *standard, slightly angled, 8-mm blade, Titanium alloy,* *Mizuho America, Inc., Beverly, MA*	Safe	1.5	
Sugita Titanium Aneurysm Clip *standard, slightly curved (165), 11-mm blade, Titanium alloy,* *Mizuho America, Beverly, MA*	Safe	1.5	
Sugita Titanium Aneurysm Clip *standard, slightly curved (170), 11-mm blade, Titanium alloy,* *Mizuho America, Beverly, MA*	Safe	1.5	
Sugita Titanium Aneurysm Clip *standard, slightly curved, 18-mm blade, Titanium alloy,* *Mizuho America, Inc., Beverly, MA*	Safe	1.5	
Sugita Titanium Aneurysm Clip *standard, slightly curved, 9-mm blade, Titanium alloy,* *Mizuho America, Inc., Beverly, MA*	Safe	1.5	
Sugita Titanium Aneurysm Clip *standard, slightly curved, small, 14-mm blade, Titanium alloy,* *Mizuho America, Beverly, MA*	Safe	1.5	
Sugita Titanium Aneurysm Clip *standard, small curved, 9-mm blade, Titanium alloy,* *Mizuho America, Inc., Beverly, MA*	Safe	1.5	
Sugita Titanium Aneurysm Clip *standard, staight (small), 12-mm blade, Titanium alloy,* *Mizuho America, Inc., Beverly, MA*	Safe	1.5	
Sugita Titanium Aneurysm Clip *standard, straight large, 18-mm blade, Titanium alloy,* *Mizuho America, Inc., Beverly, MA*	Safe	1.5	
Sugita Titanium Aneurysm Clip *standard, straight medium, 15-mm blade, Titanium alloy,* *Mizuho America, Inc., Beverly, MA*	Safe	1.5	
Sugita Titanium Aneurysm Clip *standard, straight, large, 10-mm blade, Titanium alloy,* *Mizuho America, Inc., Beverly, MA*	Safe	1.5	
Sugita Titanium Aneurysm Clip *standard, straight, small, 7-mm blade, Titanium alloy,* *Mizuho America, Inc., Beverly, MA*	Safe	1.5	

Object	Status	Field Strength (T)	Reference
Sugita Titanium Aneurysm Clip *temporary, bayonet, 7-mm blade, Titanium alloy, Mizuho America, Inc., Beverly, MA*	Safe	1.5	
Sugita Titanium Aneurysm Clip *temporary, curved, 8-mm blade, Titanium alloy, Mizuho America, Inc., Beverly, MA*	Safe	1.5	
Sugita Titanium Aneurysm Clip *temporary, slightly curved, 11-mm blade, Titanium alloy, Mizuho America, Beverly, MA*	Safe	1.5	
Sugita Titanium Aneurysm Clip *temporary, straight large, 10-mm blade, Titanium alloy, Mizuho America, Inc., Beverly, MA*	Safe	1.5	
Sugita Titanium Aneurysm Clip *temporary, straight small, 7-mm blade, Titanium alloy, Mizuho America, Inc., Beverly, MA*	Safe	1.5	
Sugita, AVM Micro Clip *Aneurysm Clip, Elgiloy, Mizuho America, Inc., Beverly, MA*	Safe	1.5	
Sugita, bent, mini aneurysm clip *for temporary occlusion, Elgiloy, Mizuho America, Inc., Beverly, MA*	Safe	1.5	
Sugita, bent, standard aneurysm clip *for temporary occlusion, Elgiloy, Mizuho America, Inc., Beverly, MA*	Safe	1.5	
Sugita, sideward CVD bayonet, standard *aneurysm clip for permanent occlusion, Mizuho America, Inc., Beverly, MA*	Safe	1.5	
Sugita, straight, large *aneurysm clip for permanent occlusion, Elgiloy, Mizuho America, Inc., Beverly, MA*	Safe	1.5	
Sugita *Fenestrated Large Fujita, Blade Deflected Type, Aneurysm Clip for Permanent Occlusion, angled, 10-mm serrated blade, Elgiloy, Mizuho America, Inc., Beverly, MA*	Safe	1.5, 3	82
Sugita *Fenestrated large, bent, Aneurysm Clip, for permanent occlusion, Elgiloy, Mizuho America, Inc., Beverly, MA*	Safe	1.5	
Sugita *Large Aneurysm Clip for Permanent Occlusion, straight, 21-mm serrated blade, Elgiloy, Mizuho America, Inc., Beverly, MA*	Safe	1.5, 3	82

Object	Status	Field Strength (T)	Reference
Sugita *Long Aneurysm Clip for Permanent Occlusion, straight, 19-mm nonserration blade, Elgiloy, Mizuho America, Inc., Beverly, MA*	Safe	1.5, 3	82
Sugita *Standard bent, Aneurysm Clip, 8-mm blade, Elgiloy, Mizuho America, Inc., Beverly, MA*	Safe	1.5, 3	82
Sugita *Standard curved, Aneurysm Clip, 6-mm blade, Elgiloy, Mizuho America, Inc., Beverly, MA*	Safe	1.5, 3	82
Sugita *Temporary Mini, Aneurysm Clip, bent, 7-mm blade, Elgiloy, Mizuho America, Inc., Beverly, MA*	Safe	1.5, 3	82
Sugita *Temporary standard straight, Aneurysm Clip, 7-mm blade, Elgiloy, Mizuho America, Inc., Beverly, MA*	Safe	1.5, 3	82
Sundt AVM Micro Aneurysm Clip System *MP35N, Codman & Shurtleff, Inc., a Johnson & Johnson Company, Raynham, MA*	Conditional 6	3	
SUNDT AVM MICRO CLIP *# 3, MP35N, Codman, Codman & Shurtleff, Inc., Johnson and Johnson Company, Raynham, MA*	Safe	1.5, 3	
SUNDT AVM MICRO CLIP *# 4, MP35N, Codman, Codman & Shurtleff, Inc., Johnson and Johnson Company, Raynham, MA*	Safe	1.5, 3	
SUNDT AVM MICRO CLIP *# 5, MP35N, Codman, Codman & Shurtleff, Inc., Johnson and Johnson Company, Raynham, MA*	Safe	1.5, 3	
Sundt AVM, Micro Clip *aneurysm clip, MP35N, Codman, Johnson & Johnson Professional, Inc., Raynham, MA*	Safe	1.5	
SUNDT SLIM-LINE ANEURYSM CLIP *# 6, Bayonet, MP35N, Codman, Codman & Shurtleff, Inc., Johnson and Johnson Company, Raynham, MA*	Safe	1.5, 3	

Object	Status	Field Strength (T)	Reference
SUNDT SLIM-LINE ANEURYSM CLIP *# 6, Forward Angle, MP35N,* *Codman, Codman & Shurtleff, Inc.,* *Johnson and Johnson Company, Raynham, MA*	Safe	1.5, 3	
SUNDT SLIM-LINE ANEURYSM CLIP *Fenestrated Bayonet, Straight,* *6-mm opening, 15-mm blade, MP35N,* *Codman, Codman & Shurtleff, Inc.,* *Johnson and Johnson Company, Raynham, MA*	Safe	1.5, 3	
SUNDT SLIM-LINE ANEURYSM CLIP *Fenestrated Straight, 4-mm opening, 24-mm blade, MP35N,* *Codman, Codman & Shurtleff, Inc.,* *Johnson and Johnson Company, Raynham, MA*	Safe	1.5, 3	
SUNDT SLIM-LINE ANEURYSM CLIP *Sharp Right Angle, 12-mm blade, MP35N,* *Codman, Codman & Shurtleff, Inc.,* *Johnson and Johnson Company, Raynham, MA*	Safe	1.5, 3	
SUNDT SLIM-LINE MINI ANEURYSM CLIP *# 6, Right Angle, MP35N,* *Codman, Codman & Shurtleff, Inc.,* *Johnson and Johnson Company, Raynham, MA*	Safe	1.5, 3	
SUNDT SLIM-LINE MINI ANEURYSM CLIP *# 6, Straight, MP35N,* *Codman, Codman & Shurtleff, Inc.,* *Johnson and Johnson Company, Raynham, MA*	Safe	1.5, 3	
SUNDT SLIM-LINE MINI ANEURYSM CLIP *# 7, Right Angle, MP35N,* *Codman, Codman & Shurtleff, Inc.,* *Johnson and Johnson Company, Raynham, MA*	Safe	1.5, 3	
Sundt Slim-Line Mini Aneurysm Clip *also known as Slimline, MP35N,* *Codman & Shurtleff, Inc.,* *a Johnson & Johnson Company, Raynham, MA*	Conditional 6	3	
Sundt Slim-Line Temporary Vessel Aneurysm Clip *also known as Slimline, MP35N,* *Codman & Shurtleff, Inc.,* *a Johnson & Johnson Company, Raynham, MA*	Conditional 6	3	
Sundt Slim-Line, Graft Clip *Aneurysm Clip, MP35N,* *Codman,* *Johnson & Johnson Professional, Inc., Raynham, MA*	Safe	1.5	
Sundt Slim-Line, Temporary Aneurysm Clip *10-mm blade, MP35N,* *Codman,* *Johnson & Johnson Professional, Inc., Raynham, MA*	Safe	1.5	

Object	Status	Field Strength (T)	Reference
Sundt-Kees Multi-Angle *Aneurysm Clip, 17-7PH,* *Downs Surgical, Inc., Decatur, GA*	Unsafe 1	1.89	2
Sundt-Kees Slim-Line Aneurysm Clip *also known as Slimline,* *30 Degree Forward Angle, MP35N,* *Codman & Shurtleff, Inc.,* *a Johnson & Johnson Company, Raynham, MA*	Conditional 6	3	
Sundt-Kees Slim-Line Aneurysm Clip *also known as Slimline,* *30 Degree Forward Curve, MP35N,* *Codman & Shurtleff, Inc.,* *a Johnson & Johnson Company, Raynham, MA*	Conditional 6	3	
Sundt-Kees Slim-Line Aneurysm Clip *also known as Slimline, Bayonet,* *30 Degree Curved Forward-Left, MP35N,* *Codman & Shurtleff, Inc.,* *a Johnson & Johnson Company, Raynham, MA*	Conditional 6	3	
Sundt-Kees Slim-Line Aneurysm Clip *also known as Slimline, Bayonet,* *30 Degree Curved Forward-Right, MP35N,* *Codman & Shurtleff, Inc.,* *a Johnson & Johnson Company, Raynham, MA*	Conditional 6	3	
Sundt-Kees Slim-Line Aneurysm Clip *also known as Slimline, Bayonet, Straight, MP35N,* *Codman & Shurtleff, Inc.,* *a Johnson & Johnson Company, Raynham, MA*	Conditional 6	3	
Sundt-Kees Slim-Line Aneurysm Clip *also known as Slimline, Curved, MP35N,* *Codman & Shurtleff, Inc.,* *a Johnson & Johnson Company, Raynham, MA*	Conditional 6	3	
Sundt-Kees Slim-Line Aneurysm Clip *also known as Slimline, Fenestrated 45 Degree Angle,* *6-mm Opening, MP35N,* *Codman & Shurtleff, Inc.,* *a Johnson & Johnson Company, Raynham, MA*	Conditional 6	3	
Sundt-Kees Slim-Line Aneurysm Clip *also known as Slimline, Fenestrated 45 Degree Angle,* *4-mm Opening, 30 Degree, MP35N,* *Codman & Shurtleff, Inc.,* *a Johnson & Johnson Company, Raynham, MA*	Conditional 6	3	
Sundt-Kees Slim-Line Aneurysm Clip *also known as Slimline, Fenestrated 90 Degree Angle,* *4-mm Opening, MP35N,* *Codman & Shurtleff, Inc.,* *a Johnson & Johnson Company, Raynham, MA*	Conditional 6	3	

Object	Status	Field Strength (T)	Reference
Sundt-Kees Slim-Line Aneurysm Clip *also known as Slimline, Fenestrated 90 Degree Angle,* *6-mm Opening, MP35N,* *Codman & Shurtleff, Inc.,* *a Johnson & Johnson Company, Raynham, MA*	Conditional 6	3	
Sundt-Kees Slim-Line Aneurysm Clip *also known as Slimline, Fenestrated Bayonet Straight,* *6-mm Opening, MP35N,* *Codman & Shurtleff, Inc.,* *a Johnson & Johnson Company, Raynham, MA*	Conditional 6	3	
Sundt-Kees Slim-Line Aneurysm Clip *also known as Slimline, Fenestrated Straight,* *3-mm Extended Tandem, 6-mm, MP35N,* *Codman & Shurtleff, Inc.,* *a Johnson & Johnson Company, Raynham, MA*	Conditional 6	3	
Sundt-Kees Slim-Line Aneurysm Clip *also known as Slimline, Fenestrated Straight,* *4-mm Opening, MP35N,* *Codman & Shurtleff, Inc.,* *a Johnson & Johnson Company, Raynham, MA*	Conditional 6	3	
Sundt-Kees Slim-Line Aneurysm Clip *also known as Slimline, Fenestrated Straight,* *5-mm Extended Tandem, 6-mm, MP35N,* *Codman & Shurtleff, Inc.,* *a Johnson & Johnson Company, Raynham, MA*	Conditional 6	3	
Sundt-Kees Slim-Line Aneurysm Clip *also known as Slimline, Fenestrated Straight,* *6-mm Opening, MP35N,* *Codman & Shurtleff, Inc.,* *a Johnson & Johnson Company, Raynham, MA*	Conditional 6	3	
Sundt-Kees Slim-Line Aneurysm Clip *also known as Slimline, Graft, 4-mm Diameter, MP35N,* *Codman & Shurtleff, Inc.,* *a Johnson & Johnson Company, Raynham, MA*	Conditional 6	3	
Sundt-Kees Slim-Line Aneurysm Clip *also known as Slimline, Reinforcing 30 Degree Angle,* *6-mm Wide, MP35N,* *Codman & Shurtleff, Inc.,* *a Johnson & Johnson Company, Raynham, MA*	Conditional 6	3	
Sundt-Kees Slim-Line Aneurysm Clip *also known as Slimline, Reinforcing 60 Degree Angle,* *6-mm Wide, MP35N,* *Codman & Shurtleff, Inc.,* *a Johnson & Johnson Company, Raynham, MA*	Conditional 6	3	

Object	Status	Field Strength (T)	Reference
Sundt-Kees Slim-Line Aneurysm Clip *also known as Slimline, Reinforcing Zero Degree Angle,* *6-mm Wide, MP35N,* *Codman & Shurtleff, Inc.,* *a Johnson & Johnson Company, Raynham, MA*	Conditional 6	3	
Sundt-Kees Slim-Line Aneurysm Clip *also known as Slimline, Right Angle, MP35N,* *Codman & Shurtleff, Inc.,* *a Johnson & Johnson Company, Raynham, MA*	Conditional 6	3	
Sundt-Kees Slim-Line Aneurysm Clip *also known as Slimline, Sharp Right Angle, MP35N,* *Codman & Shurtleff, Inc.,* *a Johnson & Johnson Company, Raynham, MA*	Conditional 6	3	
Sundt-Kees Slim-Line Aneurysm Clip *also known as Slimline, Sideward Angle, MP35N,* *Codman & Shurtleff, Inc.,* *a Johnson & Johnson Company, Raynham, MA*	Conditional 6	3	
Sundt-Kees Slim-Line Aneurysm Clip *also known as Slimline, Slightly curved, MP35N,* *Codman & Shurtleff, Inc.,* *a Johnson & Johnson Company, Raynham, MA*	Conditional 6	3	
Sundt-Kees Slim-Line Aneurysm Clip *also known as Slimline, Straight, MP35N,* *Codman & Shurtleff, Inc.,* *a Johnson & Johnson Company, Raynham, MA*	Conditional 6	3	
Sundt-Kees Slim-Line Aneurysm Clip *also known as Slimline, Super Bayonet, MP35N,* *Codman & Shurtleff, Inc.,* *a Johnson & Johnson Company, Raynham, MA*	Conditional 6	3	
Sundt-Kees Slim-Line *fenestrated, aneurysm clip, 9-mm blade, MP35N,* *Codman,* *Johnson & Johnson Professional, Inc., Raynham, MA*	Safe	1.5	
Sundt-Kees, Slim-Line *9-mm blade, MP35N, aneurysm clip,* *Codman,* *Johnson & Johnson Professional, Inc., Raynham, MA*	Safe	1.5	
Vari-Angle Aneurysm Clip *17-7PH,* *Codman, Randolf, MA*	Unsafe 1	1.89	5
Vari-Angle McFadden Aneurysm Clip *MP35N,* *Codman, Randolf, MA*	Safe	1.89	2

Object	Status	Field Strength (T)	Reference
Vari-Angle Micro Aneurysm Clip *17-7PH,* *Codman, Randolf, MA*	Unsafe 1	0.15	2
Vari-Angle Spring Aneurysm Clip *17-7PH,* *Codman, Randolf, MA*	Unsafe 1	0.15	2
Yasargil Aneurysm Clip *All "FD" Models, per the manufacturer,* *Aesculap, Inc., Center Valley, PA,* *http://www.aesculapusa.com*	Unsafe 1	1.5	
Yasargil Aneurysm Clip *All "FE" Models per the manufacturer,* *Aesculap, Inc., Center Valley, PA,* *http://www.aesculapusa.com*	Safe	3	
Yasargil Aneurysm Clip *All "FT" Models, per the manufacturer,* *Aesculap, Inc., Center Valley, PA,* *http://www.aesculapusa.com*	Safe	3	
Yasargil *Aneurysm Clip, 316L SS,* *Aesculap, Inc., Center Valley, PA*	Safe	1.89	5
Yasargil *Aneurysm Clip, Model FD,* *Aesculap, Inc., Center Valley, PA*	Unsafe 1	1.5	
Yasargil *Aneurysm Clip, Model FE 720T, mini, permanent,* *7-mm blade, Titanium alloy,* *Aesculap, Inc., Center Valley, PA*	Safe	1.5	
Yasargil *Aneurysm Clip, Model FE 740T, standard, permanent,* *7-mm blade, Titanium alloy,* *Aesculap, Inc., Center Valley, PA*	Safe	1.5	
Yasargil *Aneurysm Clip, Model FE 748, standard,* *9-mm blade, bayonet, Phynox,* *Aesculap, Inc., Center Valley, PA*	Safe	1.5	
Yasargil *Aneurysm Clip, Model FE 750, 9-mm blade, straight,* *Phynox,* *Aesculap, Inc., South Francisco, CA*	Safe	1.5	
Yasargil *Aneurysm Clip, Model FE 750T, standard, permanent,* *9-mm blade, Titanium alloy,* *Aesculap, Inc., Center Valley, PA*	Safe	1.5	

Object	Status	Field Strength (T)	Reference
Yasargil *Aneurysm Clip, Model FE,* *Aesculap, Inc., Center Valley, PA*	Safe	1.5	
Yasargil *Mini Clip, Titanium, Aneurysm Clip, Model FT728T,* *bayonet, 7-mm blade, Titanium alloy,* *Aesculap, Inc., Center Valley, PA*	Safe	1.5, 3	82
Yasargil *Standard Aneurysm Clip Titanium, Model FT740T,* *straight, 7-mm blade, Titanium alloy,* *Aesculap, Inc., Center Valley, PA*	Safe	1.5, 3	82
Yasargil *Standard Aneurysm Clip Titanium, Model FT758T,* *bayonet, 12-mm blade, Titanium alloy,* *Aesculap, Inc., Center Valley, PA*	Safe	1.5, 3	82
Yasargil *Standard Aneurysm Clip Titanium, Model FT760T,* *11-mm blade, Titanium alloy,* *Aesculap, Inc., Center Valley, PA*	Safe	1.5, 3	82
Yasargil *Standard Aneurysm Clip Titanium, Model FT790T,* *straight, 20-mm blade, Titanium alloy,* *Aesculap, Inc., Center Valley, PA*	Safe	1.5, 3	82
Yasargil *Standard Aneurysm Clip, Permanent, Model FE660K,* *straight, 12-mm blade, Phynox, SN FYA21,* *Aesculap, Inc., Center Valley, PA*	Safe	3	
Yasargil *Standard Aneurysm Clip, Permanent, Model FE660K,* *straight, 12-mm blade, Phynox, SN FYA46,* *Aesculap, Inc., Center Valley, PA*	Safe	3	
Yasargil *Standard Aneurysm Clip, Permanent, Model FE662K,* *angled, 10-mm blade, Phynox, SN FKJ41,* *Aesculap, Inc., Center Valley, PA*	Safe	3	
Yasargil *Standard Aneurysm Clip, Permanent, Model FE662K,* *angled, 10-mm blade, Phynox, SN FUJ53,* *Aesculap, Inc., Center Valley, PA*	Safe	3	
Yasargil *Standard Aneurysm Clip, Permanent, Model FE840K,* *straight, 25-mm blade, Phynox, SN FYR65,* *Aesculap, Inc., Center Valley, PA*	Safe	3	

Object	Status	Field Strength (T)	Reference
Yasargil *Standard Aneurysm Clip, Permanent, Model FE840K, straight, 25-mm blade, Phynox, SN FYS01, Aesculap, Inc., Center Valley, PA*	Safe	3	
Yasargil *Standard Aneurysm Clip, Permanent, Model FT650T, straight, 9-mm blade, Titanium alloy, SN CQY63, Aesculap, Inc., Center Valley, PA*	Safe	3	
Yasargil *Standard Aneurysm Clip, Permanent, Model FT650T, straight, 9-mm blade, Titanium alloy, SN CQY83, Aesculap, Inc., Center Valley, PA*	Safe	3	
Yasargil *Standard Aneurysm Clip, Permanent, Model FT662T, angled, 10-mm blade, Titanium alloy, SN CLU37, Aesculap, Inc., Center Valley, PA*	Safe	3	
Yasargil *Standard Aneurysm Clip, Permanent, Model FT662T, angled, 10-mm blade, Titanium alloy, SN CLU54, Aesculap, Inc., Center Valley, PA*	Safe	3	
Yasargil *Standard Aneurysm Clip, Permanent, Model FTD790D, straight, 20-mm blade, Titanium alloy, SN CTW58, Aesculap, Inc., Center Valley, PA*	Safe	3	
Yasargil *Standard Aneurysm Clip, Permanent, Model FTD790D, straight, 20-mm blade, Titanium alloy, SN CTW73, Aesculap, Inc., Center Valley, PA*	Safe	3	
Yasargil *Standard Aneurysm Clip, Model FE750, straight, 9-mm blade, Phynox, Aesculap, Inc., Center Valley, PA*	Safe	1.5, 3	82
Yasargil *Standard Aneurysm Clip, Model FE780, straight, 14-mm blade, Phynox, Aesculap, Inc., Center Valley, PA*	Safe	1.5, 3	82
Yasargil *Standard Aneurysm Clip, Model FE786, curved, 15.3-mm blade, Phynox, Aesculap, Inc., Center Valley, PA*	Safe	1.5, 3	82
Yasargil *Standard Aneurysm Clip, Model FE790K, straight, 20-mm blade, Phynox, Aesculap, Inc., Center Valley, PA*	Safe	1.5, 3	82

Object	Status	Field Strength (T)	Reference
Yasargil *Standard Aneurysm Clip, Model FE798, bayonet,* *20-mm blade, Phynox,* *Aesculap, Inc., Center Valley, PA*	Safe	1.5, 3	82
Yasargil *Standard Aneurysm Clip, Model FE798, bayonet,* *20-mm blade, Phynox,* *Aesculap, Inc., Center Valley, PA*	Safe	1.5, 3	82
Yasargil *Standard Aneurysm Clip, Model FE887, 7-mm blade, Phynox,* *Aesculap, Inc., Center Valley, PA*	Safe	1.5, 3	82
Yasargil *T-Bar Aneurysm Clip, Permanent, Model FE853K,* *45 degree angle, 9-mm blade, Phynox,* *Aesculap, Inc., Center Valley, PA*	Safe	3	
Yasargil *T-Bar Aneurysm Clip, Permanent, Model FE856K,* *90 degree angle, 13-mm blade, Phynox,* *Aesculap, Inc., Center Valley, PA*	Safe	3	
Yasargil *T-Bar Aneurysm Clip, Permanent, Model FT853T,* *45 degree angle, 9-mm blade, Titanium,* *Aesculap, Inc., Center Valley, PA*	Safe	3	
Yasargil *T-Bar Aneurysm Clip, Permanent, Model FT856T,* *90 degree angle, 13-mm blade, Titanium,* *Aesculap, Inc., Center Valley, PA*	Safe	3	

Biopsy Needles, Markers, and Devices

Object	Status	Field Strength (T)	Reference
Adjustable, Automated Aspiration Biopsy Gun *10, 15, and 20-mm, 304 SS,* *MD Tech, Watertown, MA*	Unsafe 1	1.5	7
Adjustable, Automated Biopsy Gun *6, 13, and 19-mm, 304 SS,* *MD Tech, Watertown, MA*	Unsafe 1	1.5	7
AOS Marker Seed *Alpha-Omega Services, Inc., Bellflower, CA*	Conditional 6	3	
ASAP 16, Automatic 16 G Core Biopsy System *19-cm length, 304 SS*	Unsafe 1	1.5	7
AspirationNeedle MRI *MRI Devices Corporation, Waukesha, WI*	Safe	1.5	
Automatic Cutting Needle with Depth Markings *14 G, 10-cm length, 304 SS, biopsy needle,* *Manan, Northbrook, IL*	Unsafe 1	1.5	7

Object	Status	Field Strength (T)	Reference
Automatic Cutting Needle with Ultrasound Tip & *Depth Markings 18 G, 16-cm length, 304 SS, biopsy needle, Manan, Northbrook, IL*	Unsafe 1	1.5	7
Automatic Cutting Needle with Ultrasound Tip & Depth Markings *18 G, 20-cm length, 304 SS, biopsy needle, Manan, Northbrook, IL*	Unsafe 1	1.5	7
Basic II Hookwire Breast Localization Needle *304 SS, MD Tech, Watertown, MA*	Unsafe 1	1.5	7
Beaded Breast Localization Wire Set *19 G, 3-1/2 inch needle with 7-7/8 inch wire, 304 SS, Inrad, Grand Rapids, MI*	Unsafe 1	1.5	7
Beaded Breast Localization Wire Set *20 G, 2 inch needle with 5-7/8 inch wire, 304 SS, Inrad, Grand Rapids, MI*	Unsafe 1	1.5	7
Biopsy Gun *13-mm, biopsy needle, Meadox, Oakland, NJ*	Unsafe 1	1.5	7
Biopsy Gun *25-mm, biopsy needle, Meadox, Oakland, NJ*	Unsafe 1	1.5	7
Biopsy Needle *17 G, 10-cm length, Meadox, Oakland, NJ*	Unsafe 1	1.5	7
Biopsy Needle *20 G, 15-cm length, Meadox, Oakland, NJ*	Unsafe 1	1.5	7
Biopsy Needle *22 G, 15-cm length, Cook, Inc., Bloomington, IN*	Unsafe 1	1.5	7
Biopsy Needle *22 G, 15-cm length, Meadox, Oakland, NJ*	Unsafe 1	1.5	7
Biopty-Cut Biopsy Needle *14 G, 10-cm length, 304 SS, C.R. Bard, Inc., Covington, GA*	Unsafe 1	1.5	7
Biopty-Cut Biopsy Needle *16 G, 16-cm length, 304 SS, C.R. Bard, Inc., Covington, GA*	Unsafe 1	1.5	7
Biopty-Cut Biopsy Needle *18 G, 18-cm length, 304 SS, C.R. Bard, Inc., Covington, GA*	Unsafe 1	1.5	7

Object	Status	Field Strength (T)	Reference
Biopty-Cut Biopsy Needle *18 G, 20-cm length, 304 SS,* *C.R. Bard, Inc., Covington, GA*	Unsafe 1	1.5	7
BoneBiopsy Set MRI *manual version, includes trocar, stylet, drill and ejector,* *MRI Devices Corporation, Waukesha, WI*	Safe	1.5	
Breast Localization Needle *20 G, 5-cm length, 304 SS,* *Manan, Northbrook, IL*	Unsafe 1	1.5	7
Breast Localization Needle *20 G, 7-cm length, 304 SS,* *Manan, Northbrook, IL*	Unsafe 1	1.5	7
Chiba Needle and HiLiter *Ultrasound Enhancement, 22 G,* *3-7/8 inch biopsy needle, 304 SS,* *Inrad, Grand Rapids, MI*	Unsafe 1	1.5	7
Coaxial Needle Set Chiba-type *22 G, 5-7/8 inch biopsy needle, 304 SS,* *Inrad, Grand Rapids, MI*	Unsafe 1	1.5	7
Coaxial Needle Set Introducer *19G, 2-15/16 inch biopsy needle, 304 SS,* *Inrad, Grand Rapids, MI*	Unsafe 1	1.5	7
CoaxNeedle MRI *MRI Devices Corporation, Waukesha, WI*	Safe	1.5	
CorMark *Tissue Marker, 14 gauge,* *Ethicon Endosurgery, Cincinnati, OH*	Safe	3	
Cutting Needle & Gun *18 G, 155-mm length, biopsy needle,* *Meadox, Oakland, NJ*	Unsafe 1	1.5	7
Cutting Needle *14 G, 9-cm length, biopsy needle,* *West Coast Medical, Laguna Beach, CA*	Unsafe 1	1.5	7
Cutting Needle *16 G, 17-mm length, 304 SS, biopsy needle,* *BIP USA, Inc., Niagara Falls, NY*	Unsafe 1	1.5	7
Cutting Needle *16 G, 19-mm length, 304 SS, biopsy needle,* *BIP USA, Inc., Niagara Falls, NY*	Unsafe 1	1.5	7
Cutting Needle *18 G, 100-mm length, biopsy needle,* *Meadox, Oakland, NJ*	Unsafe 1	1.5	7

Object	Status	Field Strength (T)	Reference
Cutting Needle *18 G, 15-cm length, biopsy needle,* *West Coast Medical, Laguna Beach, CA*	Unsafe 1	1.5	7
Cutting Needle *18 G, 150-mm length, biopsy needle,* *Meadox, Oakland, NJ*	Unsafe 1	1.5	7
Cutting Needle *18 G, 9-cm length, biopsy needle,* *West Coast Medical, Laguna Beach, CA*	Unsafe 1	1.5	7
Cutting Needle *19 G, 15-cm length, biopsy needle,* *West Coast Medical, Laguna Beach, CA*	Unsafe 1	1.5	7
Cutting Needle *19 G, 6-cm length, biopsy needle,* *West Coast Medical, Laguna Beach, CA*	Unsafe 1	1.5	7
Cutting Needle *19 G, 9-cm length, biopsy needle,* *West Coast Medical, Laguna Beach, CA*	Unsafe 1	1.5	7
Cutting Needle *20 G, 15-cm length, biopsy needle,* *West Coast Medical, Laguna Beach, CA*	Unsafe 1	1.5	7
Cutting Needle *20 G, 20-cm length, biopsy needle,* *West Coast Medical, Laguna Beach, CA*	Unsafe 1	1.5	7
Cutting Needle *20 G, 9-cm length, biopsy needle,* *West Coast Medical, Laguna Beach, CA*	Unsafe 1	1.5	7
Fully Automatic BiopsyGun MRI *MRI Devices Corporation, Waukesha, WI*	Safe	1.5	
Hawkins Blunt Needle *304 SS, biopsy needle,* *MD Tech, Watertown, MA*	Unsafe 1	1.5	7
Hawkins III Breast Localization Needle *MD Tech, Watertown, MA*	Unsafe 1	1.5	7
HydroMark Breast Biopsy Site Marker *Stainless Steel and Titanium,* *Biopsy Sciences, Tucson, AZ*	Conditional 6	3	
KMD-Mark1 *marker,* *Kent Medical Devices, Inc., Minneapolis, MN*	Conditional 6	3	
LeLoc MRI *Tumor Localizer,* *MRI Devices Corporation, Waukesha, WI*	Safe	1.5	

Object	Status	Field Strength (T)	Reference
Lufkin Aspiration Cytology Needle *20 G, 5-cm length, biopsy needle, high nickel alloy,* *E-Z-Em, Inc., Westbury, NY*	Safe	1.5	9
Lufkin Biopsy Needle *18 G, 15-cm length, high nickel alloy,* *E-Z-Em, Inc., Westbury, NY*	Safe	1.5	8
Lufkin Biopsy Needle *18 G, 5-cm length, high nickel alloy,* *E-Z-Em, Inc., Westbury, NY*	Safe	1.5	8
Lufkin Biopsy Needle *22 G, 10-cm length, high nickel alloy,* *E-Z-Em, Inc., Westbury, NY*	Safe	1.5	8
Lufkin Biopsy Needle *22 G, 15-cm length, high nickel alloy,* *E-Z-Em, Inc., Westbury, NY*	Safe	1.5	8
Lufkin Biopsy Needle *22 G, 5-cm length, high nickel alloy,* *E-Z-Em, Inc., Westbury, NY*	Safe	1.5	8
MammoMark *Tissue Marker, 8 gauge,* *Ethicon Endosurgery, Cincinnati, OH*	Safe	3	
MammoMark *Tissue Marker Deployment Device, 8 gauge,* *Ethicon Endosurgery, Cincinnati, OH*	Safe	3	
MammoMark *Tissue Marker, 11 gauge,* *Ethicon Endosurgery, Cincinnati, OH*	Safe	3	
MammoMark *Tissue Marker Deployment Device, 11 gauge,* *Ethicon Endosurgery, Cincinnati, OH*	Safe	3	
MammoMark II *Tissue Marker, 11 gauge,* *Ethicon Endosurgery, Cincinnati, OH*	Safe	3	
MammoMark II *Tissue Marker Deployment Device, 11 gauge,* *Ethicon Endosurgery, Cincinnati, OH*	Safe	3	
Micromark Clip, marking clip *316L SS, Biopsys Medical, Irvine, CA*	Safe	1.5	61
MicroMark II Clip *316L SS,* *Ethicon Endosurgery, Cincinnati, Ohio*	Safe	1.5, 3	
MReye Chiba Biopsy Needle *William Cook Europe A/S, Bjaeverskov, Denmark*	Safe	1.5	

Object	Status	Field Strength (T)	Reference
MReye Franseen Lung Biopsy Needle *William Cook Europe A/S, Bjaeverskov, Denmark*	Safe	1.5	
MReye Interventional Needle *biopsy needle,* *William Cook Europe A/S, Bjaeverskov, Denmark*	Safe	1.5	
MReye Kopans Breast Lesion *Localization Needles,* *(21, 20, 19 gauges; 5.0, 9.0, 15.0 lengths),* *William Cook Europe A/S, Bjaeverskov, Denmark*	Safe	1.5	
MR Ghiatas Beaded *Breast Localization Wire Set, needle and wire,* *Inrad Inc., Kentwood, MI*	Conditional 6	3	
MR Ghiatas *Breast Localization Wire Sets, Inconel Alloy,* *C. R. Bard, Inc., Murray Hill, NJ*	Conditional 6	3	
MRI BioGun *18 G, 10-cm length, high nickel alloy, biopsy needle,* *E-Z-Em, Inc., Westbury, NY*	Safe	1.5	8
MRI BiopsyKit *MRI Devices Corporation, Waukesha, WI*	Safe	1.5	
MRI Histology Needle *18 G, 15-cm length, high nickel alloy, biopsy needle,* *E-Z-Em, Inc., Westbury, NY*	Safe	1.5	7
MRI Histology Needle *18 G, 5-cm length, high nickel alloy, biopsy needle,* *E-Z-Em, Inc., Westbury, NY*	Safe	1.5	8
MRI Histology Needle *20 G, 10-cm length, high nickel alloy, biopsy needle,* *E-Z-Em, Inc., Westbury, NY*	Safe	1.5	8
MRI Histology Needle *20 G, 15-cm length, high nickel alloy, biopsy needle,* *E-Z-Em, Inc., Westbury, NY*	Safe	1.5	8
MRI Histology Needle *20 G, 5-cm length, high nickel alloy, biopsy needle,* *E-Z-Em, Inc., Westbury, NY*	Safe	1.5	7
MRI Histology Needle *20 G, 7.5-cm length, high nickel alloy, biopsy needle,* *E-Z-Em, Inc., Westbury, NY*	Safe	1.5	8
MRI Lesion Marking System *20 G, 7.5-cm length, high nickel alloy,* *E-Z-Em, Inc., Westbury, NY*	Safe	1.5	8
MRI Needle *surgical grade SS, biopsy needle,* *Cook, Inc., Bloomington, IN*	Safe	1.5	7

Object	Status	Field Strength (T)	Reference
mrt Biopsy Needle *all sizes, Titanium alloy,* *Daum Medical, Baltimore, MD and, Schwerin, Germany*	Safe	1.5	
NeuroCut Needle MRI *MRI Devices Corporation, Waukesha, WI*	Safe	1.5	
NeuroGate Set MRI *MRI Devices Corporation, Waukesha, WI*	Safe	1.5	
NeuroPunctureNeedle MRI *MRI Devices Corporation, Waukesha, WI*	Safe	1.5	
Percucut Biopsy Needle and Stylet *19.5 gauge x 10-cm, 316L SS,* *E-Z-Em, Inc., Westbury, NY*	Unsafe 1	1.5	7
Percucut Biopsy Needle and Stylet *21 gauge x 10-cm, 316L SS,* *E-Z-Em, Inc., Westbury, NY*	Unsafe 1	1.5	7
PunctureNeedle MRI *MRI Devices Corporation, Waukesha, WI*	Safe	1.5	
Sadowsky Breast Marking System *20 G, 5-cm length needle and 7 inch hook wire,* *316L SS,* *Ranfac Corporation, Avon, MA*	Unsafe 1	1.5	7
Semi-Automatic BiopsyGun MRI *MRI Devices Corporation, Waukesha, WI*	Safe	1.5	
SenoMark UltraCor MRI *SS, M shaped breast biopsy marker, clip,* *SenoRx, Aliso Viejo, CA*	Conditional 6	3	
SenoMark UltraCor MRI *Titanium, X shaped breast biopsy marker, clip,* *SenoRx, Aliso Viejo, CA*	Conditional 6	3	
Single Loop Titanium Marker *Tissue Marker, Titanium alloy,* *RUBICOR Medical Inc., Redwood City, CA*	Conditional 6	3	
SmartGuide CT/MRI *MRI Devices Corporation, Waukesha, WI*	Safe	1.5	
Soft Tissue Biopsy Needle Gun & Biopsy Needle *304 SS, Anchor Procducts Co., Addison, IL*	Unsafe 1	1.5	7
Spirotome Single Use 10 Standard *receiving needle, plastic trocar, Inox trocar,* *cutting cannula, biopsy device,* *MEDINVENTS, Belgium*	Condiitonal 5	3	
Surgical Mesh with X-Ray Marker *NuVasive, Inc., San Diego, CA*	Conditional 6	3	

Object	Status	Field Strength (T)	Reference
TargoGrid *positioning grid for, biopsies and punctures,* *MRI Devices Corporation, Waukesha, WI*	Safe	1.5	
Trocar Needle *304 SS, biopsy needle,* *BIP USA, Inc., Niagara Falls, NY*	Unsafe 1	1.5	7
Trocar Needle, Disposable *SS, biopsy needle,* *Cook, Inc., Bloomington, IN*	Unsafe 1	1.5	7
TumoLoc MRI *Tumor Localizer,* *MRI Devices Corporation, Waukesha, WI*	Safe	1.5	
UltraClip II *MR Tissue Marker Device, tissue marker,* *Inrad Inc., Kentwood, MI*	Conditional 6	3	
UltraClip II *MR Tissue Marker Device, Titanium Alloy,* *C. R. Bard, Inc., Murray Hill, NJ*	Conditional 6	3	
UltraClip II *Tissue Markers, Clips Only, Titanium Alloy, PVA,* *Inconel Alloy, BioDur Alloy,* *C. R. Bard, Inc., Murray Hill, NJ*	Conditional 6	3	
Ultra-Core, biopsy needle *16 G, 16-cm length, 304 SS*	Unsafe 1	1.5	7

Breast Tissue Expanders and Implants

Object	Status	Field Strength (T)	Reference
Becker Expander/Mammary Mentor H/S *Prosthesis, 316L SS, breast implant,* *Santa Barbara, CA*	Safe	1.5	10
Breast Tissue Expander *Style 133 FV, with MAGNA-SITE Injection Site,* *magnetic port,* *McGhan Medical/INAMED Aesthetics, Santa Barbara, CA*	Unsafe 1	1.5	86
Breast Tissue Expander *Style 133 LV, with MAGNA-SITE Injection Site,* *magnetic port,* *McGhan Medical/INAMED Aesthetics, Santa Barbara, CA*	Unsafe 1	1.5	86
Breast Tissue Expander *Style 133 MV, with MAGNA-SITE Injection Site,* *magnetic port,* *McGhan Medical/INAMED Aesthetics, Santa Barbara, CA*	Unsafe 1	1.5	86
Breast Tissue Expander *STYLE 133V (133 V) Series,* *MAGNA-SITE Injection Site,* *Allergan, Inc., www.allergan.com*	Unsafe 1	1.5	

Object	Status	Field Strength (T)	Reference
Breast Tissue Expander *STYLE 133 FV,* *MAGNA-SITE Injection Site,* *Allergan, Inc., www.allergan.com*	Unsafe 1	1.5	
Breast Tissue Expander *STYLE 133 FX,* *MAGNA-SITE Injection Site,* *Allergan, Inc., www.allergan.com*	Unsafe 1	1.5	
Breast Tissue Expander *STYLE 133 LV,* *MAGNA-SITE Injection Site,* *Allergan, Inc., www.allergan.com*	Unsafe 1	1.5	
Breast Tissue Expander *STYLE 133 MV,* *MAGNA-SITE Injection Site,* *Allergan, Inc., www.allergan.com*	Unsafe 1	1.5	
Breast Tissue Expander *STYLE 133 MX,* *MAGNA-SITE Injection Site,* *Allergan, Inc., www.allergan.com*	Unsafe 1	1.5	
Breast Tissue Expander *STYLE 133 SV,* *MAGNA-SITE Injection Site,* *Allergan, Inc., www.allergan.com*	Unsafe 1	1.5	
Breast Tissue Expander *STYLE 133 SX,* *MAGNA-SITE Injection Site,* *Allergan, Inc., www.allergan.com*	Unsafe 1	1.5	
Double Chamber Breast Tissue Expander *Model 20739-400,* *SILIMED, Inc., Dallas, TX*	Unsafe 1	1.5	
Infall, breast implant (inflatable with magnetic port) *3101198 Model, breast implant,* *Heyerschultzz*	Unsafe 1	1.5	
Radovan Tissue Expander *316L SS,* *Mentor H/S, Santa Barbara, CA*	Safe	1.5	10
Siltex Spectrum Post-Operatively *Adjustable Saline-Filled Mammary Prosthesis, 316L SS,* *Mentor H/S, Santa Barbara, CA*	Safe	1.5	10
Tissue expander with magnetic port *breast implant,* *McGhan Medical Corporation, Santa Barbara, CA*	Unsafe 1	1.5	

Object	Status	Field Strength (T)	Reference

Cardiac Pacemakers, ICDs, and Cardiac Monitors

Object	Status	Field Strength (T)	Reference
Advisa MRI SureScan Pacing System *not available in the U.S. (2009),* *Medtronic, Inc., www.Medtronic.com*	Conditional 5	1.5	
AngelMed Guardian *Implantable Cardiac Monitor,* *Angel Medical Systems, Shrewsbury, NJ*	Unsafe 1	1.5	
Cosmos *Model 283-01, Pacemaker,* *Intermedics, Inc., Freeport, TX*	Unsafe 1	3	85
Cosmos II *Model 283-03, Pacemaker,* *Intermedics, Inc., Freeport, TX*	Unsafe 2	3	85
Cosmos II *Model 284-05, Pacemaker,* *Intermedics, Inc., Freeport, TX*	Unsafe 1	3	85
Delta TRS *Type DDD, Model 0937, Pacemaker,* *Cardiac Pacemakers, Inc., St. Paul, MN*	Unsafe 1	3	85
EnRhythm MRI *SureScan Pacing System, Cardiac Pacemaker,* *Medtronic, Inc., Minneapolis, MN*	Condiitonal 5	3	
GEM DR 7271 *Dual Chamber Implantable, Cardioverter Defibrillator,* *Medtronic, Inc., Minneapolis, MN*	Unsafe 1	3	85
GEM II DR 7273 *Dual Chamber Implantable, Cardioverter Defibrillator,* *Medtronic, Inc., Minneapolis, MN*	Unsafe 1	3	85
KAPPA DR403 *Dual Chamber Rate, Responsive Pacemaker,* *Medtronic, Inc., Minneapolis, MN*	Unsafe 2	3	85
KAPPA DR706 *Dual Chamber Rate, Responsive Pacemaker,* *Medtronic, Inc., Minneapolis, MN*	Unsafe 1	3	85
MARQUIS DR 7274 *Implantable Cardioverter Defibrillator,* *Medtronic, Inc., Minneapolis, MN*	Unsafe 1	3	85
MICRO JEWEL II 7223CX *Implantable Cardioverter Defibrillator,* *Medtronic, Inc., Minneapolis, MN*	Unsafe 1	3	85
Nova *Model 281-01,* *Intermedics, Inc., Freeport, TX*	Unsafe 1	3	85

Object	Status	Field Strength (T)	Reference
Nova II *Model 281-05, Pacemaker,* *Intermedics, Inc., Freeport, TX*	Unsafe 2	3	85
Nova II *Model 282-04, Pacemaker,* *Intermedics, Inc., Freeport, TX*	Unsafe 2	3	85
Quantum *Model 253-19, Pacemaker,* *Intermedics, Inc., Freeport, TX*	Unsafe 1	3	85
Reveal Plus Insertable Loop Recorder *9526 Reveal Plus Insertable Loop Recorder, ILR,* *Medtronic, Inc., Minneapolis, MN*	Condiitonal 5	1.5	90, 91
Reveal DX 9528 *Insertable Loop Recorder,* *Medtronic, Inc., Minneapolis, MN*	Conditional 5	1.5, 3	
Reveal XT 9529 *Insertable Loop Recorder,* *Medtronic, Inc., Minneapolis, MN*	Conditional 5	1.5, 3	
Relay *Model 294-03, Pacemaker,* *Intermedics, Inc., Freeport, TX*	Unsafe 1	3	85
Res-Q ACE *Model 101-01, Pacemaker,* *Intermedics, Inc., Freeport, TX*	Unsafe 1	3	85
SJM Confirm *Model DM2100, Implantable Cardiac Monitor,* *St. Jude Medical, Sylmar, CA*	Unsafe 1	1.5	
SIGMA SDR306 *Dual Chamber Rate, Responsive Pacemaker,* *Medtronic, Inc., Minneapolis, MN*	Unsafe 1	3	85
THERA VDD 8968I *Dual Chamber Atrial Sensing, Ventricular Sensing,* *Pacing Pacemaker,* *Medtronic, Inc., Minneapolis, MN*	Unsafe 2	3	85

Object	Status	Field Strength (T)	Reference

Cardiovascular Catheters and Accessories

Object	Status	Field Strength (T)	Reference
Apollo Micro Catheter *15-mm Tip,* *ev3 Inc., Irvine, CA*	Conditional 8	1.5, 3	
Apollo Micro Catheter *70-mm Tip, Nitinol, Platinum Alloy,* *Teflon, Polyether Amide,* *ev3 Inc., Irvine, CA*	Conditional 8	1.5, 3	
Arrow You-Bend *Two Lumen Hemodialysis Catheter,* *Arrow International Inc., Reading, PA*	Conditional 6	3	
CliniCath Catheter *Smiths Medical, St. Paul, MN*	Safe	3	
Codman SureStream Intraspinal Catheter *0-degree connector, 90-degree connector,* *Codman,* *a Johnson and Johnson company, Raynham, MA*	Conditional 6	3	
Chronic Catheter *COVIDIEN, http://www.covidien.com*	Conditional 6	3	
FlexTip Plus Epidural Catheter *Regional Anesthesia Device,* *Teleflex Medical, Wyomissing, PA*	Conditional 5	1.5, 3	
Opticath Catheter, Model U400, catheter *Abbott Laboratories, Morgan Hill, CA*	Unsafe 2	1.5	60
Opticath PA Catheter with extra port *Abbott Laboratories, Morgan Hill, CA*	Unsafe 2	1.5	60
Opticath PA Catheter with RV Pacing Port *Abbott Laboratories, Morgan Hill, CA*	Unsafe 2	1.5	60
Opti-Q SvO2/CCO *catheter,* *Abbott Laboratories, Morgan Hill, CA*	Unsafe 2	1.5	60
Oximetric 3, SO2 *Optical Module,* *Abbott Laboratories, Morgan Hill, CA*	Unsafe 2	1.5	60
Palindrome Sapphire HD Catheter *Covidien, Mansfield, MA*	Conditional 6	3	
PolyFlow Peripherally Inserted Catheter *Smiths Medical, St. Paul, MN*	Safe	3	
RV Pacing Lead *Abbott Laboratories, Morgan Hill, CA*	Unsafe 2	1.5	60
SecurACath, PICC Catheter with Nitinol Securement *Interrad Medical, Inc., St. Paul, MN*	Conditional 5	3	

Object	Status	Field Strength (T)	Reference
StimuCath Continuous Peripheral Nerve Block (CPNB) Catheter *Regional Anesthesia Device,* *Teleflex Medical, Wyomissing, PA*	Conditional 5	1.5, 3	
Swan-Ganz thermodilution Catheter *American Edwards, Laboratories, Irvine, CA*	Unsafe 2	1.5	57
Swan-Ganz triple-lumen thermodilution catheter *American Edwards Laboratories, Irvine, CA*	Unsafe 2	1.5	60
TD Thermodilution Catheter *Flow-directed thermodilution pulmonary artery catheter,* *Abbott Laboratories, Morgan Hill, CA*	Unsafe 2	1.5	60
TDQ CCO Catheter *Flow-directed thermodilution continuous,* *cardiac output pulmonary artery catheter,* *Abbott Laboratories, Morgan Hill, CA*	Unsafe 2	1.5	60
Torque-Line Flow-directed *thermodilution pulmonary artery catheter,* *Abbott Laboratories, Morgan Hill, CA*	Unsafe 2	1.5	60
Transpac IV *Abbott Laboratories, Morgan Hill, CA*	Safe	1.5	60
TruFlow Hemodialysis Catheter *Smiths Medical, St. Paul, MN*	Safe	3	
VENTRA Percutaneous Intravenous Catheter *Smiths Medical, St. Paul, MN*	Safe	3	

Carotid Artery Vascular Clamps

Object	Status	Field Strength (T)	Reference
Crutchfield *SS, carotid artery vascular clamp,* *Codman, Randolf, MA*	Conditional 1	1.5	11
Kindt *SS, carotid artery vascular clamp,* *V. Mueller*	Conditional 1	1.5	11
Poppen-Blaylock *SS, carotid artery vascular clamp,* *Codman, Randolf, MA*	Unsafe 1	1.5	11
Salibi *SS, carotid artery vascular clamp,* *Codman, Randolf, MA*	Conditional 1	1.5	11
Selverstone *SS, carotid artery vascular clamp,* *Codman, Randolf, MA*	Conditional 1	1.5	11

Object	Status	Field Strength (T)	Reference

Cerebrospinal Fluid (CSF) Shunt Valves and Accessories

Object	Status	Field Strength (T)	Reference
ACCU FLO Connector *Right Angle, 316L SS,* *Codman & Shurtleff, Inc., Raynham, MA*	Conditional 6	3	
ACCU FLO Connector *Right Angle, Plastic,* *Codman & Shurtleff, Inc., Raynham, MA*	Safe	3	
ACCU-FLO Connector *Straight, 316L SS,* *Codman & Shurtleff, Inc., Raynham, MA*	Conditional 6	3	
ACCU-FLO Connector *Straight, Plastic,* *Codman & Shurtleff, Inc., Raynham, MA*	Safe	3	
ACCU-FLO Connector *Three Way, 316L SS,* *Codman & Shurtleff, Inc., Raynham, MA*	Conditional 6	3	
ACCU-FLO Connector *Three Way, Plastic,* *Codman & Shurtleff, Inc., Raynham, MA*	Safe	3	
Accura II *Adult Integral Shunt System,* *Phoenix Biomedical Corporation, Valley Forge, PA*	Safe	1.5	103
Accura II *Pediatric Integral Shunt System,* *Phoenix Biomedical Corporation, Valley Forge, PA*	Safe	1.5	102
BUS Device *Ventriculo-peritoneal shunt,* *Codman, Raynham, MA*	Conditional 6	3	
Cerebral ventricular shunt tube connector, *Accu-flow right angle,* *Codman, Randolf, MA*	Safe	1.5	3, 94, 95
Cerebral ventricular shunt tube connector, *Accu-Flow, straight,* *Codman, Randolf, MA*	Safe	1.5	3, 94, 95
Cerebral ventricular shunt tube connector, *Accu-flow, T-connector,* *Codman, Randolf, MA*	Safe	1.5	3, 94, 95
Codman EDS CSF *External Drainage System,* *Codman,* *a Johnson and Johnson Company, Raynham, MA*	Safe	1.5, 3	103

Object	Status	Field Strength (T)	Reference
Codman HAKIM Programmable Valve *Codman,* *a Johnson and Johnson Company, Raynham, MA*	Conditional 5	1.5, 3	110
CODMAN MEDOS Right Angle Connector *also known as CODMAN Hakim Right Angle Connector,* *Codman & Shurtleff, Inc., Raynham, MA*	Conditional 6	3	
CODMAN MEDOS Straight Connector *also known as CODMAN Hakim Straight Connector,* *Codman & Shurtleff, Inc., Raynham, MA*	Conditional 6	3	
Delta Shunt Assembly *Medtronic Neurosurgery, Goleta, CA*	Safe	3	96, 103
EDM ventricular catheter *External CSF Drainage Product,* *Medtronic Neurosurgery, Goleta, CA*	Safe	3	103
EDS 2 CSF External Drainage System *Codman,* *a Johnson and Johnson Company, Raynham, MA*	Safe	3	103
EDS 3 CSF External Drainage System *Codman,* *a Johnson and Johnson Company, Raynham, MA*	Safe	3	103
HOLTER Cerebral Catheter-Reservoir *LeRoy Design,* *Codman & Shurtleff, Inc., Raynham, MA*	Conditional 6	3	
HOLTER In Line Shunt Filter *Codman & Shurtleff, Inc., Raynham, MA*	Conditional 5	3	
HOLTER In Line Shunt Filter *Hoffman Design,* *Codman & Shurtleff, Inc., Raynham, MA*	Conditional 6	3	
HOLTER Reservoir *316L SS,* *Codman & Shurtleff, Inc., Raynham, MA*	Conditional 6	3	
HOLTER Rickham Reservoir *316L SS,* *Codman & Shurtleff, Inc., Raynham, MA*	Conditional 6	3	
HOLTER Rickham Reservoir *Plastic,* *Codman & Shurtleff, Inc., Raynham, MA*	Safe	3	
HOLTER Salmon-Rickham Ventriculostomy Reservoir *316L SS,* *Codman & Shurtleff, Inc., Raynham, MA*	Conditional 6	3	

Object	Status	Field Strength (T)	Reference
HOLTER Salmon-Rickham Ventriculostomy Reservoir *Plastic,* *Codman & Shurtleff, Inc., Raynham, MA*	Safe	3	
HOLTER Selker Ventriculostomy Reservoir *Plastic,* *Codman & Shurtleff, Inc., Raynham, MA*	Safe	3	
HOLTER Type A Connector *Codman & Shurtleff, Inc., Raynham, MA*	Conditional 6	3	
HOLTER Type B Connector *Codman & Shurtleff, Inc., Raynham, MA*	Conditional 6	3	
HOLTER Ventricular Catheter *Codman & Shurtleff, Inc., Raynham, MA*	Conditional 6	3	
HOLTER, Selker Valve *316L SS,* *Codman & Shurtleff, Inc., Raynham, MA*	Conditional 6	3	
POLARIS Adjustable Pressure Valve *Sophysa USA, Inc., Costa Mesa, CA*	Conditional 5	3	97, 103
proGAV Adjustable Valve *Aesculap, Inc., Center Valley, PA*	Conditional 5	3	104
PS Medical CSF-Flow Control Valve *Medtronic Neurosurgery, Goleta, CA*	Safe	1.5	96
PS Medical CSF-Ventricular Access Port *Medtronic Neurosurgery, Goleta, CA*	Safe	1.5	96
PS Medical CSF-Ventricular Reservoir *Medtronic Neurosurgery, Goleta, CA*	Safe	1.5	96
PS Medical CSF-Ventriculostomy Reservoir *Medtronic Neurosurgery, Goleta, CA*	Safe	1.5	96
PS Medical Strata Valve *adjustable cerebral spinal fluid valve,* *Medtronic Neurosurgery, Goleta, CA*	Conditional 5	1.5	96
Pulsar Valve *Sophysa USA, Inc., Costa Mesa, CA*	Safe	1.5	97
Rickham Reservoir *316L SS,* *Codman & Shurtleff, Inc., Raynham, MA*	Conditional 6	3	
Right Angle Connector *Nylon,* *Codman & Shurtleff, Inc., Raynham, MA*	Safe	3	
Selker Valve *316L SS,* *Codman & Shurtleff, Inc., Raynham, MA*	Conditional 6	3	

Object	Status	Field Strength (T)	Reference
Selker Valve *Nylon,* *Codman & Shurtleff, Inc., Raynham, MA*	Safe	3	
Shunt valve, Holter-Hausner type *Holter-Hausner, Inc., Bridgeport, PA*	Safe	1.5	55
Shunt valve, Holtertype *The Holter Co., Bridgeport, PA*	Unsafe 1	1.5	55
Sophy Adjustable Pressure Valve *Model SP3, Sophysa, Orsay, France*	Conditional 5	1.5	97
Sophy Adjustable Pressure Valve *Model SU8, Sophysa, Orsay, France*	Conditional 5	1.5	97
SOPHY Adjustable Pressure Valve *Sophysa USA, Inc., Costa Mesa, CA*	Conditional 5	1.5	97
Sophy Mini Monopressure Valve *Sophysa USA, Inc., Costa Mesa, CA*	Safe	1.5	97
Straight Connector *Nylon,* *Codman & Shurtleff, Inc., Raynham, MA*	Safe	3	
Strata II *Programmable CSF Shunt Valve,* *Medtronic Neurosurgery, Goleta, CA*	Conditional 5	3	
Strata NSC *Programmable CSF Shunt Valve,* *Medtronic Neurosurgery, Goleta, CA*	Conditional 5	3	
Strata *Programmable CSF Shunt Valve,* *Medtronic Neurosurgery, Goleta, CA*	Conditional 5	3	
Three Way Connector *Silicone, Nylon,* *Codman & Shurtleff, Inc., Raynham, MA*	Safe	3	

Coils, Stents, Filters, and Grafts

Object	Status	Field Strength (T)	Reference
AAA Endograft *TriVascular2, Inc., Santa Rosa, CA*	Conditional 6	3	
Absolute Biliary Stent *Abbott Vascular, www.abbottvascular.com*	Conditional 5	3	
Absolute Pro Stent *Nickel titanium with nickel titanium platinum markers,* *8-mm x 120-mm, Single version,* *Abbott Vascular, www.abbottvascular.com*	Conditional 6	3	
Absolute Pro Stent *Nickel titanium with nickel titanium platinum markers,* *8-mm x 348-mm, three overlapped version,* *Abbott Vascular, www.abbottvascular.com*	Conditional 6	3	

Object	Status	Field Strength (T)	Reference
Acculink Carotid Stent *Abbott Vascular, www.abbottvascular.com*	Conditional 5	3	
ACS MULTI-LINK Coronary Stent *Abbott Vascular, www.abbottvascular.com*	Conditional 5	3	
ACS Multi-Link RX Duet *18 x 3.0-mm, stent, 316L SS*	Safe	1.5	72
ACS MULTI-LINK DUET Coronary Stent *Abbott Vascular, www.abbottvascular.com*	Conditional 5	3	
ACS MULTI-LINK TRISTAR Coronary Stent *Abbott Vascular, www.abbottvascular.com*	Conditional 5	3	
ACS MULTI-LINK ULTRA Coronary Stent *Abbott Vascular, www.abbottvascular.com*	Conditional 5	3	
ACS RX Multi-Link *15 x 3.0-mm, stent, 316L SS*	Safe	1.5	72
ACS RX Multi-Link *15 x 4.0-mm, stent, 316L SS*	Safe	1.5	72
ACS RX Multi-Link *25 x 3.0-mm, stent, 316L SS*	Safe	1.5	72
ACS Stent *316L SS*	Safe	1.5	
ACURATE Stent *Symetis SA, Switzerland*	Conditional 6	3	
Adapt Carotid Stent *carotid artery stent, Nitinol, Tantalum,* *Endotex Interventional Systems, Inc., Cupertino, CA*	Conditional 6	3	
Advanta V12 Stent *Atrium Medical Corporation, Hudson, New Hampshire*	Conditional 6	3	
Aero Tracheal Stent *18-mm x 80-mm,* *Nickel Titanium with a polyurethane cover,* *AlveolUs, Inc., Charlotte, NC*	Conditional 6	3	
Aero Tracheal Stent *Nitinol with Polyurethane Cover,* *AlveolUs, Inc., Charlotte, NC*	Conditional 6	3	
ALIMAXX-B Covered Biliary Stent *10-mm x 80-mm, Nickel Titanium with a silicone covering,* *AlveolUs, Inc., Charlotte, NC*	Conditional 6	3	
ALIMAXX-B Uncovered Biliary Stent *10-mm x 80-mm, Nickel Titanium,* *AlveolUs, Inc., Charlotte, NC*	Conditional 6	3	
ALN Vena Cava Filter *316L SS, ALN Implants Chirurgicaux, France*	Conditional 6	3	

Object	Status	Field Strength (T)	Reference
Amplatz IVC filter *Cook, Inc., Bloomington, IN*	Safe	4.7	21
Anaconda Endovascular Device *Nitinol, Vascutek Ltd., Scotland*	Conditional 6	3	
ANCURE Endograft *stent*	Safe	1.5	
AneuRx AAA Stent Grafts System *Medtronic Vascular, Santa Rosa, CA*	Conditional 6	3	
AneuRx AAAdvantage Stent Grafts System *Medtronic Vascular, Santa Rosa, CA*	Safe	3	
AneuRx II Bifurcation Stent Graft *Medtronic Vascular, Santa Rosa, CA*	Safe	3	
Angiomed Memotherm Femoral *stent, 4-mm x 120-mm, Nitinol,* *C.R. Bard, Inc., Billerica, MA*	Safe	1.5	
Angiomed Memotherm Femoral *stent, 5-mm x 20-mm, Nitinol,* *C.R. Bard, Inc., Billerica, MA*	Safe	1.5	
Angiomed Memotherm Iliac *stent, 12-mm x 110-mm, Nitinol,* *C.R. Bard, Inc., Billerica, MA*	Safe	1.5	
Angiomed Memotherm Iliac *stent, 8-mm x 20-mm, Nitinol,* *C.R. Bard, Inc., Billerica, MA*	Safe	1.5	
AngioStent *stent, 15-mm, Platinum, iridium,* *Angiodynamics, Queensbury, NY*	Safe	1.5	
Aorfix Bifurcated Stent Graft system *Lombard Medical, www.LombardMedical.com*	Conditional 5	3	
APOLLO Cerebral Stent *316LVM SS,* *MicroPort Medical Co., Ltd., People's Republic of China*	Conditional 6	3	
aSpire Covered Stent *100 x 14-mm, Nitinol, nickel, Titanium,* *Vascular Architects, Portola, CA*	Safe	1.5	
aSpire II stent *Nitinol with an ePTFE covering,* *Vascular Architects, Inc., San Jose, CA*	Safe	3	
Assurant Cobalt Iliac Stent *single and two overlapped versions,* *Medtronic, Inc., www.Medtronic.com*	Conditional 8	1.5, 3	
Astron Biliary Stent *Nitinol, gold markers,* *BIOTRONIK GmbH & Co., Berlin, Germany*	Safe	3	

Object	Status	Field Strength (T)	Reference
AVE GFX Stent *316L SS,* *Arterial Vascular Engineering, Santa Rosa, CA*	Safe	1.5	69
AVE Micro I Stent *316L SS, Arterial Vascular Engineering, Santa Rosa, CA*	Safe	1.5	69
AVE Micro II Stent *316L SS,* *Arterial Vascular Engineering, Santa Rosa, CA*	Safe	1.5	69
AXIUM Detachable Coil *embolization coil,* *ev3, Inc., http://www.ev3.net*	Condiitional 5	3	
Axium Detachable Implant for *Neurovascular Malformation, Embolization coil,* *ev3 Neurovascular, Irvine, CA*	Conditional 6	3	
Axxess Biolimus A9 *Eluting Bifurcation Stent, coronary artery stent, Nitinol,* *Devax, Inc., Irvine, CA*	Conditional 6	3	
Axxess Stent *coronary artery stent, Nitinol,* *Devax, Inc., Irvine, CA*	Safe	3	
BARD CONFORMEXX *Biliary Stent, 12 x 120-mm, Nitinol,* *C. R. Bard, Angiomed GmbH & Co. Medizintechnik KG,* *Karlsruhe, Germany*	Safe	1.5, 3	83
Bard DeBakey Woven Graft *PET Polyester,* *Bard Peripheral Vascular, Tempe, AZ*	Safe	3	
Bard E LUMINEXX Vascular Stent *Bard Peripheral Vascular, www.bardpv.com*	Condiitional 5	3	
Bard LifeStent FlexStar XL Stent *Bard Peripheral Vascular, www.bardpv.com*	Conditional 5	1.5, 3	
Bard LUMINEXX 3 *Biliary and Vascular Stent, Nitinol, tantalum,* *14-mm x 120-mm,* *C. R. Bard, Angiomed GmbH & Co. Medizintechnik KG,* *Karlsruhe, Germany*	Safe	1.5, 3	
BARD LUMINEXX *Biliary and Vascular Stent, 12 x 120-mm, Nitinol, tantalum,* *C. R. Bard, Angiomed GmbH & Co. Medizintechnik KG,* *Karlsruhe, Germany*	Safe	1.5, 3	83
Bard Stent, bifurcated *36 x 20-mm, Nitinol*	Safe	1.5	70

Object	Status	Field Strength (T)	Reference
Bard ViVEXX Carotid Stent *Nitinol,* *C. R. Bard, Angiomed GmbH & Co. Medizintechnik KG,* *Karlsruhe, Germany*	Safe	3	
Bard XT Stent *15 x 3.0-mm, 316 LVM,* *Bard Interventional Products, Billerica, MA*	Safe	1.5	72
Bard XT Stent *316 LVM,* *Bard Limited, Ireland*	Safe	1.5	69
Bernstein Fluid Coil *embolization coil, MicroVention, Inc., Alison Viejo, CA*	Conditional 6	3	
BeStent *15 x 3.0-mm, 316L SS, stent,* *Medtronic AVE, Minneapolis, MN*	Safe	1.5	72
BeStent *25 x 3.0-mm, 316L SS, stent,* *Medtronic AVE, Minneapolis, MN*	Safe	1.5	72
BeStent *MR-safe SS, stent,* *Medtronic, Inc., Minneapolis, MN*	Safe	1.5	69
Bifurcated EXCLUDER Endoprosthesis *Nitinol, stent,* *W.L. Gore and Associates, Inc., www.goremedical.com*	Safe	1.5	
BIOFLEX Stent *coronary artery stent, 316L SS,* *Biosensors International, La Jolla, CA*	Safe	3	
BioMatrix Flex Stent *Biosensors International - USA, La Jolla, CA*	Conditional 8	1.5, 3	
Bridge Constant Stent *cobalt alloy, stent,* *Medtronic Vascular, Santa Rosa, CA*	Safe	3	
BX Stent *316L SS,* *Cordis, Miami Lakes, FL*	Safe	1.5	69
BX Velocity Balloon-Expander *Intracranial Intravascular stent, 4.0-mm x 8-mm,* *Cordis, Miami Lakes, FL*	Safe	1.5, 3	83
Carotid WALLSTENT Endoprosthesis *Boston Scientific, www.bostonscientific.com*	Conditional 5	3	
CASHMERE Microcoil *embolization coil,* *Micrus Endovascular,* *http://www.micrusendovascular.com*	Conditional 5	3	

Object	Status	Field Strength (T)	Reference
Celect Vena Cava Filter *Cook Medical Inc.,* *http://www.cookmedical.com/di/productMri.do*	Conditional 6	3	
CenterFlex Vascular Graft *Carbon-impregnated ePTFE,* *Bard Peripheral Vascular, Tempe, AZ*	Safe	3	
Chromaxx BX Stent *Cobalt Chromium Alloy (Phynox),* *Angiomed GmbH & Co.,* *Karlsruhe, Germany*	Conditional 6	3	
Cinatra Cobalt-Chromium *coronary artery stent,* *Atrium Medical Corporation, Hudson, NH*	Conditional 8	1.5, 3	
Cobra BMS *Bare Metal Stent, L605 Cobalt Chrome,* *Medlogics Device Corporation, Santa Rosa, CA*	Conditional 6	3	
Cobra Stent *MEDLOGICS Device Corporation, Santa Rosa, CA*	Conditional 6	3	
Coherex FlatStent EF *Coherex Medical, Salt Lake City, UT*	Conditional 6	3	
Complete SE Stent *Nitinol, Tantalum,* *Medtronic Vascular, Santa Rosa, CA*	Conditional 6	3	
Cook Celect Vena Cava Filter *Cook Medical, Inc.,* *http://www.cookmedical.com/di/productMri.do*	Conditional 5	3	
Cook occluding spring embolization coil *MWCE- 338-5-10,* *Cook, Inc., Bloomington, IN*	Conditional 2	1.5	
Cook-Z Stent *Gianturco-Rosch Biliary Design, 10-mm x 30-mm,* *Cook, Inc., Bloomington, IN*	Conditional 2	1.5	
Cook-Z Stent *Gianturco-Rosch Tracheobronchial Design,* *20-mm x 5-cm,* *Cook, Inc., Bloomington, IN*	Conditional 2	1.5	
CORDIS ENTERPRISE Vascular Reconstruction Device *Cordis,* *a Johnson and Johnson Co., www.cordis.com*	Conditional 5	3	
CoRectCoil *Nitinol, stent,* *Intratherapeutics, Inc., St. Paul, MN*	Safe	1.5	

Object	Status	Field Strength (T)	Reference
Corvita Endoluminal *Graft for Abdominal, Aortic Aneurysm, 27-mm x 120-mm,* *Schneider (USA) Inc.,* *Pfizer Medical Technology Group, Minneapolis, MN*	Safe	1.5	64
CoStar *Coronary Stent, Cobalt Chromium,* *Conor Medsystems, Menlo Park, CA*	Safe	3	
CoStar *Paclitaxel-Eluting Coronary Stent,* *Conor Medsystems, Menlo Park, CA*	Safe	3	
Covered UltraFlex Esophageal Stent *23-mm diameter x 12-cm length,* *Nitinol stent with polyurethane covering,* *Boston Scientific Corporation, Natick, MA*	Safe	1.5	
Covered WallFlex Biliary RX Stent *Boston Scientific Corporation, Marlborough, MA*	Conditional 6	3	
Cragg Nitinol Spiral Filter	Safe	4.7	21
Cristallo Ideale Carotid Self-Expanding Stent *Conical version, Nitinol,* *Invatec Technology Center GmbH, Thurgau, Switzerland*	Conditional 6	3	
Cristallo Ideale Carotid Self-Expanding Stent *Cylindrical version, Nitinol,* *Invatec Technology Center GmbH, Thurgau, Switzerland*	Conditional 6	3	
Crossflex Stent *316L SS,* *Cordis, Miami, FL*	Safe	1.5	69
Crown Stent *316L SS,* *Cordis, Miami, FL*	Safe	1.5	69
Crux Filter *Vena cava filter, Nitinol,* *Crux Biomedical, Inc., Portola Valley, CA*	Conditional 6	3	
Cypher Select *Sirolimus-Eluting Stent,* *Cordis, Miami Lakes, FL*	Conditional 5	3	
CYPHER Sirolimus-eluting Coronary Stent *Cordis,* *a Johnson and Johnson Co., www.cordis.com*	Conditional 5	3	
DELTAPAQ Microcoil *embolization coil,* *Micrus Endovascular,* *http://www.micrusendovascular.com*	Conditional 5	3	

Object	Status	Field Strength (T)	Reference
Diamond Colonic Stent *26-mm diameter x 10-cm length,* *Nitinol stent with Platinum/iridium markers,* *Boston Scientific Corporation, Natick, MA*	Safe	1.5	
Distaflo Bypass Graft *Carbon-impregnated ePTFE,* *Bard Peripheral Vascular, Tempe, AZ*	Safe	3	
DISTAFLO Bypass Graft *Carbon-impregnated ePTFE,* *Bard Peripheral Vascular, Tempe, AZ*	Safe	3	
Diverter Stent *8-mm x 32-mm, Elgiloy (Conichrome), Tantalum,* *MindGuard, Ltd., Israel*	Safe	1.5	
Double-J Closed Tip *Ureteral Stent, Silicone,* *Gyrus ACMI, Inc., Maple Grove, MN*	Safe	3	
Double-J II Closed Tip *Ureteral Stent, Polyurethane,* *Gyrus ACMI, Inc., Maple Grove, MN*	Safe	3	
Double Pigtail Ureteral Stent *Polyurethane,* *Gyrus ACMI, Inc., Maple Grove, MN*	Safe	3	
Double Pigtail Ureteral Stent *Hydrophilic Coated, Polyurethane,* *Gyrus ACMI, Inc., Maple Grove, MN*	Safe	3	
Driver Sprint Stent *Medtronic, Inc., www.Medtronic.com*	Conditional 5	3	
Driver Stent *Including Driver RX, Driver MXII, MicroDriver,* *MicroDriver MXII, MicroDriver RX, Coronary Stent,* *Medtronic, Inc., www.Medtronic.com,* *http://manuals.medtronic.com/en/index.htm*	Conditional 5	3	
Duraflex SE Stent *Nickel Titanium alloy, Tantalum,* *Flexible Stenting Solutions, Inc., Eatontown, NJ*	Conditional 8	1.5, 3	
Dynaflo Bypass Graft *Bard Peripheral Vascular, www.bardpv.com*	Safe	1.5	
Dynalink Biliary Stent *Abbott Vascular, www.abbottvascular.com*	Conditional 5	3	
DYNALINK Stent *10-mm x 100-mm, Nickel/Titanium*	Safe	1.5, 3	
DYNALINK Stent *5-mm x 100-mm, Nickel/Titanium*	Safe	1.5, 3	

Object	Status	Field Strength (T)	Reference
DYNALINK Stent *5 to 10-mm (OTW), Nitinol*	Safe	1.5	
DYNALINK E Stent *drug eluting stent*	Conditional 6	3	
Dynamic Biliary Stent *316L SS,* *BIOTRONIK GmBH & Co., Berlin, Germany*	Safe	3	
Dynamic Renal Stent *cobalt chromium,* *BIOTRONIK GmBH & Co., Berlin, Germany*	Conditional 6	3	
Embolization Coil *IMWCE-38-15-15, Inconel, coil,* *Cook, Inc., Bloomington, IN*	Safe	3	
Embolization Coil *IMWCE-38-20-15, Inconel, coil,* *Cook, Inc., Bloomington, IN*	Safe	3	
Embolization Coil *MWCE-38-14-12 NESTER, Platinum, Inconel, coil,* *Cook, Inc., Bloomington, IN*	Safe	3	
Embolization Coil, Stainless Steel *Cook Medical, Inc.,* *www.cookmedical.com/di/productMri.do*	Unsafe 1	1.5	
Endeavor Drug Eluting Stent *cobalt alloy, stent,* *Medtronic Vascular, Santa Rosa, CA*	Conditional 5	3	88
Endeavor Resolute Zotarolimus-Eluting Coronary Stent *Medtronic, Inc., www.Medtronic.com*	Conditional 5	3	
Endeavor Stent *Including Endeavor Sprint, Endeavor MXII,* *Endeavor Zotarolimus Eluting Coronary Stent,* *Medtronic, Inc., www.Medtronic.com*	Conditional 5	3	
EndoCoil *Nitinol, stent,* *Intratherapeutics, Inc., St. Paul, MN*	Safe	1.5	
EndoCoil-T *Nitinol, stent,* *Intratherapeutics, Inc., St. Paul, MN*	Safe	1.5	
EndoFit Endoluminal Stent Graft *Cuff(C), ENDOMED, Inc., Phoenix, AZ*	Safe	1.5	
EndoFit Endoluminal Stent Graft *Extender (E), ENDOMED, Inc., Phoenix, AZ*	Safe	1.5	
EndoFit Endoluminal Stent Graft *Occluder (O), ENDOMED, Inc., Phoenix, AZ*	Safe	1.5	

Object	Status	Field Strength (T)	Reference
EndoFit Endoluminal Stent Graft *Tapered Aortomonoiliac (A), ENDOMED, Inc., Phoenix, AZ*	Safe	1.5	
EndoFit Endoluminal Stent Graft *Thoracic (T), ENDOMED, Inc., Phoenix, AZ*	Safe	1.5	
Endurant Stent Graft *Medtronic, Inc., www.Medtronic.com,* *http://manuals.medtronic.com/en/index.htm*	Conditional 5	1.5, 3	
Enforcer Stent *316L SS, Cardiovascular Dynamics, Inc.*	Safe	1.5	
Enovus AAA Bifurcated Stent Graft *Nitinol, stent, TriVascular, Inc., Santa Rosa, CA*	Safe	3	
Enovus Iliac Stent Graft *Boston Scientific Corporation, Watertown, MA*	Conditional 6	3	
Enterprise Stent *Nitinol with tantalum markers,* *Cordis Neurovascular, Inc., Miami Lakes, FL*	Safe	3	
EsophaCoil-SR *Nitinol, stent,* *Intratherapeutics, Inc., St. Paul, MN*	Safe	1.5	
Eta-2 TA Stent *Nitinol, Tantalum, Angiomed GmbH & Co., Germany*	Conditional 6	3	
Evolution Colonic Stent *Nitinol wire, Tantalum marker bands, Silicone elastomer,* *MED Institute, West Lafayette, IN*	Conditional 6	3	
Evolution Esophageal Stent *Nitinol, Cook Endoscopy, Winston-Salem, NC*	Conditional 8	1.5, 3	
EXCLUDER Bifurcated Endoprosthesis *W.L. Gore & Associates, Inc., www.goremedical.com*	Safe	3	
Exhale Drug Eluting Stent *Broncus Technologies, Inc., Mountain View, CA*	Conditional 6	3	
Exponent Carotid Stent *Nitinol,* *Medtronic Vascular, Santa Rosa, CA*	Safe	3	
Express Biliary SD Stent *Boston Scientific, http://www.bostonscientific.com*	Conditional 5	3	
Express LD Stent *316L SS,* *http://www.bostonscientific.com*	Conditional 5	3	
Express SD Stent *316L SS,* *http://www.bostonscientific.com*	Conditional 5	3	
Express2 Coronary Stent *Boston Scientific, http://www.bostonscientific.com*	Conditional 5	3	

Object	Status	Field Strength (T)	Reference
Fanelli Laparoscopic Endobiliary Stent *Stent, Cook Surgical Products, Bloomington, IN*	Safe	1.5	
Filiform Double Pigtail *Silicone Stent, Cook Urological, Inc., Spencer, IN*	Safe	1.5	
FLAIR Endovascular Stent Graft *Bard Peripheral Vascular, www.bardpv.com*	Conditional 5	3	
Flamingo Wallstent Esophageal Endoprosthesis *Elgiloy,* *Schneider GmbH, Bulach, Switzerland*	Safe	1.5	
Flower Embolization Microcoil *Platinum,* *Target Therapeutics, San Jose, CA*	Safe	1.5	22
FLUENCY Plus Tracheobronchial Stent Graft *Nitinol with tantalum markers,* *C. R. Bard, Angiomed GmbH & Co. Medizintechnik KG,* *Karlsruhe, Germany*	Safe	3	
FLUENCY Plus Vascular Stent Graft *Nitinol with tantalum markers,* *C. R. Bard, Angiomed GmbH & Co. Medizintechnik KG,* *Karlsruhe, Germany*	Safe	3	
FLUENCY Vascular and Tracheobronchial Stent Grafts *10-mm x 80-mm, Nitinol,* *C. R. Bard, Angiomed GmbH & Co. Medizintechnik KG,* *Karlsruhe, Germany*	Safe	1.5	
Formula 418 Balloon Expandable Biliary Stent *Cook Medical, Inc.,* *http://www.cookmedical.com/di/productMri.do*	Conditional 5	3	
G2 Express Vena Cava Filter *Bard Peripheral Vascular, Tempe, AZ*	Conditional 6	3	
G2 Filter *Vena Cava Filter, Femoral Vein,* *Bard Peripheral Vascular, www.bardpv.com*	Conditional 5	1.5	
G2 X Filter *Vena Cava Filter, Femoral Vein,* *Bard Peripheral Vascular, www.bardpv.com*	Conditional 5	3	
G2 X Filter *Vena Cava Filter, Jugular Vein,* *Bard Peripheral Vascular, www.bardpv.com*	Conditional 5	3	
GDC 3D Shape *various sizes, Platinum,* *Boston Scientific/Target, Wayne, NJ*	Safe	1.5	
GDC Detachable Coil *GDC 10-3D, 3-D Shape, Platinum alloy, coil,* *Boston Scientific Corporation, Fremont, CA*	Safe	3	

Object	Status	Field Strength (T)	Reference
GDC Detachable Coil *GDC 10-Soft, Platinum alloy, coil,* *Boston Scientific Corporation, Fremont, CA*	Safe	3	
GDC Detachable Coil *GDC 10-Standard, Platinum alloy, coil,* *Boston Scientific Corporation, Fremont, CA*	Safe	3	
GDC Detachable Coil *GDC 18-2D, 2 Diameter, Platinum alloy, coil,* *Boston Scientific Corporation, Fremont, CA*	Safe	3	
GDC Detachable Coil *GDC 18-3D, 3-D Shape, Platinum alloy, coil,* *Boston Scientific Corporation, Fremont, CA*	Safe	3	
GDC Detachable Coil *GDC 18-Soft, Platinum alloy, coil,* *Boston Scientific Corporation, Fremont, CA*	Safe	3	
GDC Detachable Coil *GDC 18-Standard, Platinum alloy, coil,* *Boston Scientific Corporation, Fremont, CA*	Safe	3	
GDC Detachable Coil *GDC 2D, 2 Diameter, Platinum alloy, coil,* *Boston Scientific Corporation, Fremont, CA*	Safe	3	
GDC TriSpan Coil *14-mm, Nitinol, Platinum, coil,* *Boston Scientific Corporation-Target, Fremont, CA*	Safe	1.5, 3	
GDC TriSpan Coil *16-mm, Nitinol, Platinum, coil,* *Boston Scientific Corporation-Target, Fremont, CA*	Safe	1.5, 3	
GDC *18-Fibered VortX Shape, Platinum alloy, coil,* *Boston Scientific Corporation, Fremont, CA*	Safe	3	
GDC *Stretch Resistant Detachable Coil, GDC 10-Soft 2D SR,* *Platinum alloy, coil,* *Boston Scientific Corporation, Fremont, CA*	Safe	3	
GDC *Stretch Resistant Detachable Coil, GDC 10-Soft SR,* *Platinum alloy, coil,* *Boston Scientific Corporation, Fremont, CA*	Safe	3	
GDC *Stretch Resistant Detachable Coil, GDC 10-UltraSoft SR,* *Platinum alloy, coil,* *Boston Scientific Corporation, Fremont, CA*	Safe	3	
GDC *TriSpan Coil, Platinum alloy, Nitinol, coil,* *Boston Scientific Corporation, Fremont, CA*	Safe	3	

Object	Status	Field Strength (T)	Reference
Genous Bio-Engineered R Stent *316L SS,* *OrbusNeich Medical, Inc., Fort Lauderdale, FL*	Conditional 6	3	
Genous Bio-engineered R Stent *coronary artery stent,* *OrbusNeich Medical, Inc., Fort Lauderdale, FL*	Conditional 6	3	
Gianturco bird nest IVC filter *Cook, Inc., Bloomington, IN*	Conditional 2	1.5	21
Gianturco zig-zag stent *Cook, Inc., Bloomington, IN*	Conditional 2	1.5	21
Gianturco-Roehm Bird's Nest Vena Cava Filter *Cook Medical Inc.,* *http://www.cookmedical.com/di/productMri.do*	Conditional 6	3	
Gianturco-Roubin II *20 x 3.0-mm, stent, 316L SS,* *Cook, Bloomington, IN*	Safe	1.5	72
Gianturco-Roubin Flex Stent *Coronary Artery Stent,* *Cook Medical, Inc.,* *http://www.cookmedical.com/di/productMri.do*	Conditional 5	3	
Gianturco-Roubin Stent *316L SS, Cook, Bloomington, IN*	Safe	1.5	69
Goldvalve Detachable Balloon *Coils, Filters, Stents,* *NFocus Neuromedical, Palo Alto, CA*	Conditional 6	3	
GORE EXCLUDER AAA Endoprosthesis *Stent Graft,* *W.L. Gore & Associates, Inc., www.goremedical.com*	Conditional 8	1.5, 3	
GORE Intering Vascular Graft *W.L. Gore & Associates, http://www.goremedical.com*	Safe	1.5	
GORE MYCROMESH Biomaterial *W.L. Gore & Associates, http://www.goremedical.com*	Safe	1.5	
GORE MYCROMESH PLUS Biomaterial *W.L. Gore & Associates, http://www.goremedical.com*	Safe	1.5	
GORE PRECLUDE Pericardial Membrane *W.L. Gore & Associates, http://www.goremedical.com*	Safe	1.5	
GORE PROPATEN Vascular Graft *W.L. Gore & Associates, http://www.goremedical.com*	Safe	1.5	
Gore TAG Thoracic Endoprosthesis *W. L. Gore & Associates, Inc., www.goremedical.com*	Conditional 6	1.5, 3	
GORE-TEX Stretch Vascular Graft *W.L. Gore & Associates, http://www.goremedical.com*	Safe	1.5	

Object	Status	Field Strength (T)	Reference
GORE-TEX Vascular Graft *W.L. Gore & Associates, http://www.goremedical.com*	Safe	1.5	
Gore TIPS Endoprosthesis *W. L. Gore & Associates, Inc., www.goremedical.com*	Safe	1.5	
Greenfield vena cava filter *SS,* *MD Tech, Watertown, MA*	Conditional 2	1.5	21
Greenfield vena cava filter *Titanium alloy,* *Ormco, Glendora, CA*	Safe	1.5	21
GTX Coronary Artery Stent *CoCr,* *Global Therapeutics, Broomfield, CO*	Conditional 8	1.5, 3	
Guglielmi detachable coil *Platinum,* *Target Therapeutics, San Jose, CA*	Safe	1.5	25
Gunther IVC Filter *William Cook, Europe*	Conditional 2	1.5	21
Gunther Tulip Vena Cava Filter *Cook Medical Inc.,* *http://www.cookmedical.com/di/productMri.do*	Conditional 6	3	
Gunther Tulip Vena Cava Filter *Conichrome, Cook Incorporated, Bloomington, IN*	Conditional 5	3	
Gunther Tulip Vena Cava MReye Filter *Conichrome,* *Cook Incorporated, Bloomington, IN*	Conditional 5	3	
HELIPAQ Microcoil *embolization coil,* *Micrus Endovascular,* *http://www.micrusendovascular.com*	Conditional 5	3	
HERCULINK ELITE *Stent*	Conditional 5	3	
Herculink Elite Biliary Stent *Abbott Vascular, www.abbottvascular.com*	Conditional 5	3	
Herculink Plus Biliary Stent *Abbott Vascular, www.abbottvascular.com*	Conditional 5	3	
Hilal Embolization Microcoils *Cook Medical, Inc.,* *http://www.cookmedical.com/di/productMri.do*	Conditional 5	3	
Horizon Prostatic Stent *Nitinol, Endocare, Irvine, CA*	Safe	1.5	
ICAST Stent *Atrium Medical Corporation, Hudson, NH*	Conditional 6	3	

Object	Status	Field Strength (T)	Reference
Iliac Wallgraft Endoprosthesis *12 x 90,* *Schneider (USA) Inc.,* *Pfizer Medical Technology Group, Minneapolis, MN*	Safe	1.5	64
Iliac Wallstent Endoprosthesis *5 x 80,* *Schneider (USA) Inc.,* *Pfizer Medical Technology Group, Minneapolis, MN*	Safe	1.5	64
Iliac Wallstent Endoprosthesis *6 X 90,* *Schneider (USA) Inc.,* *Pfizer Medical Technology Group, Minneapolis, MN*	Safe	1.5	64
IMPRA Carboflo Vascular Graft *Carbon-impregnated ePTFE,* *Bard Peripheral Vascular, Tempe, AZ*	Safe	3	
IMPRA CenterFlex Vascular Graft *Carbon-impregnated ePTFE,* *Bard Peripheral Vascular, Tempe, AZ*	Safe	3	
Inflow Gold *15 x 3.0-mm, 316L SS, gold plate, stent,* *Inflow Dynamics, Munich, Germany*	Safe	1.5	72
Inflow Gold *9 x 3.0-mm, 316L SS, gold plate, stent,* *Inflow Dynamics, Munich, Germany*	Safe	1.5	72
Inflow Stent *316L SS, stent,* *Inflow Dynamics, Munich, Germany*	Safe	1.5	69
Inflow *15 x 3.0-mm, 316L SS, stent,* *Inflow Dynamics, Munich, Germany*	Safe	1.5	72
INTERPAQ Microcoil *embolization coil,* *Micrus Endovascular,* *http://www.micrusendovascular.com*	Conditional 5	3	
IntraCoil Bronchial Endoprosthesis *Nitinol, stent,* *Intratherapeutics, Inc., St. Paul, MN*	Safe	1.5	
IntraStent Biliary Endoprosthesis *stent,* *Intratherapeutics, Inc., St. Paul, MN*	Safe	1.5	
IntraStent DoubleStrut Biliary Endoprosthesis *stent,* *Intratherapeutics, Inc., St. Paul, MN*	Safe	1.5	

Object	Status	Field Strength (T)	Reference
IntraStent LP Biliary Endoprosthesis *stent,* *Intratherapeutics, Inc., St. Paul, MN*	Safe	1.5	
IntraStent Max LD Biliary Stent *ev3, Inc., http://www.ev3.net*	Conditional 5	1.5	
IntraStent Mega LD Biliary Stent *ev3, Inc., http://www.ev3.net*	Conditional 5	1.5	
Jostent *316L SS,* *Jomed, Helsingborg, Sweden*	Safe	1.5	69
Kaneka Stent, Model GGH008 *coronary artery stent,* *Kaneka Corporation, Japan*	Conditional 6	3	
L605 Stent *Promed Medical Tech, China*	Conditional 6	3	
LEO Plus Next Generation Self-Expanding Intracranial Stent *BALT, France*	Conditional 5	1.5, 3	
LGM IVC Filter *Phynox,* *B. Braun Vena Tech, Evanston, IL*	Safe	1.5	26
Liberte Coronary Artery Stent *316L SS,* *Boston Scientific Corporation, Maple Grove, MN*	Conditional 5	3	
LifeStent FlexStar Stent *Nitinol, Tantalum,* *Edwards Lifesciences, Irvine, CA*	Conditional 6	3	
LifeStent FlexStar XL Stent *Nitinol,* *Edwards Lifesciences, Irvine, CA*	Conditional 6	3	
LifeStent XL Balloon Expandable Stent *biliary and peripheral vascular stent, 316L SS,* *Edwards Lifesciences, Irvine, CA*	Conditional 6	3	
LithoStent Ureteral Stent *Polyurethane,* *Gyrus ACMI, Inc., Maple Grove, MN*	Safe	3	
LPS Stent, bifurcated *36 x 20-mm, Nitinol,* *World Medical Manufacturing Corp., Sunrise, FL*	Safe	1.5	70
LPS Thoracic Stent *46mm, Nitinol,* *World Medical Manufacturing Corp., Sunrise, FL*	Safe	1.5	70

Object	Status	Field Strength (T)	Reference
Lubri-Flex Open Tip *Ureteral Stent, Polyurethane,* *Gyrus ACMI, Inc., Maple Grove, MN*	Safe	3	
Maas Helical Endovascular Stent *Medinvent, Lausanne, Switzerland*	Safe	4.7	21
Maas Helical IVC Filter *Medinvent, Lausanne, Switzerland*	Safe	4.7	21
MAC-Stent *17 x 3-mm, 316L SS, stent,* *AMG, Munich, Germany*	Safe	1.5	72
Magic Wallstent *Platinum and cobalt-alloy, stent,* *Schneider, Bulach, Switzerland*	Safe	1.5	69
Matrix *Detachable Coil, Matrix Extra Firm-2D, Platinum alloy, coil,* *Boston Scientific Corporation, Fremont, CA*	Safe	3	
Matrix *Detachable Coil, Matrix Extra Firm-3D, Platinum alloy, coil,* *Boston Scientific Corporation, Fremont, CA*	Safe	3	
Matrix *Detachable Coil, Matrix Firm-2D, Platinum alloy, coil,* *Boston Scientific Corporation, Fremont, CA*	Safe	3	
Matrix *Detachable Coil, Matrix Firm-3D, Platinum alloy, coil,* *Boston Scientific Corporation, Fremont, CA*	Safe	3	
Matrix *Detachable Coil, Matrix Soft Helical, Platinum alloy, coil,* *Boston Scientific Corporation, Fremont, CA*	Safe	3	
Matrix *Detachable Coil, Matrix Soft-2D, Platinum alloy, coil,* *Boston Scientific Corporation, Fremont, CA*	Safe	3	
Matrix *Detachable Coil, Matrix Standard-2D, Platinum alloy, coil,* *Boston Scientific Corporation, Fremont, CA*	Safe	3	
Matrix *Detachable Coil, Matrix Standard-3D, Platinum alloy, coil,* *Boston Scientific Corporation, Fremont, CA*	Safe	3	
Matrix *Stretch Resistant Detachable Coil, Matrix Soft-SR 2D,* *Platinum alloy, coil,* *Boston Scientific Corporation, Fremont, CA*	Safe	3	

Object	Status	Field Strength (T)	Reference
Matrix *Stretch Resistant Detachable Coil, Matrix Soft-SR, Platinum alloy, coil, Boston Scientific Corporation, Fremont, CA*	Safe	3	
Matrix *Stretch Resistant Detachable Coil, Matrix Standard-SR 2D, Platinum alloy, coil, Boston Scientific Corporation, Fremont, CA*	Safe	3	
Matrix *Stretch Resistant Detachable Coil, Matrix UltraSoft-SR, Platinum alloy, coil, Boston Scientific Corporation, Fremont, CA*	Safe	3	
MC1 L30 *coronary artery stent, magnesium alloy, BIOTRONIK GmbH & Co, Berlin, Germany*	Safe	3	
Medtronic AVE Stent *316L SS, gold, Medtronic AVE, Ireland*	Safe	1.5	70
Megalink Biliary Stent *Abbott Vascular, www.abbottvascular.com*	Conditional 5	3	
Mercury Carotid Artery Stent *Nitinol, MicroPort Medical Co., Ltd., People's Republic of China*	Conditional 6	3	
Merlin MD Aneurysm Occlusion Device (AOD) *316L SS, gold markers, polyurethane, Merlin MD Pte Ltd, Singapore*	Conditional 6	3	
Micro Stent II *24 x 3.0-mm, 316L SS, stent, Medtronic AVE, Minneapolis, MN*	Safe	1.5	72
Micro-Driver Coronary Stent *Medtronic Vascular, Santa Rosa, CA*	Conditional 6	3	
Micro-Driver *MP35N, stent, Medtronic Vascular, Santa Rosa, CA*	Conditional 5	3	
MicroNester *Cook Medical, Inc., http://www.cookmedical.com/di/productMri.do*	Conditional 5	3	
MICRUSPHERE Microcoil *embolization coil, Micrus Endovascular, http://www.micrusendovascular.com*	Conditional 5	3	
Mini-Crown Stent *316L SS, Cordis, Miami, FL*	Safe	1.5	69

Object	Status	Field Strength (T)	Reference
Mobin-Uddin IVC/umbrella filter *American Edwards, Santa Ana, CA*	Safe	4.7	21
MReye Flipper Detachable Embolization Coils *Cook Medical, Inc.,* *http://www.cookmedical.com/di/productMri.do*	Conditional 5	3	
Multi-Flex Open Tip *Ureteral Stent, Polyurethane,* *Gyrus ACMI, Inc., Maple Grove, MN*	Safe	3	
MULTI-LINK DUET *Stent, 2.5 to 4.0-mm (RX and OTW), 316L SS,* *Abbott Vascular, www.abbottvascular.com*	Conditional 5	3	
MULTI-LINK MINI VISION Coronary Stent *Abbott Vascular, www.abbottvascular.com*	Conditional 5	3	
MULTI-LINK PENTA Coronary Stent *Abbott Vascular, www.abbottvascular.com*	Conditional 5	3	
MULTI-LINK PIXEL Coronary Stent *Abbott Vascular, www.abbottvascular.com*	Conditional 5	3	
MULTI-LINK TETRA Coronary Stent *Abbott Vascular, www.abbottvascular.com*	Conditional 5	3	
MULTI-LINK TRISTAR Stent *Abbott Vascular, www.abbottvascular.com*	Conditional 5	3	
MULTI-LINK VISION Coronary Stent *Abbott Vascular, www.abbottvascular.com*	Conditional 5	3	
MULTI-LINK ULTRA Stent *Abbott Vascular, www.abbottvascular.com*	Conditional 5	3	
MULTI-LINK ZETA Coronary Stent *Abbott Vascular, www.abbottvascular.com*	Conditional 5	3	
MULTI-LINK Stent *2.5 to 4.0-mm (RX and OTW), 316L SS,* *Abbott Vascular, www.abbottvascular.com*	Conditional 5	3	
NEC Hemi Device *Coils, Filters, Stents,* *NFocus Neuromedical, Palo Alto, CA*	Conditional 6	3	
Nellix AAA Endoprosthesis *Nellix Endovascular, Palo Alto, CA*	Conditional 8	1.5, 3	
Nester Embolization Coils *Cook Medical, Inc.,* *http://www.cookmedical.com/di/productMri.do*	Conditional 5	3	
Neuroform Stent *Boston Scientific, http://www.bostonscientific.com*	Conditional 5	3	108
Neuroform3 Stent *Boston Scientific, http://www.bostonscientific.com*	Conditional 5	3	

Object	Status	Field Strength (T)	Reference
Neurolink Stent *Abbott Vascular, www.abbottvascular.com*	Conditional 5	1.5	
Neurostring Embolization Coil *Biomerix Corporation, Fremont, CA*	Conditional 6	3	
New retrievable IVC filter *Thomas Jefferson University, Philadelphia, PA*	Conditional 2	1.5	21
NexStent Carotid Stent *Nitinol, stent,* *Endotex Interventional Solutions, Cupertino, CA*	Safe	3	
Nexus Detachable Coil *embolization coil,* *ev3, Inc., http://www.ev3.net*	Conditional 5	3	
Nexus Embolization Coil *Nexus X-10-20-T10-TC, Platinum-Iridium, Nitinol,* *Micro Therapeutics, Inc., Irvine, CA*	Conditional 6	3	
NIR Stent *MR-safe metal, Medinol Ltd., Jerusalem, Israel*	Safe	1.5	69
NIR Royal Advance Stent *Boston Scientific, http://www.bostonscientific.com*	Conditional 5	1.5	
Nitinol Braided Neuro Coil Assist Stent *MicroVention, Inc., Alison Viejo, CA*	Conditional 6	3	
Nuloy Stent *Coronary Artery Stent,* *Icon Interventional Systems, Inc., Cleveland, OH*	Conditional 6	3	
NXT Detachable Coil *embolization coil,* *ev3, Inc., http://www.ev3.net*	Conditional 5	3	
NXT Tetris Detachable Coil *embolization coil,* *ev3, Inc., http://www.ev3.net*	Conditional 5	3	
Omnilink Elite Stent *Abbott Vascular Instruments Deutschland GmbH,* *Germany*	Conditional 8	1.5, 3	
Omnilink Biliary Stent *Abbott Vascular, www.abbottvascular.com*	Conditional 5	3	
OPTEASE Retrievable Vena Cava Filter *Cordis,* *a Johnson and Johnson Co., http://www.cordis.com*	Conditional 5	3	
Optimized Flair Endovascular Stent Graft *9-mm x 50-mm,* *Bard Peripheral Vascular, Tempe, AZ*	Conditional 6	3	
Option Vena Cava Filter *REX MEDICAL, Conshohocken, PA*	Conditional 5	3	

Object	Status	Field Strength (T)	Reference
Orbit Galaxy Embolization Coil *Codman and Shurtleff, Inc.* *a Johnson & Johnson Co., Raynham, MA*	Conditional 6	3	
PALMAZ BLUE Stent *Cordis,* *a Johnson and Johnson Co., http://www.cordis.com*	Conditional 5	3	
PALMAZ BLUE Transhepatic Biliary Stent *Cordis,* *a Johnson and Johnson Co., http://www.cordis.com*	Conditional 5	3	
Palmaz Endovascular Stent *Cordis,* *a Johnson and Johnson Co., http://www.cordis.com*	Conditional 5	3	
PALMAZ Genesis Stent *Cordis,* *a Johnson and Johnson Co., http://www.cordis.com*	Conditional 5	3	
Palmaz Genesis Peripheral Stent *316L SS,* *http://www.cordis.com*	Conditional 5	3	
Palmaz Genesis Transhepatic Biliary Stent *316L SS,* *Cordis,* *a Johnson and Johnson Co., http://www.cordis.com*	Conditional 5	3	
Palmaz-Schatz Stent *15 x 3.0-mm, 316L SS,* *Cordis,* *a Johnson and Johnson Co., http://www.cordis.com*	Safe	1.5	72
Palmaz-Schatz Stent *P-S 153, 316L SS,* *Cordis,* *a Johnson and Johnson Co., http://www.cordis.com*	Safe	1.5	69
Palmaz-Schatz Stent *P-S 154, 316L SS,* *Cordis,* *a Johnson and Johnson Co., http://www.cordis.com*	Safe	1.5	69
Palmaz-Shatz *balloon-expandable stent,* *Cordis,* *a Johnson and Johnson Co., http://www.cordis.com*	Conditional 2	1.5	
ParaMount Mini Biliary Stent *ev3, Inc., http://www.ev3.net*	Conditional 5	1.5	
Passager Stent *tantalum, 10-mm x 30-mm,* *Meadox Surgimed, Oakland, NJ*	Safe	1.5	

Object	Status	Field Strength (T)	Reference
Passager Stent *tantalum, 4-mm x 30-mm,* *Meadox Surgimed, Oakland, NJ*	Safe	1.5	
Percuflex Plus *Stent Graft with Suprarenal, Ureteral Stent,* *4.8 Fr. (1.6-mm x 220-mm), Microvasive,* *Boston Scientific Corporation, Watertown, MA*	Safe	1.5, 3	83
PHAROS Stent *carotid artery stent,* *BIOTRONIK AG, Switzerland*	Conditional 6	3	
Polyflex Airway Stent *silicone and polyester,* *Boston Scientific, http://www.bostonscientific.com*	Safe	1.5	
Powerlink Suprarenal *Bifurcated Stent Graft, Model 34-16-175RBL,* *Endologix, Irvine, CA*	Conditional 8	1.5, 3	
PowerLink *cobalt-alloy,* *Endologix, Inc., Irvine, CA*	Safe	1.5	70
PowerWeb, Model 1 *cobalt-alloy,* *Endologix, Inc., Irvine, CA*	Safe	1.5	70
PowerWeb *cobalt-alloy,* *Endologix, Inc., Irvine, CA*	Safe	1.5	70
Precedent Stent *Nitinol, Platinum,* *Boston Scientific, Wayne, NJ*	Safe	1.5	70
Precise Microvascular Anastomotic Device (MACD) *316L SS*	Safe	1.5	71
Precise Nitinol Stent, Carotid *Cordis,* *a Johnson and Johnson Co.,* *http://www.cordis.com, http://cordislabeling.com com*	Conditional 5	1.5	
Precise Pro RX Nitinol Stent *Cordis,* *a Johnson and Johnson Co.,* *http://www.cordis.com, http://cordislabeling.com com*	Conditional 5	1.5	
Precise RX Nitinol Stent *Cordis,* *a Johnson and Johnson Co.,* *http://www.cordis.com, http://cordislabeling.com com*	Conditional 5	1.5	

Object	Status	Field Strength (T)	Reference
PRESIDIO Microcoil *embolization coil,* *Micrus Endovascular,* *http://www.micrusendovascular.com*	Conditional 5	3	
PRIMUS Biliary Stent *ev3, Inc., http://www.ev3.net*	Conditional 5	1.5	
PRO-Kinetic Stent *coronary artery stent,* *BIOTRONIK AG, Switzerland*	Safe	3	
PROMUS Everolimus-Eluting Coronary Stent *PROMUS Stent,* *Boston Scientific, http://www.bostonscientific.com*	Conditional 5	3	
ProPass Stent *Vascular Innovations, Inc., Freemont, CA*	Conditional 6	3	
Protege EverFlex Self-Expanding Biliary Stent *ev3, Inc., http://www.ev3.net*	Conditional 5	1.5	
Protege GPS Carotid Stent *ev3, Inc., http://www.ev3.net*	Conditional 5	3	
Protege GPS Self-Expanding Biliary Stent *ev3, Inc., http://www.ev3.net*	Conditional 5	1.5	
Protege RX Carotid Stent *ev3, Inc., http://www.ev3.net*	Conditional 5	3	
Quadra-coil Ureteral Stent *Polyurethane,* *Gyrus ACMI, Inc., Maple Grove, MN*	Safe	3	
R Stent *316 LVM SS,* *Spectranetics Corporation, Colorado Springs, CO*	Safe	1.5	
R Stent *316L SS,* *Orbus Medical Technologies, Fort Lauderdale, FL*	Safe	1.5	
Racer Biliary Stent System *cobalt alloy, stent,* *Medtronic Vascular, Santa Rosa, CA*	Safe	3	
Radius Stent *4.0-mm x 31-mm, Nitinol,* *Boston Scientific Corporation, Natick, MA*	Safe	1.5, 3	
Radius Stent *Nitinol,* *Boston Scientific Corporation, Scimed, Maple Grove, MN*	Safe	1.5	69
Recovery G2 Filter *Vena Cava Filter, Femoral Vein,* *Bard Peripheral Vascular, www.bardpv.com*	Conditional 5	1.5	

Object	Status	Field Strength (T)	Reference
Recovery Nitinol Filter *Nitinol,* *C.R. Bard,* *Bard Peripheral Vascular, www.bardpv.com*	Safe	3	
Resonance Double Pigtail Ureteral Stent *MP35N,* *MED Institute Incorporated, West Lafayette, IN*	Conditional 6	3	
RX HERCULINK ELITE *Biliary Stent, 316L SS*	Conditional 6	3	
S3 Stent *L605 Cobalt-Chrome,* *Medlogics Device Corporation, Santa Rosa, CA*	Conditional 6	3	
S670 *4.0-mm x 30-mm, 316L SS, stent,* *Medtronic Vascular, Santa Rosa, CA*	Safe	3	
S7 *4.0-mm x 30-mm, 316L SS, stent,* *Medtronic Vascular, Santa Rosa, CA*	Safe	3	
SafeFlo IVC Filter *inferior vena cava filter, Nitinol, Titanium,* *Rafael Medical Technologies, Inc., Israel*	Conditional 6	3	
Sapphire Detachable Coil *embolization coil, platinum alloy,* *ev3, Inc. Neurovascular Division, Irvine, CA*	Conditional 5	1.5	
Seaquence *stent, 15 x 3.5, 316L SS,* *Nycomed Amersham, Princeton, NJ*	Safe	1.5	72
Silhouette Ureteral Patency Devices *316L SS with Tantalum,* *MRI information applies to all Silhouette Devices,* *Applied Medical Resources, Rancho Santa Margarita, CA*	Conditional 8	1.5, 3	
Silk Artery Reconstruction Device *stent, BALT, France*	Conditional 8	1.5, 3	
Single-J Urinary *Diversion Specialty Stent, Silicone,* *Gyrus ACMI, Inc., Maple Grove, MN*	Safe	3	
Simon Nitinol Filter *vena cava filter,* *C.R. Bard, Tempe, AZ*	Conditional 6	3	
S.M.A.R.T. CONTROL Nitinol Stent *Transhepatic Biliary System,* *Cordis,* *a Johnson and Johnson Co., http://www.cordis.com*	Conditional 6	3	

Object	Status	Field Strength (T)	Reference
S.M.A.R.T. *Shape Memory Alloy Recoverable Technology,* *Nitinol Stent,* *Cordis,* *a Johnson and Johnson Co., http://www.cordis.com*	Conditional 6	3	
S.M.A.R.T. Nitinol Stent *Transhepatic Biliary System,* *Cordis,* *a Johnson and Johnson Co., http://www.cordis.com*	Conditional 5	3	
Sof-Curl Ureteral Stent *Polyurethane,* *Gyrus ACMI, Inc., Maple Grove, MN*	Safe	3	
Solitaire Flow Restoration Stent *Nitinol, SS, Platinum,* *ev3 Inc., Irvine, CA*	Conditional 8	1.5, 3	
St. Jude Carotid Stent *10-7 x 40-mm taper stent, two-overlapped version,* *St. Jude Medical Cardiology Division, www.SJM.com*	Conditional 6	3	
St. Jude Carotid Stent *10-7 x 50-mm taper stent, single version,* *St. Jude Medical Cardiology Division, www.SJM.com*	Conditional 6	3	
Strecker stent *tantalum,* *MD Tech, Watertown, MA*	Safe	1.5	27
Stentys Bifurcation Stent *Stentys Inc., Princeton, NJ*	Conditional 6	3	
Strider Stent *biliary artery, iliac artery, Nitinol with tantalum markers,* *Medtronic Vascular, Santa Rosa, CA*	Safe	3	
Svelte Bare Metal Stent *single and two overlapped versions,* *Svelte Medical Systems, New Providence, NJ*	Conditional 8	1.5, 3	
T6-XR Stent *cobalt chromium, gold markers,* *BIOTRONIK GmbH & Co., Berlin, Germany*	Conditional 6	3	
TAA Endograft *TriVascular2, Inc., Santa Rosa, CA*	Conditional 6	3	
Taarget Stent Graft *LeMaitre Vascular, Burlington, MA*	Conditional 6	3	
TAG Endoprosthesis *thoracic aneurysm stent graft,* *45-mm x 20-cm endoprostheses,* *W.L Gore and Associates, www.goremedical.com*	Conditional 5	3	

Object	Status	Field Strength (T)	Reference
Talent Abdominal Stent Graft *Medtronic, Inc., www.Medtronic.com,* *http://manuals.medtronic.com/en/index.htm*	Conditional 5	3	
Talent Graft Stent *bare spring model, 16 x 8-mm, Nitinol,* *World Medical Manufacturing Corp., Sunrise, FL*	Safe	1.5	
Talent Graft Stent *bare spring model, 36 x 20-mm, Nitinol,* *World Medical Manufacturing Corp., Sunrise, FL*	Safe	1.5	
Talent Graft Stent *open web model, 16 x 8-mm, Nitinol,* *World Medical Manufacturing Corp., Sunrise, FL*	Safe	1.5	
Talent Graft Stent *open web model, 36 x 20-mm, Nitinol,* *World Medical Manufacturing Corp., Sunrise, FL*	Safe	1.5	
Talent Thoracic Graft *Medtronic, Inc., www.Medtronic.com,* *http://manuals.medtronic.com/en/index.htm*	Conditional 5	3	
TAXUS Element Stent *Boston Scientific, http://www.bostonscientific.com*	Conditional 5	3	
TAXUS Express *Paclitaxel-Eluting Coronary Stent, 316L SS,* *Boston Scientific, http://www.bostonscientific.com*	Conditional 5	3	
TAXUS Express2 Atom Stent *Boston Scientific, http://www.bostonscientific.com*	Conditional 5	3	
TAXUS Express2 Atom Paclitaxel-eluting Coronary Stent *Boston Scientific, http://www.bostonscientific.com*	Conditional 5	3	
TAXUS Liberte *Paclitaxel-Eluting Coronary Stent, 316L SS,* *Boston Scientific, http://www.bostonscientific.com*	Conditional 5	3	
TAXUS Liberte Atom Paclitaxel-Eluting Coronary Stent *TAXUS Liberte Atom Stent,* *Boston Scientific, http://www.bostonscientific.com*	Conditional 5	3	
TAXUS Liberte Long Paclitaxel-Eluting Coronary Stent *TAXUS Liberte Long Stent* *Boston Scientific, http://www.bostonscientific.com*	Conditional 5	3	
Tornado Embolization Coils *Cook Medical, Inc.,* *http://www.cookmedical.com/di/productMri.do*	Conditional 5	3	

Object	Status	Field Strength (T)	Reference
Tracheobronchial *Wallstent Endoprosthesis, 14 x 80, stent,* *Schneider (USA) Inc.,* *Pfizer Medical Technology Group, Minneapolis, MN*	Safe	1.5	64
Tracheobronchial *Wallstent Endoprosthesis, 24 x 70, stent,* *Schneider (USA) Inc.,* *Pfizer Medical Technology Group, Minneapolis, MN*	Safe	1.5	64
TRAPEASE Permanent Vena Cava Filter *Cordis,* *a Johnson and Johnson Co., http://www.cordis.com*	Conditional 5	3	
TriMaxx Coronary Stent *SS-Tantalum composite, stent,* *Abbott Vascular Devices, Redwood City, CA*	Safe	3	
TRUFILL DCS ORBIT Detachable Coil *embolization coil, Platinum, Tungsten,* *Cordis Neurovascular, Miami Lakes, FL*	Safe	3	87
TRUFILL Pushable Coils *Vascular Occlusion System, Platinum,* *Cordis Endovascular Systems, Inc., Miami Lakes, FL*	Safe	1.5	
Ultraflex *stent, Titanium alloy*	Safe	1.5	73
Uncovered WallFlex Biliary RX Stent System *Boston Scientific Corporation, Marlborough, MA*	Conditional 6	3	
Uro-Guide Open Tip *Ureteral Stent, Silicone,* *Gyrus ACMI, Inc., Maple Grove, MN*	Safe	3	
Valecor Platinum Stent *coronary artery stent, CoCr L605, Platinum,* *Cornova, Inc., Burlington, MA*	Conditional 8	1.5, 3	
Valiant Thoracic Stent Graft *Medtronic Vascular, Santa Rosa, CA*	Safe	3	
Vanguard Stent *Nitinol, Platinum,* *Boston Scientific, Wayne, NJ*	Safe	1.5	70
VBS Stent (also known as the Verdi Stent) *Synthes GmbH, Switzerland*	Conditional 6	3	
Vectra VAG *Vascular Access Graft, Thoralon,* *Bard Peripheral Vascular, Tempe, AZ*	Safe	3	
VENAFLO II Vascular Graft *Carbon-impregnated ePTFE,* *Bard Peripheral Vascular, Tempe, AZ*	Safe	3	

Object	Status	Field Strength (T)	Reference
VENAFLO Vascular Graft *Carbon-impregnated ePTFE,* *Bard Peripheral Vascular, Tempe, AZ*	Safe	3	
VIABAHN Endoprosthesis *13-mm x 10-cm, Nitinol,* *W. L. Gore & Associates, Inc., www.goremedical.com*	Conditional 5	3	
VIABAHN Endoprosthesis *8-mm x 25-cm, single version, Nitinol,* *W. L. Gore & Associates, www.goremedical.com*	Conditional 5	3	
VIABAHN Endoprosthesis *8-mm x 25-cm, two-overlapped version, Nitinol,* *W. L. Gore & Associates, www.goremedical.com*	Conditional 5	3	
VIABAHN Endoprosthesis *9-mm x 15-cm, Nitinol,* *W. L. Gore & Associates, Inc., www.goremedical.com*	Conditional 5	3	
VIABAHN Endoprosthesis *W.L. Gore & Associates, Inc., www.goremedical.com*	Conditional 5	3	
VIABIL Biliary Endoprosthesis *W.L. Gore & Associates, Inc., www.goremedical.com*	Conditional 5	3	
VIATORR Endoprosthesis *Stent, Nitinol,* *W. L. Gore and Associates, Inc., www.goremedical.com*	Conditional 5	1.5	
VIATORR TIPS Endoprosthesis *W.L. Gore & Associates, Inc., www.goremedical.com*	Conditional 5	3	
ULTIPAQ Microcoil *embolization coil,* *Micrus Endovascular,* *http://www.micrusendovascular.com*	Conditional 5	3	
Valiant Thoracic Stent Graft *Medtronic, Inc., www.Medtronic.com*	Conditional 5	3	
Vena Tech LP *vascular filter,* *B. Braun, http://www.bbraunusa.com*	Conditional 5	1.5	
Visi-Pro Biliary Stent *ev3, Inc., http://www.ev3.net*	Conditional 5	1.5	
VIVAL Coronary Stent *Avantec Vascular, Sunnyvale, CA*	Conditional 6	3	
vProtect Luminal Shield *Nitinol, Tantalum, Stent,* *Prescient Medical, Inc., Doylestown, PA*	Conditional 8	1.5, 3	
V-Track Embolization Coil *HydroCoil,* *MicroVention, Inc., Alison Viejo, CA*	Conditional 6	3	

Object	Status	Field Strength (T)	Reference
V-Track Embolization Coil *MultiPlex,* *MicroVention, Inc., Alison Viejo, CA*	Conditional 6	3	
WallFlex Biliary RX Stent *Boston Scientific, http://www.bostonscientific.com*	Conditional 5	3	
WallFlex Biliary Stent *covered version,* *Boston Scientific, http://www.bostonscientific.com*	Safe	3	
WallFlex Biliary Stent *uncovered version,* *Boston Scientific, http://www.bostonscientific.com*	Safe	3	
WallFlex Enteral Colonic Stent with Anchor Lock Delivery System *Nitinol,* *Boston Scientific, http://www.bostonscientific.com*	Safe	3	
WallFlex Enteral Duodenal Stent with Anchor Lock Delivery System *Nitinol,* *Boston Scientific, http://www.bostonscientific.com*	Safe	3	
WallFlex Partially Covered Esophageal Stent *Boston Scientific, http://www.bostonscientific.com*	Conditional 5	3	
WallGraft *Elgiloy,* *Boston Scientific, http://www.bostonscientific.com*	Safe	3	
WallStent biliary endoprosthesis *stent, high nickle SS,* *Schneider USA, Plymouth, MN*	Safe	1.5	28
WALLSTENT Endoprosthesis *Boston Scientific, http://www.bostonscientific.com*	Conditional 5	3	
WallStent Endoprosthesis *Magic Wallstent, 3.5 x 25, stent,* *Schneider (USA) Inc.,* *Pfizer Medical Technology Group, Minneapolis, MN*	Safe	1.5	64
WallStent Endoprosthesis *With Permalume covering, 8 x 80, stent,* *Schneider (USA) Inc.,* *Pfizer Medical Technology Group, Minneapolis, MN*	Safe	1.5	64
WallStent Esophageal II Endoprosthesis *20 x 130, stent,* *Schneider (USA) Inc.,* *Pfizer Medical Technology Group, Minneapolis, MN*	Safe	1.5	64
WallStent *carotid artery stent,* *Boston Scientific, http://www.bostonscientific.com*	Safe	3	

Object	Status	Field Strength (T)	Reference
WallStent *Platinum and cobalt-alloy,* *Schneider, Bulach, Switzerland*	Safe	1.5	69
WALLSTENT RX Biliary Endoprosthesis *Boston Scientific, http://www.bostonscientific.com*	Conditional 5	3	
Wiktor coronary artery stent *Medtronic Inverventional Vascular, www.Medtronic.com*	Safe	1.5	
Wiktor GX *tantalum, stent,* *Medtronic AVE, www.Medtronic.com*	Safe	1.5	72
Wilson-Cook Pancreatic Stent *stent,* *Wilson-Cook Medical, Inc., Winston-Salem, NC*	Safe	1.5	
Wilson-Cook Pancreatic Wedge Stent *stent,* *Wilson-Cook Medical, Inc., Winston-Salem, NC*	Safe	1.5	
Wingspan Stent System *Boston Scientific Corporation, Freemont, CA*	Safe	3	
Xact Stent *Nitinol,* *Abbott Vascular, www.abbottvascular.com*	Safe	3	
XactfleX Carotid Stent *Nitinol,* *Abbott Vascular, www.abbottvascular.com*	Safe	3	
Xceed Biliary Stent *Abbott Vascular, www.abbottvascular.com*	Conditional 5	3	
XIENCE PRIME Stent *Abbott Vascular, www.abbottvascular.com*	Conditional 5	3	
XIENCE V Stent *Abbott Vascular, www.abbottvascular.com*	Conditional 5	3	
Xpert Biliary Stent *Abbott Vascular, www.abbottvascular.com*	Conditional 5	3	
Xpert Stent *Nitinol,* *Abbott Vascular, www.abbottvascular.com*	Conditional 6	3	
X-Suit NIR Biliary Metallic Stent *Olympus and Medinol, http://www.medinol.com*	Conditional 5	1.5, 3	
XTENT Customizable Stent *Coronary Artery Stent, XTENT, Inc., Menlo Park, CA*	Conditional 6	3	
X-Trode, 3 segment *stent, 316 SS,* *C.R. Bard, Inc., Billerica, MA*	Safe	1.5	

Object	Status	Field Strength (T)	Reference
X-Trode, 9 segment *stent, 316 SS,* *C.R. Bard, Inc., Billerica, MA*	Safe	1.5	
Zenith AAA Endovascular Graft	Conditional 5	3	
Zenith Flex AAA, Stent, Including starting with prefix TFB, TFFB, TFLE, ELSE, ESBE, ESC, ESP, ZIP, AX1, RX1, *Cook Medical,* *http://www.cookmedical.com/di/productMri.do*	Conditional 5	3	
Zenith TX2 TAA Endovascular Graft *Cook Medical, Inc.,* *http://www.cookmedical.com/di/productMri.do*	Conditional 8	1.5, 3	
Zilver 518 Vascular *Cook Medical, Inc.,* *http://www.cookmedical.com/di/productMri.do*	Conditional 5	3	
Zilver 518 Biliary *Cook Medical, Inc.,* *http://www.cookmedical.com/di/productMri.do*	Conditional 5	3	
Zilver 635 Vascular *Cook Medical, Inc.,* *http://www.cookmedical.com/di/productMri.do*	Conditional 5	3	
Zilver 635 Biliary *Cook Medical, Inc.,* *http://www.cookmedical.com/di/productMri.do*	Conditional 5	3	
Zilver Stent *Iliac artery stent, Nitinol,* *Cook Medical, Inc.,* *http://www.cookmedical.com/di/productMri.do*	Conditional 5	3	
Zilver Stent *Nitinol, gold,* *Cook Medical,* *Inc., http://www.cookmedical.com/di/productMri.do*	Conditional 5	3	
Zilver Self-Expanding Stent *Cook Medical, Inc.,* *http://www.cookmedical.com/di/productMri.do*	Conditional 5	3	

Object	Status	Field Strength (T)	Reference

Dental Implants, Devices, and Materials

Object	Status	Field Strength (T)	Reference
Brace band *SS, dental,* *American Dental, Missoula, MT*	Conditional 1	1.5	3
Brace wire *chrome alloy, dental,* *Ormco Corp., San Marcos, CA*	Conditional 1	1.5	3
Castable alloy, dental *Golden Dental Products, Inc., Golden, CO*	Conditional 1	1.5	12
Cement-in keeper, dental *Solid State Innovations, Inc., Mt. Airy, NC*	Conditional 1	1.5	12
Dental amalgam *dental material*	Safe	1.39	1
GDP Direct Keeper *Pre-formed post, dental,* *Golden Dental Products, Inc., Golden, CO*	Conditional 1	1.5	12
Gutta Percha Points *dental device*	Safe	1.5	
Indian Head Real Silver Points, dental *Union Broach Co., Inc., New York, NY*	Safe	1.5	
Keeper, pre-formed post, dental *Parkell Products, Inc., Farmingdale, NY*	Conditional 1	1.5	1
Magna-Dent, large indirect keeper, dental *Dental Ventures of America, Yorba Linda, CA*	Conditional 1	1.5	1
Palladium clad magnet, dental *Parkell Products, Inc., Farmingdale, NY*	Unsafe 1	1.5	13
Palladium/palladium keeper, dental *Parkell Products, Inc., Farmingdale, NY*	Conditional 1	1.5	13
Palladium/Platinum casting alloy, dental *Parkell Products, Inc., Farmingdale, NY*	Conditional 1	1.5	13
Permanent crown *amalgam, dental,* *Ormco Corp.*	Safe	1.5	3
Silver point, dental *Union Broach Co., Inc., New York, NY*	Safe	1.5	3
Stainless steel clad magnet, dental *Parkell Products, Inc., Farmingdale, NY*	Unsafe 1	1.5	13
Stainless steel keeper, dental *Parkell Products, Inc., Farmingdale, NY*	Conditional 1	1.5	13
Titanium clad magnet, dental *Parkell Products, Inc., Farmingdale, NY*	Unsafe 1	1.5	13

Object	Status	Field Strength (T)	Reference

ECG Electrodes

Object	Status	Field Strength (T)	Reference
Accutac, ECG electrode *ConMed Corp., Utica, NY*	Safe	1.5	
Accutac, ECG electrode *Diaphoretic, ConMed Corp., Utica, NY*	Safe	1.5	
Adult Cloth, ECG electrode *ConMed Corp., Utica, NY*	Safe	1.5	
Adult ECG, ECG electrode *Electrode 3-Pack,* *ConMed Corp., Utica, NY*	Safe	1.5	
Adult Foam, ECG electrode *ConMed Corp., Utica, NY*	Safe	1.5	
Cleartrace 2, ECG electrode *ConMed Corp., Utica, NY*	Safe	1.5	
Dyna/Trace Diagnostic *ECG Electrode,* *ConMed Corp., Utica, NY*	Safe	1.5	
Dyna/Trace Mini, ECG electrode *ConMed Corp., Utica, NY*	Safe	1.5	
Dyna/Trace Stress, ECG electrode *ConMed Corp., Utica, NY*	Safe	1.5	
Dyna/Trace, ECG electrode *ConMed Corp., Utica, NY*	Safe	1.5	
High Demand, ECG electrode *ConMed Corp., Utica, NY*	Safe	1.5	
Holtrode, ECG electrode *ConMed Corp., Utica, NY*	Safe	1.5	
HP M2202A Radio-lucent, ECG electrode *Monitoring Electrode, Ag/AgCl,* *Hewlett-Packard, Medical Supplies, Andover, MA*	Safe	1.5	
Invisatrace Adult, ECG electrode *ConMed Corp., Utica, NY*	Safe	1.5	
Pediatric Foam, ECG electrode *ConMed Corp., Utica, NY*	Safe	1.5	
Plia Cell Diagnostic, ECG electrode *ConMed Corp., Utica, NY*	Safe	1.5	
Plia-Cell Diaphoretic, ECG electrode *ConMed Corp., Utica, NY*	Safe	1.5	
Plia-Cell, ECG electrode *ConMed Corp., Utica, NY*	Safe	1.5	
Quadtrode MRI, ECG electrode *InVivo Research, Inc., Orlando, FL*	Safe	1.5	

Object	Status	Field Strength (T)	Reference
Silvon Adult ECG Electrode *ConMed Corp., Utica, NY*	Safe	1.5	
Silvon Diaphoretic, ECG electrode *ConMed Corp., Utica,NY*	Safe	1.5	
Silvon Stress, ECG electrode *ConMed Corp., Utica, NY*	Safe	1.5	
Silvon, ECG electrode *ConMed Corp., Utica, NY*	Safe	1.5	
Snaptrace, ECG electrode *ConMed Corp., Utica, NY*	Safe	1.5	
SSE Radiotransparent ECG Electrode *ConMed Corp., Utica, NY*	Safe	1.5	
SSE, ECG electrode *ConMed Corp., Utica, NY*	Safe	1.5	

Foley Catheters With and Without Temperature Sensors

Object	Status	Field Strength (T)	Reference
Bardex I.C. Foley *Catheter with silver and hydrogel, coating,16Fr.,* *Bard Medical Division, Covington, GA*	Conditional 5	1.5	
Bardex I.C. *Temperature Sensing Foley Catheter,* *with a 6 foot cable, 16 Fr.,* *Bard Medical Division, Covington, GA*	Conditional 5	1.5	
Bardex Latex-Free *Temperature Sensing 400-Series Foley Catheter,* *C. R.Bard, Inc., Covington, GA*	Conditional 5	1.5, 3	
Bardex Lubricath *Temperature Sensing, Urotrack Plus, Foley Catheter,* *with a 6 foot cable, 16 Fr,* *Bard Medical Division, Covington, GA*	Conditional 5	1.5	
Bardex Pediatric *Temperature Sensing 400-Series,* *Urotrack Foley Catheter, with a detachable cable, 12 Fr.,* *Bard Medical Division, Covington, GA*	Conditional 5	1.5	
Extension cable for *Foley Catheter, with temperature sensor, 10 feet,* *RSP Respiratory Support Products, Inc.,* *SIMS, Smiths Industries, Irvine, CA*	Unsafe 2	1.5	
Foley catheter *Bard Medical Division, Covington, GA*	Safe	1.5	
Foley Catheter *SilverTouch Catheter,* *Medline Industries, Inc., Mundelein, IL*	Conditional 6	3	

Object	Status	Field Strength (T)	Reference
Foley Catheter with *Temperature Sensor, 10 Fr.,* *RSP Respiratory Support Products, Inc.,* *SIMS, Smiths Industries, Irvine, CA*	Conditional 5	1.5	
Foley Catheter with *Temperature Sensor, 18 Fr.,* *RSP Respiratory Support Products, Inc.,* *SIMS, Smiths Industries, Irvine, CA*	Conditional 5	1.5	
Lubri-Sil I.C. Foley Catheter *No metal version,* *C. R.Bard, Inc., Covington, GA*	Safe	3	
Lubri-Sil I.C. Foley Catheter *Temperature Sensing 400-Series Foley Catheter,* *C. R.Bard, Inc., Covington, GA*	Conditional 6	1.5, 3	

Halo Vests and Cervical Fixation Devices

Object	Status	Field Strength (T)	Reference
Ambulatory Halo System *halo and cervical fixation*	Conditional 4	1.5	14
Bremer 3D Halo Crown System *with Bremer Air Flo Vest, and Titanium Skull Pins,* *Cervical Fixation Device,* *DePuy Spine Inc., Raynham, MA*	Conditional 6	3	
Bremer Halo Crown System *with Bremer Air Flo Vest, and Titanium Skull Pins,* *Cervical Fixation Device,* *DePuy Spine Inc., Raynham, MA*	Conditional 6	3	
Closed-back halo *Titanium, halo and cervical fixation,* *DePuy ACE Medical Co., El Segundo, CA*	Safe	1.5	16
Closed Back Halo *OSSUR Reykjavik, Iceland,* *OSSUR AMERICAS, Aliso Viejo, CA*	Unsafe 1	1.5	
EXO adjustable coller *halo and cervical fixation,* *Florida Manufacturing Co., Daytona, FL*	Conditional 4	1.0	15
Generation 80 Halo System *with Generation 80 Halo Vest, and Aluminum Ring,* *and Generation 80 Titanium Halo Pins,* *OSSUR Reykjavik, Iceland,* *OSSUR AMERICAS, Aliso Viejo, CA*	Unsafe 1	3	114
Guilford cervical orthosis, modified *halo and cervical fixation,* *Guilford & Son, Ltd., Cleveland, OH*	Safe	1.0	15

Object	Status	Field Strength (T)	Reference
Guilford cervical orthosis *halo and cervical fixation,* *Guilford & Son, Ltd., Cleveland, OH*	Conditional 4	1.0	15
J-Tongs *OSSUR Reykjavik, Iceland,* *OSSUR AMERICAS, Aliso Viejo, CA*	Unsafe 1	1.5	
JTO Cervico-Thoracic Extension *OSSUR Reykjavik, Iceland,* *OSSUR AMERICAS, Aliso Viejo, CA*	Safe	3	
'LiL Angel Pediatric Halo System *with Jerome Halo Vest, and* *Resolve Glass-composite Halo Ring,* *and Resolve Ceramic-tipped Skull Pins,* *OSSUR Reykjavik, Iceland,* *OSSUR AMERICAS, Aliso Viejo, CA*	Conditional 6	3	114
'LiL Angel Pediatric Halo System *with Resolve Halo Vest,* *and Resolve Glass-composite Halo Ring,* *and Resolve Ceramic-tipped Skull Pins,* *OSSUR Reykjavik, Iceland,* *OSSUR AMERICAS, Aliso Viejo, CA*	Conditional 6	3	114
Mark III halo vest *aluminum superstructure, SS rivets, Titanium bolts,* *DePuy ACE Medical Co., El Segundo, CA*	Safe	1.5	16
Mark IV halo vest *aluminum superstructure and Titanium bolts,* *DePuy ACE Medical Co., El Segundo, CA*	Safe	1.5	16
Miami J Cervical Collar *OSSUR Reykjavik, Iceland,* *OSSUR AMERICAS, Aliso Viejo, CA*	Safe	3	
MR-compatible *halo vest and cervical fixation,* *Lerman & Son Co., Beverly Hills, CA*	Safe	1.5	
NecLoc Extrication Collar *OSSUR Reykjavik, Iceland,* *OSSUR AMERICAS, Aliso Viejo, CA*	Safe	3	
Occian Collar Back *OSSUR Reykjavik, Iceland,* *OSSUR AMERICAS, Aliso Viejo, CA*	Safe	3	
Open-back halo *aluminum,* *DePuy ACE Medical Co., El Segundo, CA*	Safe	1.5	16
Open-back halo *with Delrin inserts for skull pins, aluminum and Delrin,* *DePuy ACE Medical Co., El Segundo, CA*	Safe	1.5	16

Object	Status	Field Strength (T)	Reference
Papoos Infant Spinal Immobilization Device *OSSUR Reykjavik, Iceland,* *OSSUR AMERICAS, Aliso Viejo, CA*	Safe	3	
Patriot Extrication Collar *OSSUR Reykjavik, Iceland,* *OSSUR AMERICAS, Aliso Viejo, CA*	Safe	3	
Philadelphia Cervical Collar *OSSUR Reykjavik, Iceland,* *OSSUR AMERICAS, Aliso Viejo, CA*	Safe	3	
Philadelphia coller *Philadelphia Coller Co., Westville, NJ*	Safe	1.0	15
PMT halo cervical orthosis *PMT Corp., Chanhassen, MN*	Safe	1.0	15
PMT halo cervical orthosis *with graphite rods and halo ring,* *PMT Corp., Chanhassen, MN*	Safe	1.0	15
PMT Halo System *with Carbon Graphite Open Back Ring,* *and Titanium Skull Pins,* *PMT Corporation, Chanhassen, MN*	Conditional 5	3	
Resolve Halo System *with Jerome Halo Vest,* *and Resolve Glass-composite Halo Ring,* *and Resolve Ceramic-tipped Skull Pins,* *OSSUR Reykjavik, Iceland,* *OSSUR AMERICAS, Aliso Viejo, CA*	Conditional 6	3	114
Resolve Halo System *with Resolve Halo Vest,* *and Resolve Glass-composite Halo Ring,* *and Resolve Ceramic-tipped Skull Pins,* *OSSUR Reykjavik, Iceland,* *OSSUR AMERICAS, Aliso Viejo, CA*	Conditional 6	3	114
S.O.M.I. cervical orthosis *U.S. Manufacturing Co., Pasadena, CA*	Conditional 4	1.0	15
Trippi-Wells tong *Titanium,* *DePuy ACE Medical Co., El Segundo, CA*	Safe	1.5	16
V1 Halo System *with V1 Halo Vest, and V1 Halo Ring,* *and V1 Titanium Halo Pins,* *OSSUR Reykjavik, Iceland,* *OSSUR AMERICAS, Aliso Viejo, CA*	Conditional 6	3	114
V2 *OSSUR Reykjavik, Iceland,* *OSSUR AMERICAS, Aliso Viejo, CA*	Unsafe 1	1.5	

Object	Status	Field Strength (T)	Reference

Heart Valve Prostheses and Annuloplasty Rings

Object	Status	Field Strength (T)	Reference
AAV-2 Heart Valve *Aortic heart valve prosthesis,* *Arbor Surgical Technologies, Inc., Irvine, CA*	Conditional 6	3	
Annuloflex *Annuloplasty Ring, Size 26-mm, L001285A 26M,* *Model AF800,* *Sulzer Carbomedics, Inc., Austin, TX*	Safe	1.5, 3	
Annuloflex *Annuloplasty Ring, Size 36-mm, L004032A 36M,* *Sulzer Carbomedics, Inc., Austin, TX*	Safe	1.5, 3	
Annuloflo *Annuloplasty Ring, Size 26-mm, S011896A 26M,* *Sulzer Carbomedics, Inc., Austin, TX*	Safe	1.5, 3	
Annuloflo *Annuloplasty Ring, Size 36-mm, S013460A 36M,* *Sulzer Carbomedics, Inc., Austin, TX*	Safe	1.5, 3	
AnnuloFlo *Mitral Annuloplasty Device, Size 36,* *Model AR-736, Titanium,* *Sulzer Carbomedics, Inc., Austin, TX*	Safe	1.5, 3	83
Annuloplasty ring *Titanium,* *Sulzer Medica and Sulzer Carbomedics*	Safe	1.5	
Attune Flexible Annuloplasty Ring *St. Jude Medical, Inc., www.sjm.com*	Conditional 5	3	
AorTech *Aortic, Model 3800, Titanium, heart valve,* *Aortech Ltd., Strathclyde, U.K.*	Conditional 1	1.5	75
AorTech *Mitral, Model 4800, Titanium, heart valve,* *Aortech Ltd., Strathclyde, U.K.*	Conditional 1	1.5	75
Aortic Mitroflow Synergy PC *Aortic Pericardial Heart Valve, Size 19-mm,* *Sulzer Carbomedics, Inc., Austin, TX*	Safe	1.5, 3	
Aortic Mitroflow Synergy PC *Aortic Pericardial Heart Valve, Size 29-mm,* *Sulzer Carbomedics, Inc., Austin, TX*	Safe	1.5, 3	
Aortic SJM Regent Valve *Mechanical Heart Valve, Size 27-mm, 27AGN-751,* *Rotatable Aortic, Standard Cuff-Polyester,* *AGN, St. Jude Medical, St. Paul, MN*	Conditional 5	3	

Object	Status	Field Strength (T)	Reference
Aortic Valve *Size 16-mm, A419529D 16A,* *Sulzer Carbomedics, Inc., Austin, TX*	Safe	1.5, 3	
Apical Connector *Model 174A, heart valve,* *Medtronic Heart Valve Division, www.Medtronic.com*	Safe	1.5, 3	84
ATS Medical Open Pivot *BiLeaflet Heart Valve, Mitral, Model 500DM29,* *Standard Valve, pyrolytic carbon, heart valve,* *ATS Medical, Minneapolis, MN*	Conditional 1	1.5	75
ATS Medical Open Pivot *BiLeaflet Heart Valve, Aortic, Model 501DA18,* *Advanced Performance (AP), pyrolytic carbon,* *heart valve,* *ATS Medical, Minneapolis, MN*	Conditional 1	1.5	75
Autogenics Autologous *Model APHV, Eligoy, heart valve,* *Autogenics Europe Ltd, Glasgow, Scotland*	Safe	1.5	75
Autogenics Autologous *Model ATCV, Eligoy, heart valve,* *Autogenics Europe Ltd, Glasgow, Scotland*	Safe	1.5	75
Beall *heart valve, Coratomic Inc., Indiana, PA*	Conditional 1	2.35	17
Beall *Mitral, pyrolitic carbon, heart valve,* *Coratomic Inc., Indianapolis, IN*	Conditional 1	1.5	75
Bileaflet *Model A7760, 29-mm, heart valve,* *Medtronic Heart Valve Division, www.Medtronic.com*	Safe	1.5	
Biocor Valve *Aortic, Model H3636, heart valve,* *St. Jude Medical, www.SJM.com*	Conditional 5	3	
Biocor Valve *Mitral, Size 35-mm, Model B10-35M,* *Heart Valves and Annuloplasty Rings,* *St. Jude Medical, Inc., www.SJM.com*	Conditional 5	3	
Bjork-Shiley (convexo/concave) *heart valve, Shiley Inc., Irvine, CA*	Safe	1.5	3
Bjork-Shiley (universal/spherical) *heart valve, Shiley Inc., Irvine, CA*	Conditional 1	1.5	3
Bjork-Shiley, Model 22 MBRC 11030 *heart valve, Shiley Inc., Irvine, CA*	Conditional 1	2.35	18
Bjork-Shiley, Model MBC *heart valve, Shiley Inc., Irvine, CA*	Conditional 1	2.35	18

Object	Status	Field Strength (T)	Reference
Bjork Shiley Monostrut *Aortic, Model ABMS, chromium cobalt alloy, heart valve,* *Pfizer, Inc., Cincinnati, OH*	Safe	1.5	75
Bjork Shiley Monostrut *Mitral, Model MBRMS, chromium cobalt alloy, heart valve,* *Pfizer, Inc., Cincinnati, OH*	Safe	1.5	75
Bjork Shiley Monostrut *Mitral, Model MBUM, chromium cobalt alloy, heart valve,* *Pfizer, Inc., Cincinnati, OH*	Conditional 1	1.5	75
Bjork Shiley *Pyrolitic Carbon Conical Disc, Mitral, Model MBRP,* *chromium cobalt alloy, heart valve,* *Pfizer, Inc., Cincinnati, OH*	Conditional 1	1.5	75
Bjork Shiley *Pyrolitic Carbon Conical Disc, Mitral, Model MBUP,* *chromium cobalt alloy, heart valve,* *Pfizer, Inc., Cincinnati, OH*	Safe	1.5	75
Carbomedics Heart Valve Prosthesis *Annuloflo Annuloplasty Ring, Size 26,* *Carbomedics, Austin, TX*	Safe	1.5	
Carbomedics Heart Valve Prosthesis *Annuloflo Annuloplasty Ring, Size 36,* *CarboMedics, Austin, TX*	Safe	1.5	
CarboMedics Heart Valve Prosthesis *Aortic Reduced, Model R500, Size 19,* *CarboMedics, Austin, TX*	Safe	1.5	19
CarboMedics Heart Valve Prosthesis *Aortic Reduced, Model R500, Size 21,* *CarboMedics, Austin, TX*	Safe	1.5	19
CarboMedics Heart Valve Prosthesis *Aortic Reduced, Model R500, Size 23,* *CarboMedics, Austin, TX*	Safe	1.5	19
CarboMedics Heart Valve Prosthesis *Aortic Reduced, Model R500, Size 25,* *CarboMedics, Austin, TX*	Safe	1.5	19
CarboMedics Heart Valve Prosthesis *Aortic Reduced, Model R500, Size 27,* *CarboMedics, Austin, TX*	Safe	1.5	19
CarboMedics Heart Valve Prosthesis *Aortic Reduced, Model R500, Size 29,* *CarboMedics, Austin, TX*	Safe	1.5	19
CarboMedics Heart Valve Prosthesis *Aortic Standard, Model 500, Size 31,* *CarboMedics, Austin, TX*	Safe	1.5	19

Object	Status	Field Strength (T)	Reference
Carbomedics Heart Valve Prosthesis *Aortic Valve, Size 16,* *CarboMedics, Austin, TX*	Safe	1.5	
Carbomedics Heart Valve Prosthesis *Carboseal, Size 31,* *CarboMedics, Austin, TX*	Safe	1.5	
CarboMedics Heart Valve Prosthesis *Mitral Standard, Model 700, Size 23,* *CarboMedics, Austin, TX*	Safe	1.5	19
CarboMedics Heart Valve Prosthesis *Mitral Standard, Model 700, Size 25,* *CarboMedics, Austin, TX*	Safe	1.5	19
CarboMedics Heart Valve Prosthesis *Mitral Standard, Model 700, Size 27,* *CarboMedics, Austin, TX*	Safe	1.5	19
CarboMedics Heart Valve Prosthesis *Mitral Standard, Model 700, Size 29,* *CarboMedics, Austin, TX*	Safe	1.5	19
CarboMedics Heart Valve Prosthesis *Mitral Standard, Model 700, Size 31,* *CarboMedics, Austin, TX*	Safe	1.5	19
CarboMedics Heart Valve Prosthesis *Mitral Standard, Model 700, Size 33,* *CarboMedics, Austin, TX*	Safe	1.5	19
Carbomedics Heart Valve Prosthesis *Mitral Valve, Size 33,* *CarboMedics, Austin, TX*	Safe	1.5	
Carboseal *Ascending Aortic Prosthesis, Size 33-mm,* *Model AP 33, S/N C489492-H,* *Sulzer Carbomedics, Inc., Austin, TX*	Safe	1.5, 3	
Carboseal *Ascending Aortic Valve Conduit, Size 33-mm,* *Model AP-033, Nitinol,* *Sulzer Carbomedics, Inc., Austin, TX*	Safe	1.5, 3	83
Carboseal *Ascending Aortic Valve Conduit, Size 33-mm,* *Model AP-033, Titanium,* *Sulzer Carbomedics, Inc., Austin, TX*	Safe	1.5, 3	83
Carpentier Edwards BioPhysio Heart Valve Prosthesis *Model 3100, 29M, Nitinol, silicone,* *Edwards Lifesciences, Irvine, CA*	Safe	1.5, 3, 8	
Carpentier-Edwards *Classic Annuloplasty Ring, Mitral Model 4400, size 40-mm,* *Edwards Lifesciences, Irvine, CA*	Safe	1.5, 3	77, 83

Object	Status	Field Strength (T)	Reference
Carpentier-Edwards (porcine) heart valve, American Edwards Laboratories, Santa Ana, CA	Conditional 1	2.35	18
Carpentier-Edwards Annuloplasty Ring, Model 4400, Baxter Healthcare Corporation, Santa Ana, CA	Safe	1.5	
Carpentier-Edwards Annuloplasty Ring, Model 4500, Baxter Healthcare Corporation, Santa Ana, CA	Safe	1.5	
Carpentier-Edwards Annuloplasty Ring, Model 4600, Baxter Healthcare Corporation Santa Ana, CA	Safe	1.5	
Carpentier-Edwards Bioprosthesis, Model 2625, heart valve, Baxter Healthcare Corporation, Santa Ana, CA	Safe	1.5	
Carpentier-Edwards Bioprosthesis, Model 6625, heart valve, Baxter Healthcare Corporation, Santa Ana, CA	Safe	1.5	
Carpentier-Edwards Low Pressure Bioprosthesis, Porcine, Mitral Model 6625-LP, size 35-mm, heart valve, Edwards Lifesciences, Irvine, CA	Safe	1.5, 3	77, 83
Carpentier-Edwards Magna II Pericardial, Aortic Heart Valve Prosthesis, Model 3300/3300TFX, Elgiloy alloy, Edwards Lifesciences, Irvine, CA	Conditional 6	3	
Carpentier-Edwards Pericardial Bioprosthesis, Model 2700, heart valve, Baxter Healthcare Corporation, Santa Ana, CA	Safe	1.5	
Carpentier-Edwards PERIMOUNT, Pericardial Bioprosthesis, Mitral Model 6900, size 33-mm, heart valve, Edwards Lifesciences, Irvine, CA	Conditional 1	1.5, 3	77, 83
Carpentier-Edwards Physio Annuloplasty Ring, Mitral Model 4450, size 40-mm, Edwards Lifesciences, Irvine, CA	Conditional 1	1.5, 3	77, 83
Carpentier-Edwards Physio Annuloplasty Ring, Model 4450, Baxter Healthcare Corporation, Santa Ana, CA	Safe	1.5	77
Carpentier-Edwards Physio Annuloplasty Ring, Model 4450, Elgiloy alloy, Edwards Lifesciences, Irvine, CA	Conditional 6	3	
Carpentier-Edwards Model 2650, heart valve, American Edwards Laboratories, Santa Ana, CA	Conditional 1	2.35	18

Object	Status	Field Strength (T)	Reference
Colvin-Galloway Future Band 638B *annuloplasty device,* *Medtronic Heart Valve Division, www.Medtronic.com*	Safe	1.5, 3	84
Contegra 200 *heart valve,* *Medtronic Heart Valve Division, www.Medtronic.com*	Safe	1.5, 3	84
Contegra 200S *heart valve,* *Medtronic Heart Valve Division, www.Medtronic.com*	Safe	1.5, 3	84
CoreValve *Medtronic, Inc., www.Medtronic.com*	Conditional 5	3	
Cosgrove-Edwards Annuloplasty Ring *Model 4600,* *Baxter Healthcare Corporationl, Santa Ana, CA*	Safe	1.5	
CPHV *annuloplasty ring, pyrolytic carbon, Titanium,* *Sulzer Medica and Sulzer Carbomedics*	Safe	1.5	
Cribier Aortic Bioprosthesis *Percutaneous Heart Valve, 316LVM SS,* *Edwards Lifesciences, Irvine, CA*	Safe	3	
Cribier-Edwards *Aortic Bioprosthesis, Model 9000 (PHV1A-26),* *combined with Carpentier-Edwards Porcine Bioprosthesis,* *Model 6650, 31-mm, heart valve prostheses,* *Edwards Lifesciences, Irvine, CA*	Conditional 6	3	
Durafic *Aortic, Model AD, size 33-mm, heart valve*	Conditional 1	1.5	75
Durafic *Model MD, Mitral, heart valve*	Conditional 1	1.5	75
Duraflex Low Pressure Bioprosthesis *Model 6625E6R-LP, heart valve,* *Baxter Healthcare Corporation, Santa Ana, CA*	Safe	1.5	
Duraflex Low Pressure Bioprosthesis *Model 6625LP, heart valve,* *Baxter Healthcare Corporation, Santa Ana, CA*	Safe	1.5	
Duran Ring *Model H601H, annuloplasty device,* *Medtronic Heart Valve Division, www.Medtronic.com*	Safe	1.5, 3	84
Duran Ring *Model H608H, annuloplasty device,* *Medtronic Heart Valve Division, www.Medtronic.com*	Safe	1.5, 3	84
Duran Ring *Model 610R, annuloplasty device,* *Medtronic Heart Valve Division, www.Medtronic.com*	Safe	1.5, 3	84

Object	Status	Field Strength (T)	Reference
Duran Annuloplasty Ring *Model H601H, 35-mm,* *Medtronic Heart Valve Division, www.Medtronic.com*	Safe	1.5	
Dynamic Remodeller Annuloplasty Ring *MiCardia Corporation, Irvine, CA*	Conditional 6	3	
Dynaplasty *MiCardia Annuloplasty Device, Annuloplasty Ring,* *MiCardia Corporation, Irvine, CA*	Conditional 6	3	
Edwards MIRA *Mechanical Valve, Mitral, Model 9600,* *Size 27-mm, heart valve,* *Edwards Lifesciences, Irvine, CA*	Safe	1.5, 3	83
Edwards MIRA *Mechanical Valve, Mitral, Model 9600,* *size 33-mm, heart valve,* *Edwards Lifesciences, Irvine, CA*	Safe	1.5	
Edwards Myxo ETlogix Annuloplasty Ring *Model 5100, Titanium alloy,* *Edwards Lifesciences, Irvine, CA*	Conditional 6	3	
Edwards Prima Plus *Stentless Bioprosthesis, Model 2500P,* *aortic heart valve, porcine, polyester cloth,* *Edwards Lifesciences Corporation, Irvine, CA*	Safe	1.5	
Edwards SAPIEN *Transcatheter Heart Valve,* *Edwards Lifesciences, Irvine, CA*	Conditional 6	3	
Edwards TEKNA Bileaflet Valve *Model 3200, heart valve,* *Baxter Healthcare Corporation, Santa Ana, CA*	Safe	1.5	
Edwards TEKNA Bileaflet Valve *Model 9200, heart valve,* *Baxter Healthcare Corporation, Santa Ana, CA*	Safe	1.5	
Edwards-Duromedics Bileaflet Valve *Model 3160, heart valve,* *Baxter Healthcare Corporation, Santa Ana, CA*	Safe	1.5	
Edwards-Duromedics Bileaflet Valve *Model 9120, heart valve,* *Baxter Healthcare Corporation, Santa Ana, CA*	Safe	1.5	
Freestyle *Aortic Root, Model 995, heart valve,* *Medtronic Heart Valve Division, www.Medtronic.com*	Safe	1.5, 3	84
Freestyle *Model 995, 27-mm, heart valve,* *Medtronic Heart Valve Division, www.Medtronic.com*	Safe	1.5	

Object	Status	Field Strength (T)	Reference
Hall-Kaster, Model A7700 *heart valve,* *Medtronic Heart Valve Division, www.Medtronic.com*	Conditional 1	1.5	3
Hancock *Model 100, Pulmonic Conduit, heart valve,* *Medtronic Heart Valve Division, www.Medtronic.com*	Safe	1.5, 3	84
Hancock *Model 105, Low Porosity Conduit, heart valve,* *Medtronic Heart Valve Division, www.Medtronic.com*	Safe	1.5, 3	84
Hancock *Model 150, Pulmonic Conduit, heart valve,* *Medtronic Heart Valve Division, www.Medtronic.com*	Safe	1.5, 3	84
Hancock *Model 242, Aortic Valve, heart valve,* *Medtronic Heart Valve Division, www.Medtronic.com*	Safe	1.5, 3	84
Hancock *Model 342, Mitral Valve, heart valve,* *Medtronic Heart Valve Division, www.Medtronic.com*	Safe	1.5, 3	84
Hancock 342 *35-mm, Model 342, heart valve,* *Medtronic Heart Valve Division, www.Medtronic.com*	Safe	1.5	
Hancock Conduit *Model 100, 30-mm, heart valve,* *Medtronic Heart Valve Division, www.Medtronic.com*	Safe	1.5	
Hancock extracorporeal *Model 242R, heart valve,* *Johnson & Johnson, Anaheim, CA*	Conditional 1	2.35	19
Hancock extracorporeal *Model M 4365-33, heart valve,* *Johnson & Johnson, Anaheim, CA*	Conditional 1	2.35	19
Hancock I (porcine) *heart valve,* *Johnson & Johnson, Anaheim, CA*	Conditional 1	1.5	3
Hancock II (porcine) *heart valve,* *Johnson & Johnson, Anaheim, CA*	Conditional 1	1.5	3
Hancock II *Model T505, Aortic Valve, heart valve,* *Medtronic Heart Valve Division, www.Medtronic.com*	Safe	1.5, 3	84
Hancock II *Model T510, Mitral Valve, heart valve,* *Medtronic Heart Valve Division, www.Medtronic.com*	Safe	1.5, 3	84

Object	Status	Field Strength (T)	Reference
Hancock II *Model T510, 33-mm, heart valve,* *Medtronic Heart Valve Division, www.Medtronic.com*	Safe	1.5	
Hancock MO II *Model 250, Aortic Valve, heart valve,* *Medtronic Heart Valve Division, www.Medtronic.com*	Safe	1.5, 3	84
Hancock MO II *Model 250B, Aortic Valve, heart valve,* *Medtronic Heart Valve Division, www.Medtronic.com*	Safe	1.5, 3	84
Hancock MO II *Model 250C, Aortic Valve, heart valve,* *Medtronic Heart Valve Division, www.Medtronic.com*	Safe	1.5, 3	84
Hancock MO II *Model 250D, Aortic Valve, heart valve,* *Medtronic Heart Valve Division, www.Medtronic.com*	Safe	1.5, 3	84
Hancock MO II *Model 250E, Aortic Valve, heart valve,* *Medtronic Heart Valve Division, www.Medtronic.com*	Safe	1.5, 3	84
Hancock MO II *Model 250H, Aortic Valve, heart valve,* *Medtronic Heart Valve Division, www.Medtronic.com*	Safe	1.5, 3	84
Hancock Pericardial *Mitral, Model T410, Haynes alloy, heart valve,* *Medtronic Inc., www.Medtronic.com*	Safe	1.5	75
Hancock Vascor, Model 505 *heart valve,* *Johnson & Johnson, Anaheim, CA*	Safe	2.35	19
HLT Transcatheter Aortic Heart Valve *Heart Leaflet Technologies, Inc (HLT), Maple Grove, MN*	Conditional 6	3	
IMR Annuloplasty Ring, Model 4100 *Edwards Lifesciences, www.edwards.com*	Conditional 6	3	
Inonescu-Shiley, Universal ISM *heart valve*	Conditional 1	2.35	19
Intact *Aortic, Model A805, size 19-mm, heart valve,* *Medtronic Heart Valve Division, www.Medtronic.com*	Safe	1.5	75
Intact *Model 705, Mitral Valve, heart valve,* *Medtronic Heart Valve Division, www.Medtronic.com*	Safe	1.5, 3	84
Intact *Model 805, Aortic Valve, heart valve,* *Medtronic Heart Valve Division, www.Medtronic.com*	Safe	1.5, 3	84

Object	Status	Field Strength (T)	Reference
Intact *Mitral, Model M705, size 25-mm, heart valve,* *Medtronic Inc., www.Medtronic.com*	Safe	1.5	75
JenaValve Transapical Prosthesis *JenaValve Technology GmbH*	Conditional 6	3	
Jyros *Aortic, Model J1A, carbon alloy, heart valve,* *Axion Medical Ltd.*	Safe	1.5	75
Jyros *Mitral, Model J1M, carbon alloy, heart valve,* *Axion Medical Ltd.*	Safe	1.5	75
Lillehi-Kaster *Model 300S, heart valve,* *Medical Inc., Inver Grove Heights, MN*	Conditional 1	2.35	17
Lillehi-Kaster *Model 5009, heart valve,* *Medical Inc., Inver Grove Heights, MN*	Conditional 1	2.35	19
Liotta *Aortic, Model MA783, Delrin, heart valve,* *St. Jude Medical, www.SJM.com*	Conditional 5	3	
Magna Mitral *Model 7000, Bioprosthetic tissue valve, Heart Valve,* *Bovine pericardium, PTFE fabric, Elgiloy frame,* *polyester support,* *Edwards Lifesciences, Irvine, CA*	Conditional 6	3	
Med Hall Conduit *Model R7700, 33-mm, heart valve,* *Medtronic Heart Valve Division, www.Medtronic.com*	Safe	1.5	
Medtronic Advantage *Model A7760, Aortic Valve, heart valve,* *Medtronic Heart Valve Division, www.Medtronic.com*	Safe	1.5, 3	84
Medtronic Advantage *Model M7760, Mitral Valve, heart valve,* *Medtronic Heart Valve Division, www.Medtronic.com*	Safe	1.5, 3	84
Medtronic Hall *heart valve,* *Medtronic Heart Valve Division, www.Medtronic.com*	Conditional 1	2.35	18
Medtronic Hall *Model 7700, 33-mm, heart valve,* *Medtronic Heart Valve Division, www.Medtronic.com*	Safe	1.5	
Medtronic Hall *Model A7700, Aortic Valve, heart valve,* *Medtronic Heart Valve Division, www.Medtronic.com*	Safe	1.5, 3	84

Object	Status	Field Strength (T)	Reference
Medtronic Hall *Model A7700-D-16, heart valve, Medtronic Heart Valve Division, www.Medtronic.com*	Conditional 1	2.35	18
Medtronic Hall *Model C7700, Valved Conduit, heart valve, Medtronic Heart Valve Division, www.Medtronic.com*	Safe	1.5, 3	84
Medtronic Hall *Model M7700, Mitral Valve, heart valve, Medtronic Heart Valve Division, www.Medtronic.com*	Safe	1.5, 3	84
Medtronic Hall *Model R7700, Low Porosity Valved Conduit, heart valve, Medtronic Heart Valve Division, www.Medtronic.com*	Safe	1.5, 3	84
Medtronic Hall *Model Z7700, Low Porosity Valved Conduit, heart valve, Medtronic Heart Valve Division, www.Medtronic.com*	Safe	1.5, 3	84
Melody Transcatheter Pulmonary Valve *Medtronic, Inc., http://manuals.medtronic.com/en/index.htm*	Conditional 5	3	
MEMO 3D *Semirigid Annuloplasty Ring, Used for mitral valve repair, CarboMedics, a Sorin Group Co., Austin, TX*	Conditional 6	3	
MiCardia Annuloplasty Device *Annuloplasty Ring, MiCardia Corporation, Irvine, CA*	Conditional 6	3	
Mitral Prosthetic Heart Valve *Model 2100, heart valve, TRI Technologies, Brazil*	Safe	1.5	70
Mitral Valve *Size 33-mm, A307504F, Sulzer Carbomedics, Inc., Austin, TX*	Safe	1.5, 3	
Mitroflow *Aortic, Model 11A, Delrin, heart valve, Mitroflow Sulzer CarboMedics, U.K.*	Safe	1.5	75
Mitroflow *Aortic, Model 14A, Delrin, heart valve, Mitroflow Sulzer CarboMedics, U.K.*	Safe	1.5	75
Mitroflow *Mitral, Model 11M, Delrin, heart valve, Mitroflow Sulzer CarboMedics, U.K.*	Safe	1.5	75
Mitroflow Pericardial Heart Valve *Model 12, Sulzer-Medica and Mitroflow International, Richmond, B.C., Canada*	Safe	1.5	70
Mosaic *Model 305, Aortic Valve, heart valve, Medtronic Heart Valve Division, www.Medtronic.com*	Safe	1.5, 3	84

Object	Status	Field Strength (T)	Reference
Mosaic *Model 310, Mitral Valve, heart valve,* *Medtronic Heart Valve Division, www.Medtronic.com*	Safe	1.5, 3	84
Mosaic *Model 310, 33-mm, heart valve,* *Medtronic Heart Valve Division, www.Medtronic.com*	Safe	1.5	
Omnicarbon *Model 35231029, heart valve,* *Medical Inc., Inver Grove Heights, MN*	Conditional 1	2.35	18
Omniscience *Model 6522, heart valve,* *Medical Inc., Inver Grove Heights, MN*	Conditional 1	2.35	18
On-X Valve *Model 6816, heart valve,* *Medical Carbon Research Institute, Austin, TX*	Safe	1.5	
Open Pivot Heart Valve, Mitral (Model 500) *ATS Medical, Inc., Lake Forest, CA*	Conditional 6	3	
Open Pivot Heart Valve, Aortic AP 360 (Model 505) *ATS Medical, Inc., Lake Forest, CA*	Conditional 6	3	
Percutaneous Heart Valve *316LMV SS,* *Percutaneous Valve Technologies, Ltd., Israel*	Safe	1.5, 3	
Percutaneous Mitral Annuloplasty Device (PMAD) *Nitinol, Titanium,* *Cardiac Dimensions, Inc., Kirkland, WA*	Safe	3	
Physio II Annuloplasty Ring *Edwards Lifesciences, Irvine, CA*	Conditional 6	3	
Porcine Synergy ST *Aortic, Size 19-mm,* *Sulzer Carbomedics, Inc., Austin, TX*	Safe	1.5, 3	
Porcine Synergy ST *Mitral, Size 33-mm,* *Sulzer Carbomedics, Inc., Austin, TX*	Safe	1.5, 3	
Posterior Annuloplasty Band *annuloplasty device, Model H607,* *Medtronic Heart Valve Division, www.Medtronic.com*	Safe	1.5, 3	84
Posterior Annuloplasty Band *Model 610B, annuloplasty device,* *Medtronic Heart Valve Division, www.Medtronic.com*	Safe	1.5, 3	84
Profile 3D Annuloplasty Ring *Medtronic Heart Valve Division, www.Medtronic.com*	Conditional 5	3	

Object	Status	Field Strength (T)	Reference
Pulmonic Bioprosthesis *9000TFXP Cribier-Edwards, Pulmonic Bioprosthesis,* *and Palmaz XL P3110, Combined prostheses,* *Edwards Lifesciences, Irvine, CA*	Conditional 6	3	
Reduced Aortic CPHV *Carbomedics Prosthetic, Model R5-029, Size 29-mm,* *heart valve, Nitinol,* *Sulzer Carbomedics, Inc., Austin, TX*	Safe	1.5, 3	83
Reduced Aortic CPHV *Carbomedics Prosthetic, Model R5-029, Size 29-mm,* *heart valve, Titanium,* *Sulzer Carbomedics, Inc., Austin, TX*	Safe	1.5, 3	83
Regent Mechanical Heart Valve *Model 27AG-701, 27-mm,* *St. Jude Medical, Inc., www.SJM.com*	Conditional 5	3	
Sculptor Ring *Model 605M, annuloplasty device,* *Medtronic Heart Valve Division, www.Medtronic.com*	Safe	1.5, 3	84
Sculptor Ring *Model 605T, annuloplasty device,* *Medtronic Heart Valve Division, www.Medtronic.com*	Safe	1.5, 3	84
Sculptor Annuloplasty Ring *Model 605M, 35-mm,* *Medtronic Heart Valve Division, www.Medtronic.com*	Safe	1.5	
SIMULUS Semi-Rigid Annuloplasty Ring *ATS Medical, Inc., Lake Forest, CA*	Conditional 6	3	
SJM Masters Series Valve *Mitral, Size 37-mm, Model 37 MJ-501, heart valve,* *St. Jude Medical, Inc., www.SJM.com*	Conditional 5	3	
SJM Regent Heart Valve *Aortic, Size 29-mm, Model 29AGN-751, heart valve,* *St. Jude Medical, Inc., www.SJM.com*	Conditional 5	3	
SJM Regent Valve *Mechanical Heart Valve, Rotatable,* *Aortic Standard Cuff-Polyester, Model 25AGN-751-IDE,* *St. Jude Medical, www.SJM.com*	Conditional 5	3	
SJM Tailor *Annuloplasty Ring, Size 35-mm, Model TARP-35,* *St. Jude Medical, Inc., www.SJM.com*	Conditional 5	3	
Smelloff Cutter *Aortic, Titanium, heart valve, Sorin Biomedica, Italy*	Conditional 1	1.5	75
Smeloff-Cutter *heart valve, Cutter Laboratories, Berkeley, CA*	Conditional 1	2.35	18

Object	Status	Field Strength (T)	Reference
Sorin Allcarbon, AS *Model MTR-29AS, 29-mm, pyrolitic carbon, heart valve,* *Sorin Biomedica Cardio S.p.A., Saluggia, Italy*	Conditional 1	1.5	75
Sorin, No. 23 *heart valve*	Conditional 1	1.5	20
Sorin Pericarbon (stented) *Mitral, pyrolytic carbon, heart valve,* *Sorin Biomedica, Italy*	Conditional 1	1.5	75
St. Jude Medical *Mechanical Heart Valve, SJM Masters Series Rotatable,* *Aortic, Model 25AJ-501, heart valve,* *St. Jude Medical, www.SJM.com*	Conditional 5	3	
St. Jude Medical *Mechanical Heart Valve, Model 33MECS-602, 33-mm,* *St. Jude Medical, Inc., www.SJM.com*	Conditional 5	3	
St. Jude, Model A 100 *heart valve,* *St. Jude Medical Inc., www.SJM.com*	Conditional 1	2.35	19
St. Jude, Model M 101 *heart valve,* *St. Jude Medical Inc., www.SJM.com*	Conditional 5	3	
St. Jude Medical, Annuloplasty Rings *Models include, AFR-xx, RSAR-xx, SARP-xx, TARP-xx,* *TAB-xx, Note: "xx" denotes different sizes* *available (e.g. 23A-101),* *St. Jude Medical, www.SJM.com*	Conditional 5	3	
St. Jude Medical, Mechanical Heart Valves *Models include, xxAGN-751, xxAGFN-756,* *xxAHPJ-505 or xxMHPJ-505, xxAEHPJ-505,* *xxAFHPJ-505, xxAJ-501 or xxMJ-501,* *xxAECJ-502 or xxMECJ-502, xxATJ-503 or xxMTJ-503,* *xxMETJ-504, xxA-101 or xxM-101, xxVAVGJ-515,* *xxCAVGJ-514,* **Note: "xx" denotes different sizes available (e.g. 23A-101),* *St. Jude Medical, www.SJM.com*	Conditional 5	3	
St. Jude Medical, Tissue Valves *Models include, E100-xxA-00 or E100-xxM-00,* *ESP100-xx-00, B100-xxA-00 or B100-xxM-00,* *BSP100-xx, B10-xxA-00 or B10-xxM-00, B10SP-xx,* *Note: "xx" denotes different sizes available (e.g. 23A-101),* *St. Jude Medical, www.SJM.com*	Conditional 5	3	
Standard Mitral CPHV *Carbomedics Prosthetic, Model R5-029, Size 29-mm,* *heart valve, Nitinol,* *Sulzer Carbomedics, Inc., Austin, TX*	Safe	1.5, 3	83

Object	Status	Field Strength (T)	Reference
Standard Mitral CPHV *Carbomedics Prosthetic, Model M7-033, Size 33-mm,* *Heart Valve, Titanium,* *Sulzer Carbomedics, Inc., Austin, TX*	Safe	1.5, 3	83
Starr-Edwards, Model 1000 *heart valve,* *Baxter Healthcare Corporation, Santa Ana, CA*	Conditional 1	1.5	
Starr-Edwards, Model 1200 *heart valve,* *Baxter Healthcare Corporation, Santa Ana, CA*	Conditional 1	1.5	
Starr-Edwards, Model 1260 *heart valve,* *American Edwards Laboratories,* *Baxter Healthcare Corporation, Santa Ana, CA*	Conditional 1	2.35	17
Starr-Edwards, Model 2300 *heart valve,* *Baxter Healthcare Corporation, Santa Ana, CA*	Conditional 1	1.5	
Starr-Edwards, Model 2310 *heart valve,* *Baxter Healthcare Corporation, Santa Ana, CA*	Conditional 1	1.5	
Starr-Edwards, Model 2320 *heart valve,* *American Edwards Laboratories,* *Baxter Healthcare Corporation, Santa Ana, CA*	Conditional 1	2.35	17
Starr-Edwards, Model 2400 *heart valve,* *American Edwards Laboratories,* *Baxter Healthcare Corporation, Santa Ana, CA*	Safe	1.5	3
Starr-Edwards, Model 6000 *heart valve,* *Baxter Healthcare Corporation, Santa Ana, CA*	Conditional 1	1.5	
Starr-Edwards, Model 6120 *heart valve,* *Baxter Healthcare Corporation, Santa Ana, CA*	Conditional 1	1.5	
Starr-Edwards, Model 6300 *heart valve,* *Baxter Healthcare Corporation, Santa Ana, CA*	Conditional 1	1.5	
Starr-Edwards, Model 6310 *heart valve,* *Baxter Healthcare Corporation, Santa Ana, CA*	Conditional 1	1.5	
Starr-Edwards, Model 6320 *heart valve,* *Baxter Healthcare Corporation, Santa Ana, CA*	Conditional 1	1.5	

Object	Status	Field Strength (T)	Reference
Starr-Edwards, Model 6400 *heart valve,* *Baxter Healthcare Corporation, Santa Ana, CA*	Conditional 1	1.5	
Starr-Edwards, Model 6520 *heart valve,* *Baxter Healthcare Corporation, Santa Ana, CA*	Conditional 1	2.35	19
Starr-Edwards, Model Pre 6000 *heart valve,* *American Edwards Laboratories,* *Baxter Healthcare Corporation, Santa Ana, CA*	Conditional 1	2.35	17
Sulzer/Carbomedics Synergy PC *Pericardial Heart Valve,* *Sulzer-Medica and Mitroflow International,* *Richmond, B.C., Canada*	Safe	1.5	70
Tascon *Aortic, Elgiloy, heart valve,* *Medtronic Heart Valve Division, www.Medtronic.com*	Safe	1.5	75
THV2, Model 9300TFX-29 *Aortic Heart Valve Prosthesis,* *Edwards Lifesciences, Irvine, CA*	Conditional 6	3	
Toronto SPV Valve *Stentless Porcine, Aortic Model SPA-101-25, heart valve,* *St. Jude Medical, www.SJM.com*	Conditional 5	3	
TS 3f Enable Aortic Bioprosthesis *Model 6000, ATS Medical, Inc., Lake Forest, CA*	Conditional 6	3	
Valtech Cardinal Annuloplasty Ring, Mitral *Valtech Cardio LTD*	Conditional 6	3	
Wessex *Aortic, Model WAV10, heart valve,* *Sorin Biomedica, Italy*	Safe	1.5	75
Wessex *Mitral, Model WMV20, heart valve,* *Sorin Biomedica, Italy*	Safe	1.5	75
Xenofic *Aortic, Model AP80, size 23, SS, heart valve*	Safe	1.5	75

Object	Status	Field Strength (T)	Reference

Hemostatic Clips, Other Clips, Fasteners, and Staples

Object	Status	Field Strength (T)	Reference
Absolok Plus *large, hemostatic clip, polydioxanone,* *Ethicon, Endo-Surgery, Cincinnati, OH*	Safe	1.5	71
Absolok Plus *medium, hemostatic clip, polydioxanone,* *Ethicon, Endo-Surgery, Cincinnati, OH*	Safe	1.5	71
Absolok Plus *small, hemostatic clip, polydioxanone,* *Ethicon, Endo-Surgery, Cincinnati, OH*	Safe	1.5	71
AC2 System Clip *Anastomotic Clip System, Nitinol,* *Rox Medical, San Clemente, CA*	Conditional 6	3	
AcuClip *C.P. Titanium, hemostatic clip,* *Origin Medsystems, Menlo Park, CA*	Safe	1.5	71
Cosgrove-Gillinov Vascular Occlusion Clip *Nitinol, Titanium,* *AtriCure, Inc., West Chester, OH*	Conditional 6	3	
Endostaple *Surgical Fastener, MP35N,* *MedSource Technologies, Newton, MA*	Safe	1.5, 3	83
Endostaple *Surgical Fastener, Nitinol,* *MedSource Technologies, Newton, MA*	Safe	1.5, 3	83
EVALVE clip *Cardiovascular Valve Repair System, Elgiloy,* *EVALVE, Redwood City, CA*	Safe	3	
EVS Vascular Closure Staple *Titanium alloy, Misc.,* *AngioLINK Corporation, Tauton, MA*	Safe	3	
Fascia staple *316L SS,* *United States Surgical, North Haven, CT*	Safe	1.5, 3	83
Filshie Clip *Avalon Medical Corporation, Williston, VT*	Safe	1.5	
Gastrointestinal anastomosis clip *Auto Suture SGIA, SS, hemostatic clip,* *United States Surgical Corp., Norwalk, CT*	Safe	1.5	3
GIA 4.8 staple *Titanium,* *United States Surgical, North Haven, CT*	Safe	1.5, 3	83

Object	Status	Field Strength (T)	Reference
GIA 4.8 Formed Titanium Staple *Multifire Endo GIA 60 - 4.8,* *Covidien, North Haven, CT*	Conditional 6	3	
Hemoclip, #10 *316L SS, hemostatic clip,* *Edward Weck, Triangle Park, NJ*	Safe	1.5	3
Hemoclip *tantalum, hemostatic clip,* *Edward Weck, Triangle Park, NJ*	Safe	1.5	3
Hulka Clip *Richard Wolf Medical Instruments, Vernon Hills, IL*	Conditional 5	3	
IVC venous clip *Teflon,* *Pilling Weck Co.*	Safe	1.5	
Ligaclip Extra LT 100 *C.P. Titanium, hemostatic clip,* *Ethicon, Endo-Surgery, Cincinnati, OH*	Safe	1.5	71
Ligaclip Extra LT 200 *C.P. Titanium, hemostatic clip,* *Ethicon, Endo-Surgery, Cincinnati, OH*	Safe	1.5	71
Ligaclip Extra LT 300 *C.P. Titanium, hemostatic clip,* *Ethicon, Endo-Surgery, Cincinnati, OH*	Safe	1.5	71
Ligaclip Extra LT 400 *C.P. Titanium, hemostatic clip,* *Ethicon, Endo-Surgery, Cincinnati, OH*	Safe	1.5	71
Ligaclip *tantalum, hemostatic clip,* *Ethicon, Inc., Sommerville, NJ*	Safe	1.5	3
Ligaclip, #6 *316L SS, hemostatic clip,* *Ethicon, Inc., Sommerville, NJ*	Safe	1.5	3
Ligating clip, small *C.P. Titanium, hemostatic clip,* *Horizon Surgical, Evergreen, CO*	Safe	1.5	71
Ligating clip, medium *C.P. Titanium, hemostatic clip,* *Horizon Surgical, Evergreen, CO*	Safe	1.5	71
Long Clip HX-600-090L *Olympus Medical Systems Corporation, Japan*	Unsafe 1	1.5	
MCM 20 *C.P. Titanium, hemostatic clip,* *Ethicon, Endo-Surgery, Cincinnati, OH*	Safe	1.5	71

Object	Status	Field Strength (T)	Reference
MSM 20 *C.P. Titanium, hemostatic clip,* *Ethicon, Endo-Surgery, Cincinnati, OH*	Safe	1.5	71
MCS 20 *C.P. Titanium, hemostatic clip,* *Ethicon, Endo-Surgery, Cincinnati, OH*	Safe	1.5	71
Micro SurgiClips *Titanium,* *U.S. Surgical Corporation, North Haven, CT*	Safe	1.5	
MultApplier clip *Titanium,* *United States Surgical, North Haven, CT*	Safe	1.5, 3	83
Multapplier Titanium Clip *500-28 Endoclip Multapplier,* *Covidien, North Haven, CT*	Conditional 6	3	
Ogden Suture Anchor *Titanium,* *United States Surgical, North Haven, CT*	Safe	1.5, 3	83
OTSC Clip *Over The Scope Clip, Nitinol,* *Ovesco Endoscopy GmbH, Germany*	Conditional 6	3	
Premium SurgiClip, L-13 *C.P. Titanium, hemostatic clip,* *United States Surgical Corp., Norwalk, CT*	Safe	1.5	71
Premium SurgiClip, M-11 *C.P. Titanium, hemostatic clip,* *United States Surgical Corp., Norwalk, CT*	Safe	1.5	71
Premium SurgiClip, S-9 *C.P. Titanium, hemostatic clip,* *United States Surgical Corp., Norwalk, CT*	Safe	1.5	71
QuickClip2 Long *HX-201LR-135L,* *Olympus Medical Systems Corporation, Japan*	Unsafe 1	1.5	
QuickClip2 Long *HX-201UR-135L,* *Olympus Medical Systems Corporation, Japan*	Unsafe 1	1.5	
Resolution Clip *304 SS, 17-7PH SS, 304V SS,* *Boston Scientific, www.bostonscientific.com*	Unsafe 1	1.5	
Royal staple *316L SS,* *United States Surgical, North Haven, CT*	Safe	1.5, 3	83

Object	Status	Field Strength (T)	Reference
Starclose Surgical Clip *Nitinol,* *Abbott Vascular, Santa Clara, CA*	Conditional 6	3	
Surgiclip, M-9.5 *C.P. Titanium, hemostatic clip,* *United States Surgical Corp., Norwalk, CT*	Safe	1.5	71
Surgiclip, M-11 *C.P. Titanium, hemostatic clip,* *United States Surgical Corp., Norwalk, CT*	Safe	1.5	71
Surgiclip, Auto Suture M-9.5 *SS, hemostatic clip,* *United States Surgical Corp., Norwalk, CT*	Safe	1.5	3
Suture Anchor *with Titanium Nitride Coating, Herculon soft tissue anchor,* *Covidien, North Haven, CT*	Conditional 6	3	
TA 90-4.8 directional staples *Titanium,* *United States Surgical, North Haven, CT*	Safe	1.5, 3	83
Tacker helical fastener *Titanium,* *United States Surgical, North Haven, CT*	Safe	1.5, 3	83
Tacker Titanium Helical Clip *Tacker 5-mm Mesh Fixation Device,* *Covidien, North Haven, CT*	Conditional 6	3	
TriClip Endoscopic Clipping Device *Wilson-Cook Medical Inc., Winston-Salem, NC*	Unsafe 1	1.5	118
U-CLIP *(B180), represents largest version of following U-CLIP* *products: S15, S18, S20, S25, S35, S50, S60, V45, V50,* *V60, V100D, S70, S90, S105, S120, B140, B160, B180,* *Medtronic Cardiac Surgery, Brooklyn Park, MN*	Conditional 6	3	
Ultraclip *316 SS,* *Inrad, Inc., Grand Rapids, MI*	Safe	1.5	
Ultraclip *Titanium alloy,* *Inrad, Inc., Grand Rapids, MI*	Safe	1.5	
Vesocclude Ligating Clip *Vesocclude Medical, LLC, Mebane, NC*	Conditional 6	3	

Object	Status	Field Strength (T)	Reference

Miscellaneous

Object	Status	Field Strength (T)	Reference
"J" Hook Bracket *816, Amerex Corporation, Trussville, AL*	Conditional 7	3	
3/4" Socket Wrench *3/4"*41-mm, Newmatic Sound Systems, Inc., Petaluma, CA*	Conditional 7	3	
357 Magnum Revolver *Model 66-3, Smith and Wesson, Springfield, MA*	Unsafe 1	1.5	46
4-Leg Base IV Stand, Stainless Steel *Pryor Products, Oceanside, CA*	Conditional 7	3	
5-Leg Base IV Stand, Aluminum *Pryor Products, Oceanside, CA*	Conditional 7	3	
AB5000 Ventricle *with In-Flow Cannula, and Out-Flow Cannula, Cardiac assist device, Abiomed, Inc., Danvers MA*	Conditional 6	3	113
Accusite pH *Enteral Feeding System pH Site Locator, 10 Fr., Zinetics Medical, Salt Lake City, UT*	Unsafe 2	1.5	
ActiFlo Indwelling Bowel Catheter System *also known as Zassi Bowel Management System, Hollister Incorporated, Libertyville, IL*	Conditional 5	3	
ActiPatch *Drug delivery patch, BioElectronics Corporation, Frederick, MD*	Unsafe 1	1.5	
Acuvance Jelco (FEP Radiopaque) *intravenous (I.V.) catheter, Smiths Medical, Southington, CT*	Safe	3	
Acuvance Plus (PUR Radiopaque) *intravenous (I.V.) catheter, Smiths Medical, Southington, CT*	Safe	3	
Acuvance Plus W (PUR Radiopaque) *intravenous (I.V.) catheter, Smiths Medical, Southington, CT*	Safe	3	
Adapter used for ICP *Aesculap Inc., Center Valley, PA*	Safe	1.5, 3	
Adiana Silicone Implant *permanent female contraception device, silicone, Adiana, Inc., Redwood City, CA*	Safe	3	
Adjustable Combination Pliers *152-mm, Newmatic Sound Systems, Inc., Petaluma, CA*	Conditional 7	3	

Object	Status	Field Strength (T)	Reference
Adjustable Combination Pliers *P-30,* *Ampco Safety Tools, Garland, TX*	Conditional 7	3	
Adjustable-End Wrench, 3/4" *NGK Metals Corporation, Sweetwater, TN*	Conditional 7	3	
Adjustable-End Wrench, 1 1/8" *NGK Metals Corporation, Sweetwater, TN*	Conditional 7	3	
Adjustable Pipe Wrench *W-212AL,* *Ampco Safety Tools, Garland, TX*	Conditional 7	3	
Adjustable Pipe Wrench 10" *NGK Metals Corporation, Sweetwater, TN*	Conditional 7	3	
Adjustable Wrench *24*200-mm,* *Newmatic Sound Systems, Inc., Petaluma, CA*	Conditional 7	3	
Adjustable Wrench *W-70,* *Ampco Safety Tools, Garland, TX*	Conditional 7	3	
Adson Tissue Forcep *Ti6Al4V,* *Johnson & Johnson, Professional, Inc., Raynham, MA*	Safe	1.5	62
Adult Transport Cocoon *(also known as Thermoflect),* *Hypothermia Prevention Product,* *Encompass Group, LLC, Addison, TX*	Conditional 7	3	
Advance Implant System *Model 10403,* *Aspire Medical, Sunnyvale, CA*	Conditional 6	3	
Advantiv (PUR Radiopaque) *intravenous (I.V.) catheter,* *Smiths Medical, Southington, CT*	Safe	3	
AirLife Bypass HME *Cardinal Health, Yorba Linda, CA*	Conditional 6	3	
Allen wrench *WH-1/4,* *Ampco Safety Tools, Garland, TX*	Conditional 7	3	
AMS Acticon Neosphincter Prosthesis *American Medical Systems, Minnetonka, MN*	Safe	1.5, 3	
AMS Artificial Urinary Sphincter 791 *AMS, American Medical Systems, Minnetonka, MN*	Safe	1.5, 3	
AMS Mainstay Urologic Soft-Tissue Anchor *AMS, American Medical Systems, Minnetonka, MN*	Safe	1.5, 3	

Object	Status	Field Strength (T)	Reference
AMS Sphincter 800 *Urinary Control System,* *AMS, American Medical Systems, Minnetonka, MN*	Safe	1.5, 3	3
Anesthesia Machine *MR Magellan-2200, Model 1 Pneumatically Powered,* *Anesthesia Machine,* *Oceanic Medical Products, Inc., Atchison, KS*	Conditional 7	3	
Anesthesia Machine *MR Magellan-2200, Model-3 Pneumatically Powered,* *Anesthesia Machine,* *Oceanic Medical Products, Inc., Atchison, KS*	Conditional 7	3	
Annular Occlusion Device *AOD, AtriCure, Inc., West Chester, OH*	Safe	3	
Annular Occlusion Device *AOD1, 50-mm, Nitinol, Titanium, Polyurethane,* *Polyester,* *AtriCure, Inc., West Chester, OH*	Conditional 6	3	
Aquacel Ag Dressing *AQUACEL AG Hydrofiber Wound Dressing, with Ionic Silver,* *ConvaTec, Skillman, NJ*	Safe	3	115
Arctic Sun, Energy Transfer Pad *No metallic components,* *Medivance, Inc., Louisville, CO*	Safe	3	
ARGOS 11-mm Restrictor *Pulmonx, Palo Alto, CA*	Conditional 6	3	
Aria MRI Drill System *Stryker, www.stryker.com*	Conditional 5	3	
Aris Trans-obturator Tape *product for urinary incontinence,* *Coloplast A/S, Humlebaek, Denmark*	Safe	3	
Aspire Medical Advance Implant System *Aspire Medical, Sunnyvale, CA*	Conditional 6	3	
Atrostim Phrenic Nerve Stimulator *Neurostimulation System,* *ATROTECH OY, Tampere, Finland*	Unsafe 1	1.5	
Autoflush Device *Ref 5897.01, LOT 08 10 02 EA 2007,* *Vygon, Paris, France*	Safe	1.5	
babyPac 100 Ventilator *Smiths Medical PM Inc., Waukesha, WI*	Conditional 5	3	
BACTISEAL Antimicrobial Catheter System *Codman,* *a Johnson and Johnson Company, Raynham, MA*	Safe	3	

Object	Status	Field Strength (T)	Reference
Ball Peen Hammer *H-00FG,* *Ampco Safety Tools, Garland, TX*	Conditional 7	3	
BandIt Clip *AtriCure Inc., West Chester, OH*	Conditional 6	3	
Bard Edwards Outflow Tract Fabric *Bard Peripheral Vascular, www.bardpv.com*	Safe	1.5	
Bard Kugal Patch *polypropylene,* *Davol, A Bard Company, www.davol.com*	Safe	1.5	
Bard Mesh *Davol, A Bard Company, www.davol.com*	Safe	1.5	
Bard Sauvage Filamentous Fabric *Bard Peripheral Vascular, www.bardpv.com*	Safe	1.5	
Bard Soft Mesh *Davol, A Bard Company, www.davol.com*	Safe	1.5	
Barricaid ARD, Annular Reconstruction Device *Intrinsic Therapeutics, Inc., Woburn, MA*	Conditional 6	3	
Battery, lithium, 3.9 Volt *304 SS and 316L SS, nickle,* *Greatbatch Scientific, Clarence, NY*	Conditional 1	1.5	
Battery *Low Magnetic Signature, "C" sized,* *Spiral Wound Lithium- Bromine Chloride Cell,* *Wilson Greatbatch Technologies, Inc., Clarence NY*	Conditional 7	3	
B-D PosiFlow *needleless IV access connector,* *Becton Dickinson, Sandy, Utah*	Safe	1.5	
Beacon Transponder *Calypso Medical Technologies, Inc., Seattle, WA*	Safe	3	
BioClip *neurosurgery fixation,* *Codman,* *Johnson and Johnson, Berkshire, UK*	Safe	1.5	
Bioclip *neurosurgical implant, Titanium alloy,* *Bioplate, Inc., Los Angeles, CA*	Conditional 6	3	
BioMesh *neurosurgery fixation, C.P. Titanium,* *Johnson and Johnson, Berkshire, UK*	Safe	1.5	
BioMesh *neurosurgical implant, Titanium,* *Bioplate, Inc., Los Angeles, CA*	Conditional 6	3	

Object	Status	Field Strength (T)	Reference
Bionector Device *Ref 5897.01, LOT 08 10 02 EA 2007,* *Vygon, Paris, France*	Safe	1.5	
Biosearch endo-feeding tube	Safe	1.5	
Bipolar Coagulation Forceps *For use in intraoperative MRI systems,* *Aesculap AG & CO.KG, Tuttlingen, Germany*	Safe	1.5, 3	83
Blip Implanted Fiducial Marker *Platinum/Iridium,* *Navotek Medical Ltd., Yokneam, Israel*	Conditional 6	3	
Blood Collection Set *SS,* *United States Surgical, North Haven, CT*	Safe	1.5, 3	83
BrachySource *radioactive seed,* *Bard Brachytherapy, Inc., Carol Stream, IL*	Conditional 6	3	
Bravo pH Monitoring System *Medtronic, Inc., Minneapolis, MN*	Unsafe 1	1.5	
Bung wrench *W-56,* *Ampco Safety Tools, Garland, TX*	Conditional 7	3	
Burr Hole Cover *neurosurgery fixation, C.P. Titanium,* *Johnson and Johnson, Berkshire, UK*	Safe	1.5	
Burr hole cover *neurosurgical implant, Titanium,* *Bioplate, Inc., Los Angeles, CA*	Conditional 6	3	
B.Y. Fix Anastomotic Device *Phynox, HDH Medical Ltd, Israel*	Conditional 6	3	
B.Y. Fix Anastomotic Device *Stainless Steel,* *HDH Medical Ltd, Israel*	Conditional 6	3	
Cannon Catheter II *Chronic Hemodialysis Catheter, polyurethane, 304 SS,* *Arrow International, Inc., Reading, PA*	Safe	1.5, 3	
Caresite Luer Access Device *B. Braun Medical Inc., Allentown, PA*	Conditional 6	3	
CAREvent MRI *ventilator,* *O-Two Medical Technologies, Inc., www.otwo.com*	Conditional 5	3	
Carillon Implant *Mitral Contour System,* *Cardiac Dimensions Inc., Kirkland, WA*	Conditional 6	3	

Object	Status	Field Strength (T)	Reference
Celsius Control Accutrol Catheter *10.7 Fr.,* *INNERCOOL Therapies, San Diego, CA*	Conditional 5	1.5	
Celsius Control Accutrol Catheter *14 Fr.,* *INNERCOOL Therapies, San Diego, CA*	Conditional 5	1.5	
Celsius Control Standard Catheter *10.7 Fr.,* *INNERCOOL Therapies, San Diego, CA*	Conditional 5	1.5	
Celsius Control Standard Catheter *14 Fr.,* *INNERCOOL Therapies, San Diego, CA*	Conditional 5	1.5	
Claw Hammer, 1 lb head, 13" handle *NGK Metals Corporation, Sweetwater, TN*	Conditional 6	3	
Claw Hammer with Handle *680-g,* *Newmatic Sound Systems, Inc., Petaluma, CA*	Conditional 7	3	
Claw Hammer *H-19FG,* *Ampco Safety Tools, Garland, TX*	Conditional 7	3	
CleanScene MRI Fixture *4 x 4 LED, CSMRI44,* *Kenall Lighting, Gurnee, IL*	Conditional 7	3	
Clip Board *Newmatic Sound Systems, Inc., Petaluma, CA*	Conditional 7	3	
Codman EDS 3, CSF External Drainage System *Codman,* *a Johnson and Johnson Company, Raynham, MA*	Conditional 6	3	
Codman MicroSensor Skull Bolt *Skull Bolt,* *Codman,* *Johnson and Johnson Company, Raynham, MA*	Safe	3	
Combination Pliers, slip joint *NGK Metals Corporation, Sweetwater, TN*	Conditional 7	3	
Combination wrench *1304,* *Ampco Safety Tools, Garland, TX*	Conditional 7	3	
Common Knife *K-1,* *Ampco Safety Tools, Garland, TX*	Conditional 7	3	
COMPASS Headframe (Complete) *using fixation, carbon fiber pin, Delrin Sleeve,* *Carbon Fiber Pin, Delrin Collet w/Nut,* *COMPASS International, Inc., Rochester, MN*	Conditional 8	1.5, 3	

Object	Status	Field Strength (T)	Reference
COMPASS Headframe (Complete) *using fixation, sharp pin, Delrin Sleeve w/Titanium Tip Insert and Delrin Collet w/Nut, COMPASS International, Inc., Rochester, MN*	Conditional 8	1.5, 3	
Concealed Sprinkler *Model VK462, The Viking Corporation, Hastings, MI*	Conditional 7	3	
Contraceptive diaphragm *All Flex, Ortho Pharmaceutical, Raritan, NJ*	Conditional 1	1.5	3
Contraceptive diaphragm *Flat Spring, Ortho Pharmaceutical, Raritan, NJ*	Conditional 1	1.5	3
Contraceptive diaphragm *Gyne T*	Safe	1.5	47
Contraceptive diaphragm *Koroflex, Young Drug Products, Piscataway, NJ*	Conditional 1	1.5	3
Contraceptive IUD/IUS *MIRENA, intrauterine system (IUS), polyethylene, barium sulfate, silicone, Berlex Laboratories, Montville, NJ*	Safe	1.5, 3	
Contraceptive IUD *Multiload Cu375, copper, silver*	Safe	1.5	47
Contraceptive IUD *Nova T, copper, silver*	Safe	1.5	47
COOK-SWARTZ Doppler Flow Probe *COOK Vascular Incorporated, Vandergrift, PA*	Unsafe 1	1.5	
Cool Line Catheter *Alsius Heat Exchange Catheter, Alsius Medical Corporation, Irvine, CA*	Conditional 5	1.5	
CoolGard 3000 Thermoregulation System *Alsius Heat Exchange Catheter, Alsius Medical Corporation, Irvine, CA*	Unsafe 1	1.5	
Core Temperature Ingestible Capsule *Temperature Device, VitalSense Integrated Physiological Monitoring System, Mini Mitter Company, Inc., Bend, OR*	Unsafe 1	1.5	
CORFLO Ultra *Non-weighted, Feeding Tube, Stylet Removed, Polyurethange, Viasys Healthcard Systems, Wheeling, IL*	Conditional 6	3	

Object	Status	Field Strength (T)	Reference
CORFLO, ULTRA 7 *Enteral Feeding Tube,* *Viasys MedSystems, Wheeling, IL*	Conditional 6	3	
Craftsman's Knife, 4 1/4" blade *NGK Metals Corporation, Sweetwater, TN*	Conditional 7	3	
Cranial Ceramic Drill bit *ceramic,* *MicroSurgical Techniques Inc., Fort Collins, CO*	Safe	1.5	48
Cranial Screw *neurosurgery fixation, size 1.9 x 4.5-mm, Titanium alloy,* *Johnson and Johnson, Berkshire, UK*	Safe	1.5	
Cranial Screw *neurosurgery fixation, size, 1.5 x 4.5-mm, Titanium alloy,* *Johnson and Johnson, Berkshire, UK*	Safe	1.5	
CranioFix *bone flap fixation system, Titanium alloy,* *Aesculap, Inc., Center Valley, PA*	Safe	1.5	50
CranioFix *Burr Hole Clamp, FF0997, 20-mm, Titanium,* *Aesculap, Inc., Center Valley, PA*	Safe	1.5, 3	83
CranioFix *Burr Hole Clamp, FF100T, 11-mm, Titanium,* *Aesculap, Inc., Center Valley, PA*	Safe	1.5, 3	83
CranioFix *Burr Hole Clamp, FF101T, 16-mm, Titanium,* *Aesculap, Inc., Center Valley, PA*	Safe	1.5, 3	83
CranioFix Titanium Clamps *Models including FF099T, FF100T, FF101T, FF490T,* *FF491T, FF492T,* *Aesculap, Inc., Center Valley, PA*	Safe	3	
CranioFix2 Titanium Clamps *Models including FF099T, FF100T, FF101T, FF490T,* *FF491T, FF492T,* *Aesculap, Inc., Center Valley, PA*	Safe	3	
Crate Opener *70*230-mm,* *Newmatic Sound Systems, Inc., Petaluma, CA*	Conditional 7	3	
Crate Opener *CJ-1-ST,* *Ampco Safety Tools, Garland, TX*	Conditional 7	3	
CV-1 CapsoCam *Pill Camera,* *Capso Vision, Inc., Saratoga, CA*	Unsafe 1	1.5	

Object	Status	Field Strength (T)	Reference
Deck Scraper *45*300-mm,* *Newmatic Sound Systems, Inc., Petaluma, CA*	Conditional 7	3	
Deck Scraper *S-11G,* *Ampco Safety Tools, Garland, TX*	Conditional 7	3	
Deponit, nitroglycerin *transdermal delivery system, aluminized plastic,* *Schwarz Pharma, Milwaukee, WI*	Conditional 3	1.5	
Diagonal Cutting Pliers *200-mm,* *Newmatic Sound Systems, Inc., Petaluma, CA*	Conditional 7	3	
Disetronic Pumps *Disetronic Medical Systems, Inc., St. Paul, MN*	Unsafe 1	1.5	
Disposable Sterile, Non-magnetic scalpel #11, MRDS11 *Newmatic Sound Systems, Inc., Petaluma, CA*	Conditional 7	3	
Disposable Sterile, Non-magnetic scalpel #21, MRDS21 *Newmatic Sound Systems, Inc., Petaluma, CA*	Conditional 7	3	
DISTFLO MINI-CUFF Bypass Graft *Bard Peripheral Vascular, www.bardpv.com*	Safe	1.5	
DOBHOFF Gastro-Jejunal System *COVIDIEN, Hazelwood, MO*	Conditional 6	3	
Double Box End Wrench *W-3130,* *Ampco Safety Tools, Garland, TX*	Conditional 7	3	
Double Box Ended Wrench *14*15-mm,* *Newmatic Sound Systems, Inc., Petaluma, CA*	Conditional 7	3	
Double Open Ended Wrench *18*19-mm,* *Newmatic Sound Systems, Inc., Petaluma, CA*	Conditional 7	3	
Double Open Ended Wrench *5.5*7-mm,* *Newmatic Sound Systems, Inc., Petaluma, CA*	Conditional 7	3	
Double Open-end wrench *WO-17X19,* *Ampco Safety Tools, Garland, TX*	Conditional 7	3	
Double Step Stool *Newmatic Sound Systems, Inc., Petaluma, CA*	Conditional 7	3	
Dry Pad 9 x 9 with Silver Antimicrobial Agent *Newmatic Sound Systems, Inc., Petaluma, CA*	Conditional 7	3	

Object	Status	Field Strength (T)	Reference
Duet External Drainage System *Model 46914,* *Medtronic Neurosurgery, Goleta, CA*	Conditional 7	3	
DVS *Dose Verification System,* *implantable radiation dosimeter,* *Sicel Technologies, Inc., Morrisville, NC*	Conditional 5	1.5	
E Cylinder Aluminum Construction *Newmatic Sound Systems, Inc., Petaluma, CA*	Conditional 7	3	
E/D Cylinder Rack 6 *Newmatic Sound Systems, Inc., Petaluma, CA*	Conditional 7	3	
E/D Dual Cylinder Hand Cart *Newmatic Sound Systems, Inc., Petaluma, CA*	Conditional 7	3	
EEG electrodes, Adult E-6-GH *gold plated silver,* *Grass Co., Quincy, MA*	Safe	0.3	51
EEG electrodes, Pediatric E-5-GH *gold plated silver,* *Grass Co., Quincy, MA*	Safe	0.3	51
Elana Ring *Platinum,* *ELANA BV, Utrecht, The Netherlands*	Safe	3	
Emergency Medical Cot *Model 30-NM,* *Ferno-Washington, Inc., Wilmington, OH*	Conditional 7	3	
Emergency Medical Cot *Model 33-NM,* *Ferno-Washington, Inc., Wilmington, OH*	Conditional 7	3	
Emergency Medical Cot *Model 35-ANM,* *Ferno Washington Inc., Wilmington, OH*	Conditional 7	3	
Endo Capsule *Capsule Endoscope System,* *Olympus Medical Systems Corporation, Japan*	Unsafe 1	1.5	
Endobronchial Valve *EBV-6.5,* *Emphasys Medical Inc., Redwood City, CA*	Safe	3	
Endoscope, rigid, 2.7-mm (Sinuscope) *Greatbatch Scientific, Clarence, NY*	Safe	1.5	59
Endoscope, rigid, 8.0-mm (Laryngoscope) *Greatbatch Scientific, Clarence, NY*	Safe	1.5	59
EndoSure s2 Wireless AAA *(Abdominal Aortic Aneurysm) Pressure Sensor,* *CardioMEMS, Inc., Atlanta, GA*	Conditional 5	1.5, 3	

Object	Status	Field Strength (T)	Reference
EndoSure Wireless AAA *(Abdominal Aortic Aneurysm) Pressure Sensor, CardioMEMS, Inc., Atlanta, GA*	Conditional 5	1.5, 3	
Endotracheal (ET) Tube *polyurethane coating with silver, C.R. Bard, Inc., Covington, GA*	Safe	1.5	
Endotracheal tube with metal ring marker *Trachmate*	Safe	1.5	
Endotracheal Tube *Agento IC, Silver Coated Endotracheal Tube, Bard Medical Division, Covington, GA*	Conditional 6	3	
ENDO-TUBE *Naso-Jejunal Feeding Tube, COVIDIEN, Hazelwood, MO*	Conditional 6	3	
Engineer Hammer *H-14FG, Ampco Safety Tools, Garland, TX*	Conditional 7	3	
ENTRI-FLEX *Nasogastric (NG) Feeding Tube, COVIDIEN, Hazelwood, MO*	Conditional 6	3	
ESTRING *Estradiol Vaginal Ring, Pfizer, www.pfizer.com*	Safe	1.5	
ENTRISTAR *Jejunum Feeding Tube/Gastric Depression Tube, COVIDIEN, Hazelwood, MO*	Conditional 6	3	
ESSURE Device *316L SS, Platinum, iridium, nickel, Titanium, Conceptus, San Marcos, CA*	Safe	1.5, 3	76, 83
ESSURE Device *Nickel-Titanium outer and inner coils, Conceptus, Inc., Mountain View, CA*	Conditional 6	3	
ESSURE Device *Nickel-Titanium outer coil, with a SS inner coil, Conceptus, Inc., Mountain View, CA*	Conditional 6	3	
Essure Micro-insert *Permanent contraception device, Conceptus, Inc., Mountain View, CA*	Conditional 6	3	
eSVS Mesh *Kips Bay Medical, Plymouth, MN*	Conditional 8	1.5, 3	
Extension Set with Caresite Luer Access Device and Spin-Lock Connector *B. Braun Medical Inc., Allentown, PA*	Conditional 6	3	

Object	Status	Field Strength (T)	Reference
Extension Set with ULTRASITE Injection Site and Spin-Lock Connector *B. Braun Medical Inc., Allentown, PA*	Conditional 6	3	
Eyelid weight *gold*	Safe	1.5	52
EZ Huber Safety Infusion Set *PFM Medical, Inc., Oceanside, CA*	Conditional 6	3	
Fastrac Device *long-term enteral feeding management device,* *316LVM SS, silicone,* *Bard Access Systems, Inc., Salt Lake City, UT*	Conditional 6	3	
Fastrac Gastric Access Port *silicone, 316LVM SS,* *Bard Endoscopic Technologies, Billerica, MA*	Safe	1.5	
Feeding Tube *C-FMT-8.0-120, Frederick Miller Feeding Tube, Misc.,* *Cook, Inc., Bloomington, IN*	Safe	3	
Feeding Tube *C-FMT-8.0-70, Frederick Miller Feeding Tube, Misc.,* *Cook, Inc., Bloomington, IN*	Safe	3	
Feeding Tube *Gastrostomy Feeding Tube, jejunal,* *Kimberly-Clark, Draper, UT*	Safe	3	
Fiber-Optic Cardiac Pacing Lead *photonic device,* *Biophan Technologies, Inc., Rochester, NY*	Safe	1.5, 3	81
Fiber-optic Intubating *Laryngoscope Blade,* *Greatbatch Scientific, Clarence, NY*	Safe	1.5	
Fiber-optic Intubating *Laryngoscope Handle,* *Greatbatch Scientific, Clarence, NY*	Safe	1.5	
Fire Extinguisher *Model 322, 5.0 lb. CO2,* *Amerex Corporation, Trussville, AL*	Safe	3	
Fire Extinguisher *Model B270NM, 1 3/4 gallon Water Mist,* *Amerex Corporation, Trussville, AL*	Safe	3	
Fire Extinguisher *Model B272NM, 2 1/2 gallon Water Mist,* *Amerex Corporation, Trussville, AL*	Safe	3	
Firestar *9-mm semiautomatic,* *Star Bonifacio Echeverria, Eibar, Spain*	Unsafe 1	1.5	46

Object	Status	Field Strength (T)	Reference
Flex-tip Plus Epidural Catheter *304V SS,* *Arrow International Inc., Reading, PA*	Unsafe 2	1.5	
Flowmeter *Quick Click, CFMXXX-XX,* *Western Scott Fetzer, Inc., Westlake, OH*	Conditional 7	3	
Flowmeter *Slim-Line Flowmeter, FMAX0X,* *Western Scott Fetzer, Inc., Westlake, OH*	Conditional 7	3	
Flowmeter *Slim-Line Flowmeter, FMEX0X,* *Western Scott Fetzer, Inc., Westlake, OH*	Conditional 7	3	
Flowmeter *Slim-Line Flowmeter, FMR100,* *Western Scott Fetzer, Inc., Westlake, OH*	Conditional 7	3	
Forceps, ceramic *MicroSurgical Techniques Inc., Fort Collins, CO*	Safe	1.5	48
Forceps, Titanium	Safe	1.39	1
Fortius Catheter *Alsius Heat Exchange Catheter,* *Alsius Medical Corporation, Irvine, CA*	Conditional 5	1.5	
FREEHAND System *Implantable Functional Neurostimulator (FNS),* *NeuroControl Corporation, Cleveland, OH*	Conditional 5	1.5	
FREKA Intestinal Tube *Long term intestinal feeding,* *Animech Technologies AB, Uppsala, Sweden*	Conditional 6	3	
Gabriel Feeding Tube *Magnetically-Guided Feeding Tube, 12-Fr, GFT112,* *Neo-dymium magnets, imbedded in distal tip of the tube,* *Syncro Medical Innovations, Inc., Canton, OH*	Unsafe 1	3	
Gel pad *various shapes,* *AADCO Medical, Inc., Randolph, VT*	Conditional 7	3	
Grab 'n Go Heliox *portable medical heliox system, aluminum cylinder,* *CAUTION: DO NOT USE STEEL CYLINDERS,* *Praxair Healthcare Services, Burr Ridge, IL*	Conditional 7	3	
Grab 'n Go Vantage *portable oxygen system, aluminum D cylinder,* *CAUTION: DO NOT USE STEEL CYLINDERS,* *Praxair Healthcare Services, Burr Ridge, IL*	Conditional 7	3	

Object	Status	Field Strength (T)	Reference
Grab 'n Go Vantage *portable oxygen system, aluminum E cylinder,* *CAUTION: DO NOT USE STEEL CYLINDERS,* *Praxair Healthcare Services, Burr Ridge, IL*	Conditional 7	3	
Grab 'n Go Vantage *regulator/pressure gauge,* *CAUTION: DO NOT USE STEEL CYLINDERS,* *Praxair Healthcare Services, Burr Ridge, IL*	Conditional 7	3	
Grab 'n Go Vantage *D cylinder, oxygen tank,* *CAUTION: DO NOT USE STEEL CYLINDERS,* *Praxair Healthcare Services, Burr Ridge, IL*	Conditional 7	3	
Grab 'n Go Vantage *E cylinder, oxygen tank,* *CAUTION: DO NOT USE STEEL CYLINDERS,* *Praxair Healthcare Services, Burr Ridge, IL*	Conditional 7	3	
Groove Joint Pliers, 2 1/2" *NGK Metals Corporation, Sweetwater, TN*	Conditional 7	3	
Groove Joint Pliers, 10" *Newmatic Sound Systems, Inc., Petaluma, CA*	Conditional 7	3	
Groove Joint Pliers *300-mm,* *Newmatic Sound Systems, Inc., Petaluma, CA*	Conditional 7	3	
Groove Joint Pliers *P-39,* *Ampco Safety Tools, Garland, TX*	Conditional 7	3	
Gurney with IV Pole *Newmatic Sound Systems, Inc., Petaluma, CA*	Conditional 7	3	
Gurney *Newmatic Sound Systems, Inc., Petaluma, CA*	Conditional 7	3	
Hamper *HAMPF,* *Newmatic Sound Systems, Inc., Petaluma, CA*	Conditional 7	3	
Hand Tool Kit *six piece, NF-240, Standard screw driver,* *Philips screw driver, Wrench, Pliers, Adjustable pliers,* *Crate opener,* *AADCO Medical, Inc., Randolph, VT*	Conditional 7	3	
Heine Gamma Sphygmomanometer *Newmatic Sound Systems, Inc., Petaluma, CA*	Conditional 7	3	
Hemashield Finesse *Ultra-Thin, Knitted, Cardiovascular Patch,* *vascular graft, Polyester,* *Boston Scientific Corporation, Quincy, MA*	Safe	3	

Object	Status	Field Strength (T)	Reference
Hemashield Gold Microvel *Knitted Double Velour, Vascular Graft, Polyester,* *Boston Scientific Corporation, Quincy, MA*	Safe	3	
Hex Key Wrench *1.5-mm,* *Newmatic Sound Systems, Inc., Petaluma, CA*	Conditional 7	3	
Hex Key Wrench *1-1/16",* *Newmatic Sound Systems, Inc., Petaluma, CA*	Conditional 7	3	
HoverMatt, HM34DC - 34"x78" *heat-sealed air mattress,* *nylon twill with polyurethane coating,* *HoverTech International, Bethlehem, PA*	Conditional 6	3	
HoverMatt, HM34HS - 34"x78" *heat-sealed air mattress, nylon twill,* *HoverTech International, Bethlehem, PA*	Conditional 6	3	
IBV Valve *Nitinol, Spiration Inc., Redmond, WA*	Conditional 6	3	
Icy Catheter *Alsius Heat Exchange Catheter,* *Alsius Medical Corporation, Irvine, CA*	Conditional 5	1.5	
IMPLANON *etonogestrel implant, contraceptive implant,* *flexible plastic rod,* *Organon USA Inc., Roseland, NJ*	Safe	1.5	109
Implantable Spinal Fusion Stimulator *Bone Fusion Stimulator, Model SpF-100,* *Electro-Biology, Inc. (EBI), Parsippany, NJ*	Conditional 5	1.5	63
Implantable Spinal Fusion Stimulator *Bone Fusion Stimulator,* *Electro-Biology, Inc. (EBI), Parsippany, NJ*	Conditional 5	1.5	
In-Fast Bone Screw *Titanium alloy,* *American Medical Systems, Minnetonka, MN*	Safe	3	
In-Fast Loop Screw *Titanium alloy,* *American Medical Systems, Minnetonka, MN*	Safe	3	
In-Fast Sling System *AMS, American Medical Systems, Minnetonka, MN*	Safe	1.5, 3	
In-Fast Swivel Screw *Titanium alloy,* *American Medical Systems, Minnetonka, MN*	Safe	3	
In-Fast Ultra Sling System *AMS, American Medical Systems, Minnetonka, MN*	Safe	1.5, 3	

Object	Status	Field Strength (T)	Reference
Infusion Set *MMT-11X,* *Medtronic MiniMed Inc., Northridge, CA*	Safe	1.5	
Infusion Set *MMT-31X,* *Medtronic MiniMed Inc., Northridge, CA*	Safe	1.5	
Infusion Set *MMT-32X,* *Medtronic MiniMed Inc., Northridge, CA*	Safe	1.5	
Infusion Set *MMT-37X,* *Medtronic MiniMed Inc., Northridge, CA*	Safe	1.5	
Infusion Set *MMT-39X,* *Medtronic MiniMed Inc., Northridge, CA*	Safe	1.5	
Infusion Set *Polyfin, MMT-106,* *Medtronic MiniMed Inc., Northridge, CA*	Unsafe 1	1.5	
Infusion Set *Polyfin, MMT-107,* *Medtronic MiniMed Inc., Northridge, CA*	Unsafe 1	1.5	
Infusion Set *Polyfin, MMT-16X,* *Medtronic MiniMed Inc., Northridge, CA*	Unsafe 1	1.5	
Infusion Set *Polyfin, MMT-30X,* *Medtronic MiniMed Inc., Northridge, CA*	Unsafe 1	1.5	
Infusion Set *Polyfin, MMT-36X,* *Medtronic MiniMed Inc., Northridge, CA*	Unsafe 1	1.5	
Insulin Pump *Animas 2020 Insulin Pump,* *Animas Corporation,* *a Johnson & Johnson Company, www.animascorp.com*	Unsafe 1	1.5	
Insulin Pump *IR 1000 Insulin Pump,* *Animas Corporation,* *a Johnson & Johnson Company, www.animascorp.com*	Unsafe 1	1.5	
Insulin Pump *IR 1100 Insulin Pump,* *Animas Corporation,* *a Johnson & Johnson Company, www.animascorp.com*	Unsafe 1	1.5	

Object	Status	Field Strength (T)	Reference
Insulin Pump *IR 1200 Insulin Pump,* *Animas Corporation,* *a Johnson & Johnson Company, www.animascorp.com*	Unsafe 1	1.5	
Insulin Pump *IR Animas 1200,* *Animas Corporation,* *a Johnson and Johnson Company, www.animascorp.com*	Unsafe 1	1.5	
Intima-II I.V. Catheter System *BD Medical Systems, Becton Dickinson, Sandy, Utah*	Safe	1.5	
Intracranial depth electrodes *for EEG recordings, nickle- chromium alloy,* *Superior Tube Company, Norristown, NY*	Safe	1.5	53
Intracranial Pressure Monitor (ICP) *Pressio ICP Monitoring Device,* *SOPHYSA, France*	Unsafe 1	1.5	
Intraflex Feeding Tube *tungstun weight, plastic*	Safe	1.5	
Intrauterine contraceptive device (IUD) *Copper T, copper,* *Searle Pharmaceuticals, Chicago, IL*	Safe	1.5	54
Intrauterine Contraceptive Device *Copper T 380A, ParaGard,* *FEI, North Tanawanda, NY*	Conditional 5	3	111
Intrauterine contraceptive device (IUD) *Lippey loop, plastic*	Safe	1.5	
Intrauterine contraceptive device (IUD) *Perigard, Gyne Pharmaceuticals*	Safe	1.5	
InVance Male Sling System *AMS, American Medical Systems, Minnetonka, MN*	Safe	1.5, 3	
IsoMed *implantable drug infusion system,* *Medtronic, Inc., Minneapolis, MN*	Conditional 5	1.5	
IUD, LCS *Ultra Low Dose Levonorgestrel, Contraceptive System,* *Bayer Schering Pharma Oy, Turku, Finland*	Conditional 6	3	
IV Pole *HD NM, Model 513-10,* *Ferno Washington Inc., Wilmington, Ohio*	Conditional 7	3	
IV Pole, PN R&D#0556 *Pryor Products, Oceanside, CA*	Conditional 7	3	
IV Stand 4 Hook with Casters, Aluminum *Newmatic Sound Systems, Inc., Petaluma, CA*	Conditional 7	3	

Object	Status	Field Strength (T)	Reference
IV Stand 4 Hook with Casters *Newmatic Sound Systems, Inc., Petaluma, CA*	Conditional 7	3	
Janitorial Cleaning Cart *Continental Commercial Products, Bridgeton, MO*	Conditional 7	3	
Jelco (FEP Radiopaque) *intravenous (I.V.) catheter,* *Smiths Medical, Southington, CT*	Safe	3	
Jelco (FEP) *intravenous (I.V.) catheter,* *Smiths Medical, Southington, CT*	Safe	3	
Jelco 2 (FEP) *intravenous (I.V.) catheter,* *Smiths Medical, Southington, CT*	Safe	3	
Jelco W (FEP) *intravenous (I.V.) catheter,* *Smiths Medical, Southington, CT*	Safe	3	
Ladder 8-foot *Newmatic Sound Systems, Inc., Petaluma, CA*	Conditional 7	3	
Langenbeck Periosteal Elevator *304 SS,* *Johnson & Johnson Professional, Inc., Raynham, MA*	Safe	1.5	62
Laparoscopic Graspers *Greatbatch Scientific, Clarence, NY*	Safe	1.5	
LAP-BAND (LAPBAND) *adjustable gastric band,* *INAMED, Goleta, CA*	Safe	3	
LAP-BAND (LAPBAND) AP System *Adjustable Gastric Banding System* *with OMNIFORM Design,* *Allergan, Inc., www.allergan.com*	Conditional 5	3	
Large Flexible Burr Hole Cover *neurosurgery fixation, C.P. Titanium,* *Johnson and Johnson, Berkshire, UK*	Safe	1.5	
Large Rigid Burr Hole Cover *neurosurgery fixation, C.P. Titanium,* *Johnson and Johnson, Berkshire, UK*	Safe	1.5	
Laryngoscope Blade, Fiber-Optic *Sun-Flex, MAC 4, 304 SS, PriMedCo*	Conditional 7	3	
Laryngoscope Blade, Fiber-Optic *Straight, 304 SS, PriMedCo*	Conditional 7	3	
Laryngoscope Blade Miller 00, LRYM00 *Newmatic Sound Systems, Inc., Petaluma, CA*	Conditional 7	3	
Laryngoscope Blade Miller 04, LRYM4 *Newmatic Sound Systems, Inc., Petaluma, CA*	Conditional 7	3	

Object	Status	Field Strength (T)	Reference
Laryngoscope Fiber Optic Blade *Size Mac 2, Scope Medical, India*	Conditional 7	3	
Laryngoscope Fiber Optic Blade *Size Mac 3, Scope Medical, India*	Conditional 7	3	
Laryngoscope Fiber Optic Blade *Size Mac 4, Scope Medical, India*	Conditional 7	3	
Laryngoscope Fiber Optic Blade *Size Mill 1, Scope Medical, India*	Conditional 7	3	
Laryngoscope Fiber Optic Blade *Size Mill 2, Scope Medical, India*	Conditional 7	3	
Laryngoscope Fiber Optic Blade *Size Mill 3, Scope Medical, India*	Conditional 7	3	
Laryngoscope Fiber Optic *Handle Medium Size, Scope Medical, India*	Conditional 7	3	
Laryngoscope Handle *Model 15-MRI-HMED-1, Blade - Mac 3,* *Model 15-MRI-MAC3, Lithium Battery, Model 15-MRI-L1,* *NovaMed, LLC, Rye, New York*	Conditional 7	3	
Laryngoscope Handle Standard, LRYH *Newmatic Sound Systems, Inc., Petaluma, CA*	Conditional 7	3	
LED Downlight Fixture *MRIDL6VL, Kenall Lighting, Gurnee, Illinois*	Conditional 7	3	
Licox CC1.P1 Oxygen and Temperature Probe *Brain Tissue Oxygen Monitoring System,* *Integra NeuroSciences, Plainsboro, NJ*	Conditional 5	1.5	
LifeGuard Safety Infusion Set *ANGIODYNAMICS Inc., Manchester, GA*	Conditional 6	3	
Lightweight Aluminum Gurney *Newmatic Sound Systems, Inc., Petaluma, CA*	Conditional 7	3	
Lineman Pliers *200-mm,* *Newmatic Sound Systems, Inc., Petaluma, CA*	Conditional 7	3	
Lineman's pliers *P-35,* *Ampco Safety Tools, Garland, TX*	Conditional 7	3	
Linen Hamper 18-inch D-Casters *Newmatic Sound Systems, Inc., Petaluma, CA*	Conditional 7	3	
LINX Reflux Management System *Torax Medical, www.toraxmedical.com*	Unsafe 1	1.5	
LMA Fastrach Endotracheal Tube *size 8-mm, endotracheal tube,* *LMA North America, Inc., San Diego, CA*	Conditional 5	1.5	

Object	Status	Field Strength (T)	Reference
LMA-Classic *size 5, large adult, laryngeal mask airway,* *LMA North America, Inc., San Diego, CA*	Conditional 5	1.5	
LMA-Flexible *size 2, larygeal mask airway,* *LMA North America, Inc., San Diego, CA*	Conditional 5	1.5	
LMA-ProSeal *endotracheal tube,* *LMA North America, Inc., San Diego, CA*	Conditional 5	1.5	
Long nose side cut pliers *P-326,* *Ampco Safety Tools, Garland, TX*	Conditional 7	3	
Low Magnetic Signature *Lithium Battery (C size),* *Greatbatch Scientific, Clarence, NY*	Safe	1.5	
Low magnetic Signature Lithium Battery, Part # BTRY *Newmatic Sound Systems, Inc., Petaluma, CA*	Conditional 7	3	
LUNA PVO *NFOCUS Neuromedical, Palo Alto, CA*	Conditional 6	3	
Mac 4 *15-MRI-FOD-Mac 4, Plastic, Laryngoscope part,* *NovaMed, LLC, Rye, New York*	Conditional 7	3	
Mac 5 *15-MRI-Mac 5, SS, Laryngoscope part,* *NovaMed, LLC, Rye, New York*	Conditional 7	3	
Maestro Neuroregulator *Model 1002, Neurostimulator, Obesity Treatment,* *EnteroMedics Inc., St. Paul, MN*	Unsafe 1	1.5	
Manometer *NF-121, for mounting on IV pole,* *AADCO Medical, Inc., Randolph, VT*	Conditional 7	3	
Manual Jet Ventilator (P/N 00-325-MRI) *Anesthesia Associates, Inc., San Marcos, CA*	Conditional 7	3	
May Hegar Needle *Holder, Ti6Al-4V,* *Johnson & Johnson Professional, Inc., Raynham, MA*	Safe	1.5	62
Mayo Stand 16-inch x 21-inch *Newmatic Sound Systems, Inc., Petaluma, CA*	Conditional 7	3	
Mechanical Ventilator *MR Magellan, Pneumatically Powered,* *Mechanical Ventilator,* *Oceanic Medical Products, Inc., Atchison, KS*	Conditional 7	3	

Object	Status	Field Strength (T)	Reference
Medex 3000 Series MRI Syringe Infusion Pump *Medex, Dublin, OH*	Conditional 5	1.5	
Medfusion 3500 Syringe Pump *Smiths Medical, http://www.smiths-medical.com*	Conditional 5	3	
Medical M Cylinder Hand Cart *Newmatic Sound Systems, Inc., Petaluma, CA*	Conditional 7	3	
Medium Handle *15-MRI-HMED-2, Laryngoscope part,* *NovaMed, LLC, Rye, New York*	Conditional 7	3	
Medium Handle *15-MRI-HMED-3, Laryngoscope part,* *NovaMed, LLC, Rye, New York*	Conditional 7	3	
Medivance Nasogastric Sump Tube *with YSI Series 400 Temperature Sensor,* *Medivance, Inc., Louisville, CO*	Conditional 5	3	
MEDRAD Continuum MR Infusion System *MEDRAD, Inc., Indianola, PA*	Conditional 5	1.5, 3	
Mercury Duotube-feeding, feeding tube	Safe	1.5	
Micro Needle Holder *Greatbatch Scientific, Clarence, NY*	Safe	1.5	
Micro Round Handled Scissors *Greatbatch Scientific, Clarence, NY*	Safe	1.5	
Micro Tissue Forceps *Greatbatch Scientific, Clarence, NY*	Safe	1.5	
Micro Tying Forceps *Greatbatch Scientific, Clarence, NY*	Safe	1.5	
Mil 4 *15-MRI-FOMD-Mil 4, SS, plastic, Laryngoscope part,* *NovaMed, LLC, Rye, New York*	Conditional 7	3	
MiniMed 2007 *Implantable Insulin Pump,* *Medtronic MiniMed Inc., Northridge, CA*	Unsafe 1	1.5	
MiniMed 407C *Infusion Pump,* *Medtronic MiniMed Inc., Northridge, CA*	Unsafe 1	1.5	
MiniMed 508 *Insulin Pump,* *Medtronic MiniMed Inc., Northridge, CA*	Unsafe 1	1.5	
Mitek anchor *Miteck Products, Westood, MA*	Safe	1.5	
Mobile lead acrylic barrier *S-602 NF, for use in MRI and, Image Guided Therapy,* *AADCO Medical, Inc., Randolph, VT*	Conditional 7	3	

Object	Status	Field Strength (T)	Reference
MONARC System *Edwards Lifesciences, www.Edwards.com*	Conditional 5	3	
Monkey Wrench *58*305-mm,* *Newmatic Sound Systems, Inc., Petaluma, CA*	Conditional 7	3	
MR Bone Punch *Dismantalable,* *Aesculap, Inc., Center Valley, PA*	Safe	1.5	74
MR Compatible Laryngoscope Handle *short size handle,* *MINRAD INC., Buffalo, NY*	Conditional 7	3	
MR Compatible Laryngoscope Handle *standard size handle,* *MINRAD INC., Buffalo, NY*	Conditional 7	3	
MR Compatible WISCONSIN 4 Laryngoscope Blade *short size handle,* *MINRAD INC., Buffalo, NY*	Conditional 7	3	
MR Currette *Curved, 90 degree Blunt Ring,* *Aesculap, Inc., Center Valley, PA*	Safe	1.5	74
MR Suction Cannula *with Suction Stop,* *Aesculap, Inc., Center Valley, PA*	Safe	1.5	74
MR-Brain Spatula with Silicone *Model FF408K,* *Aesculap AG & CO.KG, Tuttlingen, Germany*	Safe	1.5, 3	83
MRI Conditional Flashlight, FLSH *Newmatic Sound Systems, Inc., Petaluma, CA*	Conditional 7	3	
MRI Conditional Pen, Part # MRPEN2 *Newmatic Sound Systems, Inc., Petaluma, CA*	Conditional 7	3	
MRI Conditional Roller Ball Pen, Part # MRPEN1 *Newmatic Sound Systems, Inc., Petaluma, CA*	Conditional 7	3	
MRI Disposable Scalpel *Titanium,* *QSUM Biopsy Disposables LLC, Boulder, CO*	Conditional 7	3	
MRidium 3850 MRI IV Pump *MRidium Corporation, www.iradimed.com*	Conditional 5	3	
MRidium 3860 MRI IV Pump *MRidium Corporation, www.iradimed.com*	Conditional 5	3	
MRI FastSystem Retractor System *Omni-Tract Surgical, Minneapolis, MN*	Safe	1.5	83
MRI IV Pole *adjustable, NF-110,* *AADCO Medical, Inc., Randolph, VT*	Conditional 7	3	

Object	Status	Field Strength (T)	Reference
MRI Needle *Inconel,* *QSUM Biopsy Disposables LLC, Boulder, CO*	Conditional 7	3	
MRI Wheelchair 18 " wide *NF-500,* *AADCO Medical, Inc., Randolph, VT*	Conditional 7	3	
MR-Kocher-Langenbeck Retractor *70 X 14-mm,* *Aesculap, Inc., Center Valley, PA*	Safe	1.5	74
MR-Mallet with Alloy Handle *50 grams,* *Aesculap, Inc., Center Valley, PA*	Safe	1.5	74
MR IV Pole *MRidium Corporation, www.iradimed.com*	Conditional 5	3	
MR-Septum Speculum, 75 X 7 Resp. *60 X 7-mm,* *Aesculap, Inc., Center Valley, PA*	Safe	1.5	74
MR-Weil-Blakesley Ethmoid Forceps *Aesculap, Inc., Center Valley, PA*	Safe	1.5	74
Neurostimulation System *Activa PC Deep Brain Neurostimulator (Model 37601),* *DBS System,* *Medtronic, Inc.*	Conditional 5	1.5	
Neurostimulation System *Activa RC Deep Brain Neurostimulator (Model 37612),* *DBS System,* *Medtronic, Inc.*	Conditional 5	1.5	
Neurostimulation System *deep brain stimulation, Activa System, includes* *Model 7426 Soletra and Model 7424 Itrel II neurostimulators,* *Model 3387 and Model 3389 DBS leads,* *Medtronic, Inc., Minneapolis, MN*	Conditional 5	1.5	79, 80, 100
Neurostimulation system *deep brain stimulation, Itrel II,* *Medtronic, Inc., Minneapolis, MN*	Conditional 5	1.5	99, 101
Neurostimulation system *deep brain stimulation, Kinetra,* *Medtronic, Inc., Minneapolis, MN*	Conditional 5	1.5	99, 100
Neurostimulation system *deep brain stimulation, Soletra,* *Medtronic, Inc., Minneapolis, MN*	Conditional 5	1.5	92, 99
Neurostimulation System *Enterra Therapy,* *Gastric Electrical Stimulation (GES) System,* *Medtronic, Inc., Minneapolis, MN*	Unsafe 1	1.5	

Object	Status	Field Strength (T)	Reference
Neurostimulation System *Eon (IPG), Spinal Cord Stimulation,* *St. Jude Medical*	Unsafe 1	1.5	
Neurostimulation System *Eon C, Spinal Cord Stimulation,* *St. Jude Medical, www.sjm.com*	Unsafe 1	1.5	
Neurostimulation System *Eon Mini, Spinal Cord Stimulation,* *St. Jude Medical, www.sjm.com*	Unsafe 1	1.5	
Neurostimulation System *Genesis, Spinal Cord Stimulation,* *St. Jude Medical, www.sjm.com*	Unsafe 1	1.5	
Neurostimulation System *GenesisRC, Spinal Cord Stimulation,* *St. Jude Medical, www.sjm.com*	Unsafe 1	1.5	
Neurostimulation System *GenesisXP, Spinal Cord Stimulation,* *St. Jude Medical, www.sjm.com*	Unsafe 1	1.5	
Neurostimulation System *InterStim Therapy,* *Sacral Nerve Stimulation for Urinary Control,* *Medtronic, Inc., Minneapolis, MN*	Unsafe 1	1.5	99
Neurostimulation System *PrimeAdvanced Spinal Cord Neurostimulator,* *PrimeAdvanced, Model 37702,* *Medtronic, Inc., www.Medtronic.com*	Conditional 5	1.5	
Neurostimulation System *Reclaim Deep Brain Neurostimulator (Model 37601),* *DBS System,* *Medtronic, Inc., www.Medtronic.com*	Conditional 5	1.5	
Neurostimulation System *Renew, Spinal Cord Stimulation,* *St. Jude Medical, www.sjm.com*	Unsafe 1	1.5	
Neurostimulation System *Renova Cortical Stimulation System,* *Northstar Neuroscience, Seattle, WA*	Unsafe 1	1.5	
Neurostimulation System *RestoreAdvanced Spinal Cord Neurostimulator,* *RestoreAdvanced, Model 37713,* *Medtronic, Inc., www.Medtronic.com*	Conditional 5	1.5	
Neurostimulation System *RestoreUltra Spinal Cord Neurostimulator,* *RestoreUltra, Model 37712,* *Medtronic, Inc., www.Medtronic.com*	Conditional 5	1.5	

Object	Status	Field Strength (T)	Reference
Neurostimulation system *spinal cord stimulation, chronic pain, Itrel 3,* *Medtronic, Inc., Minneapolis, MN*	Conditional 5	1.5	99
Neurostimulation system *spinal cord stimulation, chronic pain, Mattrix,* *Medtronic, Inc., Minneapolis, MN*	Unsafe 1	1.5	99
Neurostimulation system *spinal cord stimulation, chronic pain, Restore,* *Medtronic, Inc., Minneapolis, MN*	Conditional 5	1.5	99
Neurostimulation system *spinal cord stimulation, chronic pain, Synergy,* *Medtronic, Inc., Minneapolis, MN*	Conditional 5	1.5	99
Neurostimulation system *spinal cord stimulation, chronic pain, SynergyCompact,* *Medtronic, Inc., Minneapolis, MN*	Conditional 5	1.5	99
Neurostimulation system *spinal cord stimulation, chronic pain, SynergyPlus,* *Medtronic, Inc., Minneapolis, MN*	Conditional 5	1.5	99
Neurostimulation system *spinal cord stimulation, chronic pain, Versitrel,* *Medtronic, Inc., Minneapolis, MN*	Conditional 5	1.5	99
Neurostimulation system *Vagus Nerve Stimulation, Vagal Nerve Stimulator,* *VNS Therapy, NeuroCybernetic Prosthesis (NCP) System,* *Cyberonics, Inc., http://www.vnstherapy.com,*	Conditional 5	1.5	
NeuroVentriClear *Ventricular Drainage Catheter Set,* *Cook Neurological, Inc., Leechburg, PA*	Safe	3	
Nextus/Raz *Soft Tissue Anchor, Straight, Titanium alloy,* *American Medical Systems, Minnetonka, MN*	Safe	3	
Nextus/Raz *Soft Tissue Anchor, Curved, Titanium alloy,* *American Medical Systems, Minnetonka, MN*	Safe	3	
Non-Magnetic Adjustable Chair *Newmatic Sound Systems, Inc., Petaluma, CA*	Conditional 7	3	
Non-Magnetic Cylinder Cart *Newmatic Sound Systems, Inc., Petaluma, CA*	Conditional 7	3	
Non-magnetic Floor Sweeper, SWPR *Newmatic Sound Systems, Inc., Petaluma, CA*	Conditional 7	3	
Non-Magnetic Prism Glasses *Newmatic Sound Systems, Inc., Petaluma, CA*	Conditional 7	3	
Non-Magnetic Sprague Rappaport Stethoscope *Newmatic Sound Systems, Inc., Petaluma, CA*	Conditional 7	3	

Object	Status	Field Strength (T)	Reference
NovaSilk *synthetic mesh,* *Coloplast A/S, Humlebaek, Denmark*	Safe	3	
NuvaRing *Contraceptive device,* *Schering Corporation, Kenilworth, NJ*	Safe	1.5	
ON-Q Pain Relief System *I-Flow Corporation, www.iflo.com*	Safe	1.5	
ON-Q SilverDressing *I-Flow Corporation, www.iflo.com*	Conditional 6	3	
Opti-Flo Tube Attachment Device (T.A.D.) *ConvaTec Wound Therapeutics, United Kingdom*	Conditional 6	3	
Optistar MR Contrast Delivery System *Mallinckrodt, St. Louis, MO*	Safe	1.5	
Optiva (PUR Radiopaque) *intravenous (I.V.) catheter,* *Smiths Medical, Southington, CT*	Safe	3	
Optiva 2 (PUR Radiopaque) *intravenous (I.V.) catheter,* *Smiths Medical, Southington, CT*	Safe	3	
Optiva W (PUR Radiopaque) *intravenous (I.V.) catheter,* *Smiths Medical, Southington, CT*	Safe	3	
P140 System Implant *HeartNet,* *Paracor Medical, Inc., Sunnyvale, CA*	Conditional 6	3	
P150 System Implant *HeartNet,* *Paracor Medical, Inc., Sunnyvale, CA*	Conditional 6	3	
Palatal System Implant Assembly *Pavad Medical, Inc., Fremont, CA*	Conditional 5	1.5	
PAS-Port Proximal *Anastomosis System Implant,* *Cardica, Redwood City, CA*	Conditional 6	3	
Patient Scoop *Model 65 EXL,* *Ferno-Washington, Inc., Wilmington, OH*	Conditional 7	3	
PEDI-TUBE *Pediatric Nasogastric (NG) Feeding Tube,* *COVIDIEN, Hazelwood, MO*	Conditional 6	3	
Penfield Dissector *304 SS,* *Johnson & Johnson Professional, Inc., Raynham, MA*	Safe	1.5	62

Object	Status	Field Strength (T)	Reference
Percutaneous Intraspinal Catheter *Model 8516,* *Medtronic, Inc.*	Unsafe 2	1.5	
Pericardial Patch *Hancock, Model 710,* *Medtronic Heart Valve Division, Minneapolis, MN*	Safe	1.5, 3	84
Pericardial Patch *Hancock, Model 710L,* *Medtronic Heart Valve Division, Minneapolis, MN*	Safe	1.5, 3	84
Peripheral Nerve Stimulator *MR-STIM, Model GN-013,* *Greatbatch Scientific, Clarence, NY*	Safe	1.5	
Phillips Screwdriver *200-mm,* *Newmatic Sound Systems, Inc., Petaluma, CA*	Conditional 7	3	
PillCam M2A Capsule Endoscopy Device *Ingestible Capsule,* *Given Imaging Inc., Norcross, GA*	Unsafe 1	1.5	
PillCam ESO Capsule Endoscopy Device *Ingestible Capsule,* *Given Imaging Inc., Norcross, GA*	Unsafe 1	1.5	
PillCam ESO2 Capsule Endoscopy Device *Ingestible Capsule,* *Given Imaging Inc., Norcross, GA*	Unsafe 1	1.5	
PillCam SB Capsule Endoscopy Device *Ingestible Capsule,* *Given Imaging Inc., Norcross, GA*	Unsafe 1	1.5	
Pipe Wrench *50-mm,* *Newmatic Sound Systems, Inc., Petaluma, CA*	Conditional 7	3	
Polyform Mesh *Polypropylene,* *Boston Scientific, www.bostonscientific.com*	Safe	1.5	
Portex Bivona Flextend Tracheostomy Tube *All similar products, Tracheostomy,* *Smiths Medical International, England*	Conditional 6	3	
Portex Bivona Laryngectomy Tube *All similar products, Laryngectomy Tube,* *Smiths Medical International, England*	Safe	3	
Portex Bivona Non-Wire *Reinforced Cuffed Tracheostomy Tube,* *All similar products, Tracheostomy,* *Smiths Medical International, England*	Conditional 6	3	

Object	Status	Field Strength (T)	Reference
Portex Bivona Sleep Apoea (Apnea) Tube	Safe	3	
All similar products, Sleep Apoea (Apnea) Tube, Smiths Medical International, England			
Portex Bivona Uncuffed	Safe	3	
Non-Reinforced Endotracheal Tube, All similar products, Smiths Medical International, England			
Portex Bivona Uncuffed	Safe	3	
Non-Wire Reinforced Tracheostomy Tube, All similar products, Tracheostomy, Smiths Medical International, England			
Portex Bivona Wire	Conditional 6	3	
Reinforced Endotracheal Tube, All similar products, Endotracheal, Smiths Medical International, England			
Portex Bivona Wire	Conditional 6	3	
Reinforced, Tracheostomy Tube, All similar products, Tracheostomy, Smiths Medical International, England			
Portex Cricothyroidotomy Tube	Conditional 6	3	
Cricothyroidotomy, Smiths Medical International, England			
Portex Cuffed Endotracheal Tube	Conditional 6	3	
All similar products, Smiths Medical International, England			
Portex Guedel Airway	Safe	3	
Airway, All similar products, Smiths Medical International, England			
Portex Heat and Moisture Exchanger	Safe	3	
All similar products, Smiths Medical International, England			
Portex Mini-Trach	Safe	3	
Tracheostomy, Smiths Medical International, England			
Portex Nasal Oxygen Set	Safe	3	
All similar products, Nasal Oxygen Set, Smiths Medical International, England			
Portex Non-Wire	Conditional 6	3	
Reinforced Cuffed Tracheostomy Tube, All similar products, Tracheostomy, Smiths Medical International, England			
Portex Orator Speaking Valve	Safe	3	
All similar products, Speaking Valve, Smiths Medical International, England			

Object	Status	Field Strength (T)	Reference
Portex Tracheal Tube Holder *All similar products, Endotracheal Tube Holder,* *Smiths Medical International, England*	Safe	3	
Portex Uncuffed Non-Wire *Reinforced Endotracheal Tube,* *All similar products, Endotracheal,* *Smiths Medical International, England*	Safe	3	
Portex Uncuffed *Non-reinforced Tracheostomy Tube,* *All similar products, Tracheostomy,* *Smiths Medical International, England*	Safe	3	
Portex, UniPerc Tracheostomy Tube *Tracheostomy,* *Smiths Medical, www.smiths-medical.com*	Conditional 5	3	
Portex Wire Reinforced Endotracheal Tube *All similar products,* *Smiths Medical International, England*	Conditional 6	3	
Post Valve and Aluminum E Cylinder *PX-8703-1CW,* *Western Scott Fetzer, Inc., Westlake, OH*	Conditional 7	3	
Post Valve *MPV-5870,* *Western Scott Fetzer, Inc., Westlake, OH*	Conditional 7	3	
Precision Spinal Cord Stimulation System *Neurostimulation System,* *Boston Scientific Corporation, www.BostonScientific.com*	Unsafe 1	1.5	
ProAct, Male Adjustable Continence Therapy *Uromedica Inc., Plymouth, MN*	Conditional 6	3	
Protectiv (FEP Radiopaque) *intravenous (I.V.) catheter,* *Smiths Medical, Southington, CT*	Safe	3	
Protectiv Acuvance 2 (PUR Radiopaque) *intravenous (I.V.) catheter,* *Smiths Medical, Southington, CT*	Safe	3	
Protectiv Jelco (FEP Radiopaque) *intravenous (I.V.) catheter,* *Smiths Medical, Southington, CT*	Safe	3	
Protectiv Plus (PUR Radiopaque) *intravenous (I.V.) catheter,* *Smiths Medical, Southington, CT*	Safe	3	
Protectiv Plus W (PUR Radiopaque) *intravenous (I.V.) catheter,* *Smiths Medical, Southington, CT*	Safe	3	

Object	Status	Field Strength (T)	Reference
Protectiv W (FEP Radiopaque) *intravenous (I.V.) catheter,* *Smiths Medical, Southington, CT*	Safe	3	
Putty Knife *40*200-mm,* *Newmatic Sound Systems, Inc., Petaluma, CA*	Conditional 7	3	
Putty Knife *K-20,* *Ampco Safety Tools, Garland, TX*	Conditional 7	3	
Putty Knife, Wooden Handle *NGK Metals Corporation, Sweetwater, TN*	Conditional 7	3	
PVC Sling Bariatric Gurney *Newmatic Sound Systems, Inc., Petaluma, CA*	Conditional 7	3	
Ratchet Wrench *3/4"*320-mm,* *Newmatic Sound Systems, Inc., Petaluma, CA*	Conditional 7	3	
Realize Adjustable Gastric Band *also known as Swedish Adjustable Gastric Band,* *Ethicon Endosurgery, Inc., www.e-ifu.com*	Conditional 5	3	
REALIZE Adjustable Gastric Band-C *Ethicon Endo-Surgery, Inc., www.e-ifu.com*	Conditional 5	3	
Rebound HRD *Hernia Repair Device, Nitinol,* *Minnesota Medical, Plymouth, MN*	Conditional 6	3	
Regulator and Aluminum Cylinder System *AirTOTE, MTS-303,* *Western Scott Fetzer, Inc., Westlake, OH*	Conditional 7	3	
Regulator and Aluminum Cylinder System *OxyTOTE, MTS-603,* *Western Scott Fetzer, Inc., Westlake, OH*	Conditional 7	3	
Regulator and Aluminum Cylinder System *OxyTOTE, MTS-803,* *Western Scott Fetzer, Inc., Westlake, OH*	Conditional 7	3	
Regulator and Aluminum Cylinder System *PediaTOTE, MTS-103,* *Western Scott Fetzer, Inc., Westlake, OH*	Conditional 7	3	
Regulator *NMR-540-15FM,* *Western Scott Fetzer, Inc., Westlake, OH*	Conditional 7	3	
Regulator *NMR-870-15FM,* *Western Scott Fetzer, Inc., Westlake, OH*	Conditional 7	3	

Object	Status	Field Strength (T)	Reference
Regulator *NMR-870-P,* *Western Scott Fetzer, Inc., Westlake, OH*	Conditional 7	3	
Relieva Stratus Microflow Spacer *Acclarent, Inc., Menlo Park, CA*	Conditional 6	3	
RF BION Microstimulator *Neurostimulation System,* *Alfred E. Mann Foundation for Scientific Research,* *Valencia, CA*	Conditional 5	1.5	89
Rheos Baroreflex System *Rheos Hypertension (HT) Therapy,* *CVRx Inc., Minneapolis, MN*	Unsafe 1	1.5	
Robotic Radiosurgery Tumor Marking Seed *Tumor marking device, Gold, Silver,* *RADONTEK LTD., Ankara, Turkey*	Conditional 6	3	
Round Wire Brush *B-399,* *Ampco Safety Tools, Garland, TX*	Conditional 7	3	
Rusch Larygoscope Handle *brass head, aluminum barrel, arbon-zinc battery, SS,* *Teleflex Medical, Durham, NC*	Conditional 7	3	
Rusch Macintosh Size 4 *Fiber-optic Laryngoscope Blade,* *Teleflex Medical, Durham, NC*	Conditional 7	3	
SAM Sling *SAM Medical Products, Portland, OR*	Conditional 6	3	
Sancuso (Granisetron Transdermal System, Transdermal Patch) *ProStrakan*	Safe	1.5	
Sand bag *12 pound, Vinyl Silica Sand Bag,* *Newmatic Sound Systems, Inc., Petaluma, CA*	Conditional 7	3	
Scalpel, Microsharp Ceramic Scalpels, *sizes #10, #11, #11c, #15, ceramic,* *MicroSurgical Techniques, Inc., Fort Collins, CO*	Safe	1.5	48
Scalpel, SS	Unsafe 1	1.5	
Scissors, Ceramic *prototype, ceramic,* *Microsurgical Techniques, Inc., Fort Collins, CO*	Safe	1.5	48
Scissors *225-mm,* *Newmatic Sound Systems, Inc., Petaluma, CA*	Conditional 7	3	

Object	Status	Field Strength (T)	Reference
Scraper *S-10G,* *Ampco Safety Tools, Garland, TX*	Conditional 7	3	
Screw driver, Philips *S-1099A,* *Ampco Safety Tools, Garland, TX*	Conditional 7	3	
Screwdriver, Slot, Flat Head *NGK Metals Corporation, Sweetwater, TN*	Conditional 7	3	
Screw driver, standard *S-49,* *Ampco Safety Tools, Garland, TX*	Conditional 7	3	
Screw *Titanium alloy,* *Bioplate, Inc., Los Angeles, CA*	Conditional 6	3	
SecurAcath Universal Version 1.1 *Interrad Medical, Inc., St. Paul, MN*	Conditional 6	3	
Seven System *Continuous Glucose Monitoring System,* *DexCom, Inc., San Diego, CA*	Unsafe 1	1.5	
Shelhigh Injectable Pulmonic Valve *pulmonic valve replacement prosthesis,* *Nitinol, bovine pericardium,* *Shelhigh Inc., Union, NJ*	Conditional 6	3	
Shoe Handle Wire-brush, 4 x 17 rows *NGK Metals Corporation, Sweetwater, TN*	Conditional 7	3	
Side cutting pliers *P-36,* *Ampco Safety Tools, Garland, TX*	Conditional 7	3	
SilverSite Access Site Dressing *4-mm opening,* *Tri-State Hospital Supply Corporation, Howell, MI*	Conditional 6	3	
Single PVC Hamper Cart *Newmatic Sound Systems, Inc., Petaluma, CA*	Conditional 7	3	
Sleuth *Implantable ECG Monitoring System,* *Model 2010 Sleuth IMD, 6.5-cm version,* *Transoma Medical, St. Paul, MN*	Conditional 5	1.5	
Sleuth AT Implantable Monitoring System *Models 9006/9008,* *Transoma Medical, St. Paul, MN*	Conditional 5	1.5	
Slot Screwdriver *11*300-mm,* *Newmatic Sound Systems, Inc., Petaluma, CA*	Conditional 7	3	

Object	Status	Field Strength (T)	Reference
Slot Screwdriver *3*50-mm,* *Newmatic Sound Systems, Inc., Petaluma, CA*	Conditional 7	3	
Spectris MR Injection System *Medrad, Inc., Indianola, PA*	Safe	1.5	
Spiegelberg System Bolt *SS,* *Aesculap, Inc., Center Valley, PA*	Safe	1.5, 3	83
Spine Fusion Stimulator *SpF PLUS-Mini,* *Biomet Spine,* *http://www.biomet.com/spine/mriInfo.cfm?pdid=3*	Conditional 5	1.5	
Spine Fusion Stimulator *SpF-XL IIb,* *Biomet Spine,* *http://www.biomet.com/spine/mriInfo.cfm?pdid=3*	Conditional 5	1.5	
Sponge Forcep *Ti6Al-4V,* *Johnson & Johnson Professional, Inc., Raynham, MA*	Safe	1.5	62
SPRINKER *Model F4FR-NF, Non-Ferrous Quick Response* *Concealed Automatic Sprinkler,* *for MRI Type Applications,* *The Reliable Automatic Sprinkler Co., Inc., Elmsford, NY*	Conditional 7	3	
Step Stool with Handrail *Newmatic Sound Systems, Inc., Petaluma, CA*	Conditional 7	3	
Stereotactic headframe with removable mouthpiece *aluminum, 8-18 SS Delrin, Titanium,* *Compass International, Inc., Rochester, MN*	Safe	1.5	
Straight-In Sacral Colpopexy System *AMS, American Medical Systems, Minnetonka, MN*	Safe	1.5, 3	
Stretcher *1000 MR,* *Gendron, Inc., Archbold, OH*	Conditional 7	3	
Stryker PainPump 2 *Infusion Pump,* *Stryker Instruments, Kalamazoo, MI*	Unsafe 1	1.5	
Stryker PainPump *Infusion Pump,* *Stryker Instruments, Kalamazoo, MI*	Unsafe 1	1.5	
Subcutaneous Evacuating Port System, SEPS *Medtronic, Inc., www.Medtronic.com*	Unsafe	1.5	
Suction/Irrigation Handle for Sinuscope *Greatbatch Scientific, Clarence, NY*	Safe	1.5	

Object	Status	Field Strength (T)	Reference
Suction Regulator, Model Number 881VR *Genstar Technologies Co., Inc., Chino, CA*	Conditional 7	3	
Super ArrowFlex PSI *10 Fr. x 65-cm, 304V SS,* *Arrow International Inc., Reading, PA*	Unsafe 2	1.5	
Super ArrowFlex PSI *9 Fr. x 11-cm, 304 V SS,* *Arrow International Inc., Reading, PA*	Unsafe 2	1.5	
SUPPRELIN LA Implant *Histrelin acetate, subcutaneous implant,* *Endo Pharmaceuticals, www.supprelinla.com*	Safe	1.5	
Supris *Suprapubic mesh sling,* *Coloplast A/S, Humlebaek, Denmark*	Safe	3	
SureConnect Patient Connector *316L SS,* *Baxa Corporation, Englewood, CO*	Conditional 7	3	
Swedish Adjustable Gastric Band (SAGB) *Titanium, silicone,* *Ethicon Endo-Surgery, Inc., Cincinnati, OH*	Safe	1.5, 3	
SynchroMed EL *implantable drug infusion system,* *Medtronic, Inc., www.Medtronic.com*	Conditional 5	1.5, 3	
SynchroMed II *implantable drug infusion system,* *Medtronic, Inc., www.Medtronic.com*	Conditional 5	1.5, 3	
SynchroMed *implantable drug infusion system,* *Medtronic, Inc., www.Medtronic.com*	Conditional 5	1.5, 3	
Table Model Mercury Blood Pressure Manometer *Table model, NF-120,* *AADCO Medical, Inc., Randolph, VT*	Conditional 7	3	
Tantalum powder	Safe	1.39	1
Tape Mechanical Occlusive Device (TMOD) *implantable artificial urinary sphincter,* *GT Urological, LLC, Minneapolis, MN*	Conditional 7	3	
Tears Naturale Port Punctal Occluder *Alcon Research, Ltd., Fort Worth, Texas*	Safe	1.5	
Testicular prosthesis or implant *gel-filled,* *Coloplast A/S, Humlebaek, Denmark*	Safe	3	
Testicular prosthesis or implant *saline-filled,* *Coloplast A/S, Humlebaek, Denmark MR safe*	Safe	3	

Object	Status	Field Strength (T)	Reference
Testicular prosthesis or implant *Torosa,* *Coloplast A/S, Humlebaek, Denmark*	Safe	3	
TheraCath *304 V SS,* *Arrow International Inc., Reading, PA*	Unsafe 2	1.5	
TheraSeed Radioactive Seed Implant *Titanium, graphite, lead,* *Theragenics Corporation, Buford, GA*	Safe	1.5, 3	
Tin Snips *S-1144, W-212AL,* *Ampco Safety Tools, Garland, TX*	Conditional 7	3	
Titanium Adjustable Wrench *Newmatic Sound Systems, Inc., Petaluma, CA*	Conditional 7	3	
Titanium Bengolea Haemostatic Forceps *Curved,* *Newmatic Sound Systems, Inc., Petaluma, CA*	Conditional 7	3	
Titanium Gerald Dissecting Forceps *Newmatic Sound Systems, Inc., Petaluma, CA*	Conditional 7	3	
Titanium Knot *LSI Solutions Inc., Victor, NY*	Conditional 6	3	
Titanium Potts Micro Scissors *angulated 60 degrees,* *Newmatic Sound Systems, Inc., Petaluma, CA*	Conditional 7	3	
Transport Chair 20-inch *Newmatic Sound Systems, Inc., Petaluma, CA*	Conditional 7	3	
TS System Arterial Closure Device *Arterial Closure Device (ACD),* *Vasorum Ltd, Ireland*	Conditional 6	3	
TVFMI, Titanium Vocal Fold Medializing Implant (Friedrich) *Titanium (ASTM Grade F67 Medical Grade),* *Kurz Medical, Inc., Norcross, GA*	Safe	3	
Tweezers, Ceramic *prototype, ceramic,* *MicroSurgical Techniques, Inc., Fort Collins, CO*	Safe	1.5	48
Tweezers *8340,* *Ampco Safety Tools, Garland, TX*	Conditional 7	3	
ULT - Drainage Catheter *Cook Medical Inc., Bloomington, IN*	Conditional 6	3	
ULTRASITE Valve *B. Braun Medical Inc., Allentown, PA*	Conditional 6	3	

Object	Status	Field Strength (T)	Reference
UroLift Anchor *316L SS, SS,* *NeoTract, Pleasanton, CA*	Conditional 5	3	
Urolume Endoprosthesis *AMS, American Medical Systems, Minnetonka, MN*	Safe	1.5, 3	
V.A.C. GranuFoam Silver *Dressing,* *KCI USA, Inc., San Antonio, TX*	Conditional 6	3	
VANTAS Implant *Histrelin Implant,* *Endo Pharmaceuticals, www.vantasimplant.com*	Safe	1.5	
Vascular marker, O-ring washer *302 SS,* *PIC Design, Middlebury, CT*	Conditional 1	1.5	
Vectra Vascular Access Graft (VAG) *Bard Peripheral Vascular, www.bardpv.com*	Safe	1.5	
Vehicle Bracket *810NM, Amerex Corporation, Trussville, AL*	Conditional 7	3	
Venaflo II Vascular Graft *Bard Peripheral Vascular, www.bardpv.com*	Safe	1.5	
Ventricular Partitioning Implant *VPD, CardioKinetix Inc., Redwood City, CA*	Conditional 6	3	
VeriChip *Microtransponder,* *miniaturized radio frequency identification device,* *VeriChip Corporation, Palm Beach, FL*	Conditional 5	7	
Viadur *leuprolide acetate implant, Titanium,* *Bayer HealthCare Pharmaceuticals, West Haven, CT*	Safe	1.5	
Vitallium implant	Safe	1.5	
V-Link Luer Activated Device *with VitalShield Protective Coating,* *Non-DEHP Y-Type Catheter, Extension Set,* *Non-DEHP Y-Type, Catheter Extension Set,* *Baxter Healthcare, Round Lake, IL*	Conditional 6	3	
VOCARE Bladder System *Implantable Functional Neuromuscular Stimulator (FNS),* *Neurostimulation System,* *NeuroControl Corporation, Valley View, OH*	Conditional 5	1.5	
VPASS Implant *316L SS,* *Percardia Inc., Merrimack, NH*	Safe	3	
Vygon AutoFlush *Plastic, 316L SS, Vygon Coporation, Norristown, PA*	Conditional 6	3	

Object	Status	Field Strength (T)	Reference
Vygon Bionector *Needle Access Device, Plastic, 316L SS,* *Vygon Corporation, Norristown, PA*	Conditional 6	3	
Wall Bracket *17737 (801),* *Amerex Corporation, Trussville, AL*	Conditional 7	3	
Watchman Gen 4 Implant *Atritech Inc., Plymouth, MN*	Conditional 6	3	
WATCHMAN Left Atrial Appendage Closure Device *Nitinol, Titanium,* *Atritech Inc., Plymouth, MN*	Conditional 6	3	
Wheelchair 18-inch Detachable Foot Rest *Newmatic Sound Systems, Inc., Petaluma, CA*	Conditional 7	3	
Wheelchair 22-inch Detachable Foot Rest *Newmatic Sound Systems, Inc., Petaluma, CA*	Conditional 7	3	
Wheelchair 26-inch Detachable Foot Rest *Newmatic Sound Systems, Inc., Petaluma, CA*	Conditional 7	3	
Wheelchair IV/Oxygen Tank Holder *Newmatic Sound Systems, Inc., Petaluma, CA*	Conditional 7	3	
Wheelchair *20" SS Heavy Duty Folding Aquatic Wheelchair* *Aqua Creek Products, LLC, Missoula, MT*	Conditional 7	3	
Wheelchair *Merlexi Craft Liberty MRI Synthetic Resin* *Manual Wheelchair,* *Turbo Wheelchair Co., Beaufort, SC*	Conditional 7	3	
Wheelchair *MR 18, 4000 MR, SPORTLITE,* *Gendron, Inc., Archbold, OH*	Conditional 7	3	
Winged infusion set *MRI compatible,* *E-Z-Em, Inc., Westbury, NY*	Safe	1.5	58
Woodson Elevator *304 SS,* *Johnson & Johnson Professional, Inc., Raynham, MA*	Safe	1.5	62
Zephyr Transcopic Endobronchial Valve *Emphasys Medical Inc., Redwood City, CA*	Conditional 6	3	
Zip Implant Device *Titanium alloy,* *Bioplate, Inc., Los Angeles, CA*	Conditional 6	3	

Object	Status	Field Strength (T)	Reference

Ocular Implants, Lens Implants, and Devices

Object	Status	Field Strength (T)	Reference
Ahmed glaucoma valve *glaucoma drainage implant, nonmetallic,* *New World Medical, Rancho Cucamonga, CA*	Safe	3	105
Baerveldt glaucoma drainage implant *glaucoma drainage implant, nonmetallic,* *Pharmacia Co., Kalamazoo, MI*	Safe	3	
Clip 250, double tantalum clip *tantalum, ocular,* *Mira Inc.*	Safe	1.5	29
Clip 50, double tantalum clip *tantalum, ocular,* *Mira Inc.*	Safe	1.5	29
Clip 51, single tantalum clip *tantalum, ocular,* *Mira Inc.*	Safe	1.5	29
Clip 52, single tantalum clip *tantalum, ocular,* *Mira Inc.*	Safe	1.5	29
Double tantalum clip *tantalum, ocular,* *Storz Instrument Co.*	Safe	1.5	29
Double tantalum clip style 250 *tantalum, ocular,* *Storz Instrument Co.*	Safe	1.5	29
DuraPlug *Temporary Canalicular Insert,* *EagleVision, Memphis, TN*	Safe	3	
EaglePlug *Punctum Plug,* *EagleVision, Memphis, TN*	Safe	3	
Eagle FlexPlug *Punctum Plug,* *EagleVision, Memphis, TN*	Safe	3	
Ex-PRESS Mini Glaucoma Shunt *316LVM, Optonol Ltd.BR, Israel*	Conditional 6	3	117
Fatio eyelid spring/wire *ocular*	Unsafe 1	1.5	30
Gelansert *Temporary Canalicular Insert, Memphis, TN*	Safe	3	
Gold eyelid spring *ocular*	Safe	1.5	

Object	Status	Field Strength (T)	Reference
Intraocular lens implant *Binkhorst, iridocapsular lense, Platinum-iridium loop, Platinum, iridium, ocular*	Safe	1.0	
Intraocular lens implant *Binkhorst, iridocapsular lense, Platinum-iridium loop, ocular*	Safe	1.5	31
Intraocular lens implant *Binkhorst, iridocapsular lense, Titanium loop, Titanium, ocular*	Safe	1.0	31
Intraocular lens implant *Worst, Platinum clip lense, ocular*	Safe	1.0	31
Joseph valve *glaucoma drainage implant, nonmetallic, Valve Implants Limited, Hertford, England*	Safe	3	31
Krupin-Denver eye valve to disc implant *glaucoma drainage implant, nonmetallic, E. Benson Hood Laboratories, Pembroke, MA*	Safe	3	
Lens Implant *CR5BUO, Alcon Laboratories, Inc., Fort Worth, TX*	Safe	3	
Lens Implant *CZ60BD, Alcon Laboratories, Inc., Fort Worth, TX*	Safe	3	
Lens Implant *CZ70BD, Alcon Laboratories, Inc., Fort Worth, TX*	Safe	3	
Lens Implant *LC80BD, Alcon Laboratories, Inc., Fort Worth, TX*	Safe	3	
Lens Implant *LX10BD, Alcon Laboratories, Inc., Fort Worth, TX*	Safe	3	
Lens Implant *LX90BD, Alcon Laboratories, Inc., Fort Worth, TX*	Safe	3	
Lens Implant *MA30AC, Alcon Laboratories, Inc., Fort Worth, TX*	Safe	3	
Lens Implant *MA60AC, Alcon Laboratories, Inc., Fort Worth, TX*	Safe	3	
Lens Implant *MA30BA, Alcon Laboratories, Inc., Fort Worth, TX*	Safe	3	

Object	Status	Field Strength (T)	Reference
Lens Implant *MA50BM,* *Alcon Laboratories, Inc., Fort Worth, TX*	Safe	3	
Lens Implant *MA60BM,* *Alcon Laboratories, Inc., Fort Worth, TX*	Safe	3	
Lens Implant *MA60MA,* *Alcon Laboratories, Inc., Fort Worth, TX*	Safe	3	
Lens Implant *MC30BA,* *Alcon Laboratories, Inc., Fort Worth, TX*	Safe	3	
Lens Implant *MA40BD,* *Alcon Laboratories, Inc., Fort Worth, TX*	Safe	3	
Lens Implant *MC50BD,* *Alcon Laboratories, Inc., Fort Worth, TX*	Safe	3	
Lens Implant *MC60BD,* *Alcon Laboratories, Inc., Fort Worth, TX*	Safe	3	
Lens Implant *MC50BM,* *Alcon Laboratories, Inc., Fort Worth, TX*	Safe	3	
Lens Implant *MC51BM,* *Alcon Laboratories, Inc., Fort Worth, TX*	Safe	3	
Lens Implant *MC60BM,* *Alcon Laboratories, Inc., Fort Worth, TX*	Safe	3	
Lens Implant *MC61BM,* *Alcon Laboratories, Inc., Fort Worth, TX*	Safe	3	
Lens Implant *MC60CM,* *Alcon Laboratories, Inc., Fort Worth, TX*	Safe	3	
Lens Implant *MC61CM,* *Alcon Laboratories, Inc., Fort Worth, TX*	Safe	3	
Lens Implant *MC70CM,* *Alcon Laboratories, Inc., Fort Worth, TX*	Safe	3	

Object	Status	Field Strength (T)	Reference
Lens Implant *MC71CM,* *Alcon Laboratories, Inc., Fort Worth, TX*	Safe	3	
Lens Implant *MN20BD,* *Alcon Laboratories, Inc., Fort Worth, TX*	Safe	3	
Lens Implant *MN30BD,* *Alcon Laboratories, Inc., Fort Worth, TX*	Safe	3	
Lens Implant *MN40BD,* *Alcon Laboratories, Inc., Fort Worth, TX*	Safe	3	
Lens Implant *MN60BD,* *Alcon Laboratories, Inc., Fort Worth, TX*	Safe	3	
Lens Implant *MN60D3,* *Alcon Laboratories, Inc., Fort Worth, TX*	Safe	3	
Lens Implant *MTA2UO,* *Alcon Laboratories, Inc., Fort Worth, TX*	Safe	3	
Lens Implant *MTA3UO,* *Alcon Laboratories, Inc., Fort Worth, TX*	Safe	3	
Lens Implant *MTA4UO,* *Alcon Laboratories, Inc., Fort Worth, TX*	Safe	3	
Lens Implant *MTA5UO,* *Alcon Laboratories, Inc., Fort Worth, TX*	Safe	3	
Lens Implant *MTA6UO,* *Alcon Laboratories, Inc., Fort Worth, TX*	Safe	3	
Lens Implant *MZ20BD,* *Alcon Laboratories, Inc., Fort Worth, TX*	Safe	3	
Lens Implant *MZ30BD,* *Alcon Laboratories, Inc., Fort Worth, TX*	Safe	3	
Lens Implant *MZ40BD,* *Alcon Laboratories, Inc., Fort Worth, TX*	Safe	3	

Object	Status	Field Strength (T)	Reference
Lens Implant *MZ60BD,* *Alcon Laboratories, Inc., Fort Worth, TX*	Safe	3	
Lens Implant *MZ70BD,* *Alcon Laboratories, Inc., Fort Worth, TX*	Safe	3	
Lens Implant *MZ20CD,* *Alcon Laboratories, Inc., Fort Worth, TX*	Safe	3	
Lens Implant *MZ60CD,* *Alcon Laboratories, Inc., Fort Worth, TX*	Safe	3	
Lens Implant *MZ60MD,* *Alcon Laboratories, Inc., Fort Worth, TX*	Safe	3	
Lens Implant *MZ60PD,* *Alcon Laboratories, Inc., Fort Worth, TX*	Safe	3	
Lens Implant *SA30AL,* *Alcon Laboratories, Inc., Fort Worth, TX*	Safe	3	
Lens Implant *SA30AT,* *Alcon Laboratories, Inc., Fort Worth, TX*	Safe	3	
Lens Implant *SA60AT,* *Alcon Laboratories, Inc., Fort Worth, TX*	Safe	3	
Lens Implant *SN60AT,* *Alcon Laboratories, Inc., Fort Worth, TX*	Safe	3	
Lens Implant *SA60D3,* *Alcon Laboratories, Inc., Fort Worth, TX*	Safe	3	
Lens Implant *SN60D3,* *Alcon Laboratories, Inc., Fort Worth, TX*	Safe	3	
Lens Implant *SN60T3,* *Alcon Laboratories, Inc., Fort Worth, TX*	Safe	3	
Lens Implant *SN60T4,* *Alcon Laboratories, Inc., Fort Worth, TX*	Safe	3	

Object	Status	Field Strength (T)	Reference
Lens Implant *SN60T5,* *Alcon Laboratories, Inc., Fort Worth, TX*	Safe	3	
Lens Implant *SN60WF,* *Alcon Laboratories, Inc., Fort Worth, TX*	Safe	3	
Lens Implant *SN6AD3,* *Alcon Laboratories, Inc., Fort Worth, TX*	Safe	3	
Lens Implant *SN60WS,* *Alcon Laboratories, Inc., Fort Worth, TX*	Safe	3	
Molteno drainage device *glaucoma drainage implant, nonmetallic,* *Molteno Ophthalmic Ltd., Dunedin, New Zealand*	Safe	3	
OZURDEX Implant *(dexamethasone intravitreal implant),* *Allergan, Inc., www.allergan.com*	Safe	1.5	
Retinal tack *303 SS, ocular,* *Bascom Palmer Eye Institute*	Safe	1.5	32
Retinal tack *303 SS, ocular,* *Duke*	Safe	1.5	32
Retinal tack *aluminum textraoxide, ocular,* *Ruby*	Safe	1.5	32
Retinal tack *cobalt, nickel, ocular,* *Greishaber, Fallsington, PA*	Safe	1.5	32
Retinal tack *martensitic SS, ocular,* *Western European*	Unsafe 1	1.5	32
Retinal tack *Titanium alloy, ocular,* *Coopervision, Irvine, CA*	Safe	1.5	32
Retinal tack, Norton staple *Platinum, rhodium, ocular,* *Norton*	Safe	1.5	32
Single tantalum clip *tantalum, ocular*	Safe	1.5	29
SuperEagle *Punctum Plug,* *EagleVision, Memphis, TN*	Safe	3	

Object	Status	Field Strength (T)	Reference
SuperFlex *Punctum Plug,* *EagleVision, Memphis, TN*	Safe	3	
Tapered Shaft *Flow Controller,* *EagleVision, Memphis, TN*	Safe	3	
Troutman magnetic ocular implant *ocular*	Unsafe 1	1.5	
Unitech round wire eye spring *ocular*	Unsafe 1	1.5	
Wide Angle Implantable Miniature Telescope *lens implant,* *VisionCare Ophthalmic Technologies, Inc., Saratoga, CA*	Conditional 6	3	

Orthopedic Implants, Materials, and Devices

Object	Status	Field Strength (T)	Reference
Adjustable External Fixation Device *external fixation device, carbon composite, SS,* *Biomet, Inc., Warsaw, Indiana*	Conditional 5	3	
Advent Cervical Disc *Blackstone Medical, Inc., Wayne, NJ*	Conditional 8	1.5, 3	
Aequalis Humeral Plate *and component parts, 120-mm plate,* *4.0-mm x 60-mm length self tapping,* *cancellous locking screw,* *3.5-mm x 50-mm length self tapping,* *cortical compression screw,* *3.5-mm x 40-mm length,* *self tapping cortical locking screw,* *19-gauge cerclage wire,* *Tornier, Inc., Stafford, TX*	Conditional 6	3	
Agility Total Ankle *Titanium alloy tibial, CoCrMo alloy talus,* *DePuy Orthopaedics, Warsaw, IN*	Conditional 6	3	
AML Hip Stem *CoCrMo alloy with CoCrMo alloy head,* *DePuy Orthopaedics, Warsaw, IN*	Conditional 6	3	
AML femoral component bipolar hip prothesis *orthopedic implant,* *Zimmer, Warsaw, IN*	Safe	1.5	3
A-MAV *Spinal Arthroplasty System, cobalt chromium alloy,* *Medtronic Sofamor Danek, Memphis, TN*	Safe	1.5	
ASR-Surface Replacement Hip *CoCrMo alloy acetabulum and head,* *DePuy Orthopaedics, Warsaw, IN*	Conditional 6	3	

Object	Status	Field Strength (T)	Reference
ATLANTIS Anterior Cervical Plate System *Medtronic, Spinal and Biologics, Memphis, TN*	Conditional 6	3	
ATLAS Cable System *Medtronic, Spinal and Biologics, Memphis, TN*	Conditional 6	3	
BioPro Great Toe M-P Joint *Cobalt Chrome, BioPro, Inc., Port Huron, MI*	Safe	1.5	
Biosymetric P.P. (Finger) Fixator *external fixation device, 316 SS, carbon composite,* *Biomet, Inc., Warsaw, Indiana*	Conditional 6	3	
Bryan Cervical Disc Prosthesis Spinal *C. P. Titanium, Titanium alloy, orthopedic implant,* *Dynamics Corporation, Mercer Island, WA*	Safe	1.5, 3	
BRYAN Cervical Disc System *Medtronic, Spinal and Biologics, Memphis, TN*	Conditional 6	3	
C-Stem with CoCrMo Head *CoCrMo, high strength SS,* *DePuy Orthopaedics, Warsaw, IN*	Conditional 6	3	
Cannulated cancellous screw *6.5 x 50-mm, Titanium alloy, orthopedic implant,* *DePuy ACE Medical Co., El Segundo, CA*	Safe	1.5	
Captured screw assembly, 100-mm *Titanium alloy, orthopedic implant,* *DePuy ACE Medical Co., El Segundo, CA*	Safe	1.5	
CD HORIZON LEGACY 6.35-mm Stainless Steel Spinal System *75-mm long spinal construct, unilateral,* *Medtronic, Spinal and Biologics, Memphis, TN*	Conditional 8	1.5, 3	
CD HORIZON LEGACY 6.35-mm Stainless Steel Spinal System *175-mm long spinal construct, bilateral,* *Medtronic, Spine and Biologics, Memphis, TN*	Conditional 8	1.5, 3	
Cervical wire, 18 gauge *316L SS, orthopedic implant*	Safe	0.3	33
CerviCore Intervertebral Disc *Stryker Spine-Summit, Summit, NJ*	Conditional 6	3	
Charite Artificial Disc *DePuy Spine,* *a Johnson and Johnson Company, Raynham, MA*	Safe	3	
Charnley-Muller hip prosthesis *Protasyl-10 alloy, orthopedic implant*	Safe	0.3	
Cobalt Chrome Staple *Cobalt Chrome, ASTM F75,* *Smith & Nephew, Inc., Orthopedic Division, Memphis, TN*	Safe	1.5, 3	83

Object	Status	Field Strength (T)	Reference
Compression Hip Screw Plate *and Lag Screw (tested as assembly), 316L SS,* *Smith & Nephew, Inc., Orthopedic Division, Memphis, TN*	Safe	1.5, 3	83
Cortical bone screw *4.5 x 36-mm, Titanium alloy, orthopedic implant,* *DePuy ACE Medical Co., El Segundo, CA*	Safe	1.5	
Cortical bone screw *large, Titanium alloy, orthopedic implant,* *Zimmer, Warsaw, IN*	Safe	1.5	34
Cortical bone screw *small, Titanium alloy, orthopedic implant,* *Zimmer, Warsaw, IN*	Safe	1.5	34
Cotrel rod *SS-ASTM, grade 2, orthopedic implant*	Safe	1.5	
Cotrel rods *with hooks, 316L SS, orthopedic implant*	Safe	0.3	33
Delta Total Shoulder *SS,* *DePuy Orthopaedics, Warsaw, IN*	Conditional 6	3	
Disposable Titanium Skull Pin *polymer body, titanium alloy pin-point,* *Integra LifeSciences, Cincinnati, Ohio*	Conditional 6	3	
Drummond wire *316L SS, orthopedic implant*	Safe	0.3	33
DTT, device *for transverse traction, 316L SS, orthopedic implant*	Safe	0.3	33
Emergency Bone Screw *Titanium alloy,* *Biomet, Inc., Warsaw, Indiana*	Conditional 6	3	
Endoscopic noncannulated *interference screw, Titanium, orthopedic implant,* *Acufex Microsurgical, Norwood, MA*	Safe	1.5	34
EOI Spinal System EPPS (Expanding Polyaxial Pedicle Screw) *Expanding Orthopedics Inc., Israel*	Conditional 8	1.5, 3	
External Fixation Device *Hoffman II MRI, External Fixation System,* *Stryker Trauma AG, Switzerland*	Conditional 5	1.5, 3	
External Fixation Device *Hoffman II (Standard), External Fixation System,* *Stryker Trauma AG, Switzerland*	Unsafe 1, 2	1.5, 3	
External Fixation Device *JET-X Fixator, Smith & Nephew, Memphis, TN*	Conditional 5	1.5	

Object	Status	Field Strength (T)	Reference
FlexiCore Intervertebral Disc *Stryker Spine-Summit, Summit, NJ*	Conditional 6	3	
Fixation staple *cobalt- chromium alloy, orthopedic implant,* *Richards Medical Co., Memphis, TN*	Safe	1.5	34
FD Tibial Intramedullary Nail *316 SS,* *Biomet, Inc., Warsaw, Indiana*	Conditional 6	3	
Femoral Head Implant *cobalt chromium,* *Biomet, Inc., Warsaw, Indiana*	Conditional 6	3	
Furlong H-AC THR System *Joint Replacement Instrumentation Limited (JRI Ltd),* *Sheffield, U.K.*	Conditional 6	3	
Furlong Modular Revision System Hemiarthroplasty *Joint Replacement Instrumentation Limited (JRI Ltd),* *Sheffield, U.K.*	Conditional 6	3	
GII Titanium Anchor *Titanium, Mitek Products, Norwood, MA*	Safe	1.5	
Global Total Shoulder *CoCrMo head and, stem/poly bearing component* *DePuy Orthopaedics, Warsaw, IN*	Conditional 6	3	
Halifax clamps *orthopedic implant,* *American Medical Electronics Richardson, TX*	Safe	1.5	
Hallmark Anterior Cervical Plate System *Blackstone Medical, Inc., Wayne, NJ*	Conditional 8	1.5, 3	
Harrington compression rod *with hooks and nuts, 316L SS, orthopedic implant*	Safe	0.3	33
Harrington distraction rod with hooks *316L SS, orthopedic implant*	Safe	0.3	33
Harris hip prosthesis *orthopedic implant,* *Zimmer, Warsaw, IN*	Safe	1.5	3
Hip implant *austenitic SS, orthopedic implant,* *DePuy Inc., Warsaw, IN*	Safe	1.5, 3	83
iForma *orthopedic implant,* *CONFORMIS, Inc., Lexington, MA*	Conditional 6	3	
IMF Wire *316 SS,* *Biomet, Inc., Warsaw, Indiana*	Conditional 6	3	

Object	Status	Field Strength (T)	Reference
Ilizarov-Taylor Spatial Frame *metal version, Smith and Nephew, Memphis, TN*	Unsafe 1	1.5	
Ionic Spine Spacer System *Titanium alloy, EBI, L.P., Parsippany, NJ*	Safe	1.5	
Jewett nail *orthopedic implant,* *Zimmer, Warsaw, IN*	Safe	1.5	3
Kirschner intermedullary rod *orthopedic implant,* *Kirschner Medical, Timonium, MD*	Safe	1.5	3
Large External Fixation System *Identified as MR Conditional, only,* *Synthes, www.synthes.com*	Conditional 5	1.5, 3	
L plate, 6-hole *Titanium alloy, orthopedic implant,* *DePuy ACE Medical Co., El Segundo, CA*	Safe	1.5	
L Rod *cobalt-nickel alloy, orthopedic implant,* *Richards Medical Co., Memphis, TN*	Safe	1.5	
LT-CAGE Lumbar Tapered Fusion Device Implant *Medtronic, Spinal and Biologics, Memphis, TN*	Conditional 6	3	
Luque Wire *orthopedic implant*	Safe	0.3	33
Mandibular Locking Bone Plate *316 SS,* *Biomet, Inc., Warsaw, Indiana*	Conditional 6	3	
MAVERICK Disc Replacement System *Medtronic, Spinal and Biologics, Memphis, TN*	Conditional 6	3	
MEDPOR ATTRACTOR Screw *17-4 SS,* *Porex Surgical, Newnan, GA*	Unsafe 1	1.5	
M. KUROSAKA ADVANTAGE CANNULATED FIXATION SCREW *DePuy Mitek* *A Johnson & Johnson Company, Raynham, MA*	Conditional 6	3	
MR Safe Clamps *for use with Large External Fixation System,* *Synthes, www.synthes.com*	Conditional 5	1.5, 3	
Moe spinal instrumentation *orthopedic implant,* *Zimmer, Warsaw, IN*	Safe	1.5	
Monoblock Neolif Intersomatic Cage *Tantalum,* *Biomet, Inc., Warsaw, Indiana*	Conditional 6	3	

Object	Status	Field Strength (T)	Reference
NGage Surgical Mesh System *Blackstone Medical, Inc., Wayne, NJ*	Conditional 8	1.5, 3	
Panalok Anchor *clear PLA polymer anchor,* *Mitek Products, Norwood, MA*	Safe	1.5	
Pedicle Screw and Locking Clip *for use in the Elaspine Implant System,* *SpineLab AG, Switzerland*	Conditional 6	3	
PRESTIGE LP Cervical Disc System *Medtronic, Spinal and Biologics, Memphis, TN*	Conditional 6	3	
PRESTIGE ST Cervical Disc System *Medtronic, Spinal and Biologics, Memphis, TN*	Conditional 6	3	
Propio Foot *OSSUR Reykjavik, Iceland,* *OSSUR AMERICAS, Aliso Viejo, CA*	Unsafe 1	1.5	
PYRAMID Anterior Lumbar Plate and Screws *Medtronic, Spinal and Biologics, Memphis, TN*	Conditional 6	3	
OSS Distal Femoral Replacement Prosthesis *Titanium alloy, cobalt chrome moly, 316 SS,* *Biomet, Inc., Warsaw, Indiana*	Conditional 6	3	
OsseoFix *Titanium, Alphatec Spine Inc., Carlsbad, CA*	Conditional 6	3	
Osseotite Dental Post Implant *Titanium alloy,* *Biomet, Inc., Warsaw, Indiana*	Conditional 6	3	
Otto Bock Microprocessor Knee *Otto Bock HealthCare, Minneapolis, MN*	Unsafe 1	1.5	
Oxidized Zirconium Knee *Femoral Component,* *Smith & Nephew, Inc., Orthopedic Division, Memphis, TN*	Safe	1.5, 3	83
Perfix interence screw *17-4 SS, orthopedic implant,* *Instrument Makar, Okemos, MI*	Conditional 1	1.5	34
Pinnacle MOM Acetabular Cup System *Titanium alloy shell, CoCrMo insert,* *DePuy Orthopaedics, Warsaw, IN*	Conditional 6	3	
Reusable Titanium Skull Pin *titanium alloy coated in titanium nitride,* *Integra LifeSciences, Cincinnati, OH*	Conditional 6	3	
Rusch Rod *orthopedic implant*	Safe	1.5	
Side plate, 6-hole *Titanium alloy, orthopedic implant,* *DePuy ACE Co., El Segundo, CA*	Safe	1.5	

Object	Status	Field Strength (T)	Reference
Sigma RP Total Knee *CoCrMo alloy and polyethylene,* *DePuy Orthopaedics, Warsaw, IN*	Conditional 6	3	
SMA Staple *Medtronic, Spinal and Biologics, Memphis, TN*	Conditional 6	3	
Small External Fixator *external fixation device, carbon composite,* *Titanium alloy, aluminum, SS,* *Biomet, Inc., Warsaw, Indiana*	Conditional 5	3	
Soteira Kyphoplasty System, Cement Director *Soteira, Inc., Natick, MA*	Conditional 6	3	
SpineAlign *Orthopedic implant, Nitinol,* *SpineWorks, Santa Clara, CA*	Conditional 6	3	
Spinal L-Rod *orthopedic implant,* *DePuy, Warsaw, IN*	Safe	1.5	
Stainless steel mesh *orthopedic implant,* *Zimmer, Warsaw, IN*	Safe	1.5	3
Stainless steel plate *orthopedic implant,* *Zimmer, Warsaw, IN*	Safe	1.5	3
Stainless steel screw *orthopedic implant,* *Zimmer, Warsaw, IN*	Safe	1.5	3
Stainless steel wire *orthopedic implant,* *Zimmer, Warsaw, IN*	Safe	1.5	3
Staple plate, large *Zimaloy, orthopedic implant,* *Zimmer, Warsaw, IN*	Safe	1.5	3
Summit Basic *CoCrMo alloy with CoCrMo alloy head,* *DePuy Orthopaedics, Warsaw, IN*	Conditional 6	3	
Summit Hip Stem *Titanium alloy with CoCrMo alloy head,* *DePuy Orthopaedics, Warsaw, IN*	Conditional 6	3	
SuperAnchor *DePuy Mitek* *A Johnson & Johnson Company, Raynham, MA*	Conditional 6	3	
Synthes AO DCP 2, 3, 4, 5 hole plate *orthopedic implant*	Safe	1.5	

Object	Status	Field Strength (T)	Reference
T2 XVBR Spinal System, Expandable Centerpiece Device *with T2 Spinal System 25 mm Extended Endcaps, 8 Degree, Medtronic, Spinal and Biologics, Memphis, TN*	Conditional 6	3	
Taylor Spatial Frame *metal version, Smith and Nephew, Memphis, TN*	Unsafe 1	1.5	
Teno Fix Tendon Repair System *Ortheon Medical, LLC, Winter Park, FL*	Safe	1.5	
TiMesh Cranial Plating System *Medtronic Neurosurgery, Goleta, CA*	Safe	1.5	
Tibial Intramedullary Nail *with Transfixation Screws, Titanium alloy, DePuy Orthopaedics, Warsaw, IN*	Conditional 6	3	
Tibial nail, 9-mm *Titanium alloy, orthopedic implant, DePuy ACE Medical Co., El Segundo, CA*	Safe	1.5	
Titanium Femoral Reconstruction Nail *Titanium alloy, Biomet, Inc., Warsaw, Indiana*	Conditional 6	3	
Titanium Intramedullary Nail *Titanium alloy, Smith & Nephew, Inc., Orthopedic Division, Memphis, TN*	Safe	1.5, 3	83
TOPS (Total Posterior Arthroplasty System) and VersaLink System *Impliant Ltd.*	Conditional 6	3	
Ultima Tri-Flange *Acetabulum Cage, Titanium alloy, DePuy Orthopaedics, Warsaw, IN*	Conditional 6	3	
UltraFix RC Suture Anchor *316L SS, Linvatec Corporation*	Safe	1.5	
Universal Reconstruction Ribbon *Titanium, orthopedic implant, DePuy ACE Medical Co., El Segundo, CA*	Safe	1.5	
Variable Angle Compression Hip Screw *316L SS, Biomet, Inc., Warsaw, Indiana*	Conditional 6	3	
VERTE-STACK VBS IMPLANT BOOMERANG *Medtronic, Spinal and Biologics, Memphis, TN*	Conditional 6	3	
WedgeLoc Suture Anchor with Opti-Fiber Sutures *MedShape Solutions, Atlanta, GA*	Conditional 6	3	
Wristore Distal Radius Fracture Fixator *external fixation device, Zimmer, Inc., Warsaw, IN*	Conditional 5	3	

Object	Status	Field Strength (T)	Reference
X STOP Interspinous Process *Decompression (IPD) Implant, Medtronic, Spinal and Biologics, Memphis, TN*	Conditional 6	3	
Zielke rod with screw *washer and nut, 316L SS, orthopedic implant*	Safe	0.3	33

Otologic and Cochlear Implants

Object	Status	Field Strength (T)	Reference
Adjustable Length Titanium Ossicular *(ALTO) Partial Prostheses, Grace Medical, www.gracemedical.com/mri.htm*	Conditional 5	1.5	
Adjustable Micron *PORP, Otologic implant, Titanium, Gyrus ACMI Inc. ENT Division, Bartlett, TN*	Conditional 5	3	
Adjustable Micron *TORP, Otologic implant, Titanium, Gyrus ACMI Inc. ENT Division, Bartlett, TN*	Conditional 5	3	
Aerial Total Dusseldorf Titanium *0.2 x 7.0-mm, middle ear implant, otologic implant, Kurz Medical, Inc., Norcross, GA*	Safe	3	
Aerial Total Tuebingen Titanium *0.2 x 7.0-mm, middle ear implant, otologic implant, Kurz Medical, Inc., Norcross, GA*	Safe	3	
Austin Tytan Piston *Titanium, otologic implant, Treace Medical, Nashville, TN*	Safe	1.5	35
Baha, Bone Conduction Implant *Cochlear Americas, Englewood, CO*	Conditional 5	1.5	
Bell Partial Dusseldorf Titanium *0.2 x 4.5-mm, middle ear implant, otologic implant, Kurz Medical, Inc., Norcross, GA*	Safe	3	
Bell Partial Tuebingen Titanium *0.2 x 3.5-mm, middle ear implant, otologic implant, Kurz Medical, Inc., Norcross, GA*	Safe	3	
Berger V Bobbin *Ventilation tube, Titanium, otologic implant, Richards Medical Co., Memphis, TN*	Safe	1.5	35
Berger V Bobbin VT *Ventilation tube, Otologic implant, Titanium, Gyrus ACMI Inc. ENT Division, Bartlett, TN*	Conditional 5	3	
Blue Bobbin VT *Ventilation tube, Otologic implant, Titanium, Gyrus ACMI Inc. ENT Division, Bartlett, TN*	Conditional 5	3	

Object	Status	Field Strength (T)	Reference
Bobbin VT *Ventilation tube, Otologic implant, Titanium,* *Gyrus ACMI Inc. ENT Division, Bartlett, TN*	Conditional 5	3	
Bucket Handle *Stapes Prosthesis, Otologic implant, Titanium,* *Gyrus ACMI Inc. ENT Division, Bartlett, TN*	Conditional 5	3	
Causse Flex H/A *partial ossicular prosthesis, Titanium, otologic implant,* *Microtek Medical, Inc., Memphis, TN*	Safe	1.5	36
Causse Flex H/A *total ossicular prosthesis, Titanium, otologic implant,* *Microtek Medical Inc., Memphis, TN*	Safe	1.5	36
Chicago Bucket Handle *Stapes Prosthesis, Otologic implant, Titanium,* *Gyrus ACMI Inc. ENT Division, Bartlett, TN*	Conditional 5	3	
Classic SS *Otologic Implant, 316L SS,* *Gyrus ACMI Inc. ENT Division, Bartlett, TN*	Conditional 5	3	
Classic Stapes Prosthesis *Otologic implant, Titanium,* *Gyrus ACMI Inc. ENT Division, Bartlett, TN*	Conditional 5	3	
Classic Stapes Prostheses *Otologic Implant, Titanium,* *Gyrus ACMI Inc. ENT Division, Bartlett, TN*	Conditional 5	3	
CliP Partial Prosthesis Titanium *(Dresden type), 0.2 x 3.5-mm, middle ear implant,* *otologic implant,* *Kurz Medical, Inc., Norcross, GA*	Safe	3	
CliP Piston Wengen Titanium *0.6 x 5.5-mm, middle ear implant, otologic implant,* *Kurz Medical, Inc., Norcross, GA*	Safe	3	
Cochlear Implant *HiRes 90K Cochlear Implant,* *Advanced Bionics Corporation, Sylmar, CA*	Conditional 5	0.3, 1.5	
Cochlear implant *Nucleus 24 ABI Cochlear Implant System,* *otologic implant,* *Cochlear Corporation, Engelwood, CO*	Conditional 5	1.5	
Cochlear implant *Nucleus Mini 20-channel, otologic implant,* *Cochlear Corporation, Engelwood, CO*	Unsafe 1	1.5	38
Cochlear implant *3M/House*	Unsafe 1	0.6	37

Object	Status	Field Strength (T)	Reference
Cochlear implant *3M/Vienna*	Unsafe 1	0.6	37
Cody tack *otologic implant*	Safe	0.6	37
Collar Bobbin VT *Ventilation tube, Otologic implant, Titanium,* *Gyrus ACMI Inc. ENT Division, Bartlett, TN*	Conditional 5	3	
Custom Classic Stapes *Otologic Implant, 316L SS,* *Gyrus ACMI Inc. ENT Division, Bartlett, TN*	Conditional 5	3	
De La Cruz *Fluoroplastic, Platinum, Piston,* *Medtronic Xomed, Jacksonville, TN*	Conditional 5	1.5	
Dornhoffer Footplate Shoe *Otologic implant, Titanium,* *Gyrus ACMI Inc. ENT Division, Bartlett, TN*	Conditional 5	3	
Dornhoffer Malleable PORP *Otologic Implant, 316L SS,* *Gyrus ACMI Inc. ENT Division, Bartlett, TN*	Conditional 5	3	
Dornhoffer Titanium *Otologic implant, Titanium,* *Gyrus ACMI Inc. ENT Division, Bartlett, TN*	Conditional 5	3	
Ehmke hook stapes prosthesis *Platinum, otologic implant,* *Richards Medical Co., Memphis, TN*	Safe	1.5	35
Fisch Piston *Teflon, SS, otologic implant,* *Richards Medical Co., Memphis, TN*	Safe	1.5	38
Fisch Piston *Otologic Implant, 316L SS,* *Gyrus ACMI Inc. ENT Division, Bartlett, TN*	Conditional 5	3	
Fisch Teflon Piston *Otologic Implant, 316L SS,* *Gyrus ACMI Inc. ENT Division, Bartlett, TN*	Conditional 5	3	
Flex H/A notched *offset total ossicular prosthesis, 316L SS, otologic implant,* *Microtek Medical, Inc., Memphis, TN*	Safe	1.5	36
Flex H/A offset partial *ossicular prosthesis, 316L SS,* *Microtek Medical, Inc., Memphis, TN*	Safe	1.5	36
FLPL Malleable Piston *Otologic Implant, 316L SS,* *Gyrus ACMI Inc. ENT Division, Bartlett, TN*	Conditional 5	3	

Object	Status	Field Strength (T)	Reference
FLPL/Titanium VT *Ventilation tube, Otologic implant, Titanium,* *Gyrus ACMI Inc. ENT Division, Bartlett, TN*	Conditional 5	3	
Goldenberg Mal Porp *Otologic Implant, 316L SS,* *Gyrus ACMI Inc. ENT Division, Bartlett, TN*	Conditional 5	3	
Gyrus All Titanium Centered *PORP, partial ossicular replacement prosthesis, Titanium,* *Gyrus ENT, Bartlett, TN*	Safe	3	106
Gyrus All Titanium Monolithic Centered *(TORP, total ossicular replacement prosthesis), Titanium,* *Gyrus ENT, Bartlett, TN*	Safe	3	106
Gyrus *PORP, partial ossicular replacement prosthesis, Titanium,* *Gyrus ENT, Bartlett, TN*	Safe	3	106
Gyrus *TORP, total ossicular replacement prosthesis, Titanium,* *Gyrus ENT, Bartlett, TN*	Safe	3	106
Gyrus SMart Stapes Piston *Titanium,* *Gyrus ENT, Bartlett, TN*	Safe	3	106
House double loop *ASTM-318- 76 Grade 2 SS, otologic implant,* *Storz, St. Louis, MO*	Safe	1.5	35
House double loop *tantalum, otologic implant,* *Storz, St. Louis, MO*	Safe	1.5	35
House single loop *ASTM-318- 76, Grade 2 SS, otologic implant,* *Storz, St. Louis, MO*	Safe	1.5	31
House single loop *tantalum, otologic implant,* *Storz, St. Louis, MO*	Safe	1.5	35
House Wire Loop *Otologic Implant, 316LVM SS,* *Gyrus ACMI Inc. ENT Division, Bartlett, TN*	Conditional 5	3	
House wire *SS, otologic implant,* *Otomed*	Safe	0.5	39
House wire *tantalum, otologic implant,* *Otomed*	Safe	0.5	39
House-type incus prosthesis *otologic implant*	Safe	0.6	

Object	Status	Field Strength (T)	Reference
House-type SS *piston and wire, ASTM-318-76 Grade 2 SS, otologic implant, Xomed-Treace Inc., A Bristol-Myers Squibb Co.*	Safe	1.5	35
House-type wire loop *stapes prosthesis, 316L SS, otologic implant, Richards Medical Co., Memphis, TN*	Safe	1.5	35
InSound XT Series *InSound Medical, Newark, CA*	Unsafe 1	1.5	
K Piston Titanium *0.6 x 10.0-mm, middle ear implant, otologic implant, Kurz Medical, Inc., Norcross, GA*	Safe	3	
Kurz Aerial *Titanium, Kurz Medical, Dusslingen, Germany*	Safe	3	106
Kurz Aerial-Total-Dusseldorf-Titanium *TORP, total ossicular replacement prosthesis, Kurz Medical, Dusslingen, Germany*	Safe	3	106
Kurz Bell *Titanium, Kurz Medical, Dusslingen, Germany*	Safe	3	106
Kurz Bell-Partial-Dusseldorf-Titanium *PORP, partial ossicular replacement prosthesis, Titanium, Kurz Medical, Dusslingen, Germany*	Safe	3	106
Kurz Piston *Titanium, Kurz Medical, Dusslingen, Germany*	Safe	3	106
Kurz Piston-Titanium *stapes, Titanium, Kurz Medical, Dusslingen, Germany*	Safe	3	106
Lippy Modified Bucket Handle *Stapes Prosthesis, Otologic implant, Titanium, Gyrus ACMI Inc. ENT Division, Bartlett, TN*	Conditional 5	3	
Lippy Modified Stapes Prostheses *Otologic Implant, Titanium, Gyrus ACMI Inc. ENT Division, Bartlett, TN*	Conditional 5	3	
Lyric Hearing Device *InSound Medical, Newark, CA*	Unsafe 1	1.5	
McGee Piston *Otologic Implant, 316LVM SS, Gyrus ACMI Inc. ENT Division, Bartlett, TN*	Conditional 5	3	
McGee piston stapes prosthesis *316L, SS, otologic implant, Richards Medical Co., Memphis, TN*	Safe	1.5	35

Object	Status	Field Strength (T)	Reference
McGee piston stapes prosthesis *Platinum, 316L SS, otologic implant,* *Richards Medical Co., Memphis, TN*	Safe	1.5	35
McGee piston stapes prosthesis *Platinum, chromium-nickel alloy, SS, otologic implant,* *Richards Medical Co., Memphis, TN*	Unsafe 1	1.5	38
McGee Shepard's Crook Pistons *Otologic Implant, SS,* *Gyrus ACMI Inc. ENT Division, Bartlett, TN*	Conditional 5	3	
McGee Sheperd's Crook stapes prosthesis *316L SS, otologic implant,* *Richards Medical Co., Memphis, TN*	Safe	1.5	35
MED-EL COMBI 40+ *MED-EL Cochlear Implant System,* *MED-EL Corporation, Durham, NC* *COMBI 40+ is MRI safe* *at 0.2, 1.0 and 1.5 Tesla depending on regulatory* *approval in different countries. Contact MED-EL* *prior to MRI examination for important guidelines* *MED-EL Corporation, www.medel.com*	Conditional 5	0.2, 1, 1.5	98
Medtronic-Xomed *PORP, partial ossicular replacement prosthesis, Titanium,* *Medtronic-Xomed, Jacksonville, FL*	Safe	3	106
Medtronic-Xomed *TORP, total ossicular replacement prosthesis, Titanium,* *Medtronic-Xomed, Jacksonville, FL*	Safe	3	106
MEY Modified Lippy *Otologic Implant, 316L SS,* *Gyrus ACMI Inc. ENT Division, Bartlett, TN*	Conditional 5	3	
Micron Bobbin Blue VT *Ventilation tube, Otologic implant, Titanium,* *Gyrus ACMI Inc. ENT Division, Bartlett, TN*	Conditional 5	3	
Micron Bobbin VT *Ventilation tube, Otologic implant, Titanium,* *Gyrus ACMI Inc. ENT Division, Bartlett, TN*	Conditional 5	3	
Micron II Modular *PORP, Otologic implant, Titanium,* *Gyrus ACMI Inc. ENT Division, Bartlett, TN*	Conditional 5	3	
Micron II Modular *TORP, Otologic implant, Titanium,* *Gyrus ACMI Inc. ENT Division, Bartlett, TN*	Conditional 5	3	
Micron II Monolithic *PORP, Otologic implant, Titanium,* *Gyrus ACMI Inc. ENT Division, Bartlett, TN*	Conditional 5	3	

Object	Status	Field Strength (T)	Reference
Micron II Monolithic *TORP, Otologic implant, Titanium,* *Gyrus ACMI Inc. ENT Division, Bartlett, TN*	Conditional 5	3	
Micron Plus VT *Ventilation tube, Otologic implant, Titanium,* *Gyrus ACMI Inc. ENT Division, Bartlett, TN*	Conditional 5	3	
Micron Spoon Bobbin VT *Ventilation tube, Otologic implant, Titanium,* *Gyrus ACMI Inc. ENT Division, Bartlett, TN*	Conditional 5	3	
Modified Lippy *Otologic Implant, 316L SS,* *Gyrus ACMI Inc. ENT Division, Bartlett, TN*	Conditional 5	3	
Moretz Type VT *Ventilation tube, Otologic implant, Titanium,* *Gyrus ACMI Inc. ENT Division, Bartlett, TN*	Conditional 5	3	
Nucleus 22, Cochlear Implant *Without removable magnet,* *Cochlear LTD,* *http://professionals.cochlearamericas.com*	Unsafe 1	1.5	
Nucleus 22, Cochlear Implant *With removable magnet,* *Cochlear LTD,* *http://professionals.cochlearamericas.com*	Conditional 5	1.5	
Nucleus 24 Series, Cochlear Implant *Cochlear LTD,* *http://professionals.cochlearamericas.com*	Conditional 5	1.5	
Nucleus Freedom, Cochlear Implant *Cochlear LTD,* *http://professionals.cochlearamericas.com*	Conditional 5	1.5	
Pediatric VT *Ventilation tube, Otologic implant, Titanium,* *Gyrus ACMI Inc. ENT Division, Bartlett, TN*	Conditional 5	3	
Piston Teflon Wire *Otologic Implant, 316L SS,* *Gyrus ACMI Inc. ENT Division, Bartlett, TN*	Conditional 5	3	
Plasti-pore piston *316L SS, Plasti-pore material, otologic implant,* *Richards Medical Co., Memphis, TN*	Safe	1.5	35
Platinum ribbon loop stapes prosthesis *Platinum, otologic implant,* *Richards Medical Co., Memphis, TN*	Safe	1.5	35
Pulsar Cochlear Implant *PULSARCI100, MedEl Corporation, Durham, NC*	Conditional 5	0.2	98

Object	Status	Field Strength (T)	Reference
Reuter Bobbin *Ventilation tube, 316L SS, otologic implant,* *Richards Medical Co., Memphis, TN*	Safe	1.5	35
Reuter Bobbin VT *Ventilation tube, Otologic implant, Titanium,* *Gyrus ACMI Inc. ENT Division, Bartlett, TN*	Conditional 5	3	
Reuter Bobbin Vent Tube *Ventilation tube, Otologic Implant, 316L SS,* *Gyrus ACMI Inc. ENT Division, Bartlett, TN*	Conditional 5	3	
Reuter drain tube *otologic implant*	Safe	1.5	35
Richards bucket handle stapes prosthesis *316L SS, otologic implant,* *Richards Medical Co., Memphis, TN*	Safe	1.5	35
Richard's Bucket Handle *Otologic Implant, Tantalum,* *Gyrus ACMI Inc. ENT Division, Bartlett, TN*	Conditional 5	3	
Richards piston stapes prosthesis *Platinum, fluoroplastic, otologic implant,* *Richards Medical Co., Memphis, TN*	Safe	1.5	35
Richards Plasti-pore *with Armstrong-style, Platinum ribbon, Platinum,* *otologic implant,* *Richards Medical Co., Memphis, TN*	Safe	1.5	35
Richards Platinum Teflon piston *0.6-mm, Teflon, Platinum, otologic implant,* *Richards Medical Co., Memphis, TN*	Safe	1.5	38
Richards Platinum Teflon piston *0.8-mm, Teflon, Platinum, otologic implant,* *Richards Medical Co., Memphis, TN*	Safe	1.5	38
Richards Shepherd's crook *Platinum, otologic implant,* *Richards Medical Co., Memphis, TN*	Safe	0.5	39
Richards Teflon piston *Teflon, otologic implant,* *Richards Medical Co., Memphis, TN*	Safe	1.5	38
Roberson Stapes Prosthesis *Titanium,* *Medtronic Xomed, Inc.*	Safe	3	
Roberts Universal Prosthesis *PORP, Otologic implant, Titanium,* *Gyrus ACMI Inc. ENT Division, Bartlett, TN*	Conditional 5	3	

Object	Status	Field Strength (T)	Reference
Roberts Universal Prosthesis *TORP, Otologic implant, Titanium,* *Gyrus ACMI Inc. ENT Division, Bartlett, TN*	Conditional 5	3	
Robinson incus replacement prosthesis *ASTM-318-76 Grade 2 SS, otologic implant,* *Storz, St. Louis, MO*	Safe	1.5	35
Robinson stapes prosthesis *ASTM-318-76 Grade 2 SS, otologic implant,* *Storz, St. Louis, MO*	Safe	1.5	35
Robinson-Moon offset *stapes prosthesis, ASTM-318-76 Grade 2 SS,* *otologic implant,* *Storz, St. Louis, MO*	Safe	1.5	35
Robinson-Moon-Lippy offset *stapes prosthesis, ASTM- 318-76 Grade 2 SS,* *otologic implant,* *Storz, St. Louis, MO*	Safe	1.5	35
Ronis Piston *Stapes prosthesis, 316L SS, fluoroplastic,* *otologic implant,* *Richards Medical Co., Memphis, TN*	Safe	1.5	35
Ronis Piston *Otologic Implant, 316L SS,* *Gyrus ACMI Inc. ENT Division, Bartlett, TN*	Conditional 5	3	
Ronis Wire Piston *Otologic Implant, 316L SS,* *Gyrus ACMI Inc. ENT Division, Bartlett, TN*	Conditional 5	3	
Schea cup piston stapes prosthesis *Platinum, fluoroplastic, otologic implant,* *Richards Medical Co., Memphis, TN*	Safe	1.5	35
Schea malleus attachment piston *Teflon, otologic implant,* *Richards Medical Co., Memphis, TN*	Safe	1.5	38
Schea SS *and Teflon wire prosthesis, Teflon, 316L SS,* *otologic implant,* *Richards Medical Co., Memphis, TN*	Safe	1.5	38
Scheer FLPL Wire *Otologic Implant, 316L SS,* *Gyrus ACMI Inc. ENT Division, Bartlett, TN*	Conditional 5	3	
Scheer piston *Teflon, 316L SS, otologic implant,* *Richards Medical Co., Memphis, TN*	Safe	1.5	33

Object	Status	Field Strength (T)	Reference
Scheer piston stapes prosthesis *316L SS, fluoroplastic, otologic implant,* *Richards Medical Co., Memphis, TN*	Safe	1.5	35
Schuk Wire Piston *Otologic Implant, 316L SS,* *Gyrus ACMI Inc. ENT Division, Bartlett, TN*	Conditional 5	3	
Schuknecht gelfoam and wire *prosthesis, Armstrong style, 316L SS, otologic implant,* *Richards Medical Co., Memphis, TN*	Safe	1.5	40
Schuknecht piston stapes prosthesis *316L SS, fluoroplastic, otologic implant,* *Richards Medical Co., Memphis, TN*	Safe	1.5	35
Schuknecht Tef-wire incus attachment *ASTM-318-76 Grade 2 SS, otologic implant,* *Storz, St. Louis, MO*	Safe	1.5	35
Schuknecht Tef-wire malleus attachment *ASTM-318-76 Grade 2 SS, otologic implant,* *Storz, St. Louis, MO*	Safe	1.5	35
Schuknecht Teflon wire piston *0.6-mm, Teflon, 316L SS, otologic implant,* *Richards Medical Co., Memphis, TN*	Safe	1.5	38
Schuknecht Teflon wire piston *0.8-mm, Teflon, 316L SS, otologic implant,* *Richards Medical Co., Memphis, TN*	Safe	1.5	38
Sheehy incus replacement *ASTM-318-76 Grade 2 SS, otologic implant,* *Storz, St. Louis, MO*	Safe	1.5	35
Sheehy incus strut *316L SS, otologic implant,* *Richards Medical Co., Memphis, TN*	Safe	1.5	38
Sheehy Stapes *Replacement strut, Otologic Implant, 316L SS,* *Gyrus ACMI Inc. ENT Division, Bartlett, TN*	Conditional 5	3	
Sheehy-Type Incus *Replacement strut, Teflon, 316L SS, otologic implant,* *Richards Medical Co., Memphis, TN*	Safe	1.5	35
Sheehy-Type Incus *Replacement strut, Otologic Implant, 316L SS,* *Gyrus ACMI Inc. ENT Division, Bartlett, TN*	Conditional 5	3	
Shepherd Crook Piston *Otologic Implant, 316L SS,* *Gyrus ACMI Inc. ENT Division, Bartlett, TN*	Conditional 5	3	

Object	Status	Field Strength (T)	Reference
Shipp Modified Berger VT *Ventilation tube, Otologic implant, Titanium,* *Gyrus ACMI Inc. ENT Division, Bartlett, TN*	Conditional 5	3	
Silverstein malleus clip, ventilation tube *Teflon, 316L SS, otologic implant,* *Richards Medical Co., Memphis, TN*	Safe	1.5	38
SMart De La Cruz Piston *Otologic Implant, Nitinol/Fluoroplastic,* *Gyrus ACMI Inc. ENT Division, Bartlett, TN*	Conditional 5	3	
SMart Malleus Piston *Otologic Implant, Nitinol/Fluoroplastic,* *Gyrus ACMI Inc. ENT Division, Bartlett, TN*	Conditional 5	3	
SMart Piston *Otologic Implant, Fluoroplastic/Nitinol,* *Gyrus ACMI Inc. ENT Division, Bartlett, TN*	Conditional 5	3	
SOUNDTEC Direct Drive Hearing System *SOUNDTEC, Inc., Oklahoma City, OK*	Unsafe 1	1.5	
Spoon Bobbin *Ventilation tube, 316L SS, otologic implant,* *Richards Medical Co., Memphis, TN*	Safe	1.5	35
Spoon-Bobbin Vent Tube *Ventilation tube, Otologic Implant, 316L SS,* *Gyrus ACMI Inc. ENT Division, Bartlett, TN*	Conditional 5	3	
Stainless Steel Vent Tube & Stainless Steel Wire *VT-1400-0, because the size of the metallic mass* *associated with this product, the MRI test findings* *apply to all of the following products from Micromedics, Inc.,* *VT-0205-, Fluoroplastic with stainless steel wire,* *VT-0702-, Silicone with stainless steel wire,* *VT-1402-, Stainless Steel with stainless steel wire,* *VT-1412-, Titanium with stainless steel wire,* *VT-1505-, Polyethylene with stainless steel wire,* *Micromedics, Inc., Eagan, MN*	Conditional 6	3	
Stapes, fluoroplastic/Platinum, piston *otologic implant,* *Microtek Medical, Inc., Memphis, TN*	Safe	1.5	36
Stapes, fluoroplastic/SS piston *316L SS, otologic implant,* *Microtek Medical, Inc., Memphis, TN*	Safe	1.5	36
Stapes Grommet *Replacement strut, Otologic Implant, 316L SS,* *Gyrus ACMI Inc. ENT Division, Bartlett, TN*	Conditional 5	3	
Tantalum Wire Loop *Otologic Implant, Tantalum,* *Gyrus ACMI Inc. ENT Division, Bartlett, TN*	Conditional 5	3	

Object	Status	Field Strength (T)	Reference
Tantalum wire loop *Stapes prosthesis, Tantalum, Otologic implant,* *Richards Medical Co., Memphis, TN*	Safe	1.5	35
Teflon Malleable Piston *Otologic Implant, 316L SS,* *Gyrus ACMI Inc. ENT Division, Bartlett, TN*	Conditional 5	3	
Teflon Piston *Otologic Implant, 316L SS,* *Gyrus ACMI Inc. ENT Division, Bartlett, TN*	Conditional 5	3	
Teflon Wire Piston *Otologic Implant, 316L SS,* *Gyrus ACMI Inc. ENT Division, Bartlett, TN*	Conditional 5	3	
Tef-Platinum piston *Platinum, otologic implant,* *Xomed-Treace Inc., A Bristol-Myers Squibb Co.*	Safe	1.5	35
Touma Modified Crook Piston *Otologic Implant, 316L SS,* *Gyrus ACMI Inc. ENT Division, Bartlett, TN*	Conditional 5	3	
The Big Easy Piston *Titanium, Platinum,* *Medtronic Xomed, Jacksonville, TN*	Conditional 5	3	
Total ossicular replacement *prosthesis (TORP), 316L SS, otologic implant,* *Richards Medical Co., Memphis, TN*	Safe	1.5	38
Trapeze ribbon loop *stapes prosthesis, Platinum, otologic implant,* *Richards Medical Co., Memphis, TN*	Safe	1.5	35
TTP Aerial Vario Titanium *0.2 x 7.0-mm, middle ear implant, otologic implant,* *Kurz Medical, Inc., Norcross, GA*	Safe	3	
TTP Bell Vario Titanium *0.2 x 4.5-mm, middle ear implant, otologic implant,* *Kurz Medical, Inc., Norcross, GA*	Safe	3	
UniBobbin VT *Ventilation tube, Otologic implant, Titanium,* *Gyrus ACMI Inc. ENT Division, Bartlett, TN*	Conditional 5	3	
Venturi Plus VT *Ventilation tube, Otologic implant, Titanium,* *Gyrus ACMI Inc. ENT Division, Bartlett, TN*	Conditional 5	3	
Venturi VT *Ventilation tube, Otologic implant, Titanium,* *Gyrus ACMI Inc. ENT Division, Bartlett, TN*	Conditional 5	3	
Vibrant Soundbridge *Symphonix Devices, Inc., San Jose, CA*	Unsafe 1	1.5	

Object	Status	Field Strength (T)	Reference
Williams Microclip *316L SS, otologic implant,* *Richards Medical Co., Memphis, TN*	Safe	1.5	35
Williams Microclip *Wire clip, Otologic Implant, 316L SS,* *Gyrus ACMI Inc. ENT Division, Bartlett, TN*	Conditional 5	3	
Winkel Partial Plester Titanium *0.2 x 3.5-mm, middle ear implant, otologic implant,* *Kurz Medical, Inc., Norcross, GA*	Safe	3	
Xomed Baily stapes implant *otologic implant*	Safe	1.5	35
Xomed ceravital *partial ossicular prosthesis, otologic implant*	Safe	1.5	
Xomed stapes prosthesis *Robinson-style, otologic implant,* *Richard's Co., Nashville, TN*	Safe	1.5	35
Xomed stapes *ASTM-318-76 Grade 2 SS, otologic implant,* *Xomed-Treace Inc., A Bristol-Myers Squibb Co.*	Safe	1.5	35

Patent Ductus Arteriosus (PDA), Atrial Septal Defect (ASD), Ventricular Septal Defect (VSD) Occluders, and Patent Foramen Ovale (PFO) Closure Devices

Object	Status	Field Strength (T)	Reference
AMPLATZER Cardiac Plug *(also known as ACP device), Nitinol, SS,* *Platinum/iridium, Polyester,* *AGA Medical Corporation, Plymouth, MN*	Conditional 6	3	
AMPLATZER Muscular VSD PI Occluder *AGA Medical Corporation,* *http://international.amplatzer.com*	Conditional 6	3	
AMPLATZER PFO Occluder *Nitinol, SS, Platinum/iridium, Polyester,* *AGA Medical Corporation, Plymouth, MN*	Conditional 6	3	
AMPLATZER Post Infarction *Muscular Ventricular Septal Device, Nitinol,* *SS, Platinum/iridium, Polyester,* *AGA Medical Corporation, Plymouth, MN*	Conditional 6	3	
AMPLATZER Septal Occluder *Nitinol, SS, Platinum/iridium, Polyester,* *AGA Medical Corporation, Plymouth, MN*	Conditional 6	3	
AMPLATZER Transcatheter Occlusion Device *AGA Medical Corporation, Golden Valley, MN*	Conditional 6	3	

Object	Status	Field Strength (T)	Reference
AMPLATZER Vascular Plug 4 *AVP4 device,* *AGA Medical Corporation,* *http://international.amplatzer.com*	Conditional 6	3	
Atrial Septal Defect Occluder *Guardian Angel, 12-mm, occluder,* *Microvena Corporation, White Bear Lake, MN*	Safe	1.5	
Atrial Septal Defect Occluder *Guardian Angel, 40-mm, occluder,* *Microvena Corporation, White Bear Lake, MN*	Safe	1.5	
Atriasept Closure Device *Cardia, Inc., Eagan, MN*	Conditional 6	3	
Bard Clamshell Septal Umbrella *17-mm, occluder, MP35N,* *C.R. Bard, Inc., Billerica, MA*	Safe	1.5	41
Bard Clamshell Septal Umbrella *23-mm, occluder, MP35N,* *C.R. Bard, Inc., Billerica, MA*	Safe	1.5	41
Bard Clamshell Septal Umbrella *28-mm, occluder, MP35N,* *C.R. Bard, Inc., Billerica, MA*	Safe	1.5	41
Bard Clamshell Septal Umbrella *33-mm, occluder, MP35N,* *C.R. Bard, Inc., Billerica, MA*	Safe	1.5	41
Bard Clamshell Septal Umbrella *40-mm, occluder, MP35N,* *C.R. Bard, Inc., Bellerica, MA*	Safe	1.5	41
BioTREK *patent foramen ovale (PFO) closure device,* *Tungsten, polymer,* *NMT Medical, Boston, MA*	Safe	3	
CardioSEAL Septal Occluder *17-mm, MP35N,* *NMT Medical, Inc., Boston, MA*	Safe	1.5	
CardioSEAL Septal Occluder *23-mm, MP35N,* *NMT Medical, Inc., Boston, MA*	Safe	1.5	
CardioSEAL Septal Occluder *28-mm, MP35N,* *NMT Medical, Inc., Boston, MA*	Safe	1.5	
CardioSEAL Septal Occluder *33-mm, MP35N,* *NMT Medical, Inc., Boston, MA*	Safe	1.5	

Object	Status	Field Strength (T)	Reference
CardioSEAL Septal Occluder *40-mm, MP35N,* *NMT Medical, Inc., Boston, MA*	Safe	1.5	
CardioSEAL Septal Repair Implant *MP35N,* *NMT Medical, Inc., Boston, MA*	Safe	3	107
Cocoon Septal Occluder *Nitinol, Platinum,* *Vascular Innovations Co. Ltd, Nonthaburi, Thailand*	Conditional 6	3	
GORE HELEX Septal Occluder *W.L. Gore & Associates, www.goremedical.com*	Conditional 6	3	
HELEX *ASD closure device, occluder, size 15-mm, Nitinol,* *W. L. Gore and Associates, Inc., www.goremedical.com*	Conditional 5	3	
HELEX *ASD closure device, occluder, size 35-mm, Nitinol,* *W. L. Gore and Associates, Inc., www.goremedical.com*	Conditional 5	3	
HELEX Septal Occluder *Nitinol,* *W. L. Gore & Associates, Inc., www.goremedical.com*	Conditional 5	3	
Intrasept *patent foramen ovale (PFO) closure device,* *Nitinol, Titanium, Cardia Inc., Burnsville, MN*	Conditional 6	3	
Lock Clamshell Septal Occlusion Implant *17-mm, occluder, 304 V SS,* *C.R. Bard, Inc., Billerica, MA*	Conditional 2	1.5	41
Lock Clamshell Septal Occlusion Implant *23-mm, occluder, 304 V SS,* *C.R. Bard, Inc., Billerica, MA*	Conditional 2	1.5	41
Lock Clamshell Septal Occlusion Implant *28-mm, occluder, 304 V SS,* *C.R. Bard, Inc., Billerica, MA*	Conditional 2	1.5	41
Lock Clamshell Septal Occlusion Implant *33-mm, occluder, 304 V SS,* *C.R. Bard, Inc., Billerica, MA*	Conditional 2	1.5	41
Lock Clamshell Septal Occlusion Implant *40-mm, occluder, 304 V SS,* *C.R. Bard, Inc., Billerica, MA*	Conditional 2	1.5	41
Nit-Occlud Spiral Coil *PFM Medical, Inc., Oceanside, CA*	Conditional 6	3	
Rashkind PDA Occlusion Implant *12-mm, occluder, 304V SS,* *C.R. Bard, Inc., Billerica, MA*	Conditional 2	1.5	41

Object	Status	Field Strength (T)	Reference
Rashkind PDA Occlusion Implant *17-mm, occluder, 304 V SS,* *C.R. Bard, Inc., Billerica, MA*	Conditional 2	1.5	41
STARFlex Septal Repair Implant *MP35N, Nitinol,* *NMT Medical, Inc., Boston, MA*	Safe	3	107

Pellets and Bullets

Object	Status	Field Strength (T)	Reference
BBs (Crosman)	Unsafe 1	1.5	
BBs (Daisy)	Unsafe 1	1.5	
Bullet, .357 inch *aluminum, lead, pellets and bullets,* *Winchester*	Safe	1.5	42
Bullet, .357 inch *bronze, plastic, pellets and bullets,* *Patton-Morgan*	Safe	1.5	42
Bullet, .357 inch *copper, lead, pellets and bullets,* *Cascade*	Safe	1.5	42
Bullet, .357 inch *copper, lead, pellets and bullets,* *Hornady*	Safe	1.5	42
Bullet, .357 inch *copper, lead, pellets and bullets,* *Patton-Morgan*	Safe	1.5	42
Bullet, .357 inch *lead, pellets and bullets,* *Remington*	Safe	1.5	42
Bullet, .357 inch *nickel, copper, lead, pellets and bullets,* *Winchester*	Safe	1.5	42
Bullet, .357 inch *nylon, lead, pellets and bullets,* *Smith & Wesson*	Safe	1.5	42
Bullet, .357 inch *steel, lead, pellets and bullets,* *Fiocchi*	Safe	1.5	42
Bullet, .380 inch *copper, nickel, lead, pellets and bullets,* *Winchester*	Unsafe 1	1.5	42
Bullet, .380 inch *copper, plastic, lead, pellets and bullets,* *Glaser*	Safe	1.5	42

Object	Status	Field Strength (T)	Reference
Bullet, .44 inch *Teflon, bronze, pellets and bullets,* *North American Ordinance*	Safe	1.5	42
Bullet, .45 inch *copper, lead, pellets and bullets,* *Samson*	Safe	1.5	42
Bullet, .45 inch *steel, lead, pellets and bullets,* *Evansville Ordinance*	Unsafe 1	1.5	42
Bullet, 7.62 x 39-mm *copper, steel, pellets and bullets,* *Norinco*	Unsafe 1	1.5	42
Bullet, 9-mm *copper, lead, pellets and bullets,* *Norma*	Unsafe 1	1.5	42
Bullet, 9-mm *copper, lead, pellets and bullets,* *Remington*	Safe	1.5	42
Shot, 00 buckshot *lead, pellets and bullets*	Safe	1.5	42
Shot, 12 gauge, size: 00 *copper, lead, pellets and bullets,* *Federal*	Safe	1.5	42
Shot, 4 *lead, pellets and bullets*	Safe	1.5	42
Shot, 7 1/2 *lead, pellets and bullets*	Safe	1.5	42

Penile Implants

Object	Status	Field Strength (T)	Reference
Penile implant, 700 Ultrex Plus *AMS, American Medical Systems, Minnetonka, MN*	Safe	1.5, 3	
Penile implant, AMS 700 Ultrex Preconnected *AMS, American Medical Systems, Minnetonka, MN*	Safe	1.5, 3	
Penile implant, AMS 700 CX Inflatable *AMS, American Medical Systems, Minnetonka, MN*	Safe	1.5	43
Penile implant, AMS 700 CX/CXM *AMS, American Medical Systems, Minnetonka, MN*	Safe	1.5, 3	
Penile implant, AMS 700CXR *AMS, American Medical Systems, Minnetonka, MN*	Safe	3	
Penile implant, AMS 700 Inflate/Deflated Pump *AMS, American Medical Systems, Minnetonka, MN*	Safe	3	
Penile implant, AMS Tactile Pump *AMS, American Medical Systems, Minnetonka, MN*	Safe	3	

Object	Status	Field Strength (T)	Reference
Penile implant, AMS 700 Ultrex *AMS, American Medical Systems, Minnetonka, MN*	Safe	1.5, 3	
Penile implant, AMS Ambicor *AMS, American Medical Systems, Minnetonka, MN*	Safe	1.5, 3	
Penile implant, AMS Dynaflex *AMS, American Medical Systems, Minnetonka, MN*	Safe	1.5, 3	
Penile implant, AMS Hydroflex *AMS, American Medical Systems, Minnetonka, MN*	Safe	1.5, 3	
Penile implant, AMS Malleable 600 *AMS, American Medical Systems, Minnetonka, MN*	Safe	1.5, 3	43
Penile implant, AMS Malleable 600M *AMS, American Medical Systems, Minnetonka, MN*	Safe	1.5, 3	
Penile implant, AMS Malleable 650 *AMS, American Medical Systems, Minnetonka, MN*	Safe	1.5, 3	
Penile Implant, DURA II Penile Prosthesis *AMS, American Medical Systems, Minnetonka, MN*	Safe	1.5, 3	
Penile implant, Duraphase	Unsafe 1	1.5	
Penile Implant *Excel Inflatable Penile Prosthesis, Model 90-95XXSC,* *MP35N, Urethane, silicone, Polysulfone,* *Coloplast Corporation, Minneapolis, MN*	Conditional 6	3	
Penile implant, Flex-Rod II (Firm) *Surgitek, Medical Engineering Corp., Racine, WI*	Safe	1.5	43
Penile implant, Flexi-Flate *Surgitek, Medical Engineering Corp., Racine, WI*	Safe	1.5	43
Penile implant, Flexi-Rod (Standard) *Surgitek, Medical Engineering Corp., Racine, WI*	Safe	1.5	43
Penile Implant *Genesis Malleable Penile Implant,* *Coloplast, UCC - Surgical Urology, Minneapolis, MN*	Conditional 6	3	
Penile implant, Jonas *Dacomed Corp., Minneapolis, MN*	Safe	1.5	43
Penile implant, Mentor Flexible *Mentor Corp, Minneapolis, MN*	Safe	1.5	43
Penile implant, Mentor Inflatable *Mentor Corp., Minneapolis, MN*	Safe	1.5	43
Penile implant, OmniPhase *Dacomed Corp., Minneapolis, MN*	Unsafe 1	1.5	43
Penile implant, Osmond, external	Safe	1.5	
Penile Implant *Spectra Penile Implant,* *American Medical Systems, Minnetonka, MN*	Conditional 6	3	

Object	Status	Field Strength (T)	Reference
Penile Implant *Titan Inflatable Penile Prosthesis, Model 90-98XXIC,* *MP35N, Urethane, silicone, Polysulfone,* *Coloplast Corporation, Minneapolis, MN*	Conditional 6	3	
Penile Implant *Titan Inflatable Penile Prosthesis, Model 90-98XXIC,* *MP35N, Urethane, silicone, Polysulfone,* *Coloplast Corporation, Minneapolis, MN*	Conditional 6	3	
Penile Implant *Titan Inflatable Penile Prosthesis, Model 90-98XXIC,* *MP35N, Urethane, silicone, Polysulfone,* *Coloplast Corporation, Minneapolis, MN*	Conditional 6	3	
Penile Implant *Titan Inflatable Penile Prosthesis, Model 90-98ICOTR,* *MP35N, Urethane, silicone, Polysulfone,* *Coloplast Corporation, Minneapolis, MN*	Conditional 6	3	
Penile Implant *Titan Inflatable Penile Prosthesis, Model 90-99SCOTR,* *MP35N, Urethane, silicone, Polysulfone,* *Coloplast Corporation, Minneapolis, MN*	Conditional 6	3	
Penile implant, Uniflex 1000	Safe	1.5	

Pessaries

Object	Status	Field Strength (T)	Reference
95% Rigid Silicone *Pessary,* *CooperSurgical, Inc., Trumbull, CT*	Safe	3	
Cube (with drainage holes) *Pessary,* *CooperSurgical, Inc., Trumbull, CT*	Safe	3	
Cube with Drain *EvaCare, Pessary, Silicone,* *Coloplast Corporation, Minneapolis, MN*	Safe	3	
Cube *EvaCare, Pessary, Silicone,* *Coloplast Corporation, Minneapolis, MN, MN*	Safe	3	
Cube *Pessary,* *CooperSurgical, Inc., Trumbull, CT*	Safe	3	
Cube *Pessary, silicone,* *Bioteque America, Inc., Fremont, CA*	Safe	3	
Cup Pessary *EvaCare, Pessary, Silicone,* *Coloplast Corporation, Minneapolis, MN*	Safe	3	

Object	Status	Field Strength (T)	Reference
Cup *Pessary, silicone,* *Bioteque America, Inc., Fremont, CA*	Safe	3	
Dish Pessary with Support *EvaCare, Pessary, Silicone,* *Coloplast Corporation, Minneapolis, MN*	Safe	3	
Dish *Pessary, silicone,* *Bioteque America, Inc., Fremont, CA*	Safe	3	
Donut *EvaCare, Pessary, Silicone,* *Coloplast Corporation, Minneapolis, MN*	Safe	3	
Donut *Pessary,* *CooperSurgical, Inc., Trumbull, CT*	Safe	3	
Donut *Pessary, silicone,* *Bioteque America, Inc., Fremont, CA*	Safe	3	
Gehrung with Support *EvaCare, Pessary, Silicone,* *Coloplast Corporation, Minneapolis, MN*	Safe	3	
Gelhorn *Pessary, silicone,* *Bioteque America, Inc., Fremont, CA*	Safe	3	
Gellhorn with Drain *EvaCare, Pessary, Silicone,* *Coloplast Corporation, Minneapolis, MN*	Safe	3	
Gellhorn/95% Rigid *Pessary,* *CooperSurgical, Inc., Trumbull, CT*	Safe	3	
Gellhorn/Flexible - Short Stem *Pessary,* *CooperSurgical, Inc., Trumbull, CT*	Safe	3	
Gellhorn/Flexible *Pessary,* *CooperSurgical, Inc., Trumbull, CT*	Safe	3	
Gellhorn/Flexible *Pessary,* *CooperSurgical, Inc., Trumbull, CT*	Safe	3	
Hodge with Support *EvaCare, Pessary, Silicone,* *Coloplast Corporation, Minneapolis, MN*	Safe	3	

Object	Status	Field Strength (T)	Reference
Hodge *EvaCare, Pessary, Silicone,* *Coloplast Corporation, Minneapolis, MN*	Safe	3	
Incontinence Dish With Support/Folding *Pessary,* *CooperSurgical, Inc., Trumbull, CT*	Safe	3	
Incontinence Dish/Folding *Pessary,* *CooperSurgical, Inc., Trumbull, CT*	Safe	3	
Inflatoball *Pessary,* *CooperSurgical, Inc., Trumbull, CT*	Safe	3	
Marland Pessary *Pessary, silicone,* *Bioteque America, Inc., Fremont, CA*	Safe	3	
Marland with Support *EvaCare, Pessary, Silicone,* *Coloplast Corporation, Minneapolis, MN*	Safe	3	
Marland *EvaCare, Pessary, Silicone,* *Coloplast Corporation, Minneapolis, MN*	Safe	3	
Oval with Support *EvaCare, Pessary, Silicone,* *Coloplast Corporation, Minneapolis, MN*	Safe	3	
Oval *Pessary, silicone,* *Bioteque America, Inc., Fremont, CA*	Safe	3	
Regular/Folding *Pessary,* *CooperSurgical, Inc., Trumbull, CT*	Safe	3	
Rigid Acrylic Gelhorn *Pessary,* *CooperSurgical, Inc., Trumbull, CT*	Safe	3	
Ring Pessary with Knob *EvaCare, Pessary, Silicone,* *Coloplast Corporation, Minneapolis, MN*	Safe	3	
Ring With Knob/Folding *Pessary,* *CooperSurgical, Inc., Trumbull, CT*	Safe	3	
Ring with Knob *Pessary, also known as Knobbed Ring, silicone,* *Bioteque America, Inc., Fremont, CA*	Safe	3	

Object	Status	Field Strength (T)	Reference
Ring With Nylon Pegs *Pessary,* *CooperSurgical, Inc., Trumbull, CT*	Safe	3	
Ring With Support With Knob *Pessary,* *CooperSurgical, Inc., Trumbull, CT*	Safe	3	
Ring With Support *and Knob/Folding, Pessary,* *CooperSurgical, Inc., Trumbull, CT*	Safe	3	
Ring with Support *EvaCare, Pessary, Silicone,* *Coloplast Corporation, Minneapolis, MN*	Safe	3	
Ring *EvaCare, Pessary, Silicone,* *Coloplast Corporation, Minneapolis, MN*	Safe	3	
Ring *Pessary, silicone,* *Bioteque America, Inc., Fremont, CA*	Safe	3	
Schatz/Folding *Pessary,* *CooperSurgical, Inc., Trumbull, CT*	Safe	3	
Shaatz *EvaCare, Pessary, Silicone,* *Coloplast Corporation, Minneapolis, MN*	Safe	3	
Shaatz *Pessary, silicone,* *Bioteque America, Inc., Fremont, CA*	Safe	3	
Silicone Flexible Gelhorn *Pessary,* *CooperSurgical, Inc., Trumbull, CT*	Safe	3	
Tandem-Cube *Pessary,* *CooperSurgical, Inc., Trumbull, CT*	Safe	3	

Sutures

Object	Status	Field Strength (T)	Reference
Suture *Biosyn, Needle removed, glycomer 631,* *United States Surgical, North Haven, CT*	Safe	1.5, 3	83
Suture *Chromic gut, Needle removed, gut,* *United States Surgical, North Haven, CT*	Safe	1.5, 3	83
Suture *Flexon, Needle removed, SS coated with FEP,* *United States Surgical, North Haven, CT*	Safe	1.5, 3	83

Object	Status	Field Strength (T)	Reference
Suture *Flexon, Stainless Braid with Teflon Coating,* *Flexon Multifilament Stainless Steel, Needle removed,* *Covidien, North Haven, CT*	Conditional 6	3	
Suture *Maxon, Needle removed, polyglyconate,* *United States Surgical, North Haven, CT*	Safe	1.5, 3	83
Suture *Monosof, Needle removed, nylon, lead weight,* *with latex bolster,* *United States Surgical, North Haven, CT*	Safe	1.5, 3	83
Suture *Novafil, Needle removed, polybutester,* *United States Surgical, North Haven, CT*	Safe	1.5, 3	83
Suture *Plain gut, Needle removed, gut,* *United States Surgical, North Haven, CT*	Safe	1.5, 3	83
Suture *Polysorb, Needle removed, lactomer 9-1,* *United States Surgical, North Haven, CT*	Safe	1.5, 3	83
Suture *SecureStrand, Needle removed, UHMW polyethylene,* *United States Surgical, North Haven, CT*	Safe	1.5, 3	83
Suture *Sofsilk, Needle removed, silk,* *United States Surgical, North Haven, CT*	Safe	1.5, 3	83
Suture *Steel, Needle removed, 316L SS,* *United States Surgical, North Haven, CT*	Safe	1.5, 3	83
Suture *Steel Suture, Size 7 Metric, 316L SS Suture,* *Needle removed,* *Covidien, North Haven, CT*	Conditional 6	3	
Suture *Surgilon, Needle removed, braided nylon,* *United States Surgical, North Haven, CT*	Safe	1.5, 3	83
Suture *Surgipro, Needle removed, polypropylene,* *United States Surgical, North Haven, CT*	Safe	1.5, 3	83

Vascular Access Ports, Infusion Pumps, and Catheters

A Port Implantable Access System *Titanium,* *Therex Corporation, Walpole, MA*	Safe	1.5	44

Object	Status	Field Strength (T)	Reference
Access Implantable *Titanium, plastic,* *Celsa, Cedex, France*	Safe	1.5	44
AccuRx Constant Flow Implantable Pump *Titanium, silicone,* *Advanced Neuromodulation Systems, Plano, TX*	Safe	1.5	
Acuvance Jelco *FEP Radiopaque, Intravenous (I.V.) catheter,* *Smiths Medical ASD, Inc., Southington, CT*	Conditional 6	3	
Acuvance Plus *PUR Radiopaque, Intravenous (I.V.) catheter,* *Smiths Medical ASD, Inc., Southington, CT*	Conditional 6	3	
Acuvance Plus-W *PUR Radiopaque, Intravenous (I.V.) catheter,* *Smiths Medical ASD, Inc., Southington, CT*	Conditional 6	3	
AdvantIV *PUR Radiopaque, Intravenous (I.V.) catheter,* *Smiths Medical ASD, Inc., Southington, CT*	Conditional 6	3	
Ambulatory Infusion System *CADD - 1, Ambulatory Infusion Pump,* *Smiths Medical, St. Paul, MN*	Unsafe 1	1.5	
Ambulatory Infusion System *CADD - Legacy 1, Ambulatory Infusion Pump,* *Smiths Medical, St. Paul, MN*	Unsafe 1	1.5	
Ambulatory Infusion System *CADD - Legacy PCA, Ambulatory Infusion Pump,* *Smiths Medical, St. Paul, MN*	Unsafe 1	1.5	
Ambulatory Infusion System *CADD - Legacy PLUS, Ambulatory Infusion Pump,* *Smiths Medical, St. Paul, MN*	Unsafe 1	1.5	
Ambulatory Infusion System *CADD - Legacy, Ambulatory Infusion Pump,* *Smiths Medical, St. Paul, MN*	Unsafe 1	1.5	
Ambulatory Infusion System *CADD - Micro, Ambulatory Infusion Pump,* *Smiths Medical, St. Paul, MN*	Unsafe 1	1.5	
Ambulatory Infusion System *CADD - MS 3, Ambulatory Infusion Pump,* *Smiths Medical, St. Paul, MN*	Unsafe 1	1.5	
Ambulatory Infusion System *CADD - PCA, Ambulatory Infusion Pump,* *Smiths Medical, St. Paul, MN*	Unsafe 1	1.5	

Object	Status	Field Strength (T)	Reference
Ambulatory Infusion System *CADD - PLUS, Ambulatory Infusion Pump,* *Smiths Medical, St. Paul, MN*	Unsafe 1	1.5	
Ambulatory Infusion System *CADD - Prizm PCS II, Ambulatory Infusion Pump,* *Smiths Medical, St. Paul, MN*	Unsafe 1	1.5	
Ambulatory Infusion System *CADD - Prizm PCS, Ambulatory Infusion Pump,* *Smiths Medical, St. Paul, MN*	Unsafe 1	1.5	
Ambulatory Infusion System *CADD - Prizm VIP, Ambulatory Infusion Pump,* *Smiths Medical, St. Paul, MN*	Unsafe 1	1.5	
Ambulatory Infusion System *CADD - Solis, Ambulatory Infusion Pump,* *Smiths Medical, St. Paul, MN*	Unsafe 1	1.5	
Ambulatory Infusion System *CADD - TPN, Ambulatory Infusion Pump,* *Smiths Medical, St. Paul, MN*	Unsafe 1	1.5	
ambIT Epidural Pump *external pump, Model 22028,* *Medtronic, Inc. and Sorensen Medical, Inc.*	Unsafe 1	1.5	
Broviac catheter single lumen *silicone, barium sulfate,* *Bard Access Systems, Salt Lake City, UT*	Safe	1.5	
Button *Vascular Access Port, polysulfone polymer, silicone,* *Infusaid Inc., Norwood, MA*	Safe	1.5	45
CathLink LP *Titanium,* *Bard Access Systems, Salt Lake City, UT*	Safe	1.5	44
CathLink SP *Titanium,* *Bard Access Systems, Salt Lake City, UT*	Safe	1.5	45
Cathlon *FEP, Intravenous (I.V.) catheter,* *Smiths Medical ASD, Inc., Southington, CT*	Conditional 6	3	
Celsite Port and Catheter *Titanium,* *B. Braun Medical, Bethlehem, PA*	Safe	1.5	45
Chemosite Port I, Low Profile, Single Lumen Vascular Access Port *Covidien, North Haven, CT*	Conditional 6	3	

Object	Status	Field Strength (T)	Reference
CODMAN 3000 Infusion Pump *CODMAN 3000 Implantable Infusion Pump,* *Codman, www.codmanpumps.com*	Conditional 5	3	
Cozmo Pump *Insulin Pump,* *Deltec Diabetes Division, St. Paul, MN*	Safe	1.5	44
Deltec 3000 *Large Volume Infusion Pump,* *Smiths Medical, St. Paul, MN*	Unsafe 1	1.5	
Deltec Micro 3100 *Large Volume Infusion Pump,* *Smiths Medical, St. Paul, MN*	Unsafe 1	1.5	
Dome Port *Vascular Access Port, Titanium,* *Davol Inc., Subsidiary of C.R. Bard, Inc.,* *Salt Lake City, UT*	Safe	1.5	
Dual MacroPort *polysulfone polymer, silicone,* *Infusaid Inc., Norwood, MA*	Safe	1.5	44
Dual MicroPort *Vascular Access Port, polysulfone polymer, silicone,* *Infusaid Inc., Norwood, MA*	Safe	1.5	44
Dual-Lumen PORT-A-CATH *Portal and Wing-Lock Connector, Vascular Access Port,* *Smiths Medical MD, Inc., St. Paul, MN*	Safe	1.5	44
DuraCath Intraspinal Catheter *316L SS, silicone,* *Advanced Neuromodulation Systems, Plano, TX*	Conditional 6	3	
GRIPPER PLUS Needle *SS needle, 19 gauge, 1 - inch,* *Smiths Medical MD, Inc., St. Paul, MN*	Conditional 5	3	
GRIPPER PLUS Safety Needle *Deltec, Inc., Minneapolis, MN*	Conditional 5	3	
GRIPPER PLUS Safety Needle *Smiths Medical MD, Inc., St. Paul, MN*	Safe	3	
Groshong Catheter	Conditional 1	1.5	
Groshong Catheter, dual lumen, 9.5 Fr. *silicone, barium sulfate, tungsten,* *Bard Access Systems, Salt Lake City, UT*	Safe	1.5	45
Groshong Catheter, single lumen, 8 Fr. *silicone, barium sulfate, tungsten,* *Bard Access Systems, Salt Lake City, UT*	Safe	1.5	45

Object	Status	Field Strength (T)	Reference
HeRO Vascular Access Device *HeRO Graft Component,* *HeRO Outflow Catheter Component,* *GRAFTcath, Inc., Eden Prairie, MN*	Conditional 6	3	
Hickman Catheter, dual lumen, 10.0 Fr. *silicone, barium sulfate,* *Bard Access Systems, Salt Lake City, UT*	Safe	1.5	45
Hickman Catheter, single lumen, 3.0 Fr. *Bard Access Systems, Salt Lake City, UT*	Safe	1.5	45
Hickman Port, Pediatric *Vascular Access Port, Titanium,* *Davol, Inc., Subsidiary of C.R. Bard, Inc.,* *Salt Lake City, UT*	Safe	1.5	44
Hickman Port *Vascular Access Port, 316L SS,* *Davol Inc., Subsidiary of C.R. Bard, Inc.,* *Salt Lake City, UT*	Conditional 1	1.5	44
Hickman subcutaneous port *Vascular Access Port, SS, Titanium, plastic,* *Davol, Inc., Subsidiary of C.R. Bard, Inc., Salt Lake City, UT*	Safe	1.5	45
Hickman subcutaneous port *Vascular Access Port, venous catheter, Titanium,* *Davol Inc., Subsidiary of C.R. Bard, Inc.,* *Salt Lake City, UT*	Safe	1.5	44
HMP-Port *Vascular Access Port, plastic,* *Horizon Medical Products, Atlanta, GA*	Safe	1.5	44
Implantable Infusion Pump *Model 3000-16, Titanium,* *Codman, Raynham, MA*	Safe	1.5, 3	83
Implantable Infusion Pump *Model 3000-30, Titanium,* *Codman, Raynham, MA*	Safe	1.5, 3	83
Implantable Infusion Pump *Model 3000-50, Titanium,* *Codman, Raynham, MA*	Safe	1.5, 3	83
Implantofix II *Vascular Access Port, polysulfone,* *Burron Medical Inc., Bethlehem, PA*	Safe	1.5	44
Infusaid, Model 400 *Vascular Access Port, Titanium,* *Infusaid Inc., Norwood, MA*	Safe	1.5	44
Infusaid, Model 600 *Vascular Access Port, Titanium,* *Infusaid Inc., Norwood, MA*	Safe	1.5	44

Object	Status	Field Strength (T)	Reference
Infuse-A-Kit *plastic,* *Infusaid, Norwood, MA*	Safe	1.5	44
Jelco 2 *FEP Radiopaque, Intravenous (I.V.) catheter,* *Smiths Medical ASD, Inc., Southington, CT*	Conditional 6	3	
Jelco *FEP, Intravenous (I.V.) catheter,* *Smiths Medical ASD, Inc., Southington, CT*	Conditional 6	3	
Jelco-W *FEP Radiopaque, Intravenous (I.V.) catheter,* *Smiths Medical ASD, Inc., Southington, CT*	Conditional 6	3	
Jet Port Plus *Vascular Access Port,* *Clinical Plastic Products SA, La Chaux-de-Fonds,* *Switzerland*	Conditional 6	3	
LifePort Vascular Access System *attachable catheter and bayonet lock ring, plastic,* *Strato Medical Group, Beverly, MA*	Safe	1.5	44
LifePort Vascular Access System *attachable catheter, plastic,* *Strato Medical Group, Beverly, MA*	Safe	1.5	44
LifePort Vortex LVTX 5213 *Dual Titanium Vascular Access Port,* *Angiodynamics, Inc., Manchester, GA*	Conditional 6	3	
Lifeport, Model 1013 *Vascular Access Port, Titanium,* *Strato Medical Corp., Beverly, MA*	Safe	1.5	44
LifePort, Model 6013 *Vascular Access Port, Delrin,* *Strato Medical Corporation, Beverly, MA*	Safe	1.5	44
Low Profile MRI Port *Vascular Access Port, Delrin,* *Davol, Inc., Subsidiary of C.R. Bard, Inc.,* *Salt Lake City, UT*	Safe	1.5	44
Low Profile MRI Port *Vascular Access Port, Titanium,* *Davol, Inc. Subsidiary of C.R. Bard, Inc.,* *Salt Lake City, UT*	Safe	1.5	45
Macroport *Vascular Access Port, polysulfone, Titanium,* *Infusaid Inc., Norwood, MA*	Safe	1.5	
Mediport *Vascular Access Port,* *Cormed*	Safe	1.5	

Object	Status	Field Strength (T)	Reference
MedStream Programmable Infusion Pump *Codman and Shurtleff, Inc.,* *a Johnson & Johnson Company, Raynham, MA*	Conditional 5	3	112
Medtronic MiniMed 2007 *Implantable Insulin Pump System,* *Medtronic MiniMed, Northridge, CA*	Unsafe 1	1.5	
MicroPort *Vascular Access Port, polysulfone, polymersilicone,* *Infusaid Inc., Norwood, MA*	Safe	1.5	44
MiniMed Paradigm REAL-Time Insulin Pump *Continuous Glucose Monitoring System,* *522 and 722 Insulin Pumps,* *Medtronic Minimed, Northridge, CA*	Unsafe 1	1.5	
MRI Hard Base Implanted Port *Vascular Access Port, plastic,* *Davol, Inc., Salt Lake City, UT*	Safe	1.5	44
MRI Port *Vascular Access Port, Delrin, silicone,* *Davol, Inc., Subsidiary of C.R. Bard, Inc.,* *Salt Lake City, UT*	Safe	1.5	44
M.R.I. Vital Port Systems *Standard Size, Vascular Access Port,* *Cook Medical, Inc.,* *http://www.cookmedical.com/di/productMri.do*	Conditional 5	3	
Non-Coring (Huber) Needle *Medi-tech,* *Boston Scientific, Watertown, MA*	Safe	1.5, 3	83
Norport-AC *Vascular Access Port, Titanium,* *Norfolk Medical, Skokie, IL*	Safe	1.5	44
Norport-DL *Vascular Access Port, 316L SS,* *Norfolk Medical, Skokie, IL*	Safe	1.5	44
Norport-LS *Vascular Access Port, 316L SS,* *Norfolk Medical, Skokie, IL*	Safe	1.5	44
Norport-LS *Vascular Access Port, polysulfone,* *Norfolk Medical, Skokie, IL*	Safe	1.5	44
Norport-LS *Vascular Access Port, Titanium,* *Norfolk Medical, Skokie, IL*	Safe	1.5	44
Norport-PT *Vascular Access Port, Titanium,* *Norfolk Medical, Skokie, IL*	Safe	1.5	44

Object	Status	Field Strength (T)	Reference
Norport-SP *Vascular Access Port, polysulfone, silicone rubber, Dacron, Norfolk Medical, Skokie, IL*	Safe	1.5	44
OmegaPort Access System *Vascular Access Port, Titanium, 316L SS, Norfolk Medical, Skokie, IL*	Safe	1.5	44
OmegaPort-SR Access System *Vascular Access Port, Titanium, 316L SS, Norfolk Medical, Skokie, IL*	Safe	1.5	44
Open-ended Catheter, single lumen, 6 Fr. (ChronoFlex) *Davol, Inc., Subsidiary of C.R. Bard, Inc., Salt Lake City, UT*	Safe	1.5	45
Open-ended Catheter, single lumen, 8 Fr. (ChronoFlex) *Davol, Inc., Subsidiary of C.R. Bard, Inc., Salt Lake City, UT*	Safe	1.5	45
OptiPort Catheter, single lumen *silicone, Simms-Deltec, St. Paul, MN*	Safe	1.5	45
Optiva *PUR Radiopaque, Intravenous (I.V.) catheter, Smiths Medical ASD, Inc., Southington, CT*	Conditional 6	3	
Optiva-W *PUR Radiopaque, Intravenous (I.V.) catheter, Smiths Medical ASD, Inc., Southington, CT*	Conditional 6	3	
Optiva 2 *PUR Radiopaque, Intravenous (I.V.) catheter, Smiths Medical ASD, Inc., Southington, CT*	Conditional 6	3	
P.A.S. PORT Elite with *PolyFlow Polyurethane Catheter, Vascular Access Systems Division, Deltec, Inc., St. Paul, MN*	Safe	1.5, 3	83
Percutaneous Vascular Access System (PVAS) *DermaPort, Santa Clarita, CA*	Conditional 6	3	
PeriPort *Vascular Access Port, polysulfone, Titanium, Infusaid, Inc., Norwood, MA*	Safe	1.5	44
Phantom *Vascular Access Port, Norfolk Medical, Skokie, IL*	Safe	1.5	44
Plastic Port *Vascular Access Port, polysulfone, Titanium, Cardial, Saint-Etienne, France*	Safe	1.5	44

Object	Status	Field Strength (T)	Reference
PORT-A-CATH GRIPPER Needle *Vascular Access Systems Division,* *Deltec, Inc., St. Paul, MN*	Safe	1.5, 3	83
PORT-A-CATH I *Standard Portal with Ultra-Lock Connector,* *Vascular Access Port,* *Smiths Medical MD, Inc., St. Paul, MN*	Conditional 6	3	
PORT-A-CATH II Dual-Lumen *Low Profile with PolyFlow, Polyurethane Catheter,* *Deltec, Inc., St. Paul, MN*	Safe	1.5, 3	83
PORT-A-CATH II Dual-Lumen *with Silicone Catheter,* *Vascular Access Systems Division,* *Deltec, Inc., St. Paul, MN*	Safe	1.5, 3	83
PORT-A-CATH II Single-Lumen *Low Profile with PolyFlow, Polyurethane Catheter,* *Deltec, Inc., St. Paul, MN*	Safe	1.5, 3	83
PORT-A-CATH II Single-Lumen *with PolyFlow Polyurethane Catheter,* *Deltec, Inc., St. Paul, MN*	Safe	1.5, 3	83
PORT-A-CATH II *Low Profile Intraspinal Portal, Vascular Access Port,* *Smiths Medical MD, Inc., St. Paul, MN*	Conditional 6	3	
PORT-A-CATH Needle *Vascular Access Systems Division,* *Deltec, Inc., St. Paul, MN*	Conditional 5	1.5, 3	83
PORT-A-CATH Titanium Dual Lumen Portal *Titanium,* *Pharmacia Deltec, St. Paul, MN*	Safe	1.5	44
PORT-A-CATH Titanium Peritoneal Portal *Titanium,* *Pharmacia Deltec, St. Paul, MN*	Safe	1.5	44
PORT-A-CATH Titanium *Venous Low Profile Portal, Titanium,* *Pharmacia Deltec, St. Paul, MN*	Safe	1.5	44
PORT-A-CATH Titanium *Venous Portal, Titanium,* *Pharmacia Deltec, St. Paul, MN*	Safe	1.5	44
PORT-A-CATH, P.S.A. Port Portal *Titanium,* *Pharmacia Deltec, St. Paul, MN*	Safe	1.5	44
PORT-A-CATH *Epidural Portal and Cath-Shield Connector,* *Vascular Access Port,* *Smiths Medical MD, Inc., St. Paul, MN*	Conditional 6	3	

Object	Status	Field Strength (T)	Reference
PORT-A-CATH *Metal Hub 90° Bent Needle,* *Smiths Medical MD, Inc., St. Paul, MN*	Safe	3	
PORT-A-CATH *Metal Hub Straight Needle,* *Smiths Medical MD, Inc., St. Paul, MN*	Safe	3	
PORT-A-CATH *Peritoneal Portal with Ultra-Lock Connector,* *Vascular Access Port,* *Smiths Medical MD, Inc., St. Paul, MN*	Conditional 6	3	
PORT-A-CATH *Plastic Hub 90° Bent Needle,* *Smiths Medical MD, Inc., St. Paul, MN*	Conditional 5	3	
PORT-A-CATH *Plastic Hub Straight Needle,* *Smiths Medical MD, Inc., St. Paul, MN*	Conditional 5	3	
PowerPort M.R.I. *Vascular Access Port, Titanium,* *Bard Access Systems, Salt Lake City, UT*	Conditional 5	3	
PowerPort *Vascular Access Port, Titanium,* *Bard Access Systems, Salt Lake City, UT*	Conditional 5	3	
PowerPort isp Implanted Port *Vascular Access Port,* *Bard Access Systems, www.bardaccess.com*	Conditional 5	3	
PowerPort isp M.R.I. Implanted Port *Vascular Access Port,* *Bard Access Systems, www.bardaccess.com*	Conditional 5	3	
PowerPort M.R.I. Implanted Port *Vascular Access Port,* *Bard Access Systems, www.bardaccess.com*	Conditional 5	3	
ProFuse Dignity Infusion Port *Titanium, silicone port, polyurethane catheter,* *Medcomp, Harleysville, PA*	Conditional 6	3	
ProtectIV *FEP Radiopaque, Intravenous (I.V.) catheter,* *Smiths Medical ASD, Inc., Southington, CT*	Conditional 6	3	
ProtectIV Acuvance 2 *PUR Radiopaque, Intravenous (I.V.) catheter,* *Smiths Medical ASD, Inc., Southington, CT*	Conditional 6	3	
ProtectIV Plus *PUR Radiopaque, Intravenous (I.V.) catheter,* *Smiths Medical ASD, Inc., Southington, CT*	Conditional 6	3	

Object	Status	Field Strength (T)	Reference
ProtectIV Plus-W *PUR Radiopaque, Intravenous (I.V.) catheter,* *Smiths Medical ASD, Inc., Southington, CT*	Conditional 6	3	
ProtectIV-W *FEP Radiopaque, Intravenous (I.V.) catheter,* *Smiths Medical ASD, Inc., Southington, CT*	Conditional 6	3	
Purple JPP-HP *Vascular Access Port,* *Clinical Plastic Products SA, La Chaux-de-Fonds,* *Switzerland*	Conditional 6	3	
Purple TJL-HP *Vascular Access Port,* *Clinical Plastic Products SA, La Chaux-de-Fonds,* *Switzerland*	Conditional 6	3	
Q-Port *Vascular Access Port, 316L SS,* *Quinton Instrument Co., Seattle, WA*	Conditional 1	1.5	44
Rhapsody Vascular Access System *Vascular Access Port, 316 Stainless, Silicone, Titanium,* *GrantAdler Corporation, Naperville, IL*	Conditional 6	3	
R-Port Premier *Vascular Access Port, silicone, plastic, SS, Medi-tech,* *Boston Scientific, www.bostonscientific.com*	Safe	1.5, 3	83
S.E.A. *Vascular Access Port, Titanium,* *Harbor Medical Devices, Inc., Boston, MA*	Safe	1.5	44
Snap-Lock *Vascular Access Port, Titanium, polysulfone polymer,* *silicone,* *Infusaid Inc., Norwood, MA*	Safe	1.5	44
Solo MicroPump *Insulin Pump,* *Medingo US, Inc., www.Medingo.com*	Unsafe 1	1.5	
Standard M.R.I. Single Chamber System *Polysulfone Port, Titanium Connector, Silicone Catheter,* *COOK Vascular Incorporated, Vandergrift, PA*	Conditional 6	3	
Standard Titanium Dual Chamber System *Titanium Port, Titanium Connector, Silicone Catheter,* *COOK Vascular Incorporated, Vandergrift, PA*	Conditional 6	3	
Synchromed *Model 8500-1, Titanium, thermoplastic, silicone,* *Medtronic, Inc., www.Medtronic.com*	Conditional 5	1.5, 3	44
Tesio Catheter *SS, polyurethane,* *Medcomp, Harleysville, PA*	Conditional 6	3	

Object	Status	Field Strength (T)	Reference
Tita Jet Light Arterial II	Conditional 6	3	
Vascular Access Port,			
Clinical Plastic Products SA, La Chaux-de-Fonds,			
Switzerland			
Tita Jet Light	Conditional 6	3	
Vascular Access Port,			
Clinical Plastic Products SA, La Chaux-de-Fonds,			
Switzerland			
TitanPort	Safe	1.5	
Titanium, Vascular Access Port,			
Norfolk Medical, Skokie, IL			
T-Port	Conditional 6	3	
Vascular Access Port,			
Clinical Plastic Products SA, La Chaux-de-Fonds,			
Switzerland			
Triple Lumen	Safe	1.5	
Arrow International, Inc., Reading, PA			
Vascular Access Catheter With Repair Kit	Safe	1.5	
Vasport	Safe	1.5	44
Vascular Access Port, Titanium, fluoropolymer,			
Gish Biomedical, Inc., Santa Ana, CA			
Vaxcel Implantable Access System	Safe	3	
Plastic Low Profile Port,			
Boston Scientific, www.bostonscientific.com			
Vaxcel Implantable Vascular Access System	Safe	3	
with PASV Valve Technology,			
Titanium Mini Port With PASV valve,			
Boston Scientific, Natick, MA			
Vaxcel Implantable Vascular Access System	Safe	3	
with PASV Valve Technology,			
Titanium Standard Port With PASV valve,			
Boston Scientific, Natick, MA			
Vaxess, Titanium Mini-Port	Safe	1.5, 3	83
with silicone catheter, Vascular Access Port,			
Titanium, silicone, Medi-tech,			
Boston Scientific, Watertown, MA			
Vaxess, Titanium	Safe	1.5, 3	83
Vascular Access Port, Titanium, polyurethane, Medi-tech,			
Boston Scientific, Watertown, MA			
Vaxess	Safe	1.5, 3	83
Vascular Access Port, 19 gauge x 1/2", 90 degree hub,			
plastic, polyurethane,			
Medi-tech, Watertown, MA			

Object	Status	Field Strength (T)	Reference
Vaxess *Vascular Access Port, plastic, polyurethane, Medi-tech, Boston Scientific, Watertown, MA*	Safe	1.5, 3	83
Vital-Port, Dual *Vascular Access Port, polysulfone, Titanium, Cook Corp., Leechburg, PA*	Safe	1.5	45
Vital-Port System *Dual Chamber, Titanium Petite, Vascular Access Port, Cook Medical, Inc., http://www.cookmedical.com/di/productMri.do*	Conditional 5	3	
Vital-Port System *Dual Chamber, Titanium Standard, Vascular Access Port, Cook Medical, Inc., http://www.cookmedical.com/di/productMri.do*	Conditional 5	3	
Vital-Port System *MRI Petite, Vascular Access Port, Cook Medical, Inc., http://www.cookmedical.com/di/productMri.do*	Conditional 5	3	
Vital-Port System *MRI Standard, Vascular Access Port, Cook Medical, Inc., http://www.cookmedical.com/di/productMri.do*	Conditional 5	3	
Vital-Port System *Titanium Mini, Vascular Access Port, Cook Medical, Inc., http://www.cookmedical.com/di/productMri.do*	Conditional 5	3	
Vital-Port System *Titanium Petite, Vascular Access Port, Cook Medical, Inc., http://www.cookmedical.com/di/productMri.do*	Conditional 5	3	
Vital-Port System *Titanium Petite Standard, Vascular Access Port, Cook Medical, Inc., http://www.cookmedical.com/di/productMri.do*	Conditional 5	3	
Vital-Port System *Titanium for Peripheral Placement Mini, Vascular Access Port, Cook Medical, Inc., http://www.cookmedical.com/di/productMri.do*	Conditional 5	3	
Vital-Port Vascular Access Port *polysulfone, Titanium, Cook Corp., Leechburg, PA*	Safe	1.5	45

THE LIST

REFERENCES

1. New PFJ, Rosen BR, Brady TJ, et al. Potential hazards and artifacts of ferromagnetic and nonferromagnetic surgical and dental materials and devices in nuclear magnetic resonance imaging. Radiology 1983;147:139-148.

2. Becker RL, Norfray JF, Teitelbaum GP, et al. MR imaging in patients with intracranial aneurysm clips. Am J Roentgenol 1988;9:885-889.

3. Shellock FG, Crues JV. High-field strength MR imaging and metallic biomedical implants: an ex vivo evaluation of deflection forces. Am J Roentgenol 1988;151:389-392.

4. Brown MA, Carden JA, Coleman RE, et al. Magnetic field effects on surgical ligation clips. Magn Reson Imaging 1987;5:443-453.

5. Dujovny M, Kossovsky N, Kossowsky R, et al. Aneurysm clip motion during magnetic resonance imaging: in vivo experimental study with metallurgical factor analysis. Neurosurgery 1985;17:543-548.

6. Barrafato D, Henkelman RM. Magnetic resonance imaging and surgical clips. Can J Surg 1984;27:509-512.

7. Moscatel M, Shellock FG, Morisoli S. Biopsy needles and devices: assessment of ferromagnetism and artifacts during exposure to a 1.5 Tesla MR system. J Magn Reson Imaging 1995;5:369-372.

8. Shellock FG, Shellock VJ. Additional information pertaining to the MR-compatibility of biopsy needles and devices. J Magn Reson Imaging 1996;6:441.

9. Hathout G, Lufkin RB, Jabour B, et al. MR-guided aspiration cytology in the head and neck at high field strength. J Magn Reson Imaging 1992;2:93-94.

10. Fagan LL, Shellock FG, Brenner RJ, Rothman B. Ex vivo evaluation of ferromagnetism, heating, and artifacts of breast tissue expanders exposed to a 1.5 T MR system. J Magn Reson Imaging 1995;5:614-616.

11. Teitelbaum GP, Lin MCW, Watanabe AT, et al. Ferromagnetism and MR imaging: safety of carotid vascular clamps. Am J Neuroradiol 1990;11:267-272.

12. Gegauff A, Laurell KA, Thavendrarajah A, et al. A potential MRI hazard: forces on dental magnet keepers. J Oral Rehabil 1990;17:403-410.

13. Shellock FG. Ex vivo assessment of deflection forces and artifacts associated with high-field strength MRI of "mini-magnet" dental prostheses. Magn Reson Imaging 1989;7 (Suppl 1):38.

14. Shellock FG, Slimp G. Halo vest for cervical spine fixation during MR imaging. Am J Roentgenol 1990;154:631-632.

15. Clayman DA, Murakami ME, Vines FS. Compatibility of cervical spine braces with MR imaging. A study of nine nonferrous devices. Am J Neuroradiol 1990;11:385-390.

16. Shellock FG. MR imaging and cervical fixation devices: assessment of ferromagnetism, heating, and artifacts. Magn Reson Imaging 1996;14:1093-1098.

17. Soulen RL, Budinger TF, Higgins CB. Magnetic resonance imaging of prosthetic heart valves. Radiology 1985;154:705-707.

18. Shellock FG, Morisoli SM. Ex vivo evaluation of ferromagnetism, heating, and artifacts for heart valve prostheses exposed to a 1.5 Tesla MR system. J Magn Reson Imaging 1994;4:756-758.

19. Hassler M, Le Bas JF, Wolf JE, et al. Effects of magnetic fields used in MRI on 15 prosthetic heart valves. J Radiol 1986;67:661-666.

20. Frank H, Buxbaum P, Huber L, et al. In vitro behavior of mechanical heart valves in 1.5 T superconducting magnet. Eur J Radiol 1992;2:555-558.

21. Teitelbaum GP, Bradley WG, Klein BD. MR imaging artifacts, ferromagnetism, and magnetic torque of intravascular filters, stents, and coils. Radiology 1988;166:657-664.

22. Marshall MW, Teitelbaum GP, Kim HS, et al. Ferromagnetism and magnetic resonance artifacts of platinum embolization microcoils. Cardiovasc Intervent Radiol 1991;14:163-166.

23. Watanabe AT, Teitelbaum GP, Gomes AS, et al. MR imaging of the bird's nest filter. Radiology 1990;177:578-579.

24. Leibman CE, Messersmith RN, Levin DN, et al. MR imaging of inferior vena caval filter: safety and artifacts. Am J Roentgenol 1988;150:1174-1176.

25. Shellock FG, Detrick MS, Brant-Zawadski M. MR-compatibility of the Guglielmi detachable coils. Radiology 1997;203:568-570.

26. Kiproff PM, Deeb DL, Contractor FM, Khoury MB. Magnetic resonance characteristics of the LGM vena cava filter: technical note. Cardiovasc Intervent Radiol 1991;14:254-255.

27. Teitelbaum GP, Raney M, Carvlin MJ, et al. Evaluation of ferromagnetism and magnetic resonance imaging artifacts of the Strecker tantalum vascular stent. Cardiovasc Intervent Radiol 1989;12:125-127.

28. Girard MJ, Hahn P, Saini S, Dawson SL, Goldberg MA, Mueller PR. Wallstent metallic biliary endoprosthesis: MR imaging characteristics. Radiology 1992;184:874-876.

29. Shellock FG, Myers SM, Schatz CJ. Ex vivo evaluation of ferromagnetism determined for metallic scleral "buckles" exposed to a 1.5 T MR scanner. Radiology 1992;185:288-289.

30. de Keizer RJ, Te Strake L. Intraocular lens implants (pseudophakoi) and steelwire sutures: a contraindication for MRI? Doc Ophthalmol 1984;61:281-284.

31. Albert DW, Olson KR, Parel JM, et al. Magnetic resonance imaging and retinal tacks. Arch Ophthalmol 1990;108:320-321.

32. Joondeph BC, Peyman GA, Mafee MF, et al. Magnetic resonance imaging and retinal tacks [Letter]. Arch Ophthalmol 1987;105:1479-1480.

33. Lyons CJ, Betz RR, Mesgarzadeh M, et al. The effect of magnetic resonance imaging on metal spine implants. Spine 1989;14:670-672.

34. Shellock FG, Mink JH, Curtin S, et al. MRI and orthopedic implants used for anterior cruciate ligament reconstruction: assessment of ferromagnetism and artifacts. J Magn Reson Imaging 1992;2:225-228.

35. Shellock FG, Schatz CJ. High-field strength MR imaging and metallic otologic implants. Am J Neuroradiol 1991;12:279-281.

36. Nogueira M, Shellock FG. Otologic bioimplants: ex vivo assessment of ferromagnetism and artifacts at 1.5 Tesla. Am J Roentgenol 1995;163:1472-1473.

37. Mattucci KF, Setzen M, Hyman R, et al. The effect of nuclear magnetic resonance imaging on metallic middle ear prostheses. Otolaryngol Head Neck Surg 1986;94:441-443.

38. Applebaum EL, Valvassori GE. Further studies on the effects of magnetic resonance fields on middle ear implants. Ann Otol Rhinol Laryngol 1990;99:801-804.

39. White DW. Interaction between magnetic fields and metallic ossicular prostheses. Am J Otol 1987;8:290-292.

40. Leon JA, Gabriele OF. Middle ear prosthesis: significance in magnetic resonance imaging. Magn Reson Imaging 1987;5:405-406.

41. Shellock FG, Morisoli SM. Ex vivo evaluation of ferromagnetism and artifacts for cardiac occluders exposed to a 1.5 Tesla MR system. J Magn Reson Imaging 1994;4:213-215.

42. Teitelbaum GP, Yee CA, Van Horn DD, et al. Metallic ballistic fragments: MR imaging safety and artifacts. Radiology 1990;175:855-859.

43. Shellock FG, Crues JV, Sacks SA. High-field magnetic resonance imaging of penile prostheses: in vitro evaluation of deflection forces and imaging artifacts [Abstract]. In: Book of Abstracts, Society of Magnetic Resonance in Medicine. Berkeley, CA, Society of Magnetic Resonance in Medicine 1987;3:915.

44. Shellock FG, Nogueira M, Morisoli S. MR imaging and vascular access ports: ex vivo evaluation of ferromagnetism, heating, and artifacts at 1.5 T. J Magn Reson Imaging 1995;4:481-484.

45. Shellock FG, Shellock VJ. Vascular access ports and catheters tested for ferromagnetism, heating, and artifacts associated with MR imaging. Magn Reson Imaging 1996;14:443-447.

46. Kanal E, Shaibani A. Firearm safety in the MR imaging environment. Radiology 1994;193:875-876.

47. Hess T, Stepanow B, Knopp MV. Safety of intrauterine contraceptive devices during MR imaging. Eur Radiol 1996;6:66-68.

48. Shellock FG, Shellock VJ. Evaluation of MR compatibility of 38 bioimplants and devices. Radiology 1995;197:174.

49. Shellock FG, Shellock VJ. Ceramic surgical instruments: ex vivo evaluation of compatibility with MR imaging. J Magn Reson Imaging 1996;6:954-956.

50. Shellock FG, Shellock VJ. Evaluation of cranial flap fixation clamps for compatibility with MR imaging. Radiology 1998;822-825.

51. Lufkin R, Jordan S, Lylcyk M. MR imaging with topographic EEG electrodes in place. Am J Neuroradiol 1988;9:953-954.

52. Marra S, Leonetti JP, Konior RJ, Raslan W. Effect of magnetic resonance imaging on implantable eyelid weights. Ann Otol Rhinol Laryngol 1995;104:448-452.

53. Zhang J, Wilson CL, Levesque MF, Behnke EJ, Lufkin RB. Temperature changes in nickel-chromium intracranial depth electrodes during MR scanning. Am J Neuroradiol 1993;14:497-500.

54. Mark AS, Hricak H. Intrauterine contraceptive devices: MR imaging. Radiology 1987;162:311-314.

55. Go KG, Kamman RL, Mooyaart EL. Interaction of metallic neurosurgical implants with magnetic resonance imaging at 1.5 Tesla as a cause of image distortion and of hazardous movement of the implant. Clin Neurosurg 1989;91:109-115.

56. Fransen P, Dooms G, Thauvoy. Safety of the adjustable pressure ventricular valve in magnetic resonance imaging: problems and solutions. Neuroradiology 1992;34:508-509.

57. ECRI, Health devices alert. A new MRI complication? May 27, 1988.

58. To SYC, Lufkin RB, Chiu L. MR-compatible winged infusion set. Comput Med Imaging Graph 1989;13:469-472.

59. Shellock FG. MR-compatibility of an endoscope designed for use in interventional MRI procedures. Am J Roentgenol 1998;71:1297-1300.

60. Shellock FG, Shellock VJ. Cardiovascular catheters and accessories: Ex vivo testing of ferromagnetism, heating, and artifacts associated with MRI. J Magn Reson Imaging 1998;8:1338-1342.

61. Shellock FG, Shellock VJ. Metallic marking clips used after stereotactic breast biopsy: ex vivo testing of ferromagnetism, heating, and artifacts associated with MRI. Am J Roentgenol 1999;172:1417-1419.

62. Shellock FG. MRI safety of instruments designed for interventional MRI: assessment of ferromagnetism, heating, and artifacts. Workshop on New Insights into Safety and Compatibility Issues Affecting In Vivo MR, Syllabus 1998; pp. 39.

63. Shellock FG, Hatfield M, Simon BJ, Block S, Wamboldt J, Starewicz PM, Punchard WFB. Implantable spinal fusion stimulator: assessment of MRI safety. J Magn Reson Imaging 2000;12:214-223.

64. Shellock FG, Shellock VJ. Stents: Evaluation of MRI safety. Am J Roentgenol 1999;173:543-546.

65. Teissl C, Kremser C, Hochmair ES, Hochmair-Desoyer IJ. Cochlear implants: in vitro investigation of electromagnetic interference at MR imaging-compatibility and safety aspects. Radiology 1998;208:700-708.

66. Teissl C, Kremser C, Hochmair ES, Hochmair-Desoyer IJ. Magnetic resonance imaging and cochlear implants: compatibility and safety aspects. J Magn Reson Imaging 1999;9:26-38.

67. Ortler M, Kostron H, Felber S. Transcutaneous pressure-adjustable valves and magnetic resonance imaging: an ex vivo examination of the Codman-Medos programmable valve and the Sophy adjustable pressure valve. Neurosurgery 1997;40:1050-1057.

68. Shellock FG, Shellock VJ. MR-compatibility evaluation of the Spetzler titanium aneurysm clip. Radiology 1998;206:838-841.

69. Jost C, Kuman V. Are current cardiovascular stents MRI safe? J Invasive Cardiol 1998;10:477-479.

70. Shellock FG, Shellock VJ. MRI Safety of cardiovascular implants: evaluation of ferromagnetism, heating, and artifacts. Radiology 2000;214:P19H.

71. Weishaupt D, Quick HH, Nanz D, Schmidt M, Cassina PC, Debatin JF. Ligating clips for three-dimensional MR angiography at 1.5 T: In vitro evaluation. Radiology 2000;214:902-907.

72. Hug J, Nagel E, Bornstedt A, Schackenburg B, Oswald H, Fleck E. Coronary arterial stents: safety and artifacts during MR imaging. Radiology 2000;216:781-787.

73. Taal BG, Muller SH, Boot H, Koop W. Potential risks and artifacts of magnetic resonance imaging of self-expandable esophageal stents. Gastrointestinal Endoscopy 1997;46:424-429.

74. Shellock FG. Metallic surgical instruments for interventional MRI procedures: evaluation of MR safety. J Magn Reson Imaging 2001;13:152-157.

75. Edwards, M-B, Taylor KM, Shellock FG. Prosthetic heart valves: evaluation of magnetic field interactions, heating, and artifacts at 1.5 Tesla. J Magn Reson Imaging 2000;12:363-369.

76. Shellock FG. New metallic implant used for permanent female contraception: evaluation of MR safety. Am J Roentgenol 2002;178:1513-1516.

77. Shellock FG. Prosthetic heart valves and annuloplasty rings: assessment of magnetic field interactions, heating, and artifacts at 1.5-Tesla. Journal of Cardiovascular Magnetic Resonance. 2001;3:159-169.

78. Shellock FG. Metallic neurosurgical implants: evaluation of magnetic field interactions, heating, and artifacts at 1.5 Tesla. J Magn Reson Imaging 2001;14:295-299.

79. Rezai AR, Finelli D, Ruggieri P, Tkach J, Nyenhuis JA, Shellock FG. Neurostimulators: Potential for excessive heating of deep brain stimulation electrodes during MR imaging. J Magn Reson Imaging 2001;14:488-489.

80. Finelli DA, Rezai AR, Ruggieri P, Tkach J, Nyenhuis J, Hridlicka G, Sharan A, Stypulkowski PH, Shellock FG. MR-related heating of deep brain stimulation electrodes: an *in vitro* study of clinical imaging sequences. Am J Neuroradiol 2002;23:1795-1802.

81. Greatbatch W, Miller V, Shellock FG. Magnetic resonance safety testing of a newly-developed, fiber-optic cardiac pacing lead. J Magn Reson 2002;16:97-103.

82. Shellock FG, Tkach JA, Ruggieri PM, Masaryk T, Rasmussen P. Aneurysm clips: evaluation of magnetic field interactions and translational attraction using "long-bore" and "short-bore" 3.0-Tesla MR systems. Am J Neuroradiol 2003;24:463-471.

83. Shellock FG. Biomedical implants and devices: assessment of magnetic field interactions with a 3.0-Tesla MR system. J Magn Reson Imaging 2002;16:721-732.

84. Medtronic Heart Valves, Medtronic, Inc., Minneapolis, MN, Permission to publish 3-Tesla MR testing information for Medtronic Heart Valves provided by Kathryn M. Bayer, Senior Technical Consultant, Medtronic Heart Valves, Technical Service, 1-800-328-2518, extension -42861 or 763-514-2861.

85. Shellock FG, Tkach JA, Ruggieri PM, Masaryk TJ. Cardiac pacemakers, ICDs, and loop recorder: Evaluation of translational attraction using conventional ("long-bore") and "short-bore" 1.5- and 3.0-Tesla MR systems. Journal of Cardiovascular Magnetic Resonance 2003;5:387-397.

86. Product Information, Style 133 Family of Breast Tissue Expanders with Magna-Site Injection Sites, McGhan Medical/INAMED Aesthetics, Santa Barbara, CA.

87. Shellock FG, Gounis M, Wakhloo A, Detachable coil for cerebral aneurysms: *In vitro* evaluation of magnet field interactions, heating, and artifacts at 3-Tesla. American Journal of Neuroradiology 2005;26:363-366.

88. Shellock FG. Forder J. Drug eluting coronary stent: *In vitro* evaluation of magnet resonance safety at 3-Tesla. Journal of Cardiovascular Magnetic Resonance 2005;7:415-419.

89. Shellock FG, Cosendai G, Park S-M, Nyenhuis JA. Implantable microstimulator: magnetic resonance safety at 1.5-Tesla. Investigative Radiology 2004;39:591-594.

90. Shellock FG. MR safety and the Reveal Insertable Loop Recorder. Signals, No. 49, Issue 3, pp. 8, 2004

91. Reveal Plus Insertable Loop Recorder, http://www.medtronic.com/physician/reveal/mri.html, Medtronic, Inc., Minneapolis, MN.

92. Kinetra Dual Program Neurostimulator for Deep Brain Simulation, 7428 (Medtronic, Inc.), Kinetra MRI labeling. www.Medtronic.com

93. RF BION Microstimulator, Alfred E. Mann Foundation, Valencia, CA; http://www.aemf.org and Advanced Bionics Corporation, Sylmar, CA; http://www.advancedbionics.com/

94. Codman, a Johnson and Johnson Company, Raynham, MA; Cerebrospinal Fluid Shunt Valves and Accessories, http://www.codmanjnj.com/CSFshunting.asp

95. Codman, a Johnson and Johnson Company, Raynham, MA; Cerebrospinal Fluid Shunt Valves and Accessories, http://www.codmanjnj.com/PDFs/Prog_ProcedureGuide.pdf

96. Medtronic Neurosurgery, Goleta, CA; Cerebrospinal Fluid Shunt Valves and Accessories, http://www.medtronic.com/neurosurgery/shunts.html

97. Sophysa USA, Inc., Costa Mesa, CA; Cerebrospinal Fluid Shunt Valves and Accessories, http://www.sophysa.com

98. MED-EL Corporation, Durham, NC; http://www.MEDEL.com

99. Medtronic Neurological Technical Services Department, Tech Note. MRI Guidelines for Neurological Products, Issue No. NTN 04-03 Rev 2, July, 2005, Important Note: Before scanning a patient with this implant or device, obtain the latest MRI safety information by contacting Medtronic, Neurological Technical Services Department (800) 707-0933 or visit www.Medtronic.com.

100. Henderson J, Tkach J, Phillips M, Baker K, Shellock FG, Rezai A. Permanent neurological deficit related to magnetic resonance imaging in a patient with implanted deep brain stimulation electrodes for Parkinson's disease: Case report. Neurosurgery 2005;57:E1063.

101. Rezai AR, Baker K, Tkach J, Phillips M, Hrdlicka G, Sharan A, Nyenhuis J, Ruggieri P, Henderson J, Shellock FG. Is magnetic resonance imaging safe for patients with neurostimulation systems used for deep brain stimulation (DBS)? Neurosurgery 2005;57:1056-1062.

102. Shellock FG. MR Safety at 3-Tesla: Bare Metal and Drug Eluting Coronary Artery Stents. Signals No. 53, Issue 2, pp. 26-27, 2005.

103. Shellock FG. MR safety and Cerebral Spinal Fluid Shunt (CSF) Valves. Signals, No. 51, Issue 4, pp. 10, 2004.

104. Shellock FG, Habibi R, Knebel J. Programmable CSF shunt valve: *In vitro* assessment of MRI safety at 3-Tesla. American Journal of Neuroradiology. 2006;27:661-665.

105. Ceballos EM, Parrish RK. Plain film imaging of Baerveldt glaucoma drainage implants. American Journal of Neuroradiology 2002;23;935-937.

106. Martin AD, Driscoll CL, Wood CP, Felmlee JP. Safety evaluation of titanium middle ear prostheses at 3.0 Tesla. Otolaryngol Head Neck Surg 2005;132:537-42.

107. Shellock FG, Valencerina S. Septal repair implants: evaluation of MRI safety at 3-Tesla. Magnetic Resonance Imaging 2005;23:1021-1025.

108. Nehra A, Moran CJ, Cross DT, Derdeyn CP. MR safety and imaging of Neuroform Stents at 3-T. Am J Neuoradiol 2004;25:1476-1478.

109. Westerway SC, Picker R, Christie J. Implanon implant detection with ultrasound and magnetic resonance imaging. Aust NZ Obstet Gynaecol 2003;43:346-350.

110. Shellock FG, Wilson SF, Mauge CP. Magnetically programmable shunt valve: MRI at 3-Tesla. Magnetic Resonance Imaging 2007;25:1116-21.

111. Zieman M, Kanal E. Copper T 380A IUD and magnetic resonance imaging. Contraception.2007;75:93-5.

112. Shellock FG, Crivelli R, Venugopalan R. Programmable infusion pump and catheter: evaluation using 3-Tesla MRI. Neuromodulation 2008;11:163-170.

113. Shellock FG, Valencerina S. Ventricular assist implant (AB5000): *In Vitro* assessment of MRI issues at 3-Tesla. Journal of Cardiovascular Magnetic Resonance 2008;10:23-30.

114. Diaz F, Tweardy L, Shellock FG. Cervical fixation devices: MRI issues at 3-Tesla. Spine (In Press)

115. Nyenhuis J, Duan L. An evaluation of MRI safety and compatibility of a silver-impregnated antimicrobial wound dressing. J Am Coll Radiol. 2009;6:500-5.

116. Shellock FG. Valencerina S. *In vitro* evaluation of MRI issues at 3-Tesla for aneurysm clips: findings and information that pertain to 154 additional aneurysm clips. American Journal of Neuroradiology (In Press)

117. Geffen N, Trope GE, et al. Is the Ex-PRESS Glaucoma Shunt Magnetic Resonance Imaging Safe? J Glaucoma. 2009 Aug 5. [Epub ahead of print]

118. Gill KR, Pooley RA, Wallace MB. Magnetic resonance imaging compatibility of endoclips. Gastrointest Endosc. 2009;70:532-6.

APPENDIX I

GUIDANCE FOR INDUSTRY AND FDA STAFF

CRITERIA FOR SIGNIFICANT RISK INVESTIGATIONS OF MAGNETIC RESONANCE DIAGNOSTIC DEVICES

Document issued on: July 14, 2003

This document supersedes "Guidance for Magnetic Resonance Diagnostic Devices – Criteria for Significant Risk Investigations" issued n September 29, 1997

U.S. Department of Health and Human Services
Food and Drug Administration
Center for Devices and Radiological Health
Radiological Devices Branch
Division of Reproductive, Abdominal, and Radiological Devices
Office of Device Evaluation

PREFACE

Public Comment

Written comments and suggestions may be submitted at any time for Agency consideration to Division of Dockets Management, Food and Drug Administration, 5630 Fishers Lane, Room 1061, (HFA-305), Rockville, MD, 20852. When submitting comments, please refer to the exact title of this guidance document. Comments may not be acted upon by the Agency until the document is next revised or updated.

Additional Copies

Additional copies are available from the Internet at: http://www.fda.gov/cdrh/ode/guidance/793.pdf or to receive this document by fax, call the CDRH Facts-On-Demand system at 800-899-0381 or 301-827-0111 from a touch-tone telephone. Press 1 to enter the system. At the second voice prompt, press 1 to order a document. Enter the document number (793) followed by the pound sign (#). Follow the remaining voice prompts to complete your request.

This guidance represents the Food and Drug Administration's (FDA's) current thinking on this topic. It does not create or confer any rights for or on any person and does not operate to bind FDA or the public. You can use an alternative approach if the approach satisfies the requirements of the applicable statutes and regulations. If you want to discuss an alternative approach, contact the FDA staff responsible for implementing this guidance. If you cannot identify the appropriate FDA staff, call the appropriate number listed on the title page of this guidance.

INTRODUCTION

This guidance describes the device operation conditions for magnetic resonance diagnostic devices that FDA considers significant risk for the purposes of determining whether a clinical study requires Agency approval of an Investigation Device Exemption (IDE). Magnetic resonance diagnostic devices are class II devices described under 21 CFR 892.1000. The product codes for these devices are:

LNH Magnetic Resonance Imaging System

LNI Magnetic Resonance Spectroscopic System

This guidance supersedes Guidance for Magnetic Resonance Diagnostic Devices - Criteria for Significant Risk Investigations, issued September 29, 1997. We have revised our recommendation for the main static magnetic field strength, increasing it to 8 Tesla for most populations. This is based on ongoing experience in the field and numerous literature reviews (1, 2).

FDA's guidance documents, including this guidance, do not establish legally enforceable responsibilities. Instead, guidances describe the Agency's current thinking on a topic and should be viewed only as recommendations, unless specific regulatory or statutory requirements are cited. The use of the word should in Agency guidances means that something is suggested or recommended, but not required.

THE LEAST BURDENSOME APPROACH

We believe we should consider the least burdensome approach in all areas of medical device regulation. This guidance reflects our careful review of the relevant scientific and legal requirements and what we believe is the least burdensome way for you to comply with those requirements. However, if you believe that an alternative approach would be less burdensome, please contact us so we can consider your point of view. You may send your written comments to the contact person listed in the preface to this guidance or to the CDRH Ombudsman. Comprehensive information on CDRH's Ombudsman, including ways to contact him, can be found on the Internet at http://www.fda.gov/cdrh/ombudsman/

STUDIES OF MAGNETIC RESONANCE DIAGNOSTIC DEVICES

If a clinical study is needed to demonstrate substantial equivalence, i.e., conducted prior to obtaining 510(k) clearance of the device, the study must be conducted under the IDE regulation (21 CFR Part 812). FDA believes that a magnetic resonance diagnostic device used under any one of the operating conditions listed below is a significant risk device as defined in 21 CFR 812.3(m)(4) and, therefore, that studies involving such a device do not qualify for the abbreviated IDE requirements of 21 CFR 812.2(b). In addition to the requirement of having an FDA-approved IDE, sponsors of significant risk studies must comply with the regulations governing institutional review boards (21 CFR Part 56) and informed consent (21 CFR Part 50).

SIGNIFICANT RISK MAGNETIC RESONANCE DIAGNOSTIC DEVICES

You should consider the following operating conditions when assessing whether a study may be considered significant risk:

- main static magnetic field
- specific absorption rate (SAR)
- gradient fields rate of change
- sound pressure level

Generally, FDA deems magnetic resonance diagnostic devices significant risk when used under any of the operating conditions described below.

Main Static Magnetic Field

Population	Main static magnetic field greater than (Tesla)
adults, children, and infants aged > 1 month	8
neonates i.e., infants aged 1 month or less	4

Specific Absorption Rate (SAR)

Site	Dose	Time (min) equal to or greater than:	SAR (W/kg)
whole body	averaged over	15	4
head	averaged over	10	3
head or torso	per gram of tissue	5	8
extremities	per gram of tissue	5	12

Gradient Fields Rate of Change

Any time rate of change of gradient fields (dB/dt) sufficient to produce severe discomfort or painful nerve stimulation

Sound Pressure Level

Peak unweighted sound pressure level greater than 140 dB.

A-weighted root mean square (rms) sound pressure level greater than 99 dBA with hearing protection in place.

These criteria apply only to device operating conditions. Other aspects of the study may involve significant risks and the study, therefore, may require IDE approval regardless of operating conditions. See Blue Book Memorandum entitled Significant Risk and Non-significant Risk Medical Device Studies, http://www.fda.gov/cdrh/d861.html for further discussion.

After FDA determines that the device is substantially equivalent, clinical studies conducted in accordance with the indications reviewed in the 510(k), including clinical design validation studies conducted in accordance with the quality systems regulation, are exempt from the investigational device exemptions (IDE) requirements. However, such studies must be performed in conformance with 21 CFR 56 and 21 CFR 50.

(1) Kangarlu A, Burgess RE, Zu H, et al. Cognitive, cardiac and physiological studies in ultra high field magnetic resonance imaging. Magnetic Resonance Imaging, 1999;17:1407-1416.

(2) Schenck John F, Safety of strong, static magnetic fields. Journal of Magnetic Resonance Imaging, 2000;12:2-19.

APPENDIX II

WEB SITES FOR MRI SAFETY, BIOEFFECTS, AND PATIENT MANAGEMENT

There are two web sites devoted to MRI safety, bioeffects, and patient management: www.MRIsafety.com and www.IMRSER.org

www.MRIsafety.com

The international information resource for MRI safety, bioeffects, and patient management.®

This web site provides up-to-date, concise information for healthcare providers and patients seeking answers to questions on MRI safety-related topics. The latest information is also provided for screening patients with implants, materials, and medical devices.

Key Features

- The List: a searchable database that contains information for implants, devices, and other objects tested for MRI issues.
- Safety Information: concise information that pertains to the latest recommendations and guidelines for patient care and management in the MR environment.
- Research Summary: a presentation and summary of peer-reviewed articles on MRI bioeffects and safety.
- Screening Forms: information and forms for screening patients and other individuals available to imaging facilities in a "downloadable" format.

www.IMRSER.org

The web site of the Institute for Magnetic Resonance Safety, Education, and Research (IMRSER)

The Institute for Magnetic Resonance Safety, Education, and Research (IMRSER) was formed in response to the growing need for information on matters pertaining to magnetic resonance (MR) safety. The IMRSER is the first independent, multidisciplinary, professional organization devoted to promoting awareness, understanding, and communication of MR safety issues through education and research.

The functions and activities of the IMRSER involve development of MR safety guidelines and dissemination of this information to the MR community. This is accomplished through the efforts of the two Advisory Boards: the Medical, Scientific, and Technology Advisory Board and the Corporate Advisory Board.

The Medical, Scientific, and Technology Advisory Board consists of recognized leaders in the field of MR including diagnostic radiologists, clinicians, research scientists, physicists, MRI technologists, MR facility managers, and other allied healthcare professionals involved in MR technology and safety. The members of the Medical, Scientific, and Technology Advisory Board represent academic, private, research, and institutional MR facilities utilizing scanners operating at static magnetic field strengths ranging from 0.2-Tesla (including dedicated-extremity and interventional MR systems) to 8-Tesla. In addition, the Food and Drug Administration has assigned a Federal Liaison to the IMRSER.

The Corporate Advisory Board is comprised of representatives from the medical industry including MR system manufacturers, contrast agent pharmaceutical companies, RF coil manufacturers, MR accessory vendors, medical product manufacturers, and other related corporate organizations.

The Institute for Magnetic Resonance Safety, Education, and Research develops MR safety guidelines utilizing the pertinent peer-reviewed literature and by relying on each board member's extensive clinical, research, or other appropriate experience. Notably, documents developed by the IMRSER consider and incorporate MR safety guidelines and recommendations created by the International Society for Magnetic Resonance in Medicine (ISMRM), the American College of Radiology (ACR), the Food and Drug Administration (FDA), the National Electrical Manufacturers Association (NEMA), the Medical Devices Agency (MDA), the International Electrotechnical Commission (IEC), the International Commission on Non-Ionizing Radiation Protection (ICNIRP), and other organizations.

The MR Safety Papers section of this website includes wide selection of peer-reviewed articles that are available to site visitors as PDF files, posted with permission from the Journal of Magnetic Resonance Imaging, the International Society for Magnetic Resonance in Medicine, Radiology, the Journal of Cardiovascular Magnetic Resonance, the

Institute for Electrical and Electronics Engineers, IEEE Transactions on Magnetics, the Journal of the American College of Cardiology, and Concepts in Magnetic Resonance. Notably, the majority of these papers were published by members of the Medical, Scientific, and Technology Advisory Board of the Institute for Magnetic Resonance Safety, Education, and Research.

APPENDIX III

WEBSITES FOR BIOMEDICAL COMPANIES

AADCO Medical, Inc. -	www.aadcomed.com
Abbott Vascular Devices -	www.abbott.com
ABIOMED, Inc. -	www.abiomed.com
Acclarent, Inc. -	www.acclarent.com
Advanced Bionics Corporation -	www.bionicear.com
Advanced Neuromodulation Systems -	www.ans-medical.com
Aesculap, Inc. -	www.aesculap.com
AGA Medical Corporation -	www.amplatzer.com
Alcon Research, Ltd. -	www.alconlabs.com
Alphatec Spine -	www.alphatecspine.com/
Alpha-Omega Services, Inc. -	www.alpha-omegaserv.com
Alveolus, Inc. -	www.alveolus.com
Alsius Corporation -	www.alsius.com
Amerex Corporation -	amerex-fire.com
Ampco Safety Tools -	www.ampcosafetytools.com
American Medical Systems -	www.americanmedicalsystems.com
Angiodynamics, Inc. -	www.angiodynamics.com
Animas Corporation -	www.Animascorp.com
Arbor Surgical Technologies, Inc. -	www.arborsurgical.com
Applied Medical -	www.appliedmed.com
Aspire Medical -	www.aspiremedical.com
AtriCure, Inc. -	www.atricure.com
Atritech, Inc. -	www.atritech.com
Atrium Medical Corporation -	www.atriummed.com
ATS Medical -	www.atsmedical.com
B. Braun Medical Inc. -	www.bbraunusa.com
Baxa Corporation -	www.baxa.com
Becton, Dickinson, and Co. -	www.bd.com
Berlex Laborotories -	www.berlex.com
Biomerix Corporation -	www.Biomerix.com
Biomet, Inc. -	www.biomet.com
Bioplate, Inc. -	www.bioplate.com
Biosensors International -	www.biosensorsintl.com

Biopsy Sciences -	www.biopsysciences.com
BIOTRONIK AG -	www.biotronik.ch
Blackstone Medical, Inc. -	www.blackstonemedical.com
Bolton Medical, Inc. -	www.boltonmedical.com
Boston Scientific Corporation -	www.bostonscientific.com
Bracco Diagnostics Inc. -	www.Bracco.com
Bronchus Technologies, Inc. -	www.bronchus.com
Calypso Medical Technologies -	www.calypsomedical.com
Cardia, Inc. -	www.cardia.com
Cardica -	www.cardica.com
Cardiac Dimensions -	www.cardiacdimensions.com
Cardinal Health -	www.cardinal.com
CardioKinetix Inc. -	www.cardiokinetix.com
CardioMEMS, Inc. -	www.cardiomems.com
Coaxia, Inc. -	www.coaxia.com
Codman, a Johnson and Johnson Company -	www.codman.com
Coherex Medical-	www.coherex.com
Coloplast Corporation -	www.coloplast.com
Conceptus Inc.-	www.conceptus.com
Conor Medsystems -	www.conormed.com
ConvaTec Wound Therapeutics -	www.convatec.com
Cook, Inc. -	www.cook-inc.com
Cordis -	www.crdus.jnj.com
Cornova, Inc. -	www.cornova.com
COVIDIEN -	www.covidien.com
C.R. Bard, Inc. -	www.crbard.com
Crux Biomedical, Inc. -	www.cruxbiomedical.com
Cyberkinetics Neurotechnology Systems, Inc. -	www.cyberkineticsinc.com
Cyberonics, Inc. -	www.cyberonics.com
Datascope Corporation -	www.datascope.com
DePuy Products, Inc. -	www.dpyus.jnj.com
DermaPort -	www.dermaport.net
DeRoyal Technologies -	www.deroyal.com
Devax, Inc. -	www.devax.net
DexCom, Inc. –	www.dexcom.com
Edwards Lifeciences -	www.edwards.com
Emphasys Medical Inc. -	www.emphasysmedical.com
Endologix, Inc. -	www.endologix.com
EndoMed, Inc. -	www.endomedinc.com
EnteroMedics, Inc. -	www.enteromedics.com

Endotex Interventional Systems, Inc. -	www.endotex.com
ev3 The Endovascular Company -	www.ev3.net
Ethicon Endo-Surgery -	www.eesus.jnj.com
Evalve, Inc. -	www.evalveinc.com
Ferno -	www.ferno.com
Hitachi Medical Systems America, Inc. -	www.hitachimed.com
Hollister -	www.hollister.com
HoverTech International -	www.hovermatt.com
Gendron, Inc. -	www.gendroninc.com
General Electric Healthcare -	www.gehealthcare.com
Genstar Technologies -	www.genstartech.com
Glaukos Corporation -	www.glaukos.com
GrantAdler Corporation -	www.grantadler.com
GT Urological -	www.gturological.com
Glaukos Corporation -	www.glaukos.com
Gyrus -	www.gyrusacmi.com
Hollister Inc. -	www.hollister.com
Health Beacons Inc. -	www.healthbeacons.com
Hisamitsu Pharmaceutical Co., Inc. -	www.hisamitsu.co.jp/english
Icon Interventional Systems, Inc. -	www.icon-us.com
I-Flow Corporation -	www.iflo.com
Impliant Ltd. -	www.Impliant.com
INAMED -	www.inamed.com
INNERCOOL Therapies -	www.innercool.com
INRAD, Inc. -	www.inrad-inc.com
InSound Medical -	www.insoundmedical.com
Integra Lifesciences Corporation -	www.integra-ls.com
Interrad Medical, Inc. -	www.interradmedical.com
Intrinsic Therapeutics, Inc. -	www.intrinsic-therapeutics.com
Intuitive Surgical, Inc. -	www.intuitivesurgical.com
Invatec -	www.invatec.com
JenaValve Technology -	www.jenavalve.de
Joint Replacement Instrumentation Limited (JRI Ltd.) -	www.jri-ltd.co.uk
Kaneka Corporation -	www.kaneka.co.jp
KCI USA, Inc. -	www.kci1.com
KFx Medical Corporation -	www.kfxmedical.com
Kips Bay Medical, Inc. -	www.kipsbaymedical.com
LeMaitre Vascular -	www.lemaitre.com
LMA North America -	www.lmana.com
LSI Solutions, Inc. -	www.lsisolutions.com

Magmedix -	www.Magmedix.com
Medcomp -	www.medcompnet.com
MED-EL -	www.medel.com
Medivance, Inc. -	www.medivance.com
Medline Industries, Inc. -	www.medline.com
Medlogics -	www.medlogicsdc.com
MEDRAD, INC. -	www.Medrad.com
Medtronic, Inc. -	www.medtronic.com
Medtronic Xomed -	xomed.com
Mentor Corporation -	www.mentorcorp.com
Micardia Corporation -	www.micardiac.com
MicroVention-	www.microvention.com
MiniMed, Inc. -	www.minimed.com
Minrad, Inc. -	www.minrad.com
Mylan Technologies Inc. -	www.mylantech.com
Navotek Medical Ltd. -	www.navotek.com
NeuroVASx, Inc. -	www.neurovasx.com
Newmatic Sound Systems, Inc. -	www.newmaticsound.com
Nfocus Neuromedical, Inc. -	www.nfocusneuro.com
NGK Metals Corporation -	www.ngkmetals.com
NMT Medical, Inc. -	www.nmtmedical.com
NuVasive, Inc. -	www.nuvasive.com
Optonol Ltd. -	www.optonol.com
OrbusNeich Medical, Inc. -	www.orbusneich.co
OSSUR AMERICAS -	www.ossur.com
Otto Bock HealthCare –	www.ottobockus.com
Paracor Medical, Inc. -	www.paracor.com
Percardia Inc. -	www.percardia.com
Phoenix Biomedical Corporation -	www.phoenixbiomedical.com
PMT Corporation -	www.pmtcorp.com
Praxair Healthcare Services -	www.praxair.com
Prescient Medical -	www.prescientmedical.com
ProStrakan -	www.prostrakan.com
Pulmonx -	www.pulmonx.com
QSUM -	www.qsum.net
Radianse, Inc. -	www.radianse.com
Rafael Medical Technologies, Inc. -	www.rafaelmedical.com
Rex Medical -	www.rexmedical.com
Rhythmlink International, LLC -	www.rhythmlink.com
Rubicor Medical, Inc. -	www.rubicor.com

SAM Medical Products -	www.sammedical.com
Shelhigh Inc. -	www.shelhigh.com
Sicel Technologies, Inc. -	www.siceltech.com
Siemens Medical Solutions -	www.siemens.com
Smith & Nephew, Inc. -	www.smithnephew.com
Smiths Medical -	www.smiths-medical.com
Sorin Group -	www.sorin.com
Spiration Inc. -	www.spiration.com
St. Jude Medical, Inc. -	www.sjm.com
Stryker Instruments -	www.stryker.com
Sulzer Carbomedics, Inc. -	www.sulzercarbomedics.com
Syncro Medical Innovations, Inc. -	www.syncromedicalinnovations.com
Teleflex Medical -	www.teleflexmedical.com
The Viking Corporation -	www.vikingcorp.com
Theragenics Corporation -	www.theragenics.com
Torax Medical -	www.toraxmedical.com
Transoma Medical, Inc. -	www.transomamedical.com
TriVascular, Inc. -	www.trivascular.com
Uromedica Inc. -	www.uromedica-inc.com
U.S. Surgical Corporation -	www.ussurg.com
ValleyLab/Tyco -	www.tycohealthcare.com
Vascular Architects, Inc. -	www.vasculararchitects.com
Vascutek Ltd. -	www.vascutek.com
VisionCare Ophthalmic Technologies Ltd. -	www.visioncare.co.il
Vygon Ltd. -	www.vygonus.com
Western Enterprises -	www.westernenterprises.com
W.L. Gore and Associates, Inc. -	www.wlgore.com
XTENT -	www.xtent.com
Zimmer -	www.Zimmer.com

APPENDIX IV

Guidance for Industry and FDA Staff Establishing Safety and Compatibility of Passive Implants in the Magnetic Resonance (MR) Environment

Document issued on: August 21, 2008

For questions regarding this document, contact Terry O. Woods, Ph.D. at 301-796-2503 or by email at terry.woods@fda.hhs.gov

U.S. Department of Health and Human Services
Food and Drug Administration
Center for Devices and Radiological Health
Division of Solid and Fluid Mechanics
Office of Science & Engineering Laboratories

Preface
Public Comment

Written comments and suggestions may be submitted at any time for Agency consideration to the Division of Dockets Management, Food and Drug Administration, 5630 Fishers Lane, Room 1061, (HFA-305), Rockville, MD, 20852.

When submitting comments, please refer to the exact title of this guidance document. Comments may not be acted upon by the Agency until the document is next revised or updated.

Additional Copies

Additional copies are available from the Internet at:
http://www.fda.gov/cdrh/osel/guidance/1685.pdf. You may also send an e-mail request to dsmica@fda.hhs.gov to receive an electronic copy of the guidance or send a fax request to 240-276-3151 to receive a hard copy. Please use the document number (1685) to identify the guidance you are requesting.

This guidance represents the Food and Drug Administration's (FDA's) current thinking on this topic. It does not create or confer any rights for or on any person and does not operate to bind FDA or the public. You can use an alternative approach if the approach satisfies the requirements of the applicable statutes and regulations. If you want to discuss an alternative approach, contact the FDA staff responsible for implementing this guidance. If you cannot identify the appropriate FDA staff, call the appropriate number listed on the title page of this guidance.

1. Introduction

This guidance addresses testing and labeling of passive implants for safety and compatibility in the magnetic resonance (MR) environment. In preparing a premarket approval application (PMA), Investigational Device Exemption (IDE), and premarket notification (510(k)) submission, this guidance document applies to MR devices that serve their function without the supply of electronic power. Active implants or devices that are not implants do not fall within the scope of this guidance.

The information in this guidance supplements the Agency's related publications on PMA's, IDE's, and 510(k)s and is not intended to describe or substitute the information otherwise required in the following premarket submissions:

-Premarket Approval Application (PMA) Information

For general information about PMA applications, refer to 21 CFR 814 or "Application Methods," at
http://www.fda.gov/cdrh/devadvice/pma/app_methods.html.

-Investigational Device Exemption (IDE) Information

For general IDE information, refer to 21 CFR Part 812 or to the "Introduction IDE Overview," at
http://www.fda.gov/cdrh/devadvice/ide/index.shtml.

-Premarket Notification (510(k)) Information

For general information on 510(k), refer to 21 CFR 807.87, the guidance entitled "Format for Traditional and Abbreviated 510(k)s" and "Premarket Notification 510(k)" in the (Center for Devices and Radiological Health) CDRH Device Advice at
http://www.fda.gov/cdrh/devadvice/314.html.

A manufacturer who intends to market a passive implant must conform to the general controls of the Federal Food, Drug, and Cosmetic Act (the act).

The Least Burdensome Approach
We believe we should consider the least burdensome approach in all areas of medical device regulation. This guidance reflects our careful review of the relevant scientific and legal requirements and what we believe is the least burdensome way for you to comply with those requirements. However, if you believe that an alternative approach would be less burdensome, please contact us so we can consider your point of view. You may send your written comments to the contact person listed in the preface to this guidance or to the CDRH Ombudsman. Comprehensive information on CDRH's Ombudsman, including ways to contact him, can be found on the Internet at http://www.fda.gov/cdrh/ombudsman/.

FDA's guidance documents, including this guidance, do not establish legally enforceable responsibilities. Instead, guidances describe the Agency's current thinking on a topic and should be viewed only as recommendations, unless specific regulatory or statutory requirements are cited. The use of the word should in Agency guidances means that something is suggested or recommended, but not required.

2. MR Testing
The main issues affecting the safety and compatibility of passive implants in the MR environment concern magnetically induced displacement force and torque, radio frequency (RF) heating, and image artifacts. The MR static field induces displacement forces and torques on magnetic materials. Patients have been killed by the projectile effect on devices and by the rotations produced by magnetically induced force and torque (1). RF heating in the body is created by currents induced by the RF excitation pulses applied during MR scanning. Patients have been severely burned as a result during an MR scan (2). The presence of an implant may produce an image artifact that may appear as a void region or as a geometric distortion of the true image. If the image artifact is near the area of interest, the artifact may make the MR scan uninformative or may lead to an inaccurate clinical diagnosis, potentially resulting in inappropriate medical action.

We recommend that you provide the nonclinical testing described below in your PMA, IDE or 510(k) to establish the safety and compatibility of your passive implant in the MR environment. Testing should encompass the range of sizes of the device you intend to market. If you do not test all sizes of the device you intend to market, we recommend you test a size or combination of sizes that represent the worst-case scenario for each test.

We recommend you explain the rationale for determining why the size(s) you selected represent the worst-case scenario for each test.

We suggest you present data in a clear tabular or graphical form. We also recommend you describe all testing protocols. Each protocol description should include:

-test objective
-equipment used
-acceptance criteria
-rationale for test conditions
-rationale for the acceptance criteria
-number of devices tested
-description of devices tested, including device size
-description of any differences between test sample and final product, and justification for why differences would not impact the applicability of the test to the final product
-results (summarized and raw form).

Terminology
Terminology for defining the safety of items in the MR environment is provided in ASTM F2503 Standard Practice for Marking Medical Devices and Other Items for Safety in the Magnetic Resonance Environment. We recognize implementing new terminology may be challenging, but FDA believes this new terminology will help reduce the possibility of injuries involving passive implants related to MRI (Magnetic Resonance Imaging). We recommend using the terminology MR Safe, MR Conditional, and MR Unsafe, defined in ASTM F2503. If you label your device as "MR Safe," your submission should include a scientific rationale or the testing described below. If you label your device as "MR Conditional," your submission should include the testing described below. If you label your device as "MR Unsafe," your submission should include a scientific rationale or the testing described below.

MR Safe based on scientific rationale
A scientifically based rationale rather than test data may be sufficient to support identifying an implant as "MR Safe," for example, a

nonconducting or a nonmagnetic item, such as a plastic Petri dish, poses no known hazards in all MR environments.

If you intend to use a scientific rationale to support identifying your device as "MR Safe," we recommend that you provide a scientific rationale that addresses the following issues.
-magnetically induced displacement force
-magnetically induced torque
-heating of your device by RF (radio frequency) fields.

MR Unsafe based on scientific rationale
A scientifically based rationale rather than test data, may be sufficient to support identifying an item as "MR Unsafe."

If you intend to use a scientific rationale to support identifying your device as "MR Unsafe," we recommend that you provide a scientific rationale to address:
-magnetically induced displacement force
-magnetically induced torque
-heating of your device by RF (radio frequency) fields.

MR Conditional, MR Safe, or MR Unsafe based on experimental data
If you identify your device as "MR Conditional," we recommend you provide experimental data as described below. You may also choose to provide experimental data to support identifying your device as "MR Safe" or "MR Unsafe." In each case, we recommend you follow the methods described in the standards below or equivalent methods.

-Magnetically Induced Displacement Force
ASTM F2052, Standard Test Method for Measurement of Magnetically Induced Displacement Force on Medical Devices in the Magnetic Resonance Environment

-Magnetically Induced Torque
ASTM F2213, Standard Test Method for Measurement of Magnetically Induced Torque on Medical Devices in the Magnetic Resonance Environment

-Heating by RF Fields
ASTM F2182, Standard Test Method for Measurement of Radio Frequency Induced Heating Near Passive Implants During Magnetic Resonance Imaging

-Image Artifact
ASTM F2119, Standard Test Method for Evaluation of MR Image
Artifacts from Passive Implants

Although commercial 1.5-T MR systems are currently the most common,
3-T MR systems are becoming more common. A medical device that is
MR Safe or MR Conditional in a 1.5-T scanner may not be MR Safe or
MR Conditional in an MR system with a higher or lower field strength.
The amount of RF heating can vary depending on the system geometry,
MR system and scan conditions, and the conductive length of the device.
The critical length for a specific device during a particular MR scan
cannot be calculated precisely, so we recommend you evaluate a range of
lengths and conditions to determine the worst case conditions for RF
induced heating. To achieve worst-case heating conditions in the
phantom, you should pay attention to the local electric and magnetic field
distribution near the implant inside the phantom. These fields need to be
similar to the local electric and magnetic field distribution near the
implant inside the patient so the heating of the implant in the phantom is
comparable to the heating inside the patient. Anatomical positioning of
the implant in the phantom does not reliably predict the implant heating
in the patient. Therefore, we recommend you describe the field
conditions and system geometry under which you tested your device and
demonstrate that your test conditions are comparable to worst-case
clinical conditions. Accurate assessment of the whole body averaged
specific absorption rate (WB-SAR) used in your testing is critical to
determining whether your testing represents reasonable worst-case
heating conditions. Therefore, we recommend that you base WB-SAR
assessments upon calorimetry measurements rather than relying on the
MR scanner display, which may not have adequate accuracy. See also **3.
Labeling for the MR Environment**

3. Labeling for the MR Environment
General labeling requirements for medical devices are described in 21
CFR Part 801. See CDRH Device Advice
(http://www.fda.gov/cdrh/devadvice/33.html) for additional information.
In accordance with 21 CFR 814.20(b)(10), you must submit all proposed
labeling in a PMA. A 510(k) must include labeling in sufficient detail to
satisfy the requirements of 21 CFR 807.87(e). An IDE must include
labeling to satisfy the requirements of 21 CFR 812.5. The following
suggestions may assist you in preparing labeling that satisfies the
requirements of 21 CFR Part 8013 (3).

MR Labeling
We recommend you consider using the MR terminology in ASTM
F2503, Standard Practice for Marking Medical Devices and Other Items
for Safety in the Magnetic Resonance Environment. See **Section 2**. **MR
Testing** for information describing the process to determine the
appropriate MR safety term for your device.

MR Safe
The following statement may be used in your labeling for a MR Safe
device: The (insert device name) is MR Safe.

MR Unsafe
The following statement may be used in your labeling for an MR Unsafe
device: The (insert device name) is MR Unsafe.

Labeling for an MR Unsafe implant should recommend that patients
register their implant information with the MedicAlert Foundation
(www.medicalert.org) or equivalent organization.

MR Conditional
Labeling for MR Conditional devices should indicate the device was
tested under non-clinical conditions and list the conditions under which
the device can be safely scanned, for example:

Non-clinical testing has demonstrated the (insert device name) is MR
Conditional. It can be scanned safely under the following conditions:

-static magnetic field of ___ Tesla
-spatial gradient field of ___ Gauss/cm
-maximum whole body averaged specific absorption rate (SAR) of
__W/kg for __ minutes of scanning.

In non-clinical testing, the (insert device name) produced a temperature
rise of less than __ °C at a maximum whole body averaged specific
absorption rate (SAR) of ___ W/kg, as assessed by calorimetry for ___
minutes of MR scanning in a (field strength _____) (model _____)
(manufacturer _____) (software version _____) MR scanner.

Image Artifact – General

We also recommend your labeling indicate the amount of image artifact
and that you acquire MR images using standard sequences (e.g., as
described in ASTM F2119) or an equivalent method. We recommend
your labeling indicate the extent of the artifact for one or more of the
sequences used in your testing. The labeling should also include

information about the shape and extent of the artifact. For devices with a lumen, the labeling should indicate whether the lumen is obscured by the artifact. A dimensioned figure showing the implant in its typical implant site and the extent of the artifact in at least one plane may be included. It may be helpful to provide a separate dimensioned drawing of the implant and a figure showing the typical implant site.

Image Artifact – Special Examples
Devices with Slight (1-2-mm) Artifact
The following statement may be used for a device with an image artifact that extends only slightly (1-2 mm) beyond the device:

MR image quality may be compromised if the area of interest is in the same area or relatively close to the position of the device. Therefore, it may be necessary to optimize MR imaging parameters for the presence of this implant.

Devices with a Lumen
For devices with a lumen, we recommend you specify whether the lumen is obscured by the artifact, for example:

The image artifact extends approximately ___ mm from the device, both inside and outside the device lumen when scanned in nonclinical testing using the sequence: _____ in a (Field Strength) (Model)(Manufacturer)(software version) MR system with _____ coil.

We also recommend that the device labeling for an MR Conditional implant recommend that patients register the conditions under which the implant can be scanned safely with the MedicAlert Foundation (www.medicalert.org) or equivalent organization.

REFERENCES
(1) Woods, T.O. "MRI Safety" in Wiley Encyclopedia of Biomedical Engineering (Metin Akay, ed.) Hoboken: John Wiley & Sons, Inc., 2006, pp. 2360-2371.
(2) Ibid.
(3) Although final labeling is not required for 510(k) clearance, labeling is reviewed in a 510(k) and the final labeling must comply with the requirements of 21 CFR Part 801 before a medical device is introduced into interstate commerce. In addition, final labeling for prescription medical devices must comply with 21 CFR 801.109. Labeling recommendations in this guidance are consistent with the requirements of Part 801.

Frank G. Shellock, Ph.D. is a physiologist with 25 years of experience conducting laboratory and clinical investigations in the field of magnetic resonance imaging. He is an Adjunct Clinical Professor of Radiology and Medicine at the Keck School of Medicine, University of Southern California, Adjunct Professor of Clinical Physical Therapy, Division of Biokinesiology and Physical 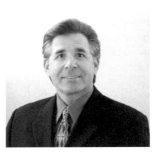 Therapy, School of Dentistry, University of Southern California and the Director of MRI Studies at the Biomimetic Microelectronic Systems, National Science Foundation (NSF) - Engineering Research Center, University of Southern California, and the Founder of the Institute for Magnetic Resonance Safety, Education, and Research (www.IMRSER.org). As a commitment to the field of MRI safety, bioeffects, and patient management, he created and maintains the internationally popular web site, www.MRIsafety.com.

Dr. Shellock has authored or co-authored more than 200 publications in the peer-reviewed literature. He co-authored the MRI safety section of the Cardiovascular MR Self-Assessment Program (CMR-SAP) for the American College of Cardiology and three of his medical textbooks are considered best sellers, having sold more than 10,000 copies each.

Dr. Shellock is a member of the Sub-Committee on MRI safety issues for the American Society for Testing and Materials (ASTM) International. Additionally, he serves in advisory roles to government, industry, and other policy-making organizations. Dr. Shellock is an Associate Editor for the Journal of Magnetic Resonance Imaging and a Reviewing Editor for several medical and scientific journals including Radiology, Investigative Radiology, Magnetic Resonance in Medicine, Magnetic Resonance Imaging, the American Journal of Roentgenology, the Journal of Cardiovascular Magnetic Resonance, and the Journal of the American College of Cardiology.

Memberships in professional societies include the American College of Radiology, the International Society for Magnetic Resonance in Medicine (ISMRM), the Radiological Society of North America, the California Radiological Society, the Hawaii Radiological Society, the Society for Cardiovascular Magnetic Resonance, and the American Heart Association. He is also a Fellow and member of the American College of Cardiology and the American College of Sportsmedicine.

In 2004, the International Society for Magnetic Resonance in Medicine recognized the significant contributions Dr. Shellock has made to the scientific and educational mission of the ISMRM by designating him a Fellow of the Society. The American College of Radiology awarded him a Distinguished Committee Service Award for years of dedicated service to the *Practice Guidelines and Technical Standards Committee – Body MRI*.

Dr. Shellock is a recipient of a National Research Service Award from the National Institutes of Health, National Heart, Lung, and Blood Institute and has received numerous grants from governmental agencies and private organizations. He is currently participating in research to define safety for cardiac pacemakers, implantable cardioverter defibrillators, neurostimulation systems, and other electronic devices.

Dr. Shellock has lectured both nationally and internationally and has provided plenary lectures to numerous organizations including the Radiological Society of North America, the International Society for Magnetic Resonance in Medicine, the American College of Radiology, the American Roentgen Ray Society, the American Society of Neuroradiology, the Environmental Protection Agency, the Oklahoma Heart Institute, the Head and Neck Radiology Society, the Center for Devices and Radiological Health (FDA), the Magnetic Resonance Managers Society, the American Heart Association, the American College of Cardiology, the American Society of Neuroimaging, the Society for Cardiovascular Magnetic Resonance, the Heart Rhythm Society, the Finnish Radiological Society, the International Congress of Radiology, the Japanese Society of Neuroradiology, the British Chapter of the International Society for Magnetic Resonance in Medicine, and the British Chapter of the International Society for Magnetic Resonance in Medicine, and the Royal Australian and New Zealand College of Radiologists.

Dr. Shellock's company, Magnetic Resonance Safety Testing Services, specializes in the assessment of MRI safety for implants and devices as well as the evaluation of electromagnetic field-related bioeffects and the development of new clinical MR imaging applications for low-field (0.2-Tesla), high-field, and very-high-field strength MR systems (www.MagneticResonanceSafetyTesting.com).